HYPOXIA AND HUMAN DISEASES

Edited by **Jing Zheng** and **Chi Zhou**

Hypoxia and Human Diseases
http://dx.doi.org/10.5772/62960
Edited by Jing Zheng and Chi Zhou

Contributors

Raja El Hasnaoui, Veronica Carroll, Nicoletta Charolidi, Guomin Shen, Xiaobo Li, DaLiao Xiao, Jun Ke, Lei Wang, Payaningal R. Somanath, Shahrzad Movafagh, Deepak Bhatia, Mohammad Sanaei Ardekani, Qiwen Shi, Paola Casanello, Bernardo Krause, Emilio A Herrera, W. Keung Leung, Bassam Janji, Nassera Aouali, Manon Bosseler, Delphine Sauvage, Kris Van Moer, Guy Berchem, Susana Pilar Gaytán, Rosario Pasaro, Carlos Salomon, Miharu Kobayashi, Shayna Sharma, Gregory Edward Rice, Richard Kline, Mona Alharbi, Katrina Wade, Andrew Lai, Kazuhiro Kaneko, Tomonori Yano, Sergei Orlov, Yulia Birulina, Svetlana Gusakova, Liudmila Smaglii, Wahyu Widowati, Dwi Davidson Rihibiha, M Aris Widodo, Sutiman B Sumitro, Indra Bachtiar, Monica Banita, Ana Marina Andrei, Anca Berbecaru-Iovan, Felix Rares Ioan Din-Anghel, Camelia Stanciulescu, Sorin Berbecaru-Iovan, Catalina Pisoschi, Markus Mandl, Reinhard Depping, Mohamed Ghorbel, Dominga Iacobazzi, Massimo Caputo, Mitchell Huber, Yuchuan Ding, Xiaokun Geng, Hong-Lian Duan, Christopher B Wolff, Flávio Reis, Sandra Ribeiro, Luís Belo, Alice Santos-Silva, Domokos Gero

Published by InTech

Janeza Trdine 9, 51000 Rijeka, Croatia

Publishing Process Manager Dajana Pemac

Technical Editor SPi Global

Cover InTech Design team

First published February, 2017
Printed in Croatia

Additional hard copies can be obtained from orders@intechopen.com

Hypoxia and Human Diseases , Edited by Jing Zheng and Chi Zhou
p. cm.
Print ISBN 978-953-51-2895-3
Online ISBN 978-953-51-2896-0

For EU product safety concerns:
IN TECH d.o.o., Prolaz Marije Krucifikse Kozulić 3, 51000 Rijeka, Croatia,
info@intechopen.com or visit our website at intechopen.com.

Meet the editors

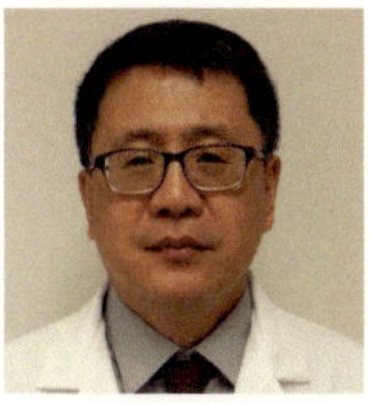

Dr. Zheng is a professor in the Department of Obstetrics and Gynecology at the University of Wisconsin-Madison. He received his PhD in Reproductive Physiology. Over the last two decades, his research interests are in the cellular and molecular mechanisms governing endothelial functions. Dr. Zheng's laboratory has been continuously funded by AHA, NIH, and private foundations, and he has served as a regular and ad hoc member of several NIH and AHA study sections. He has also been actively involved in training students and other young scientists.

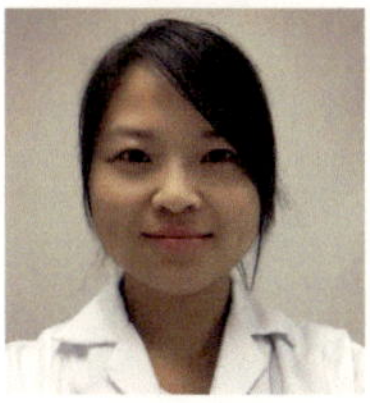

Dr. Zhou is a research associate in the Department of Obstetrics and Gynecology at the University of Wisconsin-Madison. She obtained her PhD in Reproductive Physiology, primarily in functional genomics and embryonic development. Currently, her research focuses on exploring mechanisms regulating human placental/fetal vascular growth and development relevant to human pregnancy complications using functional genomics and bioinformatics approaches.

Contents

Preface

Hypoxia refers to a state in which oxygen supply to the whole body or a region of the body is inadequate. To date, after extensive and systemic research, it is clear that chronic and severe hypoxia could be detrimental to human health and is related to many pathological conditions such as cardiovascular disorders and cancers. Additionally, we should also recognize that under physiological conditions, most cells within the tissue actually reside in low O_2 environments (~3–16% O_2) relative to ambient O_2 (~ 21% O_2). This physiological low O_2 is critical to many essential cellular functions.

This book aims to provide a comprehensive and most updated overview of our current understanding of physiological (i.e., at high altitude) and pathological hypoxia's roles in various aspects of human diseases. It also concludes with current advances and future directions of therapeutics of human hypoxic diseases. We hope that this book will become useful and attractive to medical students, practicing clinicians, and biomedical researchers who are working or are interested in the biology of hypoxia.

It has been an extraordinarily exciting and rewarding experience to put this book together. We wish to express our deep gratitude to all contributors for their hard work and scholarly efforts in preparation of each individual chapter. We also would like to thank our publishing managers, Ms. Dajana Pemac and Ms. Maja Bozicevic at InTech, for making this book available.

Chi Zhou, PhD and Jing Zheng, PhD
Department of Obstetrics and Gynecology,
University of Wisconsin-Madison,
Madison, WI, USA

Chapter 1

The Multifaceted Role of Hypoxia-Inducible Factor 1 (HIF1) in Lipid Metabolism

Guomin Shen and Xiaobo Li

Additional information is available at the end of the chapter

http://dx.doi.org/10.5772/65340

Abstract

Hypoxia-inducible factor 1 (HIF1) is a master transcription factor and regulates expression of a large number of genes involving many aspects of biology. In addition to HIF1's roles in glucose metabolism and angiogenesis, numerous studies have revealed an emerging role of HIF1 in controlling lipid homeostasis. In this chapter, we discuss that lipid accumulation is related to HIF1's activity in several diseases and the growing evidence demonstrating the functional importance of HIF1 in controlling lipid metabolism. The functions include lipid uptake and trafficking, fatty acid metabolism, sterol metabolism, triacylglycerol synthesis, phospholipid metabolism, lipid droplet biogenesis, and lipid signaling. Defining the role of HIF1 in lipid metabolism is crucial to understand the pathophysiology of lipid in disease and may help us to identify additional target sites for drug development. This review would shed light on our understanding of the critical role of HIF1 in lipid metabolism.

Keywords: hypoxia-inducible factor 1, lipid accumulation, lipid metabolism

1. Introduction

Hypoxia has been identified as a common symptom in many diseases, such as cancer [1, 2], obesity [3], atherosclerosis [4], and ischemic heart disease (IHD) [5]. Adaptation to hypoxia involves hypoxia-inducible factor 1 (HIF1) and requires reprogramming of essential elements of cellular metabolism [6]. HIF1 was described about 20 years ago [7]. It is a heterodimeric transcription factor that is composed of an oxygen-regulated HIF1α subunit and a constitutively expressed HIF1β subunit [7, 8]. HIF1α is mainly regulated by protein degradation. Under normoxic conditions, HIF1α is subjected to oxygen-dependent hydroxylation by three prolyl hydroxylase domain proteins (PHD1–3) on two proline residues in the oxygen-dependent degradation (ODD) domain [9]. The prolyl-hydroxylated HIF1α is targeted for degradation by the tumor suppressor protein von Hippel-Lindau (VHL), an E3 ubiquitin-protein ligase [10, 11]. HIF1α is also regulated in an oxygen-dependent manner by factor inhibiting HIF1 (FIH1) [12, 13]. In this case, FIH1 mediates the hydroxylation of an asparagine residue in the C-terminal trans-activation domain, which prevents the binding of HIF1α with coactivators p300 and CBP [13–15]. Hydroxylation of proline and asparagine is inhibited under hypoxic conditions causing HIF1α to rapidly accumulate [12, 13]. HIF1α subsequently heterodimerizes with HIF1β, and the complex binds to hypoxic responsive elements (HREs) within the promoter regions of target genes, and allows for recruitment of coactivators and activation of transcription [16]. In addition to hypoxia, HIF1 accumulation can also be induced by growth-factor stimulation, gene mutations, and intermediate metabolites [17] (**Figure 1**).

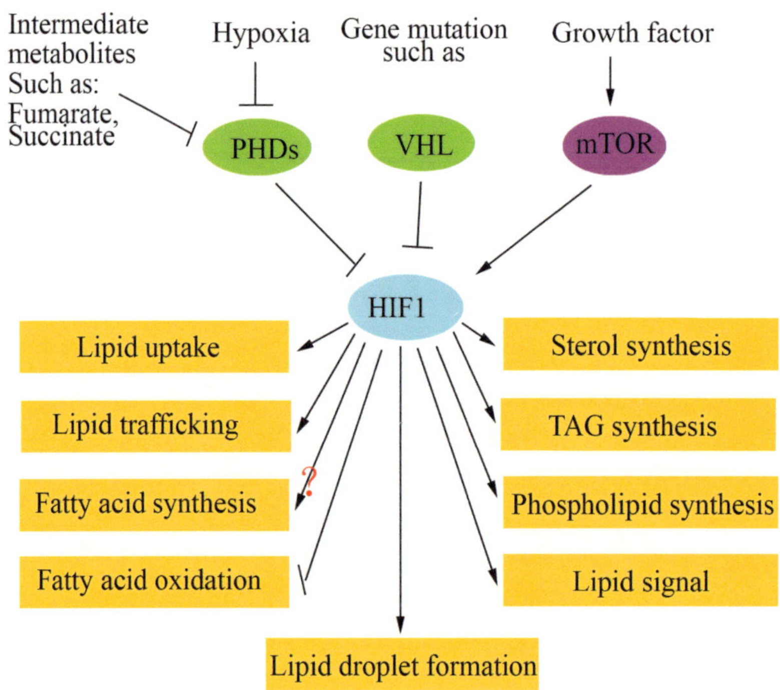

Figure 1. Regulation of HIF1 and its downstream roles related to lipid metabolism. HIF1 accumulation can be induced by hypoxia, gene mutations, intermediate metabolites, and growth factors. HIF1 plays a pivotal role in lipid metabolism. It can increase lipid uptake and trafficking, fatty acid synthesis, sterol synthesis, TAG synthesis, lipid droplet biogenesis, and lipid signal production, and suppress fatty acid β-oxidation. Lipid droplet accumulation may be the final result of HIF1 in lipid metabolism. It is unclear about its role in phospholipids metabolism.

It has been reported that HIF1 regulates the transcription of hundreds of genes involving many aspect of biology, especially energy metabolism and vascularization [16]. The role of HIF1 in glucose metabolism had been well established [17]. Most of genes involving glucose uptake and glycolysis are directly regulated by HIF1 [17]. Recent studies demonstrated that HIF1 also plays an important role in lipid metabolism [1, 2, 18–21]. Currently, our understanding of HIF1 in regulating lipid metabolism has lagged behind that of glucose metabolism. Lipids, structurally and functionally important in all organisms, are not only one of the major components of cellular membrane systems, but also the source of energy storage. Moreover, signal molecules, such as prostaglandin E2 (PGE2), hydroxyeicosatetraenoic acid (HETE), and steroid hormones, are derived from lipids. This review would focus on the HIF1's activity related to dysregulation of lipid metabolism in several diseases, including atherosclerosis [4], fatty liver disease (FLD) [19], heart failure diseases [5], obesity [3], and cancer [1, 2] as well as the involvement of HIF1 in lipid metabolism, including lipid uptake and trafficking, fatty acid metabolism, sterol metabolism, triacylglycerol (TAG) synthesis, phospholipid metabolism, lipid droplet (LD) biogenesis, and lipid signaling.

2. Lipid accumulation is associated with HIF1's activity in diseases

Most of the studies have demonstrated that HIF1's activity is associated with lipid accumulation positively [3, 18, 20–27], while few researches have indicated the opposite effect [28–31]. PHD2 inhibition or deletion, increasing HIF1's activity (**Figure 1**), decreased lipid accumulation in different animal models [28, 30, 31]. It indicated that the role of HIF1 in lipid metabolism may be different in different animal models. Details were described and discussed in the following sections.

2.1. Atherosclerosis

Hypoxia has been demonstrated in atherosclerotic plaques [4]. Arterial wall hypoxia exists in a rabbit atherosclerosis injury model [32–34], confirmed in rabbit atherosclerotic plaques [35, 36] as well as in several mouse models [23, 37, 38]. Recently, in vivo studies have demonstrated hypoxia in human atherosclerotic plaques [39]. Macrophages are the major cell types in human plaques that display signs of hypoxia. TAG-loaded foam cells derived from macrophages are characteristic of both early and late atherosclerotic plaques [40, 41]. Exposure of human macrophages to hypoxia causes an accumulation of TAG-containing lipid droplets [42]. HIF1α is expressed in various cell types of atherosclerotic lesions and is associated with lesional inflammation [43]. Knockdown of HIF1α with small interfering RNAs inhibits TAG-loaded foam cell formation in the human monoblastic cell line U937 [22]. Dyslipidemia are regarded as the key risk factors for the development of atherosclerosis, and HIF1 has been suggested to have both detrimental and beneficial roles in atherosclerosis [28, 44, 45]. In murine atherosclerosis, the hypoxia-induced accumulation of cholesterol was substantially reversed in vitro by reducing the expression of the HIF1α [23]. While in another model, PHD2 inhibition stabilized HIF1α and reduced serum cholesterol levels in low-density lipoprotein receptor-deficient mice that were fed a high-fat diet (HFD) [28]. So the role of HIF1 should be further studied in atherosclerosis lipid metabolism.

2.2. Heart failure diseases

Ischemic heart disease, systemic hypertension, and pathological cardiac hypertrophy eventually result in heart failure. Myocardial hypoxia has been associated with these clinical conditions [25, 46]. Several studies showed a correlation between TAG accumulation and heart failure [26, 47–49]. Hypoxia promotes TAG accumulation in cardiomyocytes [48, 50]. Overexpression of the constitutive active form of HIF1α in cardiomyocytes promotes intracellular lipid accumulation under normoxia [24]. The specific deletion of VHL in mice cardiac myocytes results in lipid accumulation [25, 26]. In a pathological cardiac hypertrophy mouse model, cardiac TAG accumulation in ventricles was abolished in HIF1α knockout mice [26].

2.3. Fatty liver disease (FLD)

Lipid accumulation is a common feature of fatty liver disease, whether it is alcoholic (AFLD) or nonalcoholic (NAFLD) [19]. FLD initially begins with simple hepatic steatosis, but can irreversibly progress to steatohepatitis, fibrosis, cirrhosis, or hepatocellular carcinoma [19]. Hypoxia in liver has been documented in vivo in rats on a continuous ethanol diet at a constant rate for prolonged periods [51–54]. Recent studies have demonstrated that hypoxia is also observed in NAFLD [55]. Indeed, HIF1 expression is increased in fatty liver diseases [19]. Nath and his colleagues found that ethanol feeding resulted in liver steatosis in wild-type mice compared with isocaloric diet-fed controls [27]. Constitutive activation of HIF1α in hepatocytes accelerates lipid accumulation with chronic ethanol feeding compared with wild-type mice [27]. In contrast, hepatocyte-specific deletion of HIF1α protected mice from alcohol-induced liver lipid accumulation [27]. However, another group reported that hepatocyte-specific HIF1α-null mice developed severe hyper-triglyceridemia with enhanced lipid accumulation in the liver of mice after 4 weeks of exposure to a 6% ethanol-containing liquid diet [29]. Different genetic techniques used to create specific gene expression or knockout mice in each of these studies may offer some explanation of the different results each described. The other possible explanation is that the presence of inflammation may rewire the HIF-1 pathway, which leads to a different gene expression profile compared to that observed in simple steatosis [19].

2.4. Obesity

Hypoxia has been directly demonstrated in adipose tissue of several obese mouse models, such as ob/ob mice [56, 57], KKAy obese mice [58], and high-fat diet-induced obese mice [56–58]. In HFD-induced obese mice, HIF1 activation in visceral white adipocytes is critical to maintain dietary obesity [3] and adipocyte-specific HIF1β or HIF1α knockout mice exhibit reduced fat formation compared with wild-type controls [59]. Conversely, another group, using transgenic mice with adipose tissue selective expression of a dominant negative version of HIF1, found that mice with inhibition of HIF1's activity developed a more severe obesity in HFD-induced obese mice [60]. Inactivation of PHD2 resulted in the activation of HIF1. Transgenic mice with PHD2-specific deletion in adipocyte were resistant to HFD-induced obesity and decreased lipid accumulation [30]. In another PHD2-deficient mice model, they also had improved glucose tolerance and insulin sensitivity. Whether fed normal chow or HFD, PHD2 inhibition had less adipose tissue, smaller adipocytes, and less adipose tissue inflammation than their littermates. In addition, serum cholesterol level and de novo lipid synthesis were decreased, and the mice were protected against hepatic steatosis in PHD2-deficient mice [31]. It seems that HIF1 in adipocyte of obesity had different effect on lipid metabolism compared with other models. Thus, the effect of HIF1 in lipid metabolism of obesity has yet to be defined.

2.5. Cancer

Hypoxia in the tumor microenvironment leads to the metabolic changes in cancer cells. Over 50% cellular energy is produced by glycolysis and HIF1 plays a central role in the changes [16, 61]. Recently disorders of lipid metabolism had been demonstrated in solid tumors [62, 63], such as pancreatic cancer [64], liver cancer [1], breast cancer [65], colon cancer [66], and ovarian cancer [67]. Lipid accumulation is observed in human tumor tissue [66, 68]. Accumulation of cholesterol also has been reported in prostate cancer [69]. Indeed, recent researches had demonstrated that HIF1's activity is really involved abnormal lipid metabolism of cancer cells. Hypoxia-induced lipid accumulation depends on HIF1's activity in cancer cells [18, 20, 21]. Under hypoxic condition, the flux from glutamine into fatty acid is mediated by reductive carboxylation, and HIF1α plays an important role in this metabolic shift in tumor cells [70]. HIF1α also inhibits fatty acid β-oxidation to promote lipid accumulation in human hepatocellular carcinoma [1]. Valli and his colleagues revealed that hypoxia induced many changes in lipid metabolites. Enzymatic steps in fatty acid synthesis and the Kennedy pathway were modified in an HIF1α-dependent fashion in HCT116 cell line [2]. However, the role of HIF1 in cancer lipid metabolism has not been well addressed, so more researches should be further studied.

3. The role of HIF1 in lipid metabolism

Lipid metabolism is more complicated than glucose metabolism. Besides as major components of membrane, lipids are also a source of energy storage and signal molecules. HIF1-induced genes involving lipid metabolism are listed in **Table 1**. We would discuss the role of HIF1 in lipid metabolism from the following linked aspects: lipid uptake and trafficking, fatty acid metabolism, sterol metabolism, TAG synthesis, phospholipids metabolism, lipid droplets biogenesis, and lipid signaling (**Figure 1**).

3.1. Lipid uptake and trafficking

3.1.1. Free fatty acid (FFA) uptake

At the plasma membrane, uptake of fatty acid is mainly regulated by the fatty acid transport protein family, such as CD36 [89–91], and plasma membrane-associated fatty-acid-binding proteins (FABPs). Fatty acid transporter CD36 transports long chain fatty acid (LCFA) across plasma membrane. In cardiac myocytes, acute hypoxia (15 min) induced the redistribution of CD36 from an intracellular pool to the plasma membrane [92]. Similarly, in intact Langendorff-perfused heart, a similar effect was demonstrated [92]. Thus, indicating the increased intracellular lipid accumulation in hypoxic hearts is attributable to accumulation of fatty acid in the heart [92]. CD36 also can be regulated at the transcriptional level. In neonatal mouse cardiac myocytes, phenyl-epinephrine (PE) induced free fatty acid uptake in an HIF1α -dependent fashion while inhibition of CD36 led to decreased TAG accumulation upon PE stimulation [26]. In this model, CD36 was induced through HIF1-PPARγ axis [26]. In human retinal pigment epithelial cells, CD36 is mediated by HIF1 binding on its promoter region [71]. Hypoxia also markedly induced CD36 mRNA in corneal and retinal tissue in in vivo [71].

Products of HIF1's target genes	Functions in lipid metabolism	References
CD36, PPARγ, FABP3, FABP7	Fatty acid uptake	[21, 26, 71]
VLDLR, LRP1	LDL and VLDL uptake	[18, 48, 72, 73]
CAV1, RAB20	Endocytosis and lipid trafficking	[74, 75]
PPARα*, TWIST1, Sirt2*	Fatty acid β-oxidation	[3, 76, 77]
DEC1	Fatty acid synthesis	[30, 78]
ABCA1*	Cholesterol efflux	[79]
PPARγ, Lipin1	TAG synthesis	[20, 26]
CHKA	Phospholipids synthesis	[80, 81]
ADRP, HIG2, CAV1	Lipid droplet biogenesis	[42, 74, 82–85]
COX2, PTGES1	Lipid signaling	[86–88]

PPARγ, peroxisome proliferator-activated receptor gamma; VLDLR, very-low-density lipoprotein receptor; LRP1, low-density lipoprotein receptor-related protein 1; CAV1, caveolin 1; PPARα, peroxisome proliferator-activated receptor alpha; TWIST1, twist family bHLH transcription factor 1; SIRT2, sirtuin 2; DEC1, deleted in esophageal cancer 1; ABCA1, ATP-binding cassette subfamily A member 1; LPIN1, lipin 1; HIG2, hypoxia inducible gene 2; CHKA, choline kinase alpha; COX2, cyclooxygenase 2; PTGES, prostaglandin E synthase 1.

"*" genes suppressed by HIF1.

Table 1. HIF1 targets genes that regulate lipid metabolism.

FABPs are part of a larger family of cytoplasmic proteins comprising nine members (FABP1–FABP9) [93], and are involved in reversibly binding intracellular hydrophobic ligands and trafficking them throughout cellular compartments [89]. Some evidence suggested that FABPs could interact directly with CD36 [94]. In *in vitro*, FABP3 and FABP7 were induced by hypoxia in a HIF1-dependent manner, and both are involved in fatty acid uptake [21]. Knockdown of endogenous expression of FABP3 or FABP7 significantly impaired lipids droplets formation under hypoxia [21]. More specifically, the role of FABP3 is evident from the phenotype of FABP3 knockout mice, which show a rate of palmitate uptake reduced by 50% in cardiac myocytes [95, 96]. FABP7 binds long-chain polyunsaturated FA (PUFA), allowing uptake and intracellular trafficking [97], and is involved in proliferation and invasion of melanoma cells [98] and glioblastoma cells [21]. High expression of FABP7 in glioblastomas is associated with poor prognosis and more invasive tumors [99].

3.1.2. LDL and VLDL uptake

LDL and VLDL are major source of extracellular lipid, and HIF1 has been implicated in the transport of LDL and VLDL into cells. LDL receptor (LDLR) and VLDL receptor (VLDLR) are major receptors that are responsible for LDL and VLDL uptake. It had been reported that hypoxia significantly increased LDL uptake and enhances lipid accumulation in arterial smooth muscle cells (SMCs), exclusive LDLR activity [100]. In addition, hypoxia increased VLDL uptake in cardiac myocytes, which might be partially dependent on up-regulating VLDLR expression [101]. Some studies had also reported that VLDLR could be induced under hypoxia [102]. In human cancer cell lines, we had demonstrated that HIF1-mediated VLDLR induction influenced intracellular lipid accumulation through regulating LDL and VLDL uptake under hypoxia [18]. In hepatocellular carcinoma, expression of VLDR was associated positively with HIF1 [18]. In mice, hypoxia-induced VLDLR expression in HL-1 cells was dependent on HIF1α through its interaction with an HRE in the *VLDLR* promoter. VLDLR promoted the endocytosis of lipoproteins, and causes lipid accumulation in cardiomyocytes [48].

Low-density lipoprotein receptor related protein 1 (LRP1) belongs to LDL receptor superfamily, and is a key receptor for selective cholesterol uptake in human vascular smooth muscle cells (VSMCs). Hypoxia increased LRP1 expression through HIF1α, and overexpression of LRP1 mediated hypoxia-induced aggregated LDL (agLDL) uptake in human VSMCs [72] as well as VLDL-cholesteryl ester (VLDL-CE) uptake in neonatal rat ventricular myocytes (NRVMs) [73]. In contrast to the strong impact of LRP1 inhibition on VLDL-CE uptake in hypoxic cardiomyocytes, LRP1 deficiency did not exert any significant effect on VLDL-TG uptake or VLDL-TG accumulation [73]. This indicated that VLDLR might be a key receptor for VLDL-TG uptake. Therefore, more experiments should be done to value the precise contribution of VLDLR and LRP1 in myocardial VLDL-CE and VLDL-TG uptake in pathophysiological situation in the heart.

LDL and VLDL uptake are through vesicular transport pathways [103]. The LDL receptor superfamily has NPXY motif in cytoplasmic domain that interacts with the endocytotic machinery to mediate rapid clathrin-dependent endocytosis of the receptor-ligand complex [104, 105]. Caveolaes are formed in the process of receptor-mediated endocytosis. Numerous proteins are involved in caveolae formation, including caveolins, Rabs, VAT-1, SNAP, and VAMP [106]. Caveolin-1 (CAV1) is an essential structural constituent of caveolae that is involved in constitutive endocytic vesicular trafficking. Loss of VHL function, an E3 ligase involving HIF1α degradation, was associated with increased caveolae formation [74]. CAV1, as a direct target of HIF1, accentuated the formation of caveolae [74]. Knockdown expression of CAV1 inhibited uptake of oxidized LDL (oxLDL) without changing its binding to the plasma membrane [107]. These results indicated that CAV1 was part of the pathway that allowed cells to take up oxLDL [107]. Rab20, a member of the Rab family of small GTP-binding proteins, regulating intracellular trafficking and vesicle formation, had also been characterized as an HIF-1 target [75]. Although there was no direct evidence of the involvement of CAV1 and Rab20 in hypoxia-induced LDL and VLDL uptake, we hypothesized that they might play role in hypoxia-induced LDL and VLDL uptake and/or intracellular lipid trafficking.

Taken together, HIF1 promoting lipid accumulation may increase lipid uptake and intracellular lipid trafficking by inducing related genes directly. It should be further studied if there are more genes targeted by HIF1 in the process.

3.2. Fatty acid metabolism

3.2.1. Fatty acid β-oxidation

Hypoxia increased intracellular lipid accumulation through suppression of fatty acid β-oxidation (FAO) in several models, and the molecular mechanism involvement of HIF1 in the process had been demonstrated (**Figure 2**). Under hypoxic condition, human macrophages showed in an increased TAG accumulation that was associated with a decreasing rate of FAO. The decreasing rate of FAO was shown to be partly dependent on the reduced expression of enzymes involved in FAO [42]. Peroxisome proliferator-activated receptors (PPARs), including α, γ, and β/δ, belong to the nuclear receptor family of ligand-activated transcription factors that were originally described as gene regulators of various metabolic pathways. PPARα and PPARβ/δ control expression of genes implicated in FAO. PPARγ, in contrast, is a key regulator of glucose homeostasis and adipogenesis [108].

Muscle carnitine palmitoyltransferase 1 (M-CPT1), a known PPARα target gene, catalyzes the rate-limiting step in the mitochondrial import of fatty acids for the FAO cycle [109]. In cardiomyocytes, hypoxia and adenovirus-mediated expression of a constitutively active form of HIF1α reduced the mRNA and protein levels of PPARα and M-CPT1 [24, 50, 110] as well as the DNA binding activity of PPARα [24, 50]. $CoCl_2$ treatment also decreased PPARα and M-CPT1 mRNA levels [110]. In intestinal epithelial cells, hypoxia rapidly down-regulated PPARα mRNA and protein in an HIF1-dependent manner in vitro and in vivo [76]. HIF1 could down-regulate PPARα directly through binding a functional HRE in the promoter region [76]. These results suggested that the mechanism of HIF-1 suppression of FAO involved the partial reduction of the expression of PPARα and M-CPT1.

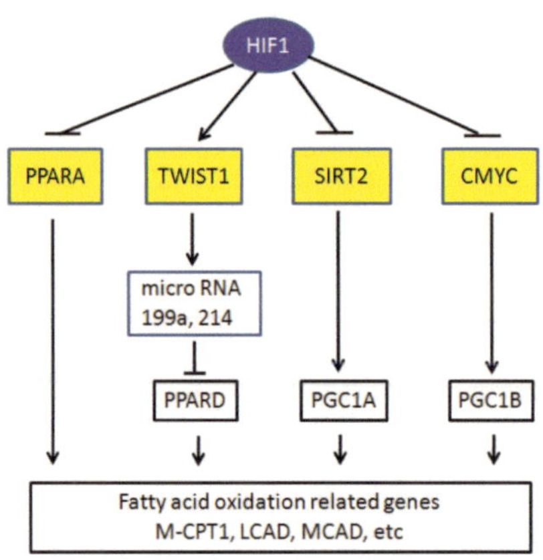

Figure 2. The molecular mechanism involving HIF1 repression of fatty acid β-oxidation. HIF1 targets PPARα, PPARδ, and Sirt2 directly and thereby suppresses the genetic expression of fatty acid β-oxidation.

HIF1 also suppressed FAO by inhibition of PPARδ's activity. In a pathological cardiac hypertrophy mouse model, myocardial hypoxia provoked Dnm3os activation and concomitantly mir-199a and mir-214 expression through the HIF1-TWIST1 axis [49]. TWIST1 is a direct target gene of HIF1 [77]. DNM3os is a noncoding RNA transcript that harbors the mi-RNA cluster mir-199a~214, for which PPARδ is a target. Increased expression of mir-199a and mir-214 decreased cardiac PPARδ expression and mitochondrial fatty acid oxidative capacity. Reduced expression of enzymes involved in FAO, for example long-chain acyl-CoA dehydrogenase (LCAD) and medium-chain acyl-CoA dehydrogenase (MCAD), was also observed. Conversely, antagomir-based silencing of miR-199a~214 in mice subjected to pressure overload derepressed cardiac PPARδ, LCAD and MCAD levels, and restored mitochondrial FAO [49].

PPARγ coactivator 1α (PGC-1α) has been prominently associated with the expression of the genes involving FAO and energy expenditure [111]. In obese mouse model, HIF1α suppressed FAO in visceral white adipocytes, in part, through transcriptional repression of sirtuin 2 (Sirt2), an NAD^+-dependent deacetylase [3]. Reduced Sirt2 function directly translated into diminished deacetylation of PGC1α and the expression of FAO genes. HIF1α negated adipocyte-intrinsic pathway of fatty acid catabolism by negatively regulating the Sirt2-PGC1α regulatory axis [3].

PPARγ coactivator 1β (PGC-1β) is a transcription factor that also plays critical roles in regulating mitochondrial function and lipid metabolism [112, 113]. PGC-1β could regulate FAO through activating medium-chain acyl-CoA dehydrogenase (MCAD) and long-chain acyl-CoA dehydrogenase (LCAD), which catalyzes the first step of FAO in mitochondria [1, 112]. It had been documented previously that hypoxia inhibited PGC-1β activity through HIF1-dependent c-Myc suppression in VHL-null RCC4 renal carcinoma cells [114]. Under hypoxic condition in Hep3B and HepG2 cells, and also in PC3 prostate cancer cells, Huang and his colleagues revealed a role of the HIF1/C-MYC/PGC-1β regulatory axis in hypoxia-mediated regulation of MCAD and LCAD by which HIF1 suppressed FAO [1]. This study confirmed that hypoxia inhibited FAO in an HIF1-dependent mechanism in cancer cells [1].

In summary, it had been confirmed by different models that hypoxia inhibits FAO depending on HIF1's activity (**Figure 2**). However, HIF1 did not target FAO-related genes directly, and it was always cross-talk with other pathway to suppress FAO indirectly. It should be further studied if HIF1 could involve cross-talk with more pathways to suppress FAO.

3.2.2. Fatty acid synthesis

De novo fatty acid synthesis begins with acetyl coenzyme A (Ac-CoA). Ac-CoA is primarily generated from glucose through tri-carboxylic acid (TCA) cycle in the mitochondrion, the citrate shuttle and ATP citrate lyase in the cytosol. Under hypoxic condition, cells converted glucose to lactate and the TCA cycle is largely disconnected from glycolysis [70, 115–117], thereby directing glucose carbon away from fatty acid synthesis. Recently, several groups had found that hypoxic tumor cells maintain proliferation by running the TCA cycle in reverse [70, 115–117]. In these cells, the source of carbon for Ac-CoA and fatty acid switched from glucose to glutamine. This hypoxic flux from glutamine to fatty acid was mediated by the reductive carboxylation of glutamine-derived α-ketoglutarate.

The reductive carboxylation of glutamine was part of the metabolic reprogramming associated with HIF1. Glutamine-derived α-ketoglutarate is reductively carboxylated by the cytosolic isocitrate dehydrogenase 1 (IDH1) [70, 115] and the mitochondrial isocitrate dehydrogenase 2 (IDH2) to form isocitrate [70, 115, 116], which could then be isomerized to citrate. The combined action of IDH1 and IDH2 was necessary and sufficient to affect the reverse TCA flux [115]. Citrate was converted into Ac-CoA by ATP citrate lyase in the cytosol. Renal cell lines deficient in the VHL preferentially used reductive glutamine metabolism for lipid biosynthesis even at normal oxygen levels [70]. Constitutive activation of HIF1 recapitulated the preferential reductive metabolism of glutamine-derived α-ketoglutarate even in normoxic condition [116]. This regulation by HIF1 of the reverse TCA cycle occurred partly through HIF1-inducing PDK1. Knocking down PDK1 suppressed reductive carboxylation [70, 118]. However, more details should be studied about the role of HIF1 in TCA cycle reverse.

The first step of fatty acid synthesis is catalyzed by AcCoA carboxylase (ACC) which converts Ac-CoA to malonyl-CoA. Then fatty-acid synthase (FASN) catalyzes acetyl-CoA and malonyl-CoA to palmitate. Further elongation and de-saturation of newly synthesized fatty acid takes place at the cytoplasmic face of the endoplasmic reticulum membrane. It had been reported that hypoxia regulated FASN expression [78, 119, 120]. However, different conclusions on hypoxia regulation of FASN had been reported. One group using human breast cancer cell lines found that FASN was significantly up-regulated by hypoxia via activation of the Akt and HIF1 followed by the induction of the SREBP1 gene [119]. Another group, using several cell lines other than breast cancer cell lines, found that hypoxia suppressed FASN expression through HIF1-DEC1 and/or DEC2-SREBP1 axis. They found that HIF1 repressed the SREBP1 gene by inducing DEC1 and DEC2, and further repressing FASN expression [78]. These results might indicate that HIF1 regulated FASN in a cell-type specific manner. In addition, it had been reported that hypoxia could induce the expression of SCD1 which introduces a double bond in the $\Delta 9$ position of palmitic acid and stearic acid to produce mono-unsaturated fatty acid [42, 121]. It is unknown if HIF1 is involved in hypoxic-induced SCD1.

Taken together, the role of HIF1 in de novo fatty acid synthesis may depend on different models and conditions, and more researches should be done in the direction.

3.3. Cholesterol metabolism

Cholesterol is an essential structural component of membrane. It modulates membrane permeability and fluidity and also forms microdomains named lipid rafts that integrate the activation of some signal transduction pathways [14]. Intermediates generated by the cholesterol biosynthesis pathway were required for the posttranslational modification of small GTPases, such as the farnesylation of Ras and the geranyl-geranylation of Rho [15]. Finally, cholesterol also serves as a precursor for the biosynthesis of steroid hormones, bile acids, and vitamin D.

Cellular cholesterol level can be modulated by three processes: cholesterol uptake, synthesis, and efflux [122]. In the preceding paragraph, we had discussed the role of HIF1 in LDL and VLDL uptake that are main source of extracellular cholesterol. Here, we discuss the cholesterol synthesis and efflux. Cholesterol biosynthesis begins with the condensation of AcCoA with acetoacetyl-CoA to form 3-hydroxy-3-methylglutaryl (HMG)-CoA. Then HMG-CoA reductase (HMGCR) reduces of HMG-CoA to mevalonate. Early research found that Hypoxia also suppressed cholesterol synthesis in cultured rabbit skin fibroblasts [123]. However, recently research indicated that hypoxia increased sterol synthesis depending on HIF1's activity [23, 124]. In hypoxic macrophages, the increase of intracellular cholesterol content was correlated with elevated HMGCR's activity and mRNA levels [23]. In HepG2 cells, HIF1α accumulation was able to increase the level and activity of HMGCR by stimulating its transcription [124]. But it was unclear if HIF1 regulated HMGCR directly.

Hypoxia suppressed the efflux of cholesterol, and this efflux was substantially reversed in vitro by reducing the expression of HIF1 [23, 123]. ATP-binding cassette transporter A1 (ABCA1) plays a major role in cholesterol efflux. Hypoxia severely reduced ABCA1-mediated cholesterol efflux, which could be explained by subcellular redistribution of ABCA1 protein under acute hypoxia and decreased protein level under prolonged hypoxia [23]. One group reported that HIF1 could repress the transcription of ABCA1 directly [79]. Hypoxia, partly mediated by HIF1α, increased intracellular cholesterol content due to the induction of cholesterol synthesis and the suppression of cholesterol efflux [23]. In addition, accumulation of cholesterol in hypoxic cells was in esterified form [23, 100]. At 2% O_2 tension, twice the total cholesteryl ester was observed compared with that at 21% O_2. At the same time, no significant difference was found in the concentration of cellular-free cholesterol [100]. Accumulation of cholesteryl ester in hypoxic cells might depend on the increased activity of AcCoA:cholesterol acyltransferases (ACATs) [123], which are important enzymes for the esterification of cholesterol. Therefore, more studies should be done to define the role of HIF1 involving the cholesterol metabolism in detail.

3.4. TAG synthesis and phospholipids metabolism

3.4.1. TAG synthesis

TAG is formed by the addition of three molecules of fatty acid to glycerol. There are two major pathways for TAG biosynthesis in mammalian cell: the glycerol phosphate pathway and the mono-acylglycerol (MG) pathway. In the glycerol phosphate pathway, two molecules of fatty acyl-CoA are esterified to glycerol-3-phosphate to yield 1,2-diacylglycerol (DAG) phosphate (commonly identified as phosphatidic acid). The phosphate is then removed to yield 1,2-diacylglycerol, which is followed by addition of the third fatty acid to form TAG. TAG accumulation under hypoxia could be mediated by HIF1-inducing Lipin1 [20], a phosphatidate phosphatase isoform that catalyzes the penultimate step in TAG biosynthesis, the removal of phosphate from diacylglycerol phosphate to yield DAG. It also had been reported that hypoxia produced a marked intracellular accumulation of diacylglycerol in different cell types [125]. DAG may also serve a feedback role regulating HIF1's activity [125]. In a mouse model of pathological hypertrophy, HIF1α promoted TAG accumulation in cardiomyocytes via the regulation of PPARγ expression. PPARγ was the principal mediator of TAG anabolism through its transcriptional regulation glycerol-3-phosphate generation (via GPD1), and downstream esterification processes (via GPAT) [26].

3.4.2. *Phospholipids metabolism*

Phospholipids are indispensable for cell growth. Phospholipids synthesis and TAG synthesis share similar steps. DAG is a precursor for phosphatidylcholine and phosphatidylethanolamine. Phosphatidic acid utilizes cytidine triphosphate (CTP) as an energy source to produce a CDP-DAG intermediate followed by conversion to phosphatidylcholine. It had been reported that the intracellular level of phosphatidic acid (PA) and DAG rose in response to hypoxia [125, 126]. However, PA accumulation in response to hypoxia was both HIF1 and VHL-independent [127]. Choline kinase α (ChKα) catalyzes the phosphorylation of choline, the first step of phosphatidylcholine synthesis. In cancer cells, one group had shown that hypoxia increased ChKα expression and this was driven by HIF1 [80]. Conversely, another group had shown that choline kinase activity and choline phosphorylation were decreased, that might be mediated via HIF1α binding to the promoter of ChKα gene [81]. Thus, further studies should be done to address the role of HIF1 in phospholipids metabolism.

3.5. Lipid droplet (LD) biogenesis and lipid signaling

Lipid droplet, also named lipid body, has been largely associated with neutral lipid storage and transport in cells [106]. The internal core of the LD is rich in neutral lipids, predominantly TAGs or cholesteryl esters, that are surrounded by an outer monolayer of phospholipids and associated proteins [128]. LD was considered to be highly regulated, dynamic and functionally active organelle [106]. Proteins on the surface of lipid droplets are crucial to the droplet structure and dynamics. Currently, the complete protein composition of LD has not been defined. The best characterized LD' proteins are the perilipin/ADRP/TIP47 (PAT) domain family. Apart from the PAT domain proteins, there are other lipid droplets associated proteins which involve the catabolism of lipids, vesicular transport, eicosanoid-forming enzymes, protein kinases, etc. [106]. Hypoxia increased LD number and size [42, 129]. Several LD-associated proteins were induced by HIF1 and might also involve HIF1-induced LD biogenesis and lipid signaling (**Figure 3**).

3.5.1. *Lipid droplet biogenesis*

Adipose differentiation-related protein (ADRP), a PAT domain protein, is a structural component of LD and had been reported by several groups to be inducible by HIF1 [42, 82–84]. Lipid accumulation was associated with high expression level of ADRP in solid tumors [68, 130], especially in clear cell lesions [131]. During the process of carcinogenesis, the ADRP expression was increased during early tumorigenesis and was associated with the proliferation rate [68]. The expression of ADRP was also correlated with atherosclerosis [132]. In mouse macrophages in vitro, ADRP expression facilitated foam cell formation induced by modified lipoproteins [132]. In apolipoprotein E-deficient mice, ADRP inactivation reduced the number of LD in foam cells in atherosclerotic lesions [132]. Under hypoxia, knockdown of ADRP in U87 and T98G or in MCF-7 and MDA-MB-231 cells significantly decreased the formation of LD, and resulted in decreased fatty acid uptake [21]. It indicated that ADRP promoted LD formation mainly through increasing FA uptake under hypoxic condition. It had been reported that ADRP can also stimulate LCFA uptake [133]. While another research reported that ADRP did not involve LDL- and VLDL-induced LD formation under hypoxia [84].

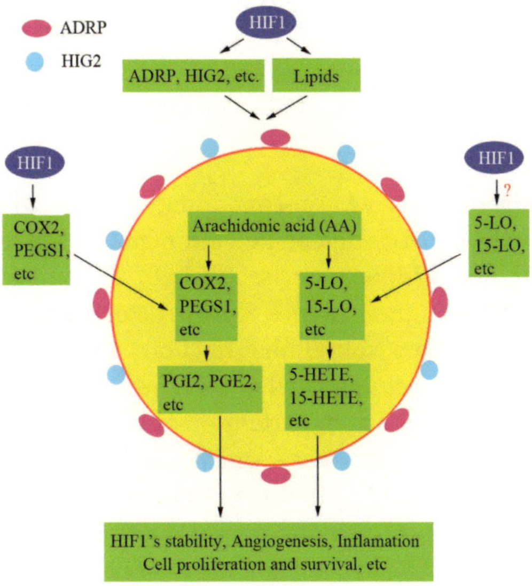

Figure 3. A hypothetical representation of molecular mechanism involving hypoxia-induced lipid droplet biogenesis and function. HIF1-induced structural proteins of the LD, such as ADRP, HIG2, combine with HIF1-increased lipids to form the LD. Enzymes involving eicosanoid production are also induced by HIF1, and are recruited to the LD. These proteins can increase lipid signaling that can involve many aspects of biology, such as HIF1α's stability, angiogenesis, inflammation, cell proliferation and survival.

Hypoxia-inducible protein 2 (HIG2), a newly identified protein associated with LD, was up-regulated by hypoxia and was a direct and specific target gene of HIF1 [85]. Overexpression of HIG2 under normoxic condition was sufficient to increase LD in HeLa cells. HIG2-driven LD might contribute to an inflammatory response. Overexpression of HIG2 stimulated cytokine expression of vascular endothelial growth factor-A (VEGFA), macrophage migration inhibitory factor (MIF), and interleukin-6 (IL-6). Increasing expression of HIG2 was also detected under several conditions of pathological lipid accumulation, such as atherosclerotic arteries and fatty liver disease [85]. We had mentioned that CAV1 was a target of HIF1. CAV1 could distribute to LD under several conditions [134–137] and the association with LD was reversible [134]. However, It is unknown if hypoxia can redistribute CAV1 to LD and CAV1 involves LD biogenesis under hypoxia.

3.5.2. Lipid signaling

Eicosanoids are signaling molecules made by oxidation of 20-carbon fatty acids, mainly from arachidonic acid. Cyclooxygenases and Lipoxygenases are two families of enzymes catalyzing fatty acid oxygenation to produce the eicosanoids. There are multiple subfamilies of eicosanoids, including prostaglandins, prostacyclins, thromboxanes, lipoxins, and leukotrienes. Prostaglandins, such as PGI_2 and PGE_2, are synthesized via cyclooxygenase (COX) by oxidation of arachidonic acid. PGE_2 is synthesized in three steps catalyzed by phospholipase (PL) A2, COX, and terminal prostaglandin E synthase (PTGES), where each catalytic activity is represented by multiple enzymes and/or isoenzymes. It had been reported that hypoxia could increase prostaglandins (PGI_2 and PGE_2) synthesis [138]. Hypoxia-induced synthesis of PGE_2 was accompanied by up-regulation of COX2, which is a direct target gene of HIF1 [86]. Several studies had indicated that LD was reservoirs of COX2 and sites of PGE_2 synthesis [66, 139, 140]. PTGES1 could also be regulated by HIF1 directly [87, 88]; however, it is unknown if PTGES1 localizes to hypoxia-induced LD.

Lipoxygenases are a family of nonheme iron-containing enzymes which dioxygenate polyunsaturated fatty acid to hydroperoxyl metabolite, and mainly include 5-lipoxygenase (5-LO), 12-lipoxygenase (12-LO), and 15-lipoxygenase (15-LO). 5-LO and 15-LO were shown by immuno-cytochemistry, immuno-fluorescence, ultrastructural postembedding immuno-gold EM and/or western blotting from subcellular fractions to localize within lipid droplets stimulated in vitro [141–144]. Increasing level of 5-LO was detected in lung tissue of rodent model of hypoxia-induced pulmonary hypertension [145]. Hypoxia increased 12-LO in rat lung and in in vitro cultured rat pulmonary artery smooth muscle cell (PASMC) and may contribute to the production of 12(S)-hydroxyeicosatetraenoic acid (12(S)-HETE) [146]. Increasing 12(S)-HETE had also been demonstrated in hypoxic macrophage cells [147]. Under hypoxia, increased levels of 15-LO had been demonstrated by different groups [147, 148] and its product, 15-hydroperoxyeicosatetraenoic acid (15-HETE), was up-regulated [147]. Up-regulation of 15-LO/15-HETE in response to hypoxia might be partially mediated by HIF1α [149]. In addition, HIF1α was shown to be regulated by 15-HETE in a positive feedback manner [149]. However, it is unknown if lipoxygenases are regulated by HIF1 directly.

4. Conclusions and perspectives

HIF1 plays an important role in lipid metabolism and a number of studies support the findings that HIF1 promotes lipid accumulation. Nevertheless, many questions remain. HIF1, as a master transcriptional factor, may target many genes directly or indirectly involved in lipid metabolism. HIF1 plays a pivotal role in glucose metabolism. Inhibition of GULT3, an HIF1 target gene, could significantly reduce both glucose uptake and hypoxia-induced de novo lipid synthesis in human monocyte-derived macrophages [150]. PGAM1, induced by hypoxia [151], catalyzes the reversible reaction of 3-phosphoglycerate (3-PGA) to 2-phosphoglycerate (2-PGA) in the glycolytic pathway. Inhibition of PGAM1 led to significantly decreased glycolysis and de novo lipid synthesis in cancer cells [152]. Thus, it is possible that glucose metabolism might couple with lipid metabolism under hypoxia. The source of carbon for fatty acid switched from glucose to glutamine under hypoxia [70]. The question thus arises. Does HIF1 induce lipid accumulation through targeting genes involving glucose metabolism, and how does glucose metabolism affect lipid metabolism under hypoxia?

HIF1 could interact with other pathways to regulate lipid metabolism besides PPARα, PPARγ, PPARδ, PGC1α, and SREBP1. There might be a pivotal role for mTOR in controlling

http://dx.doi.org/10.5772/65340

lipid homeostasis in many settings, both physiological and pathological [153]. AMPK is a cellular energy sensor that normalizes lipid, glucose, and energy imbalances [154]. Inhibition of cMYC was accompanied by accumulation of intracellular LD in tumor cells as a direct consequence of mitochondrial dysfunction [155]. Recently, p53 had also been shown to regulate lipid metabolism [156]. The role of HIF1 in these pathways and the molecular mechanism will require further investigation.

Lipid accumulation in diseases, including obesity, atherosclerosis, ALD, heart failure disease and cancer, had been associated with HIF1's activity. There may be additional pathologies with lipid metabolism disorder associated with HIF1. HIF1 is an attractive target candidate for therapeutic intervention in diseases with disorder of lipid metabolism including cancer. Its involvement in the etiology of a number of diseases and its interaction with a number of regulatory genes make it an important area for further study.

Acknowledgements

This review is supported by a National Natural Science Foundation of China (Grant No. 31301076 to G. S; Grant No. 81401961 to X. L.), We thank Gerard Moskowitz, Ph. D. (Washington University in St. Louis, St. Louis, MO) for critical reading of the manuscript. We sincerely apologize to the colleagues whose works are not covered in this review due to limitations of time and space.

Author details

Guomin Shen[1*] and Xiaobo Li[2]

*Address all correspondence to: shenba433@163.com

1 Department of Medical Genetics, Medical College, Henan University of Science and Technology, Luoyang, Henan Province, China

2 Department of Pathology & Translational Medicine Center, Harbin Medical University, Harbin, Heilongjiang Province, China

References

[1] D. Huang, T. Li, X. Li, L. Zhang, L. Sun, X. He, X. Zhong, D. Jia, L. Song, G.L. Semenza, P. Gao, H. Zhang, HIF-1-mediated suppression of acyl-CoA dehydrogenases and fatty acid oxidation is critical for cancer progression, Cell Rep 8 (2014) 1930–1942.

[2] A. Valli, M. Rodriguez, L. Moutsianas, R. Fischer, V. Fedele, H.L. Huang, R. Van Stiphout, D. Jones, M. McCarthy, M. Vinaxia, K. Igarashi, M. Sato, T. Soga, F. Buffa, J. McCullagh, O. Yanes, A. Harris, B. Kessler, Hypoxia induces a lipogenic cancer cell phenotype via HIF1alpha-dependent and -independent pathways, Oncotarget 6 (2015) 1920–1941.

[3] J. Krishnan, C. Danzer, T. Simka, J. Ukropec, K.M. Walter, S. Kumpf, P. Mirtschink, B. Ukropcova, D. Gasperikova, T. Pedrazzini, W. Krek, Dietary obesity-associated Hif1alpha activation in adipocytes restricts fatty acid oxidation and energy expenditure via suppression of the Sirt2-NAD+ system, Genes Dev 26 (2012) 259–270.

[4] E. Marsch, J.C. Sluimer, M.J. Daemen, Hypoxia in atherosclerosis and inflammation, Curr Opin Lipidol 24 (2013) 393–400.

[5] G.L. Semenza, Hypoxia-inducible factor 1 and cardiovascular disease, Annu Rev Physiol 76 (2013) 39–56.

[6] G.L. Semenza, Hypoxia-inducible factors in physiology and medicine, Cell 148 (2012) 399–408.

[7] G.L. Wang, B.H. Jiang, E.A. Rue, G.L. Semenza, Hypoxia-inducible factor 1 is a basic-helix-loop-helix-PAS heterodimer regulated by cellular O2 tension, Proc Natl Acad Sci U S A 92 (1995) 5510–5514.

[8] G.L. Wang, G.L. Semenza, Purification and characterization of hypoxia-inducible factor 1, J Biol Chem 270 (1995) 1230–1237.

[9] A.C. Epstein, J.M. Gleadle, L.A. McNeill, K.S. Hewitson, J. O'Rourke, D.R. Mole, M. Mukherji, E. Metzen, M.I. Wilson, A. Dhanda, Y.M. Tian, N. Masson, D.L. Hamilton, P. Jaakkola, R. Barstead, J. Hodgkin, P.H. Maxwell, C.W. Pugh, C.J. Schofield, P.J. Ratcliffe, C. elegans EGL-9 and mammalian homologs define a family of dioxygenases that regulate HIF by prolyl hydroxylation, Cell 107 (2001) 43–54.

[10] P.H. Maxwell, M.S. Wiesener, G.W. Chang, S.C. Clifford, E.C. Vaux, M.E. Cockman, C.C. Wykoff, C.W. Pugh, E.R. Maher, P.J. Ratcliffe, The tumour suppressor protein VHL targets hypoxia-inducible factors for oxygen-dependent proteolysis, Nature 399 (1999) 271–275.

[11] M. Ohh, C.W. Park, M. Ivan, M.A. Hoffman, T.Y. Kim, L.E. Huang, N. Pavletich, V. Chau, W.G. Kaelin, Ubiquitination of hypoxia-inducible factor requires direct binding to the beta-domain of the von Hippel-Lindau protein, Nat Cell Biol 2 (2000) 423–427.

[12] P.C. Mahon, K. Hirota, G.L. Semenza, FIH-1: a novel protein that interacts with HIF-1alpha and VHL to mediate repression of HIF-1 transcriptional activity, Genes Dev 15 (2001) 2675–2686.

[13] K.S. Hewitson, L.A. McNeill, M.V. Riordan, Y.M. Tian, A.N. Bullock, R.W. Welford, J.M. Elkins, N.J. Oldham, S. Bhattacharya, J.M. Gleadle, P.J. Ratcliffe, C.W. Pugh, C.J. Schofield, Hypoxia-inducible factor (HIF) asparagine hydroxylase is identical to factor

inhibiting HIF (FIH) and is related to the cupin structural family, J Biol Chem 277 (2002) 26351–26355.

[14] D. Lando, D.J. Peet, J.J. Gorman, D.A. Whelan, M.L. Whitelaw, R.K. Bruick, FIH-1 is an asparaginyl hydroxylase enzyme that regulates the transcriptional activity of hypoxia-inducible factor, Genes Dev 16 (2002) 1466–1471.

[15] D. Lando, D.J. Peet, D.A. Whelan, J.J. Gorman, M.L. Whitelaw, Asparagine hydroxylation of the HIF transactivation domain a hypoxic switch, Science 295 (2002) 858–861.

[16] G.L. Semenza, Defining the role of hypoxia-inducible factor 1 in cancer biology and therapeutics, Oncogene 29 (2010) 625–634.

[17] N.C. Denko, Hypoxia, HIF1 and glucose metabolism in the solid tumour, Nat Rev Cancer 8 (2008) 705–713.

[18] G.M. Shen, Y.Z. Zhao, M.T. Chen, F.L. Zhang, X.L. Liu, Y. Wang, C.Z. Liu, J. Yu, J.W. Zhang, Hypoxia-inducible factor-1 (HIF-1) promotes LDL and VLDL uptake through inducing VLDLR under hypoxia, Biochem J 441 (2012) 675–683.

[19] T. Suzuki, S. Shinjo, T. Arai, M. Kanai, N. Goda, Hypoxia and fatty liver, World J Gastroenterol 20 (2014) 15087–15097.

[20] I. Mylonis, H. Sembongi, C. Befani, P. Liakos, S. Siniossoglou, G. Simos, Hypoxia causes triglyceride accumulation by HIF-1-mediated stimulation of lipin 1 expression, J Cell Sci 125 (2012) 3485–3493.

[21] K. Bensaad, E. Favaro, C.A. Lewis, B. Peck, S. Lord, J.M. Collins, K.E. Pinnick, S. Wigfield, F.M. Buffa, J.L. Li, Q. Zhang, M.J. Wakelam, F. Karpe, A. Schulze, A.L. Harris, Fatty acid uptake and lipid storage induced by HIF-1alpha contribute to cell growth and survival after hypoxia-reoxygenation, Cell Rep 9 (2014) 349–365.

[22] G. Jiang, T. Li, Y. Qiu, Y. Rui, W. Chen, Y. Lou, RNA interference for HIF-1alpha inhibits foam cells formation in vitro, Eur J Pharmacol 562 (2007) 183–190.

[23] S. Parathath, S.L. Mick, J.E. Feig, V. Joaquin, L. Grauer, D.M. Habiel, M. Gassmann, L.B. Gardner, E.A. Fisher, Hypoxia is present in murine atherosclerotic plaques and has multiple adverse effects on macrophage lipid metabolism, Circ Res 109 (2011) 1141–1152.

[24] A.J. Belanger, Z. Luo, K.A. Vincent, G.Y. Akita, S.H. Cheng, R.J. Gregory, C. Jiang, Hypoxia-inducible factor 1 mediates hypoxia-induced cardiomyocyte lipid accumulation by reducing the DNA binding activity of peroxisome proliferator-activated receptor alpha/retinoid X receptor, Biochem Biophys Res Commun 364 (2007) 567–572.

[25] L. Lei, S. Mason, D. Liu, Y. Huang, C. Marks, R. Hickey, I.S. Jovin, M. Pypaert, R.S. Johnson, F.J. Giordano, Hypoxia-inducible factor-dependent degeneration, failure, and malignant transformation of the heart in the absence of the von Hippel-Lindau protein, Mol Cell Biol 28 (2008) 3790–3803.

[26] J. Krishnan, M. Suter, R. Windak, T. Krebs, A. Felley, C. Montessuit, M. Tokarska-Schlattner, E. Aasum, A. Bogdanova, E. Perriard, J.C. Perriard, T. Larsen, T. Pedrazzini,

W. Krek, Activation of a HIF1alpha-PPARgamma axis underlies the integration of glycolytic and lipid anabolic pathways in pathologic cardiac hypertrophy, Cell Metab 9 (2009) 512–524.

[27] B. Nath, I. Levin, T. Csak, J. Petrasek, C. Mueller, K. Kodys, D. Catalano, P. Mandrekar, G. Szabo, Hepatocyte-specific hypoxia-inducible factor-1alpha is a determinant of lipid accumulation and liver injury in alcohol-induced steatosis in mice, Hepatology 53 (2011) 1526–1537.

[28] L. Rahtu-Korpela, J. Maatta, E.Y. Dimova, S. Horkko, H. Gylling, G. Walkinshaw, J. Hakkola, K.I. Kivirikko, J. Myllyharju, R. Serpi, P. Koivunen, Hypoxia-inducible factor prolyl 4-hydroxylase-2 inhibition protects against development of atherosclerosis, Arterioscler Thromb Vasc Biol 36 (2016) 608–617.

[29] Y. Nishiyama, N. Goda, M. Kanai, D. Niwa, K. Osanai, Y. Yamamoto, N. Senoo-Matsuda, R.S. Johnson, S. Miura, Y. Kabe, M. Suematsu, HIF-1alpha induction suppresses excessive lipid accumulation in alcoholic fatty liver in mice, J Hepatol 56 (2012) 441–447.

[30] H. Matsuura, T. Ichiki, E. Inoue, M. Nomura, R. Miyazaki, T. Hashimoto, J. Ikeda, R. Takayanagi, G.H. Fong, K. Sunagawa, Prolyl hydroxylase domain protein 2 plays a critical role in diet-induced obesity and glucose intolerance, Circulation 127 (2013) 2078–2087.

[31] L. Rahtu-Korpela, S. Karsikas, S. Horkko, R. Blanco Sequeiros, E. Lammentausta, K.A. Makela, K.H. Herzig, G. Walkinshaw, K.I. Kivirikko, J. Myllyharju, R. Serpi, P. Koivunen, HIF prolyl 4-hydroxylase-2 inhibition improves glucose and lipid metabolism and protects against obesity and metabolic dysfunction, Diabetes 63 (2014) 3324–3333.

[32] J. Niinikoski, C. Heughan, T.K. Hunt, Oxygen tensions in the aortic wall of normal rabbits, Atherosclerosis 17 (1973) 353–359.

[33] C. Heughan, J. Niinikoski, T.K. Hunt, Oxygen tensions in lesions of experimental atherosclerosis of rabbits, Atherosclerosis 17 (1973) 361–367.

[34] J.F. Martin, R.F. Booth, S. Moncada, Arterial wall hypoxia following hyperfusion through the vasa vasorum is an initial lesion in atherosclerosis, Eur J Clin Invest 20 (1990) 588–592.

[35] T. Bjornheden, M. Evaldsson, O. Wiklund, A method for the assessment of hypoxia in the arterial wall, with potential application in vivo, Arterioscler Thromb Vasc Biol 16 (1996) 178–185.

[36] T. Bjornheden, M. Levin, M. Evaldsson, O. Wiklund, Evidence of hypoxic areas within the arterial wall in vivo, Arterioscler Thromb Vasc Biol 19 (1999) 870–876.

[37] J.M. Silvola, A. Saraste, S. Forsback, V.J. Laine, P. Saukko, S.E. Heinonen, S. Yla-Herttuala, A. Roivainen, J. Knuuti, Detection of hypoxia by [18F]EF5 in atherosclerotic plaques in mice, Arterioscler Thromb Vasc Biol 31 (2011) 1011–1015.

[38] B. Ramkhelawon, Y. Yang, J.M. van Gils, B. Hewing, K.J. Rayner, S. Parathath, L. Guo, S. Oldebeken, J.L. Feig, E.A. Fisher, K.J. Moore, Hypoxia induces netrin-1 and Unc5b in atherosclerotic plaques: mechanism for macrophage retention and survival, Arterioscler Thromb Vasc Biol 33 (2013) 1180–1188.

[39] J.C. Sluimer, J.M. Gasc, J.L. van Wanroij, N. Kisters, M. Groeneweg, M.D. Sollewijn Gelpke, J.P. Cleutjens, L.H. van den Akker, P. Corvol, B.G. Wouters, M.J. Daemen, A.P. Bijnens, Hypoxia, hypoxia-inducible transcription factor, and macrophages in human atherosclerotic plaques are correlated with intraplaque angiogenesis, J Am Coll Cardiol 51 (2008) 1258–1265.

[40] S. Parathath, Y. Yang, S. Mick, E.A. Fisher, Hypoxia in murine atherosclerotic plaques and its adverse effects on macrophages, Trends Cardiovasc Med 23 (2013) 80–84.

[41] L.M. Hulten, M. Levin, The role of hypoxia in atherosclerosis, Curr Opin Lipidol 20 (2009) 409–414.

[42] P. Bostrom, B. Magnusson, P.A. Svensson, O. Wiklund, J. Boren, L.M. Carlsson, M. Stahlman, S.O. Olofsson, L.M. Hulten, Hypoxia converts human macrophages into triglyceride-loaded foam cells, Arterioscler Thromb Vasc Biol 26 (2006) 1871–1876.

[43] S. Akhtar, P. Hartmann, E. Karshovska, F.A. Rinderknecht, P. Subramanian, F. Gremse, J. Grommes, M. Jacobs, F. Kiessling, C. Weber, S. Steffens, A. Schober, Endothelial hypoxia-inducible factor-1alpha promotes atherosclerosis and monocyte recruitment by upregulating MicroRNA-19a, Hypertension 66 (2015) 1220–1226.

[44] J. Ben-Shoshan, A. Afek, S. Maysel-Auslender, A. Barzelay, A. Rubinstein, G. Keren, J. George, HIF-1alpha overexpression and experimental murine atherosclerosis, Arterioscler Thromb Vasc Biol 29 (2009) 665–670.

[45] L. Gao, Q. Chen, X. Zhou, L. Fan, The role of hypoxia-inducible factor 1 in atherosclerosis, J Clin Pathol 65 (2012) 872–876.

[46] G.L. Semenza, Hypoxia-inducible Factor 1 and cardiovascular disease, Annu Rev Physiol 76 (2014) 39–56.

[47] T.S. Park, I.J. Goldberg, Sphingolipids, lipotoxic cardiomyopathy, and cardiac failure, Heart Fail Clin 8 (2012) 633–641.

[48] J.C. Perman, P. Bostrom, M. Lindbom, U. Lidberg, M. StAhlman, D. Hagg, H. Lindskog, M. Scharin Tang, E. Omerovic, L. Mattsson Hulten, A. Jeppsson, P. Petursson, J. Herlitz, G. Olivecrona, D.K. Strickland, K. Ekroos, S.O. Olofsson, J. Boren, The VLDL receptor promotes lipotoxicity and increases mortality in mice following an acute myocardial infarction, J Clin Invest 121 (2011) 2625–2640.

[49] H. El Azzouzi, S. Leptidis, E. Dirkx, J. Hoeks, B. van Bree, K. Brand, E.A. McClellan, E. Poels, J.C. Sluimer, M.M. van den Hoogenhof, A.S. Armand, X. Yin, S. Langley, M. Bourajjaj, S. Olieslagers, J. Krishnan, M. Vooijs, H. Kurihara, A. Stubbs, Y.M. Pinto, W. Krek, M. Mayr, P.A. da Costa Martins, P. Schrauwen, L.J. De Windt, The hypoxia-

inducible MicroRNA cluster miR-199a approximately 214 targets myocardial PPAR-delta and impairs mitochondrial fatty acid oxidation, Cell Metab 18 (2013) 341–354.

[50] J.M. Huss, F.H. Levy, D.P. Kelly, Hypoxia inhibits the peroxisome proliferator-activated receptor alpha/retinoid X receptor gene regulatory pathway in cardiac myocytes: a mechanism for O2-dependent modulation of mitochondrial fatty acid oxidation, J Biol Chem 56–84 (2001) 27605–27612.

[51] G.E. Arteel, Y. Iimuro, M. Yin, J.A. Raleigh, R.G. Thurman, Chronic enteral ethanol treatment causes hypoxia in rat liver tissue in vivo, Hepatology 25 (1997) 920–926.

[52] G.E. Arteel, J.A. Raleigh, B.U. Bradford, R.G. Thurman, Acute alcohol produces hypoxia directly in rat liver tissue in vivo: role of Kupffer cells, Am J Physiol 271 (1996) G494–G500.

[53] S.W. French, The role of hypoxia in the pathogenesis of alcoholic liver disease, Hepatol Res 29 (2004) 69–74.

[54] F. Bardag-Gorce, B.A. French, J. Li, N.E. Riley, Q.X. Yuan, V. Valinluck, P. Fu, M. Ingelman-Sundberg, S. Yoon, S.W. French, The importance of cycling of blood alcohol levels in the pathogenesis of experimental alcoholic liver disease in rats, Gastroenterology 123 (2002) 325–335.

[55] S.K. Mantena, D.P. Vaughn, K.K. Andringa, H.B. Eccleston, A.L. King, G.A. Abrams, J.E. Doeller, D.W. Kraus, V.M. Darley-Usmar, S.M. Bailey, High fat diet induces dysregulation of hepatic oxygen gradients and mitochondrial function in vivo, Biochem J 417 (2009) 183–193.

[56] M.E. Rausch, S. Weisberg, P. Vardhana, D.V. Tortoriello, Obesity in C57BL/6J mice is characterized by adipose tissue hypoxia and cytotoxic T-cell infiltration, Int J Obes (Lond) 32 (2008) 451–463.

[57] J. Ye, Z. Gao, J. Yin, Q. He, Hypoxia is a potential risk factor for chronic inflammation and adiponectin reduction in adipose tissue of ob/ob and dietary obese mice, Am J Physiol Endocrinol Metab 293 (2007) E1118–E1128.

[58] N. Hosogai, A. Fukuhara, K. Oshima, Y. Miyata, S. Tanaka, K. Segawa, S. Furukawa, Y. Tochino, R. Komuro, M. Matsuda, I. Shimomura, Adipose tissue hypoxia in obesity and its impact on adipocytokine dysregulation, Diabetes 56 (2007) 901–911.

[59] C. Jiang, A. Qu, T. Matsubara, T. Chanturiya, W. Jou, O. Gavrilova, Y.M. Shah, F.J. Gonzalez, Disruption of hypoxia-inducible factor 1 in adipocytes improves insulin sensitivity and decreases adiposity in high-fat diet-fed mice, Diabetes 60 (2011) 2484–2495.

[60] X. Zhang, K.S. Lam, H. Ye, S.K. Chung, M. Zhou, Y. Wang, A. Xu, Adipose tissue-specific inhibition of hypoxia-inducible factor 1{alpha} induces obesity and glucose intolerance by impeding energy expenditure in mice, J Biol Chem 285 (2010) 32869–32877.

[61] O. Warburg, On respiratory impairment in cancer cells, Science 124 (1956) 269–270.

[62] J.A. Menendez, R. Lupu, Fatty acid synthase and the lipogenic phenotype in cancer pathogenesis, Nat Rev Cancer 7 (2007) 763–777.

[63] C.R. Santos, A. Schulze, Lipid metabolism in cancer, FEBS J 279 (2012) 2610–2623.

[64] J. Swierczynski, A. Hebanowska, T. Sledzinski, Role of abnormal lipid metabolism in development, progression, diagnosis and therapy of pancreatic cancer, World J Gastroenterol 20 (2014) 2279–2303.

[65] P.L. Alo, P. Visca, G. Trombetta, A. Mangoni, L. Lenti, S. Monaco, C. Botti, D.E. Serpieri, U. Di Tondo, Fatty acid synthase (FAS) predictive strength in poorly differentiated early breast carcinomas, Tumori 85 (1999) 35–40.

[66] M.T. Accioly, P. Pacheco, C.M. Maya-Monteiro, N. Carrossini, B.K. Robbs, S.S. Oliveira, C. Kaufmann, J.A. Morgado-Diaz, P.T. Bozza, J.P. Viola, Lipid bodies are reservoirs of cyclooxygenase-2 and sites of prostaglandin-E2 synthesis in colon cancer cells, Cancer Res 68 (2008) 1732–1740.

[67] D.K. Nomura, J.Z. Long, S. Niessen, H.S. Hoover, S.W. Ng, B.F. Cravatt, Monoacylglycerol lipase regulates a fatty acid network that promotes cancer pathogenesis, Cell 140 (2010) 49–61.

[68] B.K. Straub, E. Herpel, S. Singer, R. Zimbelmann, K. Breuhahn, S. Macher-Goeppinger, A. Warth, J. Lehmann-Koch, T. Longerich, H. Heid, P. Schirmacher, Lipid droplet-associated PAT-proteins show frequent and differential expression in neoplastic steatogenesis, Mod Pathol 23 (2010) 480–492.

[69] M.H. Hager, K.R. Solomon, M.R. Freeman, The role of cholesterol in prostate cancer, Curr Opin Clin Nutr Metab Care 9 (2006) 379–385.

[70] C.M. Metallo, P.A. Gameiro, E.L. Bell, K.R. Mattaini, J. Yang, K. Hiller, C.M. Jewell, Z.R. Johnson, D.J. Irvine, L. Guarente, J.K. Kelleher, M.G. Vander Heiden, O. Iliopoulos, G. Stephanopoulos, Reductive glutamine metabolism by IDH1 mediates lipogenesis under hypoxia, Nature 481 (2011) 380–384.

[71] B.R. Mwaikambo, C. Yang, S. Chemtob, P. Hardy, Hypoxia up-regulates CD36 expression and function via hypoxia-inducible factor-1- and phosphatidylinositol 3-kinase-dependent mechanisms, J Biol Chem 284 (2009) 26695–26707.

[72] J. Castellano, R. Aledo, J. Sendra, P. Costales, O. Juan-Babot, L. Badimon, V. Llorente-Cortes, Hypoxia stimulates low-density lipoprotein receptor-related protein-1 expression through hypoxia-inducible factor-1alpha in human vascular smooth muscle cells, Arterioscler Thromb Vasc Biol 31 (2011) 1411–1420.

[73] R. Cal, J. Castellano, E. Revuelta-Lopez, R. Aledo, M. Barriga, J. Farre, G. Vilahur, L. Nasarre, L. Hove-Madsen, L. Badimon, V. Llorente-Cortes, Low-density lipoprotein receptor-related protein 1 mediates hypoxia-induced very low density lipoprotein-

cholesteryl ester uptake and accumulation in cardiomyocytes, Cardiovasc Res 94 (2012) 469–479.

[74] Y. Wang, O. Roche, C. Xu, E.H. Moriyama, P. Heir, J. Chung, F.C. Roos, Y. Chen, G. Finak, M. Milosevic, B.C. Wilson, B.T. Teh, M. Park, M.S. Irwin, M. Ohh, Hypoxia promotes ligand-independent EGF receptor signaling via hypoxia-inducible factor-mediated upregulation of caveolin-1, Proc Natl Acad Sci U S A 109 (2012) 4892–4897.

[75] T. Hackenbeck, R. Huber, R. Schietke, K.X. Knaup, J. Monti, X. Wu, B. Klanke, B. Frey, U. Gaipl, B. Wullich, D. Ferbus, G. Goubin, C. Warnecke, K.U. Eckardt, M.S. Wiesener, The GTPase RAB20 is a HIF target with mitochondrial localization mediating apoptosis in hypoxia, Biochim Biophys Acta 1813 (2011) 1–13.

[76] S. Narravula, S.P. Colgan, Hypoxia-inducible factor 1-mediated inhibition of peroxisome proliferator-activated receptor alpha expression during hypoxia, J Immunol 166 (2001) 7543–7548.

[77] M.H. Yang, M.Z. Wu, S.H. Chiou, P.M. Chen, S.Y. Chang, C.J. Liu, S.C. Teng, K.J. Wu, Direct regulation of TWIST by HIF-1alpha promotes metastasis, Nat Cell Biol 10 (2008) 295–305.

[78] S.M. Choi, H.J. Cho, H. Cho, K.H. Kim, J.B. Kim, H. Park, Stra13/DEC1 and DEC2 inhibit sterol regulatory element binding protein-1c in a hypoxia-inducible factor-dependent mechanism, Nucleic Acids Res 36 (2008) 6372–6385.

[79] P. Ugocsai, A. Hohenstatt, G. Paragh, G. Liebisch, T. Langmann, Z. Wolf, T. Weiss, P. Groitl, T. Dobner, P. Kasprzak, L. Gobolos, A. Falkert, B. Seelbach-Goebel, A. Gellhaus, E. Winterhager, M. Schmidt, G.L. Semenza, G. Schmitz, HIF-1beta determines ABCA1 expression under hypoxia in human macrophages, Int J Biochem Cell Biol 42 (2010) 241–252.

[80] K. Glunde, T. Shah, P.T. Winnard, Jr., V. Raman, T. Takagi, F. Vesuna, D. Artemov, Z.M. Bhujwalla, Hypoxia regulates choline kinase expression through hypoxia-inducible factor-1 alpha signaling in a human prostate cancer model, Cancer Res 68 (2008) 172–180.

[81] A. Bansal, R.A. Harris, T.R. DeGrado, Choline phosphorylation and regulation of transcription of choline kinase alpha in hypoxia, J Lipid Res 53 (2012) 149–157.

[82] S.T. Saarikoski, S.P. Rivera, O. Hankinson, Mitogen-inducible gene 6 (MIG-6), adipophilin and tuftelin are inducible by hypoxia, FEBS Lett 530 (2002) 186–190.

[83] X. Xia, M.E. Lemieux, W. Li, J.S. Carroll, M. Brown, X.S. Liu, A.L. Kung, Integrative analysis of HIF binding and transactivation reveals its role in maintaining histone methylation homeostasis, Proc Natl Acad Sci U S A 106 (2009) 4260–4265.

[84] G. Shen, N. Ning, X. Zhao, X. Liu, G. Wang, T. Wang, R. Zhao, C. Yang, D. Wang, P. Gong, Y. Shen, Y. Sun, Y. Jin, W. Yang, Y. He, L. Zhang, X. Jin, X. Li, Adipose differen-

tiation-related protein is not involved in hypoxia inducible factor-1-induced lipid accumulation under hypoxia, Mol Med Rep 12 (2015) 8055–8061.

[85] T. Gimm, M. Wiese, B. Teschemacher, A. Deggerich, J. Schodel, K.X. Knaup, T. Hackenbeck, C. Hellerbrand, K. Amann, M.S. Wiesener, S. Honing, K.U. Eckardt, C. Warnecke, Hypoxia-inducible protein 2 is a novel lipid droplet protein and a specific target gene of hypoxia-inducible factor-1, FASEB J 24 (2010) 4443–4458.

[86] A. Kaidi, D. Qualtrough, A.C. Williams, C. Paraskeva, Direct transcriptional up-regulation of cyclooxygenase-2 by hypoxia-inducible factor (HIF)-1 promotes colorectal tumor cell survival and enhances HIF-1 transcriptional activity during hypoxia, Cancer Res 66 (2006) 6683–6691.

[87] J.J. Lee, M. Natsuizaka, S. Ohashi, G.S. Wong, M. Takaoka, C.Z. Michaylira, D. Budo, J.W. Tobias, M. Kanai, Y. Shirakawa, Y. Naomoto, A.J. Klein-Szanto, V.H. Haase, H. Nakagawa, Hypoxia activates the cyclooxygenase-2-prostaglandin E synthase axis, Carcinogenesis 31 (2010) 427–434.

[88] C. Grimmer, D. Pfander, B. Swoboda, T. Aigner, L. Mueller, F.F. Hennig, K. Gelse, Hypoxia-inducible factor 1alpha is involved in the prostaglandin metabolism of osteoarthritic cartilage through up-regulation of microsomal prostaglandin E synthase 1 in articular chondrocytes, Arthritis Rheum 56 (2007) 4084–4094.

[89] G.S. Hotamisligil, D.A. Bernlohr, Metabolic functions of FABPs—mechanisms and therapeutic implications, Nat Rev Endocrinol 11 (2015) 592–605.

[90] A. Chabowski, J. Gorski, J.J. Luiken, J.F. Glatz, A. Bonen, Evidence for concerted action of FAT/CD36 and FABPpm to increase fatty acid transport across the plasma membrane, Prostaglandins Leukot Essent Fatty Acids 77 (2007) 345–353.

[91] R.W. Schwenk, G.P. Holloway, J.J. Luiken, A. Bonen, J.F. Glatz, Fatty acid transport across the cell membrane: regulation by fatty acid transporters, Prostaglandins Leukot Essent Fatty Acids 82 (2010) 149–154.

[92] A. Chabowski, J.C. Chatham, N.N. Tandon, J. Calles-Escandon, J.F. Glatz, J.J. Luiken, A. Bonen, Fatty acid transport and FAT/CD36 are increased in red but not in white skeletal muscle of ZDF rats, Am J Physiol Endocrinol Metab 291 (2006) E675–E682.

[93] R.L. Smathers, D.R. Petersen, The human fatty acid-binding protein family: evolutionary divergences and functions, Hum Genomics 5 (2011) 170–191.

[94] V.L. Spitsberg, E. Matitashvili, R.C. Gorewit, Association and coexpression of fatty-acid-binding protein and glycoprotein CD36 in the bovine mammary gland, Eur J Biochem 230 (1995) 872–878.

[95] F.G. Schaap, B. Binas, H. Danneberg, G.J. van der Vusse, J.F. Glatz, Impaired long-chain fatty acid utilization by cardiac myocytes isolated from mice lacking the heart-type fatty acid binding protein gene, Circ Res 85 (1999) 329–337.

[96] B. Binas, H. Danneberg, J. McWhir, L. Mullins, A.J. Clark, Requirement for the heart-type fatty acid binding protein in cardiac fatty acid utilization, FASEB J 13 (1999) 805–812.

[97] L.Z. Xu, R. Sanchez, A. Sali, N. Heintz, Ligand specificity of brain lipid-binding protein, J Biol Chem 271 (1996) 24711–24719.

[98] A. Slipicevic, K. Jorgensen, M. Skrede, A.K. Rosnes, G. Troen, B. Davidson, V.A. Florenes, The fatty acid binding protein 7 (FABP7) is involved in proliferation and invasion of melanoma cells, BMC Cancer 8 (2008) 276.

[99] G. Kaloshi, K. Mokhtari, C. Carpentier, S. Taillibert, J. Lejeune, Y. Marie, J.Y. Delattre, R. Godbout, M. Sanson, FABP7 expression in glioblastomas: relation to prognosis, invasion and EGFR status, J Neurooncol 84 (2007) 245–248.

[100] Y. Wada, A. Sugiyama, T. Yamamoto, M. Naito, N. Noguchi, S. Yokoyama, M. Tsujita, Y. Kawabe, M. Kobayashi, A. Izumi, T. Kohro, T. Tanaka, H. Taniguchi, H. Koyama, K. Hirano, S. Yamashita, Y. Matsuzawa, E. Niki, T. Hamakubo, T. Kodama, Lipid accumulation in smooth muscle cells under LDL loading is independent of LDL receptor pathway and enhanced by hypoxic conditions, Arterioscler Thromb Vasc Biol 22 (2002) 1712–1719.

[101] J. Castellano, J. Farre, J. Fernandes, A. Bayes-Genis, J. Cinca, L. Badimon, L. Hove-Madsen, V. Llorente-Cortes, Hypoxia exacerbates Ca(2+)-handling disturbances induced by very low density lipoproteins (VLDL) in neonatal rat cardiomyocytes, J Mol Cell Cardiol 50 (2011) 894–902.

[102] N. Loewen, J. Chen, V.J. Dudley, V.P. Sarthy, J.R. Mathura, Jr., Genomic response of hypoxic Muller cells involves the very low density lipoprotein receptor as part of an angiogenic network, Exp Eye Res 88 (2009) 928–937.

[103] W.A. Prinz, Lipid trafficking sans vesicles: where, why, how?, Cell 143 (2010) 870–874.

[104] Y. Li, M.P. Marzolo, P. van Kerkhof, G.J. Strous, G. Bu, The YXXL motif, but not the two NPXY motifs, serves as the dominant endocytosis signal for low density lipoprotein receptor-related protein, J Biol Chem 275 (2000) 17187–17194.

[105] L. Auderset, L.M. Landowski, L. Foa, K.M. Young, Low density lipoprotein receptor related proteins as regulators of neural stem and progenitor cell function, Stem Cells Int 2016 (2016) 1–16.

[106] P.T. Bozza, K.G. Magalhaes, P.F. Weller, Leukocyte lipid bodies – biogenesis and functions in inflammation, Biochim Biophys Acta 1791 (2009) 540–551.

[107] P.G. Frank, F. Galbiati, D. Volonte, B. Razani, D.E. Cohen, Y.L. Marcel, M.P. Lisanti, Influence of caveolin-1 on cellular cholesterol efflux mediated by high-density lipoproteins, Am J Physiol Cell Physiol 280 (2001) C1204–1214.

[108] N. Marx, H. Duez, J.C. Fruchart, B. Staels, Peroxisome proliferator-activated receptors and atherogenesis: regulators of gene expression in vascular cells, Circ Res 94 (2004) 1168–1178.

[109] J.M. Brandt, F. Djouadi, D.P. Kelly, Fatty acids activate transcription of the muscle carnitine palmitoyltransferase I gene in cardiac myocytes via the peroxisome proliferator-activated receptor alpha, J Biol Chem 273 (1998) 23786–23792.

[110] P. Razeghi, M.E. Young, S. Abbasi, H. Taegtmeyer, Hypoxia in vivo decreases peroxisome proliferator-activated receptor alpha-regulated gene expression in rat heart, Biochem Biophys Res Commun 287 (2001) 5–10.

[111] C. Handschin, B.M. Spiegelman, Peroxisome proliferator-activated receptor gamma coactivator 1 coactivators, energy homeostasis, and metabolism, Endocr Rev 27 (2006) 728–735.

[112] D.O. Espinoza, L.G. Boros, S. Crunkhorn, H. Gami, M.E. Patti, Dual modulation of both lipid oxidation and synthesis by peroxisome proliferator-activated receptor-gamma coactivator-1alpha and -1beta in cultured myotubes, FASEB J 24 (2010) 1003–1014.

[113] J. Lin, R. Yang, P.T. Tarr, P.H. Wu, C. Handschin, S. Li, W. Yang, L. Pei, M. Uldry, P. Tontonoz, C.B. Newgard, B.M. Spiegelman, Hyperlipidemic effects of dietary saturated fats mediated through PGC-1beta coactivation of SREBP, Cell 120 (2005) 261–273.

[114] H. Zhang, P. Gao, R. Fukuda, G. Kumar, B. Krishnamachary, K.I. Zeller, C.V. Dang, G.L. Semenza, HIF-1 inhibits mitochondrial biogenesis and cellular respiration in VHL-deficient renal cell carcinoma by repression of C-MYC activity, Cancer Cell 11 (2007) 407–420.

[115] F.V. Filipp, D.A. Scott, Z.A. Ronai, A.L. Osterman, J.W. Smith, Reverse TCA cycle flux through isocitrate dehydrogenases 1 and 2 is required for lipogenesis in hypoxic melanoma cells, Pigment Cell Melanoma Res 25 (2012) 375–383.

[116] D.R. Wise, P.S. Ward, J.E. Shay, J.R. Cross, J.J. Gruber, U.M. Sachdeva, J.M. Platt, R.G. DeMatteo, M.C. Simon, C.B. Thompson, Hypoxia promotes isocitrate dehydrogenase-dependent carboxylation of alpha-ketoglutarate to citrate to support cell growth and viability, Proc Natl Acad Sci U S A 108 (2011) 19611–19616.

[117] A. Le, A.N. Lane, M. Hamaker, S. Bose, A. Gouw, J. Barbi, T. Tsukamoto, C.J. Rojas, B.S. Slusher, H. Zhang, L.J. Zimmerman, D.C. Liebler, R.J. Slebos, P.K. Lorkiewicz, R.M. Higashi, T.W. Fan, C.V. Dang, Glucose-independent glutamine metabolism via TCA cycling for proliferation and survival in B cells, Cell Metab 15 (2012) 110–121.

[118] P.A. Gameiro, J. Yang, A.M. Metelo, R. Perez-Carro, R. Baker, Z. Wang, A. Arreola, W.K. Rathmell, A. Olumi, P. Lopez-Larrubia, G. Stephanopoulos, O. Iliopoulos, In vivo HIF-mediated reductive carboxylation is regulated by citrate levels and sensitizes VHL-deficient cells to glutamine deprivation, Cell Metab 17 (2013) 372–385.

[119] E. Furuta, S.K. Pai, R. Zhan, S. Bandyopadhyay, M. Watabe, Y.Y. Mo, S. Hirota, S. Hosobe, T. Tsukada, K. Miura, S. Kamada, K. Saito, M. Iiizumi, W. Liu, J. Ericsson, K.

Watabe, Fatty acid synthase gene is up-regulated by hypoxia via activation of Akt and sterol regulatory element binding protein-1, Cancer Res 68 (2008) 1003–1011.

[120] S.Y. Jung, H.K. Jeon, J.S. Choi, Y.J. Kim, Reduced expression of FASN through SREBP-1 down-regulation is responsible for hypoxic cell death in HepG2 cells, J Cell Biochem 113 (2012) 3730–3739.

[121] R.M. Young, D. Ackerman, Z.L. Quinn, A. Mancuso, M. Gruber, L. Liu, D.N. Giannoukos, E. Bobrovnikova-Marjon, J.A. Diehl, B. Keith, M.C. Simon, Dysregulated mTORC1 renders cells critically dependent on desaturated lipids for survival under tumor-like stress, Genes Dev 27 (2013) 1115–1131.

[122] J.R. Krycer, A.J. Brown, Cholesterol accumulation in prostate cancer: a classic observation from a modern perspective, Biochim Biophys Acta 1835 (2013) 219–229.

[123] J. Mukodani, Y. Ishikawa, H. Fukuzaki, Effects of hypoxia on sterol synthesis, acyl-CoA: cholesterol acyltransferase activity, and efflux of cholesterol in cultured rabbit skin fibroblasts, Arteriosclerosis 10 (1990) 106–110.

[124] V. Pallottini, B. Guantario, C. Martini, P. Totta, I. Filippi, F. Carraro, A. Trentalance, Regulation of HMG-CoA reductase expression by hypoxia, J Cell Biochem 104 (2008) 701–709.

[125] E. Temes, S. Martin-Puig, J. Aragones, D.R. Jones, G. Olmos, I. Merida, M.O. Landazuri, Role of diacylglycerol induced by hypoxia in the regulation of HIF-1alpha activity, Biochem Biophys Res Commun 315 (2004) 44–50.

[126] J. Aragones, D.R. Jones, S. Martin, M.A. San Juan, A. Alfranca, F. Vidal, A. Vara, I. Merida, M.O. Landazuri, Evidence for the involvement of diacylglycerol kinase in the activation of hypoxia-inducible transcription factor 1 by low oxygen tension, J Biol Chem 276 (2001) 10548–10555.

[127] S. Martin-Puig, E. Temes, G. Olmos, D.R. Jones, J. Aragones, M.O. Landazuri, Role of iron (II)-2-oxoglutarate-dependent dioxygenases in the generation of hypoxia-induced phosphatidic acid through HIF-1/2 and von Hippel-Lindau-independent mechanisms, J Biol Chem 279 (2004) 9504–9511.

[128] S. Martin, R.G. Parton, Lipid droplets: a unified view of a dynamic organelle, Nat Rev Mol Cell Biol 7 (2006) 373–378.

[129] L.M. Scarfo, P.F. Weller, H.W. Farber, Induction of endothelial cell cytoplasmic lipid bodies during hypoxia, Am J Physiol Heart Circ Physiol 280 (2001) H294–H301.

[130] L.M. Pawella, M. Hashani, P. Schirmacher, B.K. Straub, Lipid droplet-associated proteins in steatosis. Effects of induction and siRNA-mediated downregulation of PAT proteins in cell culture models of hepatocyte steatosis, Pathologe 31 Suppl 2 (2010) 126–131.

http://dx.doi.org/10.5772/65340

[131] D.A. Ostler, V.G. Prieto, J.A. Reed, M.T. Deavers, A.J. Lazar, D. Ivan, Adipophilin expression in sebaceous tumors and other cutaneous lesions with clear cell histology: an immunohistochemical study of 117 cases, Mod Pathol 23 (2010) 567–573.

[132] A. Paul, B.H. Chang, L. Li, V.K. Yechoor, L. Chan, Deficiency of adipose differentiation-related protein impairs foam cell formation and protects against atherosclerosis, Circ Res 102 (2008) 1492–1501.

[133] J. Gao, G. Serrero, Adipose differentiation related protein (ADRP) expressed in transfected COS-7 cells selectively stimulates long chain fatty acid uptake, J Biol Chem 274 (1999) 16825–16830.

[134] A. Pol, S. Martin, M.A. Fernandez, C. Ferguson, A. Carozzi, R. Luetterforst, C. Enrich, R.G. Parton, Dynamic and regulated association of caveolin with lipid bodies: modulation of lipid body motility and function by a dominant negative mutant, Mol Biol Cell 15 (2004) 99–110.

[135] A. Pol, R. Luetterforst, M. Lindsay, S. Heino, E. Ikonen, R.G. Parton, A caveolin dominant negative mutant associates with lipid bodies and induces intracellular cholesterol imbalance, J Cell Biol 152 (2001) 1057–1070.

[136] D.L. Brasaemle, G. Dolios, L. Shapiro, R. Wang, Proteomic analysis of proteins associated with lipid droplets of basal and lipolytically stimulated 3T3-L1 adipocytes, J Biol Chem 279 (2004) 46835–46842.

[137] D. Marchesan, M. Rutberg, L. Andersson, L. Asp, T. Larsson, J. Boren, B.R. Johansson, S.O. Olofsson, A phospholipase D-dependent process forms lipid droplets containing caveolin, adipocyte differentiation-related protein, and vimentin in a cell-free system, J Biol Chem 278 (2003) 27293–27300.

[138] A.J. North, T.S. Brannon, L.B. Wells, W.B. Campbell, P.W. Shaul, Hypoxia stimulates prostacyclin synthesis in newborn pulmonary artery endothelium by increasing cyclooxygenase-1 protein, Circ Res 75 (1994) 33–40.

[139] A.M. Dvorak, P.F. Weller, V.S. Harvey, E.S. Morgan, H.F. Dvorak, Ultrastructural localization of prostaglandin endoperoxide synthase (cyclooxygenase) to isolated, purified fractions of guinea pig peritoneal macrophage and line 10 hepatocarcinoma cell lipid bodies, Int Arch Allergy Immunol 101 (1993) 136–142.

[140] A. Arend, R. Masso, M. Masso, G. Selstam, Electron microscope immunocytochemical localization of cyclooxygenase-1 and -2 in pseudopregnant rat corpus luteum during luteolysis, Prostaglandins Other Lipid Mediat 74 (2004) 1–10.

[141] P.T. Bozza, W. Yu, J.F. Penrose, E.S. Morgan, A.M. Dvorak, P.F. Weller, Eosinophil lipid bodies: specific, inducible intracellular sites for enhanced eicosanoid formation, J Exp Med 186 (1997) 909–920.

[142] P.T. Bozza, W. Yu, J. Cassara, P.F. Weller, Pathways for eosinophil lipid body induction: differing signal transduction in cells from normal and hypereosinophilic subjects, J Leukoc Biol 64 (1998) 563–569.

[143] P. Pacheco, F.A. Bozza, R.N. Gomes, M. Bozza, P.F. Weller, H.C. Castro-Faria-Neto, P.T. Bozza, Lipopolysaccharide-induced leukocyte lipid body formation in vivo: innate immunity elicited intracellular Loci involved in eicosanoid metabolism, J Immunol 169 (2002) 6498–6506.

[144] A. Vieira-de-Abreu, E.F. Assis, G.S. Gomes, H.C. Castro-Faria-Neto, P.F. Weller, C. Bandeira-Melo, P.T. Bozza, Allergic challenge-elicited lipid bodies compartmentalize in vivo leukotriene C4 synthesis within eosinophils, Am J Respir Cell Mol Biol 33 (2005) 254–261.

[145] N.F. Voelkel, R.M. Tuder, K. Wade, M. Hoper, R.A. Lepley, J.L. Goulet, B.H. Koller, F. Fitzpatrick, Inhibition of 5-lipoxygenase-activating protein (FLAP) reduces pulmonary vascular reactivity and pulmonary hypertension in hypoxic rats, J Clin Invest 97 (1996) 2491–2498.

[146] I.R. Preston, N.S. Hill, R.R. Warburton, B.L. Fanburg, Role of 12-lipoxygenase in hypoxia-induced rat pulmonary artery smooth muscle cell proliferation, Am J Physiol Lung Cell Mol Physiol 290 (2006) L367–L374.

[147] E.K. Rydberg, A. Krettek, C. Ullstrom, K. Ekstrom, P.A. Svensson, L.M. Carlsson, A.C. Jonsson-Rylander, G.I. Hansson, W. McPheat, O. Wiklund, B.G. Ohlsson, L.M. Hulten, Hypoxia increases LDL oxidation and expression of 15-lipoxygenase-2 in human macrophages, Arterioscler Thromb Vasc Biol 24 (2004) 2040–2045.

[148] Y. Liu, X. Tang, C. Lu, W. Han, S. Guo, D. Zhu, Expression of 15-lipoxygenases in pulmonary arteries after hypoxia, Pathology 41 (2009) 476–483.

[149] L. Yao, X. Nie, S. Shi, S. Song, X. Hao, S. Li, D. Zhu, Reciprocal regulation of HIF-1alpha and 15-LO/15-HETE promotes anti-apoptosis process in pulmonary artery smooth muscle cells during hypoxia, Prostaglandins Other Lipid Mediat 99 (2012) 96–106.

[150] L. Li, B. Liu, L. Haversen, E. Lu, L.U. Magnusson, M. Stahlman, J. Boren, G. Bergstrom, M.C. Levin, L.M. Hulten, The importance of GLUT3 for de novo lipogenesis in hypoxia-induced lipid loading of human macrophages, PLoS One 7 (2012) e42360.

[151] D.R. Mole, C. Blancher, R.R. Copley, P.J. Pollard, J.M. Gleadle, J. Ragoussis, P.J. Ratcliffe, Genome-wide association of hypoxia-inducible factor (HIF)-1alpha and HIF-2alpha DNA binding with expression profiling of hypoxia-inducible transcripts, J Biol Chem 284 (2009) 16767–16775.

[152] T. Hitosugi, L. Zhou, S. Elf, J. Fan, H.B. Kang, J.H. Seo, C. Shan, Q. Dai, L. Zhang, J. Xie, T.L. Gu, P. Jin, M. Aleckovic, G. LeRoy, Y. Kang, J.A. Sudderth, R.J. DeBerardinis, C.H. Luan, G.Z. Chen, S. Muller, D.M. Shin, T.K. Owonikoko, S. Lonial, M.L. Arellano, H.J. Khoury, F.R. Khuri, B.H. Lee, K. Ye, T.J. Boggon, S. Kang, C. He, J. Chen, Phosphogly-

cerate mutase 1 coordinates glycolysis and biosynthesis to promote tumor growth, Cancer Cell 22 (2012) 585–600.

[153] S.J. Ricoult, B.D. Manning, The multifaceted role of mTORC1 in the control of lipid metabolism, EMBO Rep 14 (2013) 242–251.

[154] R.A. Srivastava, S.L. Pinkosky, S. Filippov, J.C. Hanselman, C.T. Cramer, R.S. Newton, AMP-activated protein kinase: an emerging drug target to regulate imbalances in lipid and carbohydrate metabolism to treat cardio-metabolic diseases, J Lipid Res 53 (2012) 2490–2514.

[155] H. Zirath, A. Frenzel, G. Oliynyk, L. Segerstrom, U.K. Westermark, K. Larsson, M. Munksgaard Persson, K. Hultenby, J. Lehtio, C. Einvik, S. Pahlman, P. Kogner, P.J. Jakobsson, M.A. Henriksson, MYC inhibition induces metabolic changes leading to accumulation of lipid droplets in tumor cells, Proc Natl Acad Sci U S A 110 (2013) 10258–10263.

[156] X. Wang, X. Zhao, X. Gao, Y. Mei, M. Wu, A new role of p53 in regulating lipid metabolism, J Mol Cell Biol 5 (2013) 147–150.

Chapter 2

Hypoxic Upregulation of ARNT (HIF-1β): A Cell-Specific Attribute with Clinical Implications

Markus Mandl and Reinhard Depping

Additional information is available at the end of the chapter

http://dx.doi.org/10.5772/67171

Abstract

According to the current point of view described in the literature, the transcription factor aryl hydrocarbon receptor nuclear translocator (ARNT), also designated as hypoxia-inducible factor (HIF)-1β, is constitutively expressed and not influenced by oxygen tension. However, a study published two decades ago provided early evidence regarding a hypoxia-dependent ARNT upregulation. This finding was subsequently challenged and neglected. Until now, only a limited number of publications focus on the regulation of ARNT in hypoxia. Therefore, appropriate studies and the putative mechanism mediating this cellular attribute are discussed. The advantages of an elevated ARNT expression level in tumour cells are delineated. This chapter provides an overview of hypoxia-inducible ARNT as an emerging concept in HIF biology.

Keywords: aryl hydrocarbon receptor nuclear translocator, ARNT, HIF-1β, crosstalk, cancer

1. Introduction

The name aryl hydrocarbon receptor nuclear translocator (ARNT) designates a transcription factor of the Per-ARNT-Sim family which is ubiquitously expressed. This protein is also known as hypoxia-inducible factor (HIF)-1β. The use of these two equal synonyms for the same transcription factor throughout the literature already implies its role in various signalling pathways [1]. Unfortunately, the term "hypoxia-inducible" might be misleading in this context. According to the current point of view described in the literature, ARNT expression is not affected by environmental conditions such as hypoxia. Therefore, ARNT is considered to be a constitutively expressed gene [1]. Although this notion might be true for the majority of cells/tissues investigated, numerous studies reported the capability of tumour cells to elevate

ARNT expression in response to hypoxia [1–7]. This cellular attribute was found in cells of different tumour types of both human and murine origin. These key findings clearly suggest that hypoxia-dependent ARNT upregulation might provide a certain benefit for appropriate cells [1].

ARNT and its paralogue ARNT2 [1] share a 90% identical amino acid sequence [8]. In contrast to ARNT, ARNT2 is mainly expressed in the central nervous system [8, 9]. ARNT2 expression was shown to be positively correlated with breast cancer prognosis [8]. In addition, high-ARNT2 levels in hepatocellular carcinomas are associated with a prolonged overall survival of cancer patients [8]. However, many functions of this transcription factor are still unknown [1, 8]. Moreover, the regulation of ARNT and ARNT2 varied in human hepatocellular carcinoma Hep3B cells. ARNT was elevated in hypoxia, whereas ARNT2 was not affected in this model [3].

This chapter describes the current knowledge regarding hypoxic upregulation of ARNT, which appears to be beneficial for certain types of tumour cells. Therefore, the aim of this section is to emphasise this unique cellular attribute. A potential altered ARNT expression level due to hypoxic exposure of cells should be considered and not generally excluded. In this context, the use of ARNT as loading control or as a reference gene is basically not recommended [1].

2. Regulation of ARNT

2.1. Upregulation of ARNT in response to hypoxia

First evidence for a hypoxia-dependent regulation of ARNT was provided by Wang et al. [5]. Herein, Hep3B cells were used to study the effects of HIF-1α and ARNT under hypoxic conditions. ARNT was elevated on mRNA level in this cell line due to hypoxic exposure (1% v/v O_2). In addition, treatment with hypoxia mimetics such as cobalt chloride and desferrioxamine had similar effects. Nuclear extracts prepared from Hep3B and HeLa cells were used to investigate the response of both HIF-1 subunits to oxygen deprivation. Re-oxygenation experiments were also included into the study [5]. The data revealed that both transcription factors HIF-1α and ARNT were inducible in hypoxic cells on mRNA as well as protein levels [5]. Huang et al. [10] reported that ARNT protein levels remained constant regardless of cellular oxygen tension. In this study, Hep3B, HeLa and HEK293 cells were used. Unfortunately, not all experiments were conducted with all cell lines [10], thereby making a direct comparison with the study of Wang et al. [5] complicated. Nevertheless, the latter report [10] challenged the results of the previous one [5] due to signal variations of Northern blots and discontinuities of time-course experiments [10].

However, Huang et al. [10] proposed a very graphic working model including a specific sensor for hypoxia located in the cell membrane [10]. The depicted mechanism is similar to our nowadays HIF scheme. These days the prolylhydroxylase domain enzymes (PHDs), which require O_2 as a substrate, are known to act as cellular oxygen sensors [11]. The comparison of both seminal studies conducted by Wang et al. [5] and Huang et al. [10] also requires a glance on citation frequencies of both reports. Noteworthily, the report of Wang et al. [5], which describes the upregulation of ARNT for the first time, was cited approximately four times more often as compared to Huang et al. [10]. Despite this clear distinction of citation frequencies, the opinion that ARNT is unaffected by cellular oxygen tension became a guideline in HIF biology [1].

The capability to elevate ARNT expression in hypoxia was also found in murine L929 and Hepa1 cells. Interestingly, human Hep3B cells were also used in this study conducted by Chilov et al. [7], but ARNT was unaffected by oxygen deprivation [7]. This seemingly conflicting observation compared to a previous report [5] is likely due to different experimental conditions. Obviously, a short-term exposure of Hep3B cells to hypoxia (4 h in Ref. [7]) is not sufficient to induce ARNT protein expression in this model. However, other studies clearly confirmed the hypoxia-dependent upregulation of ARNT in Hep3B cells [3, 4].

First mechanistic clues regarding the induction of ARNT under oxygen deprivation were provided by Zhong et al. [6]. Herein, the authors tested the hypothesis whether HIF-1α and ARNT are regulated by similar signalling pathways in human prostate cancer cells. Indeed, an elevated ARNT protein level was observed in hypoxic PC-3 cells. Interestingly, this effect was attenuated by inhibition of the phosphatidylinositol-3 kinase (PI3K)/AKT-pathway by Wortmannin [6]. Another hint regarding the ARNT expression pattern in cancer cells came from Skinner et al. [12]. Herein, the authors investigated the transcriptional regulation of VEGF in ovarian cancer cell lines in response to PI3K/Akt signalling. Blocking of this pathway using the compound LY294002 specifically inhibited HIF-1α expression but had no effect on ARNT. Unfortunately, the inducibility of ARNT in hypoxia was not tested in this study [12]. Most important, the observation that PI3K/Akt inhibition decreased HIF-1α but not ARNT in one model [12] whereas both transcription factors were reduced on protein level in another model [6] might suggest a HIF-dependent regulation of ARNT in certain cell lines.

The studies discussed so far clearly show that certain cell lines are capable to induce ARNT in hypoxia and that this effect is dependent on the experimental conditions (i.e. time points). Thus, one might assume that scientists became more aware of this phenomenon over time. However, ARNT was also used as a loading control in Western blot analysis [12, 13]. This application clearly demonstrates the major opinion of a complete non-hypoxic regulation of ARNT. Of note, effects of hypoxia and hypoxia mimetics on ARNT expression should be taken into consideration when studying the HIF pathway as previously proposed [1]. Such an approach will help to identify new cell types harbouring the hypoxia-inducible ARNT attribute and might provide novel mechanistic insights. The current proposed mechanism is discussed later in the chapter.

The seminal study conducted by Choi et al. shed light on ARNT expression and turnover [14]. The authors assumed that the regulation of ARNT expression or activity might significantly affect cell metabolism. Thus, ARNT should be regarded as a drug target and appropriate compounds need to be investigated. De novo synthesis of ARNT, enhanced stability of the protein and dimerisation with HIF-1α, represents three ways how this transcription factor can be controlled. Curcumin, the major component of the spice turmeric, was tested in this study for potential inhibitory effects on HIF-1. Interestingly, curcumin facilitated the degradation of ARNT and blocked HIF signalling [14]. Similar effects were reported by Ströfer et al. [15]. Curcumin-mediated ARNT depletion was observed in human HepG2, Hep3B and MCF-7 cells [15]. The half-life of ARNT was determined in Hep3B cells after cycloheximide treatment and calculated with approximately 5 h [14]. In contrast, curcumin exposure decreased ARNT half-life to roughly 2 h. It turned out that the curcumin-dependent degradation of ARNT was redox sensitive and could be reversed by antioxidants and the proteasome inhibitor MG-132 [14]. Remarkably, MG-132 did not affect ARNT protein level in the absence of curcumin. Therefore, the authors proposed the existence of two different mechanisms mediating ARNT turnover: a proteasome-independent mechanism under physiological conditions and a proteasome-dependent degradation in response to stress [14].

The elevation of ARNT protein expression under oxygen deprivation might not be an exclusive trait of cell lines. Exposure of primary mouse keratinocytes to acute hypoxia (1% O_2) resulted in an upregulation of ARNT after 4 and 5 h, respectively [16]. However, this effect was not statistically significant. Putative alterations on ARNT mRNA expression were also evaluated in this cell model. In contrast, time-course experiments revealed no apparent changes on mRNA level in murine keratinocytes cultured in hypoxia up to 48 h [16]. The selection of an inappropriate internal control in qPCR analysis can also lead to different expression levels in normoxia and hypoxia [17]. Therefore, Vavilala et al. determined the expression level of three housekeeping genes (ribosomal protein L32, β-actin and GAPDH) in normoxic and hypoxic cells, respectively [17]. The authors observed no significant changes on mRNA levels between both experimental settings. The aim of this study was to investigate inhibitory effects of Honokiol, a biphenolic phytochemical compound, on HIF signalling in several cell lines. The results presented in this report consist solely of gene expression data. Among them, the HIF-1α, HIF-2α and ARNT mRNA level were compared under normoxic and hypoxic conditions [17]. Remarkably, an approximately 7-fold increase in ARNT mRNA was observed in D407 human retinal pigment epithelial cells. In addition, a 2-fold upregulation was detected in HT-29 cells and a slight increase in the HEK293 cell line. MCF-7 cells showed no increase in ARNT mRNA due to hypoxic exposure. Unfortunately, the comparison of these effects among the cell lines tested in this study is limited because of different time points used (12 versus 24 h in D407 cells; 1% O_2) [17]. Nevertheless, the study provides clear evidence of a cell-specific transcriptional ARNT upregulation in hypoxia although these findings were not confirmed by Western blotting.

Further mechanistic insights into this cellular trait were provided by a research project investigating the regulation of ARNT in human melanoma cells [2]. Among a panel of five different cell lines, ARNT was rapidly elevated on protein level in 518A2 cells after treatment with the hypoxia mimetic cobalt chloride ($CoCl_2$). Interestingly, knockdown of HIF-1α in $CoCl_2$ stimulated and hypoxic 518A2 cells abolished the hypoxia-dependent upregulation of ARNT. Overexpression of a dominant-negative HIF mutant in this cell model indicated that ARNT expression is dependent on the HIF pathway itself. In agreement with these findings, overexpression of HIF-1α caused an elevation of ARNT protein in $CoCl_2$ treated 518A2 cells. Taken together, this study demonstrated a regulatory relationship between HIF-1α and its binding partner ARNT for the first time. In addition, it was concluded that this capability might prevent ARNT to become a limiting factor in hypoxia [2].

http://dx.doi.org/10.5772/67171

The first comprehensive study aiming to re-evaluate the regulation of ARNT was conducted by Wolff et al. [4]. Herein, numerous cell lines were exposed to 1 and 3% O_2 for different time points. In addition, hypoxia mimetics such as $CoCl_2$ and dimethyloxalylglycine (DMOG) were used and the quantity of ARNT protein determined by Western blotting. The authors found out that ARNT expression was induced in MCF-7, HeLa and Hep3B cells. Interestingly, the ARNT level was also dependent on the hypoxic environment used. A concentration of 1% O_2 led to a faster increase in ARNT protein but also to an earlier decline to basal levels as compared to 3% hypoxia. Moreover, the appropriate mRNA levels did not correlate with the amount of protein detected. In particular, in MCF-7 and Hep3B cells, a downregulation of ARNT mRNA was observed due to hypoxia. Therefore, the authors hypothesised the existence of a reciprocal feedback regulation between ARNT protein stability and de novo synthesis. This study provides convincing evidence that the predominant point of view that ARNT is unaffected by hypoxia and hypoxia mimetics cannot be applied to all cell lines in general [4].

The first review highlighting the topic of hypoxia-inducible ARNT was published by Mandl and Depping [1]. Herein, two major questions were raised: (1) How can cells acquire this attribute? and (2) What is the benefit for these cells? [1] Both issues will be discussed below. An updated list of cell lines capable to elevate ARNT in response to hypoxia is presented in **Table 1**. Among them, the human Hep3B cell line is obviously the best studied model in this context.

Cell line	Species	Origin	References
518A2	Human	Melanoma	[2]
A375	Human	Melanoma	[2]
D407*	Human	Retinal pigment epithelium	[17]
HEK-293*	Human	Embryonic kidney	[17]
HeLa	Human	Cervix adenocarcinoma	[4]
Hep3B	Human	Hepatoma	[3–5]
Hepa1	Mouse	Hepatoma	[7]
HT-29*	Human	Colorectal adenocarcinoma	[17]
L929	Mouse	Connective tissue	[7]
LNCaP*	Human	Prostate cancer	[20]
MCF-7	Human	Breast carcinoma	[4]
PC-3	Human	Prostate cancer	[20, 6]

*Only shown on mRNA level.

Table 1. Cell lines with hypoxia-inducible ARNT expression.

2.1.1. *Purpose of hypoxia-inducible ARNT*

The capability of certain tumour cells to upregulate ARNT under hypoxic conditions might provide a specific survival advantage as previously proposed [1]. Indeed, we recently discovered a relationship between ARNT and the cellular response to radiation [18]. Tumour hypoxia is associated with radioresistance and poor patient prognosis. Therefore, we investigated the effects of an altered expression of ARNT on radioresistance and performed clonogenic survival assays. As expected, silencing of ARNT in Hep3B and MCF-7 cells by siRNA rendered these models susceptible to radiation. Interestingly, overexpression of ARNT in these cell lines promoted radioresistance. Therefore, it was hypothesised that radiation treatment might provide a selection pressure and lead to an enrichment of high-ARNT expressing cells. Taken together, these findings provide evidence to consider ARNT as a drug target in order to increase radiosensitivity in tumour cells and as a predictive marker in this context [18].

As outlined above, there is evidence that HIF-1α mediates the elevation of ARNT under hypoxic conditions in certain cell lines. This regulatory relationship is the prerequisite of a feed-forward loop (FFL) as demonstrated recently in Hep3B cells. In such a network motif, one transcription factor regulates the other and both controls the expression of a target gene cooperatively. Given the fact that HIF-1α and ARNT form the transcriptional active complex HIF-1, which regulates a plethora of target genes, the FFL definition is fulfilled. By using reporter gene assays, we were able to demonstrate that overexpression of ARNT in Hep3B cells increased the luciferase signal in hypoxia. Therefore, it was concluded that augmented HIF signalling in terms of elevated target gene expression might be beneficial for tumour cells. These findings support the concept of ARNT being a limiting factor in at least certain cell models [3].

Moreover, general considerations regarding inducible gene expression are in line with the studies discussed above. In order to respond rapidly to micro-environmental alterations required genes need to be specifically activated. Inducible genes are highly regulated and must be quickly shut down to basal expression levels once the stimulus disappeared [19].

2.1.2. Mechanism of hypoxia-dependent ARNT upregulation

The mechanism(s) underlying this unique cellular attribute is (are) unclear. There is mounting evidence indicating a pivotal role of HIF-1α [2–4]. It was demonstrated that ARNT was increased in 518A2 human melanoma cells in a HIF-1α-dependent manner under hypoxic conditions [2]. A very similar mechanism was revealed in Hep3B cells [3]. Knockdown and overexpression of HIF-1α affected the ARNT protein level accordingly. Moreover, a clear transcriptional relationship between HIF-1α and its binding partner ARNT was established in this model system. Treatment with actinomycin D, an inhibitor of RNA synthesis, diminished the induction of ARNT under oxygen deprivation. In addition, appropriate gene-silencing experiments and qRT-PCR analysis confirmed this finding [3]. Another important observation might designate HIF-1α as a mediator of this cellular attribute. The PI3K/Akt inhibitor LY294002 was shown to inhibit HIF-1α expression in ovarian cancer cell lines but had no effect on ARNT protein [12]. In contrast, several independent studies have shown that the hypoxia-dependent increase in ARNT was abolished by blocking the PI3K/Akt pathway with LY294002 or similar compounds [2, 6, 20]. This finding—the susceptibility of ARNT to PI3K/Akt inhibition in certain models—might be characteristic for cells capable to induce ARNT in hypoxia. Taken together, this suggests a linear model and might imply ARNT to be a downstream target of HIF-1α.

The cellular cause of the regulatory relationship between HIF-1α and ARNT is not known. HIF-1α can act independent of its binding partner ARNT and regulate gene expression [1].

It was shown that HIF-1α can act as a co-activator or co-repressor on certain genes. In addition, an indirect regulatory connection between both transcription factors might exist [1]. HIF-regulated genes encode for growth factors, glucose transporters, glycolytic enzymes but also other transcription factors and miRNAs. Therefore, HIF-controlled transcription factors and miRNAs might influence ARNT expression [1, 3]. A general working concept is discussed below.

2.1.2.1. Working concept of hypoxia-inducible ARNT

Based on the studies mentioned above, a general working concept can be deduced (**Figure 1**). In addition to its oxygen regulation, the HIF pathway, that is, HIF-1α, is also controlled by growth factors via the PI3K/Akt signalling cascade leading to elevated translation [21, 22]. Upon activation HIF-1α induces the upregulation of its binding partner ARNT either on mRNA and/or protein level in appropriate cell lines. For instance, it was shown that hypoxic induction of ARNT in Hep3B cells is mediated by de novo synthesis [3]. This effect can be achieved either directly or indirectly. A direct mechanism might involve the recruitment of HIF-1α to the ARNT promoter, whereas an indirect mechanism might be mediated by other HIF-regulated transcription factors or miRNAs [1]. Indeed, a complex mutual regulatory relationship between miRNAs and PAS proteins exists. However, the physiological and pathophysiological mechanisms behind are unclear [23].

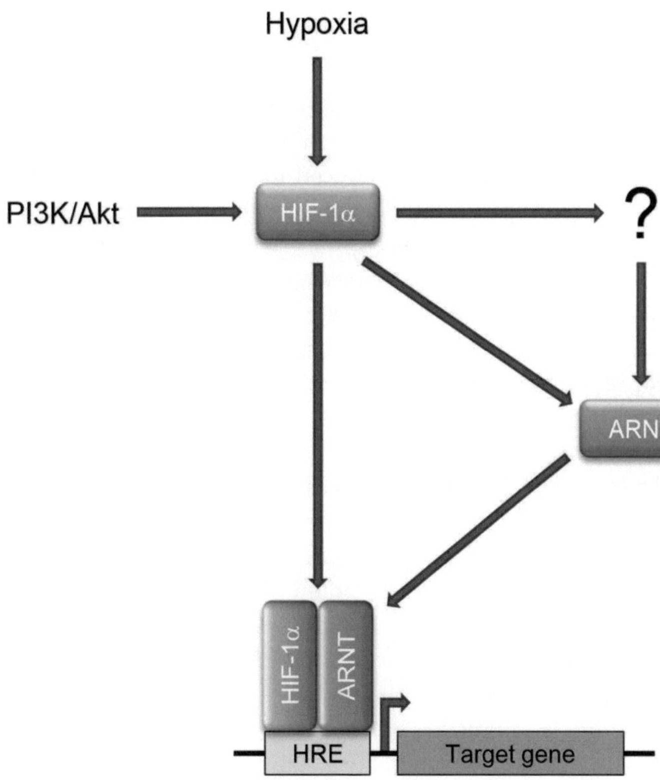

Figure 1. General working concept of hypoxia-inducible ARNT. See text for details.

Our recent experiments revealed that HIF-1α and ARNT are recruited to the ARNT gene promoter in hypoxic Hep3B cells. Deployment of CRISPR/Cas9 gene editing technology confirmed the importance of a unique genomic sequence for hypoxia-dependent ARNT upregulation. Therefore, these findings suggest a direct mechanism and render ARNT a putative HIF-1 target gene in Hep3B cells (unpublished observations; manuscript in preparation).

The regulatory relationship between HIF-1α and ARNT is part of a feed-forward loop (FFL; **Figure 1**: red arrows) as already demonstrated in Hep3B cells [3]. Subsequently, HIF-1α and its binding partner ARNT form the transcriptional active heterodimer HIF-1 and initiate the expression of various target genes. Therefore, an increased target gene expression seems to be beneficial for tumour cells [3].

2.1.3. Experimental conditions

Although the hypoxic inducibility of ARNT is described in specific cell lines by convincing data, not every study could confirm this circumstance. This obvious conflict depends mainly on the experimental conditions used. For instance, it was demonstrated that in Hep3B cells, 3% O_2 for 8 h was sufficient to elevate ARNT on protein level [3]. In contrast, a peak induction on mRNA level was observed after 5 h in the same setting [3]. Of note, these conditions need not to be appropriate in other cells. Until now, a few studies reported that ARNT mRNA and protein levels do not correlate in a number of cell lines [4, 18].

2.2. Regulation of ARNT by other factors

The regulation of ARNT or whether it responds to stimulation is poorly understood. There is evidence that ARNT expression is controlled by the NF-κB pathway in different models. It was demonstrated that ARNT mRNA was induced in HEK293 cells due to TNF-α stimulation. This effect was abrogated by pharmacological blocking or silencing of the NF-κB cascade [24]. Moreover, Per-ARNT-Sim (PAS) transcription factors belonging to different signalling circuits can compete for common binding partners such as ARNT (discussed below). Thus, misregulation of these proteins might contribute to tumour survival [9]. Noteworthily, the mutual regulation of PAS transcription factors on mRNA level was also mentioned in the literature, but appropriate citations are missing [22].

3. Crosstalk between Per-ARNT-Sim transcription factors

The HIF, AhR and BMAL1/Clock pathways respond to a decline in cellular oxygen concentration, environmental xenobiotics or govern circadian rhythms, respectively. All of these transcription factors are related. They belong to the group of Per-ARNT-Sim (PAS) transcription factors which are characterised by the presence of a PAS domain (composed of PAS-A and PAS-B subdomains) required for protein-protein interactions. Therefore, all family members are able to form homo- and heterodimers among the group [9, 25].

The transcription factor ARNT plays a pivotal role within the HIF and AhR pathways. It serves as the common binding partner for HIF-α subunits and ligands activated AhR proteins [1].

Therefore, a competition between both signalling cascades regarding the recruitment of ARNT might be obvious. Indeed, early evidence for such an antagonism was provided by Gradin et al. [26]. By using luciferase reporter gene constructs under the control of xenobiotic-responsive elements (XRE), the effect of HIF and AhR activation was studied in HepG2 cells. As expected, stimulation of cells with an appropriate AhR ligand leads to a pronounced induction of reporter gene expression. This effect was suppressed by co-treatment with the hypoxia mimetic cobalt chloride. Co-immunoprecipitation experiments clearly indicated a competition between the HIF and AhR pathway relating to ARNT binding. In addition, it was shown that HIF-1α could efficiently compete with the AhR for dimerisation with ARNT. This study provided evidence for a HIF-1α-mediated inhibition of AhR signalling by sequestration of ARNT [26]. Vorrink et al. [27] observed similar effects again in human hepatocellular carcinoma HepG2 cells and in the human keratinocyte HaCaT cell line. One major advantage of this study was the genuine hypoxic exposure of cells instead of stimulation with hypoxia mimetics such as cobalt chloride. AhR signalling was triggered by treatment with the dioxin-like compound PCB126. Again, hypoxia inhibited CYP1A1 reporter gene activity in PCB126 stimulated HepG2 cells. Importantly, ARNT overexpression caused an elevated luminescence signal under normoxic and hypoxic conditions. Moreover, forced ARNT expression was sufficient to overcome the inhibitory effect of hypoxia on AhR signalling. The authors concluded that ARNT is sequestered by HIF-1α in hypoxia thus limiting the availability of this transcription factor for AhR heterodimerisation [27]. Noteworthily, another report published nearly two decades ago claims the complete opposite [28]. This study might provide evidence for a lack of competition between HIF and AhR signalling on ARNT recruitment. Unfortunately, the presented arguments and data are not convincing at many points [28].

Furthermore, a crosstalk between AhR and BMAL1/Clock exists. Lipophilic AhR ligands such as dioxin or dietary polyphenols bind within the AhR PAS-B domain and trigger nuclear translocation. Within the nucleus activated AhR can dimerise with BMAL1 thus disrupting the autoregulatory loop of BMAL1/Clock genes. Therefore, AhR activation leads to a suppression of circadian rhythms, whereas AhR inhibition strengthens rhythm amplitude [25]. Interestingly, there is evidence that both AhR and ARNT are expressed in an oscillatory pattern in vivo [29].

4. Subcellular dynamics of ARNT and turnover

Translocation of ARNT from the cytoplasm into the nucleus is mediated by importins as also demonstrated for other HIF family members [30, 31]. Blocking of this specific process was proposed as a novel way to suppress HIF signalling [30]. Whether ARNT shuttles, back into the cytoplasm is unknown. Under these circumstances, inhibition of the putative nuclear export might prolong HIF activity. Moreover, whether ARNT is degraded, within the nucleus is not investigated in greater depth (depicted in **Figure 2**).

In general, there is evidence for two different mechanisms leading to ARNT degradation. It was found out that ARNT was not affected by the proteasome inhibitor MG-132 under physiological conditions. In contrast, proteasomal degradation of ARNT might be triggered by reactive oxygen species [3, 14].

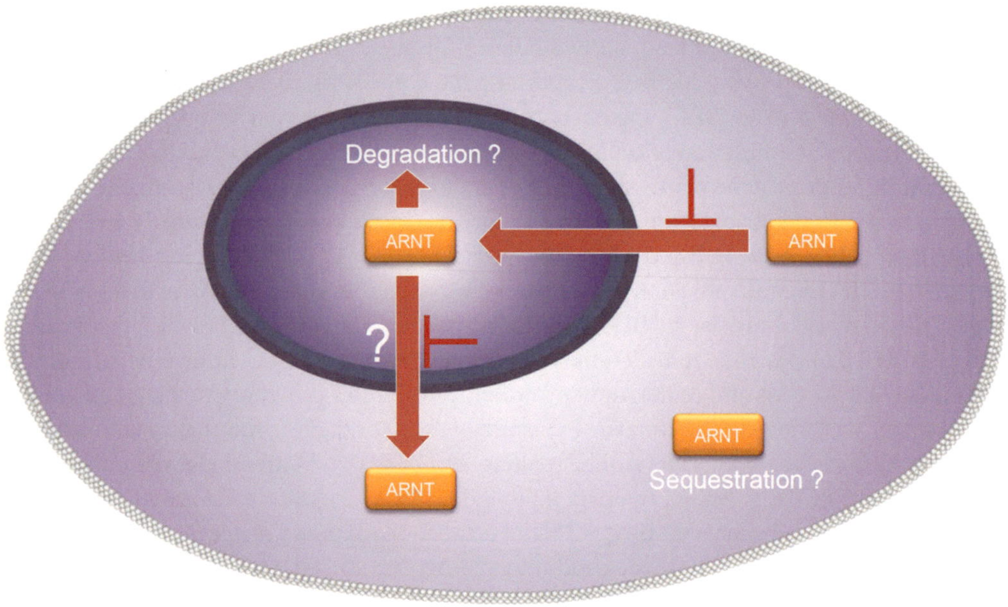

Figure 2. Subcellular logistics of ARNT. See text for details.

5. Clinical aspects

Inhibition of the HIF pathway is proposed as a treatment strategy in oncology. Several appropriate compounds have been identified and confirmed in xenograft models. These drugs are able to block different processes of the HIF signalling pathway. For instance, HIF-1α protein synthesis is diminished by rapamycin which is an inhibitor of mTOR. The antibiotic acriflavine prevents heterodimerisation of HIF-1α and ARNT subunits [32]. Moreover, a plethora of other HIF inhibitors was discovered which comprise of different chemical entities. HIF is considered as an attractive drug target, and blocking of its activity might lead to cytostatic antitumour effects. A synergistic outcome with radiotherapy is also expected [33, 34]. However, such drugs might be useful in multidrug regimes only in a subset of cancer patients. Cancers in which HIF is a strong driving force for disease progression are assumed to be susceptible for anti-HIF treatment [32].

The temporal importance of ARNT during tumour growth was investigated by Shi et al. [35]. Herein, the authors used murine hepatoma Hepa-1 cells transduced with a Tet-Off mArnt construct. Xenograft experiments conducted with these cells indicated that ARNT is particularly required during the early stage of tumour growth. The authors proposed that a profound inhibition of the HIF pathway might be achieved only by suppressing both HIF-1α and HIF-2α proteins. Therefore, it was concluded that the binding partner ARNT might represent a preferable therapeutic target rather than HIF-α subunits [35]. More convincing evidence regarding the role of ARNT in this malignancy was provided by a study using human tissue samples and cell lines [36]. ARNT expression was analysed by immunohistochemistry in hepatocellular carcinoma (HCC) and liver tissues. ARNT was found primarily in the nucleus but also in the cytoplasm in a minor fraction of cells. Interestingly, ARNT expression was significantly higher in normal liver samples as compared to appropriate HCC tissues. In addition, the impact of ARNT expression on overall survival (OS) of HCC patients was evaluated [36]. Surprisingly, a high intra-tumour ARNT level was associated with a prolonged OS. In agreement with this observation, stably lentiviral transduced ARNT-knockdown HCCLM6 cells showed a high proliferation rate, whereas overexpression of ARNT had the opposite effect. In addition, ARNT-suppressed cells formed smaller tumours in a murine xenograft model as compared to appropriate ARNT-overexpressing counterparts. This finding is in line with clinical data indicating a smaller tumour size in high-ARNT expressing hepatocellular carcinoma [36]. Moreover, the incidence of recurrence after surgery was significantly lower when a high intra-tumour ARNT level was detected. Taken together, this study describes an inhibitory role of ARNT in HCC progression. It was concluded that ARNT is a central regulator in HCC progression and a useful predictive marker regarding curative resection. The authors proposed that the relative balance of ARNT and its binding partners might be an important determinant in HCC [36]. In addition, another study demonstrated an important role of ARNT in this malignancy. Choi et al. [37] silenced ARNT expression in several human hepatoma cell lines by using siRNA and evaluated the effects on cell growth. It was shown that knockdown of this transcription factor inhibited proliferation and sensitised cells to apoptosis [37]. An elegant approach to target ARNT by small molecule inhibitors was conducted by Guo et al. [38]. Herein, nuclear magnetic resonance and biochemical screens were used in order to identify molecules selectively binding to the PAS domain of ARNT. The compound KG-548 was discovered to compete with the co-activator TACC3 for ARNT binding. The specific blocking of protein-protein interactions among transcription factors represents a novel technique to inhibit HIF signalling. Due to the shared use of ARNT among alpha subunits, targeting this protein was proposed to be more efficient as compared to its counterparts [38]. Evidence highlighting the importance of ARNT as a drug target was also provided by another study. Chan and colleagues [39] described that ARNT expression enhances cisplatin resistance in cancer cells. This phenotype was mediated by upregulation of MDR1, a multidrug efflux pump of the ABC superfamily, by a direct mechanism. Accordingly, knockdown of ARNT by siRNA transfection reduced cisplatin resistance in human cancer cells. Moreover, ARNT silencing increased the therapeutic efficacy of this cytotoxic drug in a murine xenograft model [39].

Targeting the HIF pathway in cancer therapy in order to achieve tumour control has been proposed by several reports [40–42]. Remarkably, the majority of HIF inhibitors described until now lack specificity. For instance, the drug topotecan blocks topoisomerase I activity but also diminished HIF signalling in preclinical models. This inhibitory effect on HIF was accomplished by preventing the accumulation of HIF-1α. In multihistology target-driven clinical trial, Kummar et al. [43] evaluated the oral use of this compound in a small number of cancer patients. Different tumour entities were diagnosed in these patients including ovarian cancer, sarcoma and melanoma among others. A complete inhibition of HIF-1α was detected in biopsies of a few patients, but inherent sampling and heterogeneous HIF-1α expression might limit this finding [43]. In contrast, despite the clear role of ARNT in tumour progression, its drug-ability and appropriate treatment effects need to be evaluated in a clinical setting.

6. Concluding remarks

The attribute of certain tumour cells to elevate the transcription factor ARNT in hypoxia was shown decades ago but since neglected in HIF biology. Only a small number of studies focus on the regulation of ARNT, especially under hypoxic conditions. Therefore, hypoxia-inducible ARNT is an emerging concept in this field. According to the major opinion, ARNT is a constitutively expressed gene. This means that ARNT expression is not effected by environmental factors such as hypoxia. Due to the fact that there are exceptions from this dogma, the statement of a constitutive ARNT expression should be revised and not used in general terms. Thus, ARNT should be regarded as a "cell-specific facultative gene" in tumour cells which indicates an expression as needed.

Author details

Markus Mandl and Reinhard Depping*

*Address all correspondence to: reinhard.depping@uni-luebeck.de

Institute of Physiology, Center for Structural and Cell Biology in Medicine, University of Luebeck, Luebeck, Germany

References

[1] Mandl M, Depping R. (2014). Hypoxia-inducible aryl hydrocarbon receptor nuclear translocator (ARNT) (HIF-1beta): is it a rare exception? *Molecular Medicine (Cambridge, Mass)* 20: 215–220.

[2] Mandl M, Kapeller B, Lieber R, Macfelda K. (2013). Hypoxia-inducible factor-1beta (HIF-1beta) is upregulated in a HIF-1alpha-dependent manner in 518A2 human melanoma cells under hypoxic conditions. *Biochemical and Biophysical Research Communications* 434: 166–172.

[3] Mandl M, Lieberum MK, Depping R. (2016). A HIF-1alpha-driven feed-forward loop augments HIF signalling in Hep3B cells by upregulation of ARNT. *Cell Death & Disease* 7: e2284.

[4] Wolff M, Jelkmann W, Dunst J, Depping R. (2013). The aryl hydrocarbon receptor nuclear translocator (ARNT/HIF-1beta) is influenced by hypoxia and hypoxia-mimetics. *Cellular Physiology and Biochemistry* 32: 849–858.

[5] Wang GL, Jiang BH, Rue EA, Semenza GL. (1995). Hypoxia-inducible factor 1 is a basic-helix-loop-helix-PAS heterodimer regulated by cellular O_2 tension. *Proceedings of the National Academy of Sciences of the United States of America* 92: 5510–5514.

[6] Zhong H, Hanrahan C, van der Poel H, Simons JW. (2001). Hypoxia-inducible factor 1alpha and 1beta proteins share common signaling pathways in human prostate cancer cells. *Biochemical and Biophysical Research Communications* 284: 352–356.

[7] Chilov D, Camenisch G, Kvietikova I, Ziegler U, Gassmann M, Wenger RH. (1999). Induction and nuclear translocation of hypoxia-inducible factor-1 (HIF-1): heterodimerization with ARNT is not necessary for nuclear accumulation of HIF-1alpha. *Journal of Cell Science* 112(Pt 8): 1203–1212.

[8] Kimura Y, Kasamatsu A, Nakashima D, et al. (2016). ARNT2 regulates tumoral growth in oral squamous cell carcinoma. *Journal of Cancer* 7: 702–710.

[9] Bersten DC, Sullivan AE, Peet DJ, Whitelaw ML. (2013). bHLH-PAS proteins in cancer. *Nature Reviews Cancer* 13: 827–841.

[10] Huang LE, Arany Z, Livingston DM, Bunn HF. (1996). Activation of hypoxia-inducible transcription factor depends primarily upon redox-sensitive stabilization of its alpha subunit. *The Journal of Biological Chemistry* 271: 32253–32259.

[11] Pientka FK, Hu J, Schindler SG, et al. (2012). Oxygen sensing by the prolyl-4-hydroxylase PHD2 within the nuclear compartment and the influence of compartmentalisation on HIF-1 signalling. *Journal of Cell Science* 125: 5168–5176.

[12] Skinner HD, Zheng JZ, Fang J, Agani F, Jiang BH. (2004). Vascular endothelial growth factor transcriptional activation is mediated by hypoxia-inducible factor 1alpha, HDM2, and p70S6K1 in response to phosphatidylinositol 3-kinase/AKT signaling. *The Journal of Biological Chemistry* 279: 45643–45651.

[13] Hu CJ, Wang LY, Chodosh LA, Keith B, Simon MC. (2003). Differential roles of hypoxia-inducible factor 1alpha (HIF-1alpha) and HIF-2alpha in hypoxic gene regulation. *Molecular and Cellular Biology* 23: 9361–9374.

[14] Choi H, Chun YS, Kim SW, Kim MS, Park JW. (2006). Curcumin inhibits hypoxia-inducible factor-1 by degrading aryl hydrocarbon receptor nuclear translocator: a mechanism of tumor growth inhibition. *Molecular Pharmacology* 70: 1664–1671.

[15] Strofer M, Jelkmann W, Depping R. (2011). Curcumin decreases survival of Hep3B liver and MCF-7 breast cancer cells: the role of HIF. *Strahlentherapie und Onkologie* 187: 393–400.

[16] Weir L, Robertson D, Leigh IM, Vass JK, Panteleyev AA. (2011). Hypoxia-mediated control of HIF/ARNT machinery in epidermal keratinocytes. *Biochimica et Biophysica Acta* 1813: 60–72.

[17] Vavilala DT, Ponnaluri VK, Vadlapatla RK, Pal D, Mitra AK, Mukherji M. (2012). Honokiol inhibits HIF pathway and hypoxia-induced expression of histone lysine demethylases. *Biochemical and Biophysical Research Communications* 422: 369–374.

[18] Mandl M, Lieberum MK, Dunst J, Depping R. (2015). The expression level of the transcription factor Aryl hydrocarbon receptor nuclear translocator (ARNT) determines cellular survival after radiation treatment. *Radiation Oncology (London, England)* 10: 229.

[19] Weake VM, Workman JL. (2010). Inducible gene expression: diverse regulatory mechanisms. *Nature Reviews Genetics* 11: 426–437.

[20] Huang S, Guo Y, Jacobi A, et al. (2016). Aromatic hydrocarbon receptor suppresses prostate cancer bone metastasis cells-induced vasculogenesis of endothelial progenitor cells under hypoxia. Cellular *Physiology and Biochemistry* 39: 709–720.

[21] Semenza GL. (2010). Oxygen homeostasis. *Wiley Interdisciplinary Reviews* 2: 336–361.

[22] Masoud GN, Li W. (2015). HIF-1alpha pathway: role, regulation and intervention for cancer therapy. *Acta Pharmaceutica Sinica* 5: 378–389.

[23] Li Y, Wei Y, Guo J, Cheng Y, He W. (2015). Interactional role of microRNAs and bHLH-PAS proteins in cancer (Review). *International Journal of Oncology* 47: 25–34.

[24] van Uden P, Kenneth NS, Webster R, Muller HA, Mudie S, Rocha S. (2011). Evolutionary conserved regulation of HIF-1beta by NF-kappaB. *PLoS Genetics* 7: e1001285.

[25] Jaeger C, Tischkau SA. (2016). Role of aryl hydrocarbon receptor in circadian clock disruption and metabolic dysfunction. *Environmental Health Insights* 10: 133–141.

[26] Gradin K, McGuire J, Wenger RH, et al. (1996). Functional interference between hypoxia and dioxin signal transduction pathways: competition for recruitment of the Arnt transcription factor. *Molecular and Cellular Biology* 16: 5221–5231.

[27] Vorrink SU, Severson PL, Kulak MV, Futscher BW, Domann FE. (2014). Hypoxia perturbs aryl hydrocarbon receptor signaling and CYP1A1 expression induced by PCB 126 in human skin and liver-derived cell lines. *Toxicology and Applied Pharmacology* 274: 408–416.

[28] Pollenz RS, Davarinos NA, Shearer TP. (1999). Analysis of aryl hydrocarbon receptor-mediated signaling during physiological hypoxia reveals lack of competition for the aryl hydrocarbon nuclear translocator transcription factor. *Molecular Pharmacology* 56: 1127–1137.

[29] Richardson VM, Santostefano MJ, Birnbaum LS. (1998). Daily cycle of bHLH-PAS proteins, Ah receptor and Arnt, in multiple tissues of female Sprague-Dawley rats. *Biochemical and Biophysical Research Communications* 252: 225–231.

[30] Depping R, Jelkmann W, Kosyna FK. (2015). Nuclear-cytoplasmatic shuttling of proteins in control of cellular oxygen sensing. *Journal of Molecular Medicine* 93: 599–608.

[31] Depping R, Steinhoff A, Schindler SG, et al. (2008). Nuclear translocation of hypoxia-inducible factors (HIFs): involvement of the classical importin alpha/beta pathway. *Biochimica et Biophysica Acta* 1783: 394–404.

[32] Semenza GL. (2012). Hypoxia-inducible factors in physiology and medicine. *Cell* 148: 399–408.

[33] Ban HS, Uto Y, Nakamura H. (2011). Hypoxia-inducible factor inhibitors: a survey of recent patented compounds (2004–2010). *Expert Opinion on Therapeutic Patents* 21: 131–146.

[34] Strofer M, Jelkmann W, Metzen E, Brockmeier U, Dunst J, Depping R. (2011). Stabilisation and knockdown of HIF--two distinct ways comparably important in radiotherapy. *Cellular Physiology and Biochemistry* 28: 805–812.

[35] Shi S, Yoon DY, Hodge-Bell K, Huerta-Yepez S, Hankinson O. (2010). Aryl hydrocarbon nuclear translocator (hypoxia inducible factor 1beta) activity is required more during early than late tumor growth. *Molecular Carcinogenesis* 49: 157–165.

[36] Liang Y, Li WW, Yang BW, et al. (2011). Aryl hydrocarbon receptor nuclear translocator is associated with tumor growth and progression of hepatocellular carcinoma. *International Journal of Cancer* 130: 1745–1754.

[37] Choi SH, Chung AR, Kang W, et al. (2014). Silencing of hypoxia-inducible factor-1beta induces anti-tumor effects in hepatoma cell lines under tumor hypoxia. *PLoS One* 9: e103304.

[38] Guo Y, Partch CL, Key J, et al. (2013). Regulating the ARNT/TACC3 axis: multiple approaches to manipulating protein/protein interactions with small molecules. *ACS Chemical Biology* 8: 626–635.

[39] Chan YY, Kalpana S, Chang WC, Chang WC, Chen BK. (2013). Expression of aryl hydrocarbon receptor nuclear translocator enhances cisplatin resistance by upregulating MDR1 expression in cancer cells. *Molecular Pharmacology* 84: 591–602.

[40] Milani M, Harris AL. (2008). Targeting tumour hypoxia in breast cancer. *European Journal of Cancer* 44: 2766–2773.

[41] Kizaka-Kondoh S, Tanaka S, Harada H, Hiraoka M. (2009). The HIF-1-active microenvironment: an environmental target for cancer therapy. *Advanced Drug Delivery Reviews* 61: 623–632.

[42] Wilson WR, Hay MP. (2011). Targeting hypoxia in cancer therapy. *Nature Reviews Cancer* 11: 393–410.

[43] Kummar S, Raffeld M, Juwara L, et al. (2011). Multihistology, target-driven pilot trial of oral topotecan as an inhibitor of hypoxia-inducible factor-1alpha in advanced solid tumors. *Clinical Cancer Research* 17: 5123–5131.

Chapter 3

The Hypoxia-Reoxygenation Injury Model

Domokos Gerő

Additional information is available at the end of the chapter

http://dx.doi.org/10.5772/65339

Abstract

Hypoxia-reoxygenation injury is a commonly used *in vitro* model of ischemia, which is useful to study the recovery processes following the hypoxic period. Hypoxia can be rapidly induced *in vitro* by replacing the culture atmosphere with hypoxic or anoxic gas mixture. Cellular injury mostly occurs as a result of energetic failure in this model: the lack of oxygen blocks the mitochondrial respiration and anaerobic metabolism becomes the major source of high-energy molecules in the cells. In the absence of glucose, glycolysis and pentose phosphate pathway fail to suffice the cellular energy prerequisite and longer periods of oxygen-glucose deprivation (OGD) can completely deplete the cellular NAD^+ and ATP pools. The lack of NAD^+ results in severe metabolic suppression and predisposes the cells to other injury types. This includes oxidant-induced damage, since oxidative stress activates poly(ADP-ribose) polymerase (PARP) that further depletes the cellular NAD^+ pool and leads to excessive cell death. The impaired mitochondrial respiration also leads to an increase in the mitochondrial membrane potential and augments the mitochondrial superoxide generation leading to oxidative stress. The above processes ultimately lead to necrotic cell death, but in certain cell types, mitochondrial damage can also trigger apoptosis.

Keywords: hypoxia-reoxygenation injury, poly(ADP-ribose) polymerase, energetic failure, mitochondrial dysfunction, oxidative stress

1. Introduction

This chapter gives an overview of the hypoxia-reoxygenation model, provides guidance to perform hypoxia-reoxygenation or oxygen-glucose deprivation (OGD) experiments and discusses the mechanism of cellular damage in this model.

In vivo ischemia-reperfusion models are technically simple and reproduce many aspects of ischemic diseases, but *in vitro* models are equally important, because they allow detailed study of the mechanism of cellular damage and make it possible to test large chemical libraries or sets of human small interfering RNAs (siRNAs) that are essential for early phase drug discovery [1–5]. Chemical hypoxia models that use mitochondrial uncoupling agents or respiration blockers reproduce the rapid onset of ischemia but there is no way to study the recovery processes that occur during reperfusion [6–9]. The significance of true hypoxia-reoxygenation models is in the capacity for recovery from the hypoxic phase, which makes these models especially useful for ischemia-related experiments. Oxygen-glucose deprivation is a variation of the hypoxia model to mimic the shortage of nutrients in ischemia.

2. Hypoxia-reoxygenation induction

The hypoxia/OGD models are simple experimental models that do not require expensive laboratory instruments. Regular cell culture plasticware can be placed in a gas-tight chamber and the culture atmosphere replaced with oxygen-free gas mixture using an inexpensive flow meter. In addition, OGD can be induced by replacement of the culture medium with glucose-free medium. The reoxygenation period is initiated by glucose supplementation and by returning the culture vessels to regular atmosphere. The severity of the injury can be adjusted to specific needs by varying the length of the hypoxic/OGD period. Therapeutic interventions may be delivered prior to hypoxia induction or immediately following the reoxygenation modelling preventive or reperfusion therapies.

In most hypoxia experiments, above the hypoxic and OGD groups it is essential to use normoxia controls with normal glucose concentration or to expose normoxic controls to glucose deprivation (GD). Since the normoxic and hypoxic cells must be physically separated during the hypoxic period, identical cell plates must be prepared for the hypoxia and simultaneous normoxia exposures. Culture medium is replaced with fresh medium either containing glucose or without glucose prior to the induction of hypoxia. Serum deprivation may be necessary for complete removal of glucose in OGD injury. To induce hypoxia, the culture plates are placed in gas-tight incubation chambers (Billups-Rothenberg Inc., Del Mar, CA) and the chamber is flushed with oxygen-free gas mixture at 25–30 L/min flow rate for 5–10 min to completely remove oxygen [1–5, 7, 10]. Hypoxia is maintained by clamping and incubating the chambers at 37°C for the requested period. The composition of the gas mixture may vary depending on the bicarbonate content of the culture medium and the required level of acidity change (pH level), since hypercapnia can mimic the rapid development of acidic pH of ischemic tissues [11]. The CO_2 content is typically between 5 and 20% with 80–95% N_2. This procedure removes oxygen from the atmosphere but dissolved oxygen remains in all fluids in the chamber including the culture medium and additionally in water used for humidification, thus complete anoxia is reached with a delay, following depletion of the remaining oxygen. Following the hypoxic exposure, restoration of the normal culture conditions is achieved by supplementing the culture medium with glucose and foetal bovine serum (FBS) and by reoxygenating the culture vessels in regular culture atmosphere. In most cells, the cellular ATP level is recovered during a recovery period of 16–24 hours that might be the period of interest in most experiments.

Drug treatments may be administered before the hypoxia induction to test preventive effects or following the hypoxic period to test the therapeutic potential in ischemic diseases [1–3]. For gene silencing small interfering RNAs may be added 48 hours prior to the hypoxia exposure to effectively reduce RNA and protein levels of the gene of interest at the time of the hypoxia experiment [4, 5]. Unfortunately, gene silencing cannot be selectively used to study the hypoxic or the reoxygenation phase. Pharmacological treatments using small compounds allow specific post-hypoxic treatments that permit the specific study of the recovery phase.

3. Mechanism of cellular damage in hypoxia-reoxygenation injury

3.1. Cellular energy depletion

Hypoxia and glucose deprivation cause energy depletion in the cells and may be directly responsible for the viability reduction caused by the injury. Since the lack of oxygen blocks aerobic metabolism, which is responsible for the larger part of ATP production in the cells, the cells need to use other pathways to produce sufficient ATP for survival. Most cells can adapt to low oxygen conditions in cell culture, producing ATP solely by anaerobic metabolism if adequate glucose supply is present. However, the anaerobic pathways, glycolysis and pentose phosphate pathway need to use high amounts of glucose to produce comparable output. Glycolysis produces only two ATP molecules, but oxidative phosphorylation is capable to produce ~30 ATPs per glucose molecule oxidized [12]. The typical mitochondrial ATP production is lower than the theoretical maximum, since up to 20% of the basal metabolic rate may be used to drive the proton leak [13], but it is still more than 10 times higher than the anaerobic ATP production. The compensatory increase in anaerobic metabolism would be stopped by the limited availability of NAD^+, since protons are transferred to NAD^+ by glyceraldehyde phosphate dehydrogenase to produce NADH during glycolysis, if lactate dehydrogenase (LDH) did not recycle NAD^+. This step helps maintain the higher anaerobic metabolic rate, but at the expense of metabolic acidosis (lactic acidosis).

However, in the absence of glucose, the ATP production will drop rapidly as the cellular energy storage is depleted and cell death will be induced. Most cells can survive in culture if the cellular ATP concentration will be reduced by less than 75–80% the normal ATP level [1–3, 5]. Following an OGD injury that does not reduce the cellular ATP concentration below 20% of the initial baseline value full recovery is expectable if optimal culture conditions are provided. Since the cells try to maintain normal ATP level and use all resources that can be utilized for energy production during the OGD phase, the recovery process is time-consuming: all precursor molecules need to be resynthesized in the cells. A more robust injury that decreases the cellular ATP concentration below 20% will initiate severe viability loss in the cell population [2] (**Figure 1**).

The cellular energy production remains impaired following an OGD injury: the cellular ATP production is slow even if the energy sources are provided in liberal amounts. The loss of all high-energy molecules is responsible for the diminished ATP synthesis following OGD. Not only ATP, but also adenosine diphosphate (ADP) and NAD^+ are greatly reduced in the cells to minimize the ATP loss that will sustain the metabolic suppression [5]. ATP is the central coenzyme in the cells that functions as universal energy currency to transfer chemical energy. ATP molecules are generated in large quantities by constant recycling of ADP to ATP; the daily estimated ATP synthesis is around 1000 g/kg bodyweight [14]. Organic compounds are catabolized via a series of redox reactions in the cells and ultimately generate carbon dioxide and water. During these reactions, energy is collected via transferring electrons from organic donors to the acceptor molecule NAD^+ and reducing it to NADH. Energy is retrieved from NADH in the mitochondria as the electrons are gradually transferred to oxygen through the electron transport chain and ATP is produced in the coupled oxidative phosphorylation reaction. Thus, the energy stored by NAD^+ molecules is interconvertible to ATP molecules and the lack of NAD^+ can severely limit the ATP generation.

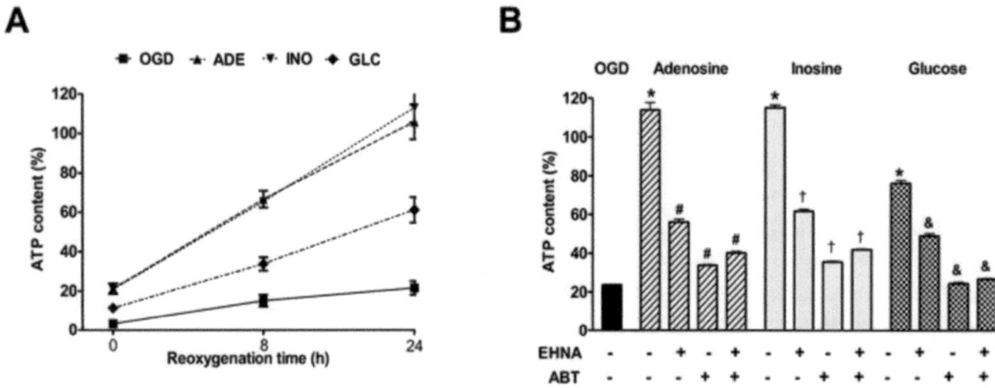

Figure 1. Post-hypoxic recovery of the cellular ATP content. (A and B) LLC-PK1 cells were subjected to hypoxia in the absence (OGD) or presence of 300 μM adenosine (ADE), inosine (INO) or glucose (GLC) to reduce the cellular ATP content to 5, 10 or 20% of normoxic controls, and ATP concentration was measured during the 24-hour-long recovery period. (A) ATP content gradually increased proportional to the hypoxic ATP depletion. (B) ATP resynthesis requires both adenosine deaminase (ADA) and adenosine kinase (AK) activity in the cells. Blockage of ADA by EHNA (10 μM) and/or AK by ABT 702 (ABT, 30μM) blocks the recovery of the cellular ATP content. (Data are shown as mean ± SD values. *$p < 0.05$ compared to OGD, #$p < 0.05$ compared to adenosine, †$p < 0.05$ compared to inosine, &$p < 0.05$ compared to glucose.) From Ref. [2].

NAD^+ biosynthesis occurs either via the *de novo* (kynurenine) pathway from tryptophan or via the *salvage* pathway using nicotinamide as substrate [15–17]. NAD^+ is not only used in cellular energy production reactions catalyzed by dehydrogenases, but it is also utilized by poly(ADP-ribose) polymerases (PARPs) in ADP-ribosylation reactions and by sirtuins in deacetylation reactions that produce nicotinamide [18, 19]. Nicotinamide can be reused for NAD^+ synthesis via the *salvage* pathway: an energy-requiring (endothermic) two-step process that uses ATP. The *salvage* pathway is considered as the main NAD^+ biosynthesis pathway in humans and the major substrate is nicotinamide, since nicotinamide deamidase, the enzyme that catalyzes the conversion of nicotinamide to nicotinic acid, is missing in humans [20]. In the first step, nicotinamide is converted to nicotinamide mononucleotide (NMN) by nicotinamide phosphoribosyltransferase (NamPRT) using phosphoribosyl pyrophosphate (PRPP) as cosubstrate and one ATP molecule (**Figure 2**). The second step is the conversion of NMN to NAD^+ by nicotinamide mononucleotide adenylyl transferases (NMNATs) that also requires one ATP molecule. This step is catalyzed by NMNAT-1 in the nucleus, NMNAT-2 in the Golgi and NMNAT-3 in the mitochondria [21, 22]. Since the conversion of ribose 5-pyrophosphate (coming from the degradation of ADP-ribose polymers) to PRPP requires a third ATP molecule, altogether three ATP molecules are necessary

http://dx.doi.org/10.5772/65339

for the resynthesis of one NAD^+ molecule [15, 16, 20]. NamPRT is recognized as the rate-limiting enzyme in NAD^+ *salvage*, partly because this step requires more energy, if PRPP synthesis is also considered, and because it relies on a single enzyme, while the cells contain multiple NMNAT isoenzymes. NAD^+ biosynthesis is an energy-requiring process, and it is further complicated by sequestered localization of NAD^+ in the cells: there are separate mitochondrial, cytoplasmic and nuclear NAD^+ pools and they are not completely exchangeable [16]. NAD^+ biosynthesis is estimated to occur at 5g/kg tissue/day [16] suggesting that nicotinamide may be recycled several times a day. Still, the recovery occurs at a slower rate following a severe OGD injury, because the lack of ATP limits the NAD^+ turnover and the low NAD^+ availability blocks the ATP generation from metabolic sources.

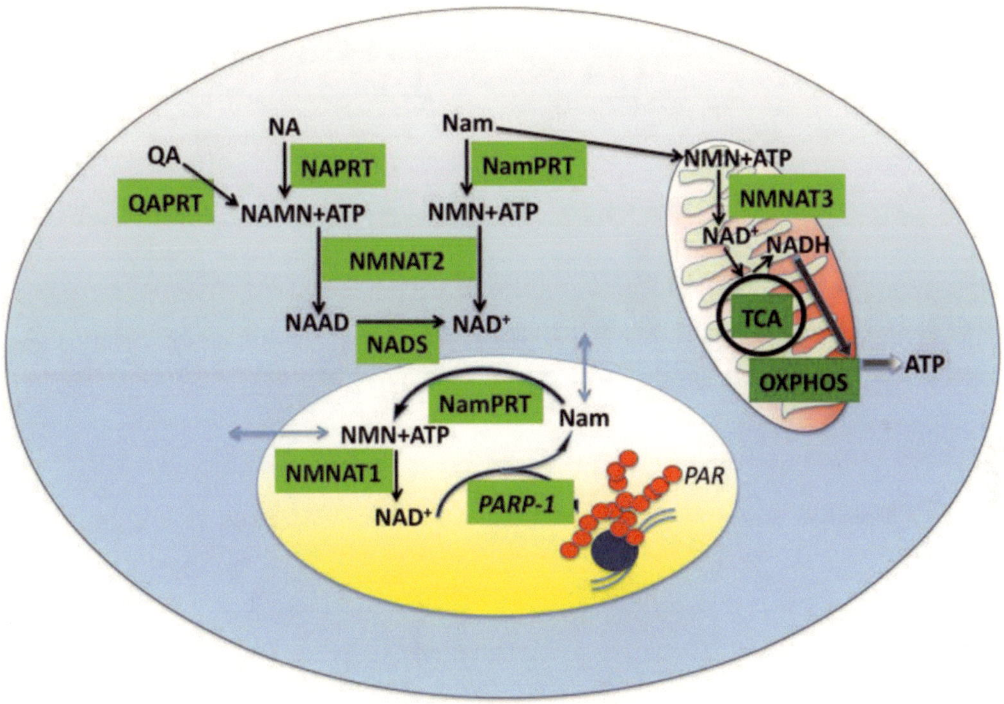

Figure 2. Compartmentalization of NAD^+ biosynthesis. The '*de novo*' synthesis of NAD^+ starts from tryptophan and produces the precursor quinolinic acid (QA), while the '*salvage*' pathway utilizes the NAD^+ break-down products nicotinamide (Nam) and nicotinic acid (NA). QA, NA and Nam are converted to nicotinic acid mononucleotide (NAMN) and nicotinamide mononucleotide (NMN) by the respective phosphoribosyltransferases (QAPRT: quinolinic acid phosphoribosyltransferase, NAPRT: nicotinic acid phosphoribosyltransferase, NamPRT: nicotinamide phosphoribosyltransferase). NAMN and NMN are converted to nicotinic acid adenine dinucleotide (NAAD) and nicotinamide adenine dinucleotide (NAD^+) by transferring the adenylate moiety of ATP to the mononucleotides by compartment-specific NMN adenylyl transferase (NMNAT) enzymes. NAAD is amidated by NAD synthetase (NADS) using glutamine as an ammonium donor. There are three NMNAT isoforms: NMNAT1 is ubiquitous and is localized to the nucleus, NMNAT2 is cytoplasmic and is predominantly expressed in the brain and NMNAT3 is present in the mitochondria. PARP-1 utilizes NAD^+ as a substrate to produce ADP-ribose polymers and nicotinamide.

The lack of NAD^+ affects both mitochondrial respiration and anaerobic metabolism following the OGD injury [5]. Severe metabolic suppression is detectable following the OGD injury if the resynthesis of NAD$^+$ is prevented by NamPRT inhibition: the mitochondrial oxygen consumption of the cells is severely reduced in the cells (**Figure 3**). The respiratory capacity of the cells is suppressed following OGD and while normal cells typically use no more than ~50–60% of their

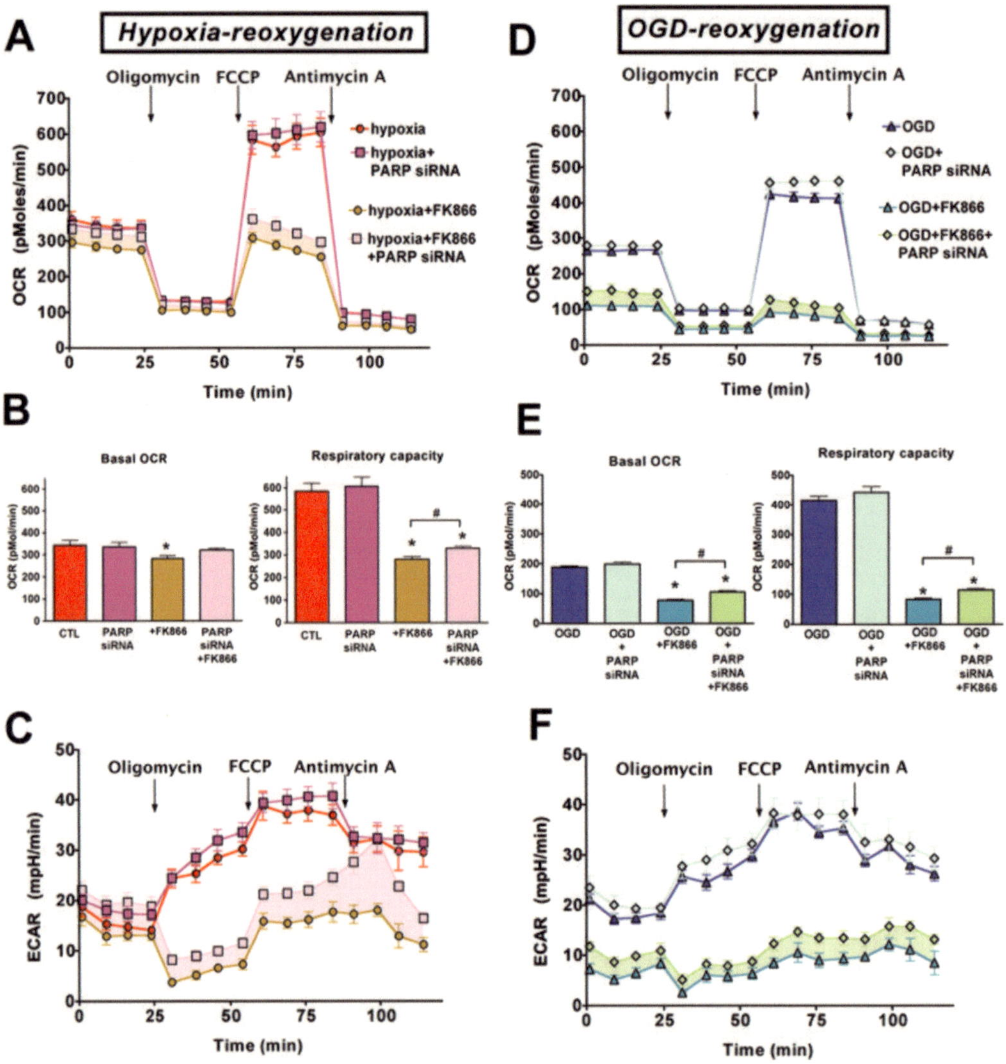

Figure 3. Suppressed cellular metabolism following oxygen-glucose deprivation (OGD). (A–F) H9c2 cells were transfected with PARP-1 (siPARP-1) or CTL siRNA and 48 hours later the cells were exposed to hypoxia or oxygen-glucose deprivation for 8 hours. Following the hypoxic phase, glucose and serum concentrations were normalized and the cells were treated with NamPRT inhibitor FK866 (10 μM) to block NAD$^+$ resynthesis (or vehicle) at normal oxygen tension for 16 hours. The metabolic profile of the cells was determined by extracellular flux analysis. (A and D) The oxygen consumption rate (OCR) and (C and F) the extracellular acidification rate (ECAR) were monitored using Oligomycin (1 μg/mL), FCCP (0.3 μM) and antimycin A (2 μg/mL) injections. (B and E) Basal oxygen consumption and total respiratory capacity were determined following the addition of FCCP. NamPRT inhibition severely blocks the recovery of the respiratory capacity and prevents the anaerobic metabolic compensation. PARP-1 silencing increases the respiratory capacity in cells with diminished NAD$^+$ content. (n = 3, $^*p$ < 0.05 compared to CTL, $\#p$ < 0.05 PARP-1 silenced cells compared to respective CTL siRNA treated cells.) From Ref. [5].

respiratory capacity under baseline conditions, the cells use their full respiratory capacity following hypoxia of OGD injury. While the basal anaerobic metabolism is less affected by the lack of NAD^+ the anaerobic compensation is reduced by 70%, which makes the cells extremely sensitive to other injuries that require excess energy. At this stage, NAD^+ is functionally shared between the mitochondrial and cytoplasmic pools, as the blockage of mitochondrial NAD^+ recycling by inhibition of ATP synthase immediately draws a halt to anaerobic metabolism. This phenomenon can help explain the vulnerability of the cells: any injury that causes mitochondrial impairment can simultaneously block the anaerobic metabolism in the cells.

3.2. Oxidative stress during reoxygenation

Oxidative stress is an important contributor to cellular damage in hypoxia- or OGD-reoxygenation injury. While it is recognized as the major cause of cellular damage in ischemia-reperfusion injury *in vivo* [23–25], reoxygenation does not induce severe oxidative stress in the *in vitro* injury. Mitochondria are the major sources of oxidants *in vitro* following OGD or hypoxia. The mitochondrial respiratory chain is turned off by the lack of oxygen during hypoxia or OGD, but the electrons and protons are fed to the mitochondria as long as possible. As a result, the protons pumped from the matrix to the intermembrane space may increase the transmembrane gradient [5]. Mitochondrial uncoupling proteins are responsible for maintaining the physiological mitochondrial membrane potential [26]. They allow reverse transfer of protons from the intermembrane space to the matrix without coupled ATP synthesis. This proton leak may reduce the efficiency of ATP production, but it also helps against mitochondrial hyperpolarization [27–29].

Superoxide is produced by the mitochondrial electron transport chain itself, most importantly at complex III: a low percentage of electrons from quinone molecules are transferred to oxygen instead of complex III even in healthy mitochondria [30–34]. The amount of ROS generation is relatively low, approximately 0.2–2% of the oxygen consumed by the mitochondria is reduced to superoxide [28]. However, this process would leave behind excess protons in the intermembrane space and increase the mitochondrial membrane potential, if mitochondria did not possess a safety mechanism against it. Uncoupling proteins and especially UCP2 are responsible for protecting against hyperpolarization. The elevated mitochondrial membrane potential directly increases the mitochondrial superoxide generation [35, 36]. This action is reversible: if the mitochondrial membrane potential is normalized, the superoxide generation will decrease to normal levels [27, 34, 37]. However, the action of UCP2 and UCP3 is regulated by reactive oxygen species (ROS) generation as their activity is affected by glutathionylation: increase in ROS production prompts the deglutathionylation and activation of proton conductivity via UCP2 and UCP3, while at low ROS levels the uncoupling proteins are glutathionylated that effectively deactivates the proton conductance process [28, 38]. During hypoxia or OGD, the absence of oxygen completely deactivates UCPs in the cell and it excludes the compensation for the hyperpolarization in the beginning of the reoxygenation phase. While an increase is detectable in the mitochondrial membrane potential, the amount of superoxide generation hardly exceeds the normal levels immediately following hypoxia or

OGD due to the suppressed mitochondrial activity [5], but increased ROS production can be detected in the cells even after full recovery of the cellular ATP and NAD^+ contents [5] (**Figure 4**).

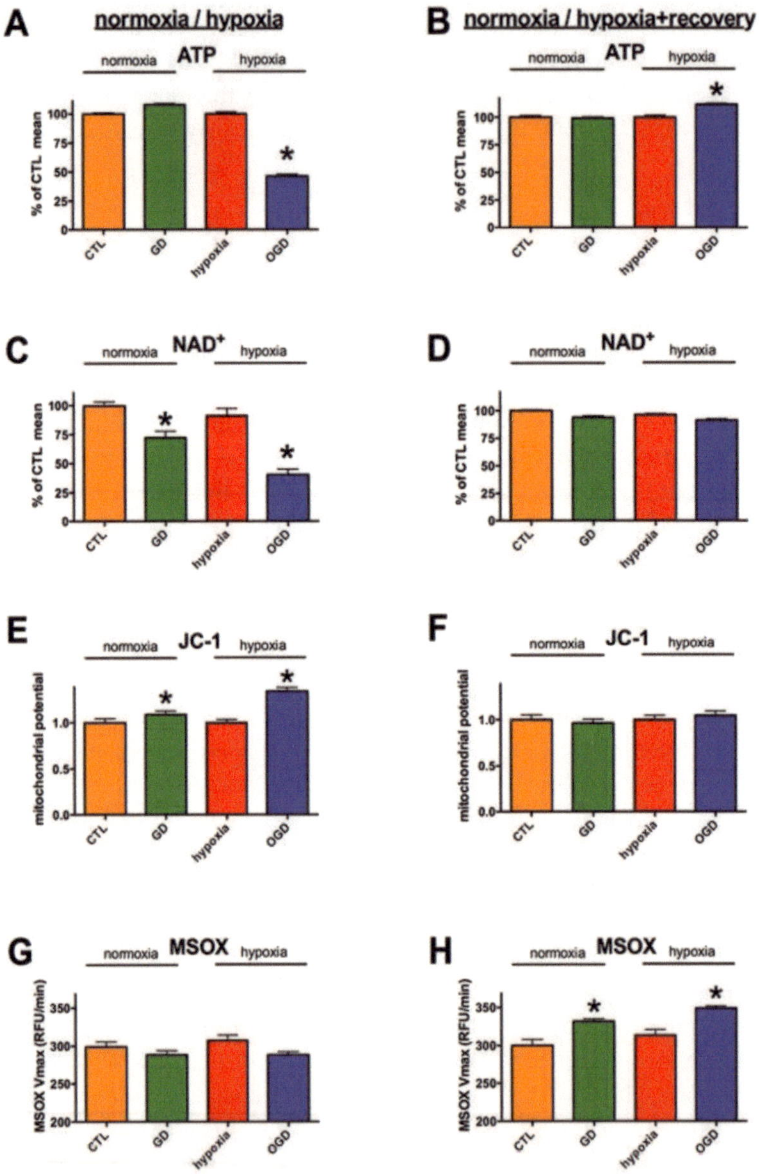

Figure 4. Mitochondrial oxidant production in hypoxia-reoxygenation injury. (A–F) H9c2 cardiomyocytes were exposed to hypoxia or oxygen-glucose deprivation (OGD) for 8 hours, followed by 16-hour-long recovery. Cells were simultaneously maintained at normoxia in glucose-containing culture medium as controls (CTL) or subjected to glucose deprivation (GD). (A and B) ATP and (C and D) NAD^+ contents were determined both at the end of the hypoxia (A and C) and following the recovery (B and D). (E and F) The mitochondrial potential and (G and H) superoxide production were measured by JC-1 and MSOX Red (MSOX) at the end of the hypoxia (E and G) and following the recovery (F and H). (n = 4, $^*p < 0.05$ compared to CTL.) From Ref. [5].

Oxidative stress damages the DNA and RNA molecules causing modified bases and strand breaks and also induces oxidative protein damage. To minimize further dysfunction caused by impaired molecules, repair processes are promptly activated in the cells and PARP-1 is the key enzyme that orchestrates this process. The activation of PARP-1 is an easily detectable sign of oxidative stress in the cells and tissues [39–41].

3.3. The function of PARP-1 and its role in oxidative stress-induced cell death

PARP-1 is the major isoform of poly(ADP-ribose) polymerases in the cells that mainly resides in the nucleus. It detects DNA strand breaks and plays a role in base excision repair by adding multiple ADP-ribose units to the DNA associated histone proteins using NAD^+ as a substrate. It promotes DNA repair by recruiting components of the repair machinery and also by providing sequestered energy source for the repair in the form of ADP-ribose. Poly(ADP-ribose) (PAR) induces conformation changes in the DNA due to its negative charge, which may serve as a surface for interaction in DNA repair. The removal of PAR is catalyzed by poly(ADP-ribose) glycohydrolase (PARG), an enzyme that is mainly localized to the cytoplasm and needs to translocate to the nucleus to counteract PARP.

While the far-reaching activity of PARP-1 in DNA repair suggests that it is essential for DNA integrity and cell survival, PARP-1 knockout mice are viable and do not exhibit high susceptibility for spontaneous tumour development [42]. There is no human 'PARP-1 deficiency syndrome'. Single nucleotide polymorphisms of the PARP gene have been identified, but only few studies found association with functional changes and increased risk of cancer, nephritis or arthritis [43–46]. DNA repair processes possibly rely on redundant actions of many other components or PARP-1 is substituted by other PARP isoforms [47, 48]. On the other hand, the principal role of PARP-1 is indisputable in cell metabolism and oxidative stress-induced cell death.

In oxidative stress, the enzyme is capable of over-activation by creating huge branching PAR polymers within minutes, thereby depleting the available NAD^+ pool of the cells and causing energetic failure [40, 49, 50]. Inhibition of PARP activity prevents necrotic cell death in oxidative stress and promotes cell survival and apoptosis, a favourable cell death form. During apoptosis PARP is inactivated by caspase cleavage that dissociates the DNA binding and catalytic domains of PARP and prevents PARP activation by DNA strand breaks. Apart from caspases, various proteases (cathepsin, calpain, granzyme B) may inactivate PARP by proteolytic cleavage following OGD or hypoxia injury [2]. PARP also catalyzes its self-PARylation and this auto-modification reduces the catalytic activity of the enzyme, thus, it also serves as a control of its activity. It was suggested that other post-translational modifications of the enzyme (phosphorylation, acetylation) are also implicated in the regulation of PARP activity [49, 51].

PARP also regulates gene transcription via interacting with other transcription factors or by directly binding to promoter regions to control cellular metabolism [52, 53]. Among others, the PAR-degrading enzyme PARG, the nuclear NAD^+ synthesis enzyme NMNAT-1 and Nuclear Respiratory Factor 1, which activates the expression of metabolic genes regulating cellular growth and mitochondrial respiration, were identified as PARP interactors [53–56]. The interplay between PARP-1 and the NAD^+ biosynthesis enzyme NMNAT-1 is particularly interesting because it suggests that under baseline conditions the nuclear NAD^+ utilization and recycling are fully coupled processes [54, 57].

PARP activation may cause mitochondrial dysfunction in cells exposed to oxidative stress that is best characterized by reduced mitochondrial reserve capacity [58]. The cellular NAD^+ pool is compartmentalized within the cells and since the NAD^+ pools are non-exchangeable between the nucleus and the mitochondria [22], the PARP-mediated nuclear NAD^+ depletion may develop mitochondrial failure via prior depletion of the cytoplasmic NAD^+ pool and inhibition of glycolysis. There seems to be a competition for substrate between PARP-1 and other NAD^+ -consuming enzymes including the sirtuins [40, 59]. The sirtuin family members use NAD^+ for their deacetylation function and are mainly implicated in the regulation of glucose and lipid metabolism [59, 60]. The various sirtuins show distinct intracellular localization profile, Sirt1, Sirt6 and Sirt7 are predominantly nuclear proteins [59]. While PARP and sirtuins share their common substrate, the NAD^+ consumption by sirtuins is hardly comparable to that of PARP, thus competition for substrate has little impact on PARP activity. Still Sirt1 may affect the action of PARP-1 via direct interaction of the two proteins and by modulating PARP activity via deacetylation [61]. On the other hand, the nuclear sirtuins are possibly affected by PARP1-mediated NAD^+ consumption under oxidative stress, since the lack of PARP-1 increases Sirt-1 activity and stimulates the mitochondrial metabolism [62]. Thus, it suggests that sirtuins and especially Sirt-1 may play a role in PARP-mediated mitochondrial suppression, as PARP-mediated NAD^+ consumption decreases Sirt-1 activity and mitochondrial metabolism.

PARP-1 activation is generally associated with necrotic cell death, but PARP-1 may be involved in other cell death forms. The obligatory trigger of PARP activation is DNA single strand break, which can be induced by a variety of oxidants. In pathophysiological conditions, reactive species capable of inducing DNA strand breakage, and thereby PARP activation, include hydroxyl radical, nitroxyl radical, as well as peroxynitrite (a reactive oxidant produced from the reaction of nitric oxide and superoxide) [63–65]. In response to DNA damage, PARP becomes activated and, using NAD^+ as a substrate, catalyzes the building of homopolymers of adenosine diphosphate ribose units. Depending of the severity of DNA damage this process can be overwhelming and it may deplete the cellular NAD^+ and ATP pools and can eventually lead to cell death via the necrotic route [39]. Hypoxia- or OGD-reoxygenation injury predisposes the cells to PARP-1 mediated NAD^+ depletion: lower level of oxidative stress and PARP-1 activity can exhaust the cellular NAD^+ pool and lead to necrosis (**Figure 5**).

The activation of PARP-1 is a regulated process and the enzyme also plays an important role in programmed cell death forms [66, 67]. PARP-1 activity level depends on the severity of oxidative stress, and its high catalytic activity is necessary to promote immediate DNA repair. This protective mechanism helps maintain genome integrity: the ADP-ribose units provide energy source for base excision repair and the negatively charged polymer recruits other repair proteins to the site of the damage [68]. Low level of PARP activity is always detectable, and it is associated with normal gene expression and physiological maintenance of DNA integrity. Severe DNA damage that occurs under pathological conditions induces excessive activation of the enzyme that can rapidly deplete the cellular NAD^+ content. Less severe oxidative damage can induce moderate PARP activation to restore the DNA integrity and if the repair process is unsuccessful, apoptosis may be induced [39, 40, 66]. The apoptotic process follows the intrinsic or mitochondrial pathway in this case [69], and it requires a nuclear-to-mitochondrial signal for initiation. The signalling molecules have not been unequivocally identified, but PARP-1 and the PAR polymer might be directly involved in this process [70]. PARP-1 can generate large PAR polymers that may escape from the nucleus. The PAR polymer itself can induce membrane damage, mitochondrial depolarization and apoptosis-inducing factor (AIF) release [70]. AIF released from the mitochondria translocates to the nucleus and plays a role in cell death progression [71]. This PAR-mediated cell death program is occasionally discriminated from necrosis and apoptosis as parthanatos, a distinct cell death form [70]. Triggering of the mitochondrial apoptotic signal leads to caspase activation, which becomes detectable 1 hour following the start of reoxygenation and remains elevated for several hours in hypoxia-reoxygenation injury [2]. During apoptosis caspase cleavage inactivates PARP-1 by removing the catalytic region of the protein from the DNA binding region to avoid unnecessary NAD^+ consumption caused by the fragmented DNA [72].

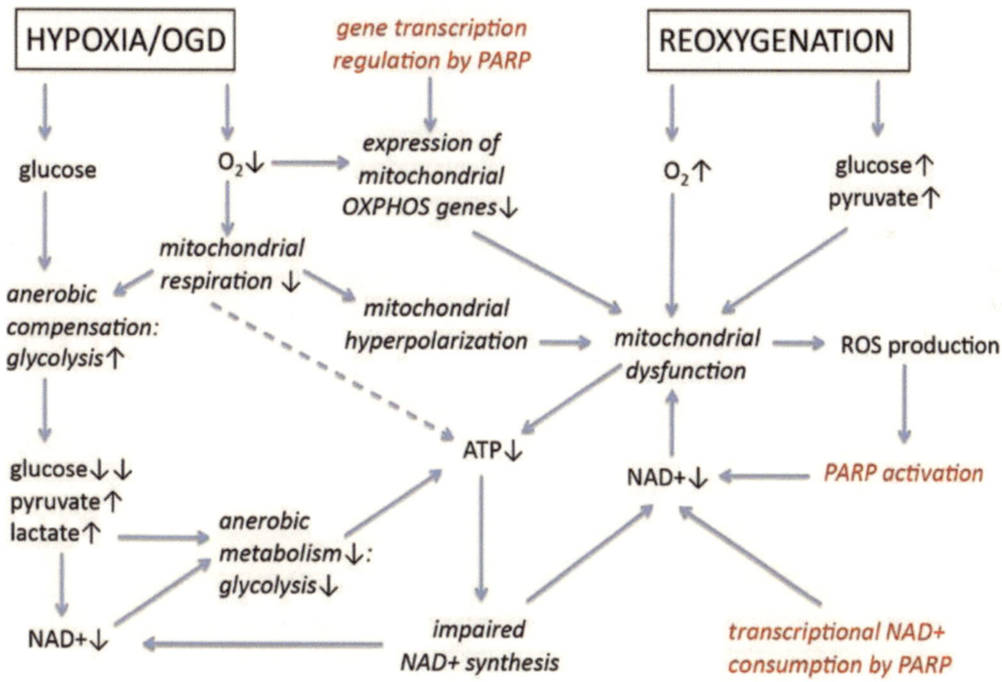

Figure 5. The mechanism of energetic failure in hypoxia-reoxygenation injury. The events of hypoxia/OGD-reoxygenation injury leading to ATP depletion with the contribution of PARP labelled in red.

PARP-1 itself can exit the nucleus in oxidative stress and interact with cytoplasmic or mitochondrial proteins [4]. Thereby, PARP-1 can have direct access to the cytoplasmic or mitochondrial NAD^+ pools and can PARylate cytoplasmic and mitochondrial proteins [73]. In this process, the PAR-binding E3 ubiquitin ligase RNF146 (ring finger protein 146, dactylidin also named Iduna) is involved [74–76], which can capture the PARP-1 protein and promote its ubiquitination and proteasomal degradation [4]. RNF146 was discovered as a neuroprotective gene product that when over-expressed exerted protection against NMDA excitotoxicity and MNNG-induced PARP-1 dependent cell death *in vitro* [77] and protects against oxidative stress-mediated neural injury in transgenic mice [78]. RNF146 is a 359 amino acid long, cytoplasmic protein that contains conserved Really Interesting New Gene (RING) and WWE domains. The special zinc finger domain (RING domain) between amino acids 38–75 is responsible for the E3 ubiquitin-protein ligase activity [79]. The WWE domain at 92–168 mediates specific interaction with ADP-ribosylated proteins (PAR-recognition sequence) and the carboxy-terminal half of the protein, which shows similarity to nucleoporin 155, a component of the nuclear pore complex, possibly plays a role in bidirectional trafficking of molecules between the nucleus and the cytoplasm [78, 79]. RNF146 can bind to the PAR polymer, thus it can recognize the auto-PARylated PARP-1 and other PARylated proteins, but their distinct subcellular localization (PARP-1 is present in the nucleus and RNF146 in the cytoplasm) prevents their direct association under physiological conditions. However, when the nuclear membrane integrity is disrupted, RNF146 can translocate to the nucleus, directly interact with PARP-1 and both proteins are rapidly degraded by the proteasome [4]. This interaction affects PARP-1 removal during cell division: PARP-1 is sequestered and degraded during the mitotic phase, and also results in rapid PARP-1 removal in oxidative stress. In the latter case, not only PARP-1 but also its targets, the PARylated proteins are affected, including the NAD^+ biosynthesis enzymes NamPRT and nicotinamide N-methyltransferase and various metabolic enzymes, e.g. lactate dehydrogenase, glyceraldehyde-3-phosphate dehydrogenase (GAPDH), pyruvate dehydrogenase and succinate dehydrogenase [80] that can slow down the recovery following OGD or hypoxic injury. A small fraction of PARP-1 is localized to the mitochondria and plays a role in mitochondrial DNA repair, but it may also be involved in degradation of interacting mitochondrial proteins [73, 81, 82]. Inhibition of PARP-1 activity renders protection against reoxygenation-induced oxidative damage and cell death in OGD injury but this effect is limited by the low concentration of cellular ATP [2, 5] and may not be comparable to the beneficial effects of PARP inhibitors observed in ischemia-reperfusion injury *in vivo* [83, 84].

3.4. Increased sensitivity to oxidative damage

Post-hypoxic cells show increased sensitivity to oxidant-induced cellular injury due to (1) diminished ATP and NAD^+ pools, (2) low mitochondrial metabolic output and (3) reduced antioxidant capacity. Hypoxia and glucose deprivation decrease the intracellular concentrations of ATP and NAD^+ that greatly reduce the tolerance to cytotoxic injuries since they are associated with enhanced energy consumption. Oxidant-induced cellular damage is further aggravated by the diminished NAD^+ and ATP synthesis due to mitochondrial dysfunction and restricted glycolytic capacity. The exposure to low oxygen atmosphere induces down-regulation of antioxidant genes that reduces the buffering capacity during the reoxygenation phase [85, 86]. Changes in oxygen supply are detected via reduced levels of oxidants and hypoxia-inducible factor-α (HIF-1α) is responsible for transcriptional regulation of the antioxidant enzymes [87, 88]. The diminished scavenging capability and the higher oxidant generation

http://dx.doi.org/10.5772/65339

during the recovery period greatly reduce the tolerance to oxidants. Overall, these factors increase the vulnerability of the cells and oxidants can induce devastating damage during the reoxygenation period.

The cells may be treated with exogenous oxidants following the *in vitro* hypoxic or OGD injury to better mimic tissue reperfusion, since (1) the infiltration and ROS production of circulating leukocytes is missing and (2) the ratio of culture volume/packed cell volume is a couple of orders of magnitude higher than the ratio of extracellular/intracellular space, thus oxidants produced by the cells are instantaneously diluted in *in vitro* hypoxia-reoxygenation injury. Oxidants induce more severe cell damage in post-OGD cells than in normal cells, since the cellular NAD^+ content is much lower following OGD exposure (**Figure 6**). The cellular NAD^+

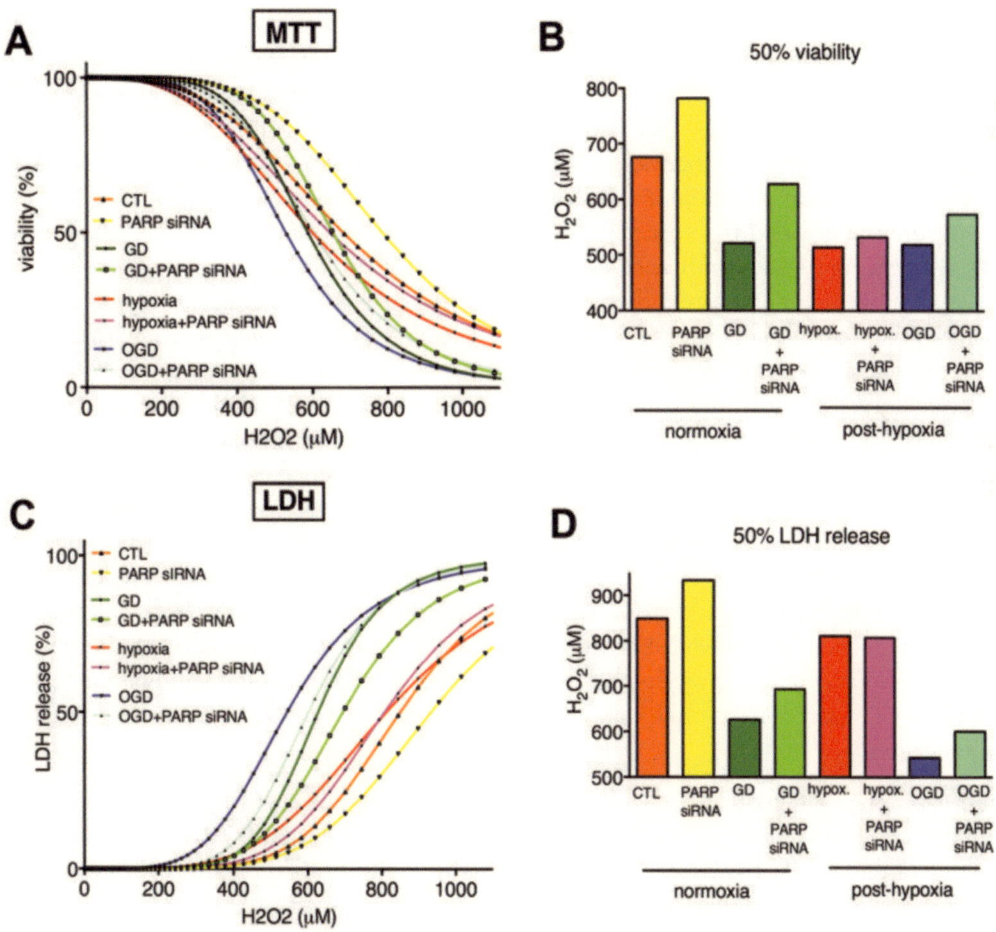

Figure 6. Hypoxia and OGD increases the sensitivity to exogenous oxidants. H9c2 cells were subjected to 8-hour-long hypoxia/OGD or GD, and then following the normalization of glucose concentration and oxygen tension the cells were exposed to various concentrations of H_2O_2 for 3 hours. (A and B) The viability of the cells was evaluated by the MTT assay. (C and D) LDH activity was measure in the supernatant. Non-linear curve-fitting was applied to the raw data (A and C) and the concentration of H2O2 that caused 50% reduction in the viability (B) or 50% increase in the LDH release (D) are shown. GD and OGD resulted in narrower range of H2O2 tolerance (steeper curves). From Ref. [5].

pools may be completely depleted by a moderate oxidative damage that hardly induces viability reduction in normal cells [5]. Cells undergoing OGD injury are less tolerant to oxidants and can survive oxidant-exposure in a narrow concentration range. PARP inhibition reduces the NAD^+ consumption and has protective effect against oxidant-induced cell damage in post-hypoxic or post-OGD cells that is in line with *in vivo* ischemia-reperfusion data [23, 67, 89–91].

4. Interventions to increase the recovery following hypoxia-reoxygenation or OGD-reoxygenation injury

In drug discovery, the ultimate goal of using *in vitro* models, like hypoxia-reoxygenation or the OGD-reoxygenation is to find novel drugs that show efficacy against ischemic diseases *in vivo*. The relative contribution of various pathways leading to cellular damage in hypoxia or OGD-injury has not been definitely established, thus it is unclear which pathways can serve as drug targets in this injury. Furthermore, there are notable differences between the hypoxia-reoxygenation model and ischemia-reperfusion injury that may result in discrepancy between the *in vitro* and *in vivo* drug efficacy [92, 93]. There are numerous factors that may account for this difference and their significance should be individually evaluated depending on the target disease for each organ or tissue type. While the organs consist of various cell types and the extracellular matrix, usually a single cell type is used in the *in vitro* model. This excludes the cells that build up the blood vessels and the circulating blood cells, and the secreted pro-inflammatory mediators and ROS produced by leukocytes are similarly absent. There are functional differences between tissues and cultured cells including muscle contraction, absorption of nutrients in the digestive system, kidney filtration, excretion and reabsorption and the detoxification function of the liver that all require lot of metabolic energy. Cultured cells may show slightly different expression profiles than their *in vivo* counterparts that may affect the expression level of drug targets and can change the observed responses. There are deficiencies of the *in vitro* model, which are associated with the differences in extracellular volume: the hypoxia induction is slower, the energy resources are more abundant and the dilutions of secreted cytotoxic or cytoprotective agents are greater than *in vivo*. On the other hand, there are no drug absorption, solubility and metabolism issues *in vitro* that may reduce the drug effects *in vivo*.

Interventions that reduce the cellular damage in hypoxia-reoxygenation injury and enhance recovery following hypoxia or OGD exposure may target (1) the metabolism and energy resources, (2) the oxidative stress pathways and antioxidant responses or (3) the proteasome and proteolytic activity. Apart from these universal cellular targets, some tissue-specific receptors were also found to have beneficial effects in some models. Energy replenishment using adenosine or inosine is effective in various cell types exposed to OGD injury since the pentose part of these nucleosides can be anaerobically metabolized through the pentose phosphate pathway [1–3]. Purine nucleosides are preferable to glucose in hypoxia since their metabolism can produce more ATP molecules than glycolysis and their utilization is more effective at low concentrations. Furthermore, they possess anti-inflammatory and weak PARP inhibitor activity that supports their activity *in vivo* [94]. Various ROS scavengers and antioxidants also exert cytoprotective effect in hypoxia-reoxygenation models [95] and inhibition of the NAD^+ consumer PARP-1 that recognizes the oxidative DNA damage is also beneficial [96, 97]. Not only the necrosis-associated PARP-1 blockage is effective in OGD-reoxygenation injury, but also caspase inhibition has protective effect in select cell types, confirming that the cell death features both apoptotic and necrotic elements in this injury [2]. Proteasome inhibition that possibly prevents the degradation of key signalling proteins and metabolic enzymes is also beneficial in hypoxia-reoxygenation injury [98, 99].

5. Conclusion

The hypoxia-reoxygenation model is a valuable tool in hypoxia and ischemia research that may be combined with other injury models to fully reproduce features of inflammatory and vascular diseases. This low-cost model does not require advanced research skills and may be optimized within a short time in the laboratory. The cellular damage mostly occurs as a consequence of energetic failure and shows necrotic characteristics in this model. Both the hypoxic phase and the post-hypoxic recovery period involve massive changes in the cellular metabolism: a characteristic suppression of mitochondrial energy production is caused by the lack of oxygen and later by the shortage of NAD^+ supply. The recovery from this state is a delicate process that recreates the balance in cellular energetics.

Acknowledgement

D.G. received funding from the People Programme (Marie Curie Actions) of the European Union's Seventh Framework Programme under the grant agreement number 628100.

Author details

Domokos Gerő

Address all correspondence to: gerodomokos@yahoo.com

University of Exeter Medical School, Exeter, UK

References

[1] Modis K, Gero D, Nagy N, Szoleczky P, Toth ZD, Szabo C. Cytoprotective effects of adenosine and inosine in an in vitro model of acute tubular necrosis. British Journal of Pharmacology. 2009;158(6):1565–1578. doi: 10.1111/j.1476-5381.2009.00432.x. PubMed PMID: 19906119; PubMed Central PMCID: PMC2795223.

[2] Szoleczky P, Modis K, Nagy N, Dori Toth Z, DeWitt D, Szabo C, et al. Identification of agents that reduce renal hypoxia-reoxygenation injury using cell-based screening: purine nucleosides are alternative energy sources in LLC-PK1 cells during hypoxia. Archives of Biochemistry and Biophysics. 2012;517(1):53–70. Epub 2011/11/22. doi: 10.1016/j.abb.2011.11.005. PubMed PMID: 22100704.

[3] Modis K, Gero D, Stangl R, Rosero O, Szijarto A, Lotz G, et al. Adenosine and inosine exert cytoprotective effects in an in vitro model of liver ischemia-reperfusion injury. International Journal of Molecular Medicine. 2013;31(2):437–446. doi: 10.3892/ijmm.2012.1203. PubMed PMID: 23232950; PubMed Central PMCID: PMC3981016.

[4] Gero D, Szoleczky P, Chatzianastasiou A, Papapetropoulos A, Szabo C. Modulation of poly(ADP-ribose) polymerase-1 (PARP-1)-mediated oxidative cell injury by ring finger protein 146 (RNF146) in cardiac myocytes. Molecular Medicine. 2014;20:313–328. doi: 10.2119/molmed.2014.00102. PubMed PMID: 24842055; PubMed Central PMCID: PMC4153837.

[5] Gero D, Szabo C. Salvage of nicotinamide adenine dinucleotide plays a critical role in the bioenergetic recovery of post-hypoxic cardiomyocytes. British Journal of Pharmacology. 2015;172(20):4817–4832. doi: 10.1111/bph.13252. PubMed PMID: 26218637; PubMed Central PMCID: PMC4621988.

[6] Lemasters JJ, Oliver C. Cell Biology of Trauma. Boca Raton, FL: CRC Press; 1995. 367 p.

[7] Wu D, Yotnda P. Induction and testing of hypoxia in cell culture. Journal of Visualized Experiments. 2011;54(e2899). doi: 10.3791/2899. PubMed PMID: 21860378; PubMed Central PMCID: PMC3217626.

[8] Roemgens A, Singh S, Beyer C, Arnold S. Inducers of chemical hypoxia act in a gender- and brain region-specific manner on primary astrocyte viability and cytochrome C oxidase. Neurotoxicity Research. 2011;20(1):1–14. doi: 10.1007/s12640-010-9213-z. PubMed PMID: 20734249.

[9] Ren L, Liu W, Wang Y, Wang JC, Tu Q, Xu J, et al. Investigation of hypoxia-induced myocardial injury dynamics in a tissue interface mimicking microfluidic device. Analytical Chemistry. 2013;85(1):235–244. doi: 10.1021/ac3025812. PubMed PMID: 23205467.

[10] Szabo G, Veres G, Radovits T, Gero D, Modis K, Miesel-Groschel C, et al. Cardioprotective effects of hydrogen sulfide. Nitric Oxide: Biology and Chemistry/Official Journal of the Nitric Oxide Society. 2011;25(2):201–210. Epub 2010/11/26. doi: 10.1016/j.niox.2010.11.001. PubMed PMID: 21094267; PubMed Central PMCID: PMC3139695.

[11] Hotter G, Palacios L, Sola A. Low O_2 and high CO_2 in LLC-PK1 cells culture mimics renal ischemia-induced apoptosis. Laboratory Investigation; a Journal of Technical Methods and Pathology. 2004;84(2):213–220. doi: 10.1038/labinvest.3700026. PubMed PMID: 14688798.

[12] Hinkle PC. P/O ratios of mitochondrial oxidative phosphorylation. Biochimica et Biophysica Acta. 2005;1706(1–2):1–11. doi: 10.1016/j.bbabio.2004.09.004. PubMed PMID: 15620362.

[13] Brand MD. The efficiency and plasticity of mitochondrial energy transduction. Biochemical Society Transactions. 2005;33(Pt 5):897–904. doi: 10.1042/BST20050897. PubMed PMID: 16246006.

[14] Buono MJ, Kolkhorst FW. Estimating ATP resynthesis during a marathon run: a method to introduce metabolism. Advances in Physiology Education. 2001;25:70–71.

[15] Massudi H, Grant R, Guillemin GJ, Braidy N. NAD+ metabolism and oxidative stress: the golden nucleotide on a crown of thorns. Redox Report. 2012;17(1):28–46. Epub 2012/02/22. doi: 10.1179/1351000212Y.0000000001. PubMed PMID: 22340513.

[16] Chiarugi A, Dolle C, Felici R, Ziegler M. The NAD metabolome—a key determinant of cancer cell biology. Nature Reviews Cancer. 2012;12(11):741–752. Epub 2012/09/29. doi: 10.1038/nrc3340. PubMed PMID: 23018234.

[17] Houtkooper RH, Canto C, Wanders RJ, Auwerx J. The secret life of NAD+: an old metabolite controlling new metabolic signaling pathways. Endocrine Reviews. 2010;31(2):194–223. Epub 2009/12/17. doi: 10.1210/er.2009-0026. PubMed PMID: 20007326; PubMed Central PMCID: PMC2852209.

[18] Hassa PO, Haenni SS, Elser M, Hottiger MO. Nuclear ADP-ribosylation reactions in mammalian cells: where are we today and where are we going? Microbiology and Molecular Biology Reviews. 2006;70(3):789–829. Epub 2006/09/09. doi: 10.1128/MMBR.00040-05. PubMed PMID: 16959969; PubMed Central PMCID: PMC1594587.

[19] Hirschey MD. Old enzymes, new tricks: sirtuins are NAD(+)-dependent de-acylases. Cell Metabolism. 2011;14(6):718–719. Epub 2011/11/22. doi: 10.1016/j.cmet.2011.10.006. PubMed PMID: 22100408; PubMed Central PMCID: PMC3830953.

[20] Rongvaux A, Andris F, Van Gool F, Leo O. Reconstructing eukaryotic NAD metabolism. Bioessays. 2003;25(7):683–690. Epub 2003/06/20. doi: 10.1002/bies.10297. PubMed PMID: 12815723.

[21] Berger F, Lau C, Dahlmann M, Ziegler M. Subcellular compartmentation and differential catalytic properties of the three human nicotinamide mononucleotide adenylyltransferase isoforms. Journal of Biological Chemistry. 2005;280(43):36334–36341. Epub 2005/08/25. doi: M508660200 [pii] 10.1074/jbc.M508660200. PubMed PMID: 16118205.

[22] Nikiforov A, Dolle C, Niere M, Ziegler M. Pathways and subcellular compartmentation of NAD biosynthesis in human cells: from entry of extracellular precursors to mitochondrial NAD generation. Journal of Biological Chemistry. 2012;286(24):21767–21778. Epub 2011/04/21. doi: M110.213298 [pii] 10.1074/jbc.M110.213298. PubMed PMID: 21504897; PubMed Central PMCID: PMC3122232.

[23] Liaudet L, Szabo G, Szabo C. Oxidative stress and regional ischemia-reperfusion injury: the peroxynitrite-poly(ADP-ribose) polymerase connection. Coronary Artery Disease. 2003;14(2):115–122. doi: 10.1097/01.mca.0000060943.08352.b7. PubMed PMID: 12655275.

[24] Szabo G, Liaudet L, Hagl S, Szabo C. Poly(ADP-ribose) polymerase activation in the reperfused myocardium. Cardiovascular Research. 2004;61(3):471–480. doi: 10.1016/j.cardiores.2003.09.029. PubMed PMID: 14962478.

[25] Szabo G, Soos P, Bahrle S, Zsengeller Z, Flechtenmacher C, Hagl S, et al. Role of poly (ADP-ribose) polymerase activation in the pathogenesis of cardiopulmonary dysfunction in a canine model of cardiopulmonary bypass. European Journal of Cardiothorac Surgery. 2004;25(5):825–832. Epub 2004/04/15. doi: 10.1016/j.ejcts.2004.01.031. PubMed PMID: 15082289.

[26] Rousset S, Alves-Guerra MC, Mozo J, Miroux B, Cassard-Doulcier AM, Bouillaud F, et al. The biology of mitochondrial uncoupling proteins. Diabetes. 2004;53(Suppl. 1):S130–S135. PubMed PMID: 14749278.

[27] Gero D, Szabo C. Glucocorticoids suppress mitochondrial oxidant production via upregulation of uncoupling protein 2 in hyperglycemic endothelial cells. PloS One. 2016;11(4):e0154813. doi: 10.1371/journal.pone.0154813. PubMed PMID: 27128320. PubMed Central PMCID: PMC4851329.

[28] Mailloux RJ, Harper ME. Uncoupling proteins and the control of mitochondrial reactive oxygen species production. Free Radical Biology and Medicine. 2011;51(6):1106–1115. doi: 10.1016/j.freeradbiomed.2011.06.022. PubMed PMID: 21762777.

[29] Pecqueur C, Alves-Guerra MC, Gelly C, Levi-Meyrueis C, Couplan E, Collins S, et al. Uncoupling protein 2, in vivo distribution, induction upon oxidative stress, and evidence for translational regulation. Journal of Biological Chemistry. 2001;276(12):8705–8712. doi: 10.1074/jbc.M006938200. PubMed PMID: 11098051.

[30] Lenaz G. The mitochondrial production of reactive oxygen species: mechanisms and implications in human pathology. IUBMB Life. 2001;52(3–5):159–164. doi: 10.1080/15216540152845957. PubMed PMID: 11798028.

[31] Lenaz G, Baracca A, Barbero G, Bergamini C, Dalmonte ME, Del Sole M, et al. Mitochondrial respiratory chain super-complex I-III in physiology and pathology. Biochimica et Biophysica Acta. 2010;1797(6–7):633–640. doi: 10.1016/j.bbabio.2010.01.025. PubMed PMID: 20116362.

[32] Quijano C, Castro L, Peluffo G, Valez V, Radi R. Enhanced mitochondrial superoxide in hyperglycemic endothelial cells: direct measurements and formation of hydrogen peroxide and peroxynitrite. American Journal of Physiology Heart and Circulatory Physiology. 2007;293(6):H3404–H3414. doi: 10.1152/ajpheart.00761.2007. PubMed PMID: 17906108.

[33] Turrens JF. Mitochondrial formation of reactive oxygen species. Journal of Physiology. 2003;552(Pt 2):335–344. doi: 10.1113/jphysiol.2003.049478. PubMed PMID: 14561818. PubMed Central PMCID: PMC2343396.

[34] Brownlee M. The pathobiology of diabetic complications: a unifying mechanism. Diabetes. 2005;54(6):1615–1625. PubMed PMID: 15919781.

[35] Korshunov SS, Skulachev VP, Starkov AA. High protonic potential actuates a mechanism of production of reactive oxygen species in mitochondria. FEBS Letters. 1997;416(1):15–18. PubMed PMID: 9369223.

[36] Suski JM, Lebiedzinska M, Bonora M, Pinton P, Duszynski J, Wieckowski MR. Relation Between Mitochondrial Membrane Potential and ROS Formation. In: Palmeira CM, Moreno AJ, editors. Mitochondrial Bioenergetics: Methods and Protocols Methods in Molecular Biology. Springer Science + Business Media, LLC New York, NY; 2012. Vol. 810, pp. 183–205.

[37] Suzuki K, Olah G, Modis K, Coletta C, Kulp G, Gero D, et al. Hydrogen sulfide replacement therapy protects the vascular endothelium in hyperglycemia by preserving mitochondrial function. Proceedings of the National Academy of Sciences of the United States of America. 2011;108(33):13829–13834. doi: 10.1073/pnas.1105121108. PubMed PMID: 21808008. PubMed Central PMCID: PMC3158211.

[38] Mailloux RJ, Seifert EL, Bouillaud F, Aguer C, Collins S, Harper ME. Glutathionylation acts as a control switch for uncoupling proteins UCP2 and UCP3. Journal of Biological Chemistry. 2011;286(24):21865–21875. doi: 10.1074/jbc.M111.240242. PubMed PMID: 21515686; PubMed Central PMCID: PMC3122241.

[39] Gero D, Szabo C. Role of the peroxynitrite-poly (ADP-ribose) polymerase pathway in the pathogenesis of liver injury. Current Pharmceutical Design. 2006;12(23):2903–2910. PubMed PMID: 16918420.

[40] Gero D, Szabo C. Poly(ADP-ribose) polymerase: a new therapeutic target? Current Opinion in Anaesthesiology. 2008;21(2):111–121. doi: 10.1097/ACO.0b013e3282f63c15. PubMed PMID: 18443476.

[41] Molnar A, Toth A, Bagi Z, Papp Z, Edes I, Vaszily M, et al. Activation of the poly(ADP-ribose) polymerase pathway in human heart failure. Molecular Medicine. 2006;12(7–8):143–152. Epub 2006/11/08. doi: 10.2119/2006-00043.Molnar. PubMed PMID: 17088946. PubMed Central PMCID: PMC1626594.

[42] Piskunova TS, Yurova MN, Ovsyannikov AI, Semenchenko AV, Zabezhinski MA, Popovich IG, et al. Deficiency in poly(ADP-ribose) polymerase-1 (PARP-1) accelerates aging and spontaneous carcinogenesis in mice. Current Gerontology and Geriatrics Research. Volume 2008:754190. Epub 2008/01/01. doi: 10.1155/2008/754190. PubMed PMID: 19415146; PubMed Central PMCID: PMC2672038.

[43] Hur JW, Sung YK, Shin HD, Park BL, Cheong HS, Bae SC. Poly(ADP-ribose) polymerase (PARP) polymorphisms associated with nephritis and arthritis in systemic lupus erythematosus. Rheumatology (Oxford). 2006;45(6):711–717. Epub 2006/02/08. doi: kei262 [pii] 10.1093/rheumatology/kei262. PubMed PMID: 16461442.

[44] Cottet F, Blanche H, Verasdonck P, Le Gall I, Schachter F, Burkle A, et al. New polymorphisms in the human poly(ADP-ribose) polymerase-1 coding sequence: lack of association with longevity or with increased cellular poly(ADP-ribosyl)ation capacity. Journal

of Molecular Medicine (Berl). 2000;78(8):431–440. Epub 2000/11/30. PubMed PMID: 11097112.

[45] Lockett KL, Hall MC, Xu J, Zheng SL, Berwick M, Chuang SC, et al. The ADPRT V762A genetic variant contributes to prostate cancer susceptibility and deficient enzyme function. Cancer Research. 2004;64(17):6344–6348. Epub 2004/09/03. doi: 10.1158/0008-5472. CAN-04-033864/17/6344 [pii]. PubMed PMID: 15342424.

[46] Roszak A, Lianeri M, Sowinska A, Jagodzinski PP. Involvement of PARP-1 Val762Ala polymorphism in the onset of cervical cancer in Caucasian women. Molecular Diagnosis and Therapy. 2013;17(4):239–245 Epub 2013/05/02. doi: 10.1007/s40291-013-0036-5. PubMed PMID: 23633189.

[47] Huber A, Bai P, de Murcia JM, de Murcia G. PARP-1, PARP-2 and ATM in the DNA damage response: functional synergy in mouse development. DNA Repair (Amst). 2004;3 (8–9):1103–1108. Epub 2004/07/29. doi: 10.1016/j.dnarep.2004.06.002S1568786404001764 [pii]. PubMed PMID: 15279798.

[48] Boehler C, Gauthier LR, Mortusewicz O, Biard DS, Saliou JM, Bresson A, et al. Poly(ADP-ribose) polymerase 3 (PARP3), a newcomer in cellular response to DNA damage and mitotic progression. Proceedings of the National Academy of Sciences of the United States of America 2011; 108(7):2783–2788. Epub 2011/01/29. doi: 1016574108 [pii] 10.1073/pnas.1016574108. PubMed PMID: 21270334; PubMed Central PMCID: PMC3041075.

[49] Luo X, Kraus WL. On PAR with PARP: cellular stress signaling through poly(ADP-ribose) and PARP-1. Genes Development. 2012;26(5):417–432. Epub 2012/03/07. doi: 26/5/417 [pii] 10.1101/gad.183509.111. PubMed PMID: 22391446. PubMed Central PMCID: PMC3305980.

[50] Kim MY, Zhang T, Kraus WL. Poly(ADP-ribosyl)ation by PARP-1: 'PAR-laying' NAD+ into a nuclear signal. Genes Development. 2005;19(17):1951–1967. Epub 2005/09/06. doi: 19/17/1951 [pii] 10.1101/gad.1331805. PubMed PMID: 16140981.

[51] Brunyanszki A, Olah G, Coletta C, Szczesny B, Szabo C. Regulation of mitochondrial poly(ADP-Ribose) polymerase activation by the beta-adrenoceptor/cAMP/protein kinase A axis during oxidative stress. Molecular Pharmacology. 2014;86(4):450–462. doi: 10.1124/mol.114.094318. PubMed PMID: 25069723. PubMed Central PMCID: PMC4164979.

[52] Krishnakumar R, Gamble MJ, Frizzell KM, Berrocal JG, Kininis M, Kraus WL. Reciprocal binding of PARP-1 and histone H1 at promoters specifies transcriptional outcomes. Science. 2008;319(5864):819–821. doi: 10.1126/science.1149250. PubMed PMID: 18258916.

[53] Kraus WL. Transcriptional control by PARP-1: chromatin modulation, enhancer-binding, coregulation, and insulation. Current Opinion in Cell Biology. 2008;20(3):294–302. doi: 10.1016/j.ceb.2008.03.006. PubMed PMID: 18450439. PubMed Central PMCID: PMC2518631.

[54] Zhang T, Berrocal JG, Yao J, DuMond ME, Krishnakumar R, Ruhl DD, et al. Regulation of poly(ADP-ribose) polymerase-1-dependent gene expression through promoter-directed

recruitment of a nuclear NAD+ synthase. Journal of Biological Chemistry. 2012;287 (15):12405–12416. doi: 10.1074/jbc.M111.304469. PubMed PMID: 22334709. PubMed Central PMCID: PMC3320990.

[55] Hossain MB, Ji P, Anish R, Jacobson RH, Takada S. Poly(ADP-ribose) polymerase 1 interacts with nuclear respiratory factor 1 (NRF-1) and plays a role in NRF-1 transcriptional regulation. Journal of Biological Chemistry. 2009;284(13):8621–8632. Epub 2009/02/03. doi: M807198200 [pii] 10.1074/jbc.M807198200. PubMed PMID: 19181665. PubMed Central PMCID: PMC2659221.

[56] Frizzell KM, Gamble MJ, Berrocal JG, Zhang T, Krishnakumar R, Cen Y, et al. Global analysis of transcriptional regulation by poly(ADP-ribose) polymerase-1 and poly(ADP-ribose) glycohydrolase in MCF-7 human breast cancer cells. Journal of Biological Chemistry. 2009;284(49):33926–33938. Epub 2009/10/09. doi: M109.023879 [pii] 10.1074/jbc.M109.023879. PubMed PMID: 19812418. PubMed Central PMCID: PMC2797163.

[57] Berger F, Lau C, Ziegler M. Regulation of poly(ADP-ribose) polymerase 1 activity by the phosphorylation state of the nuclear NAD biosynthetic enzyme NMN adenylyl transferase 1. Proceedings of the National Academy of Sciences of the United States of America. 2007;104(10):3765–3770. doi: 10.1073/pnas.0609211104. PubMed PMID: 17360427. PubMed Central PMCID: PMC1820658.

[58] Modis K, Gero D, Erdelyi K, Szoleczky P, DeWitt D, Szabo C. Cellular bioenergetics is regulated by PARP1 under resting conditions and during oxidative stress. Biochemical Pharmacology. 2012;83(5):633–643. Epub 2011/12/27. doi: 10.1016/j.bcp.2011.12.014. PubMed PMID: 22198485. PubMed Central PMCID: PMC3272837.

[59] Sack MN, Finkel T. Mitochondrial metabolism, sirtuins, and aging. Cold Spring Harbor Perspectives in Biology. 2012;4(12):1-10 doi: 10.1101/cshperspect.a013102. PubMed PMID: 23209156. PubMed Central PMCID: PMC3504438.

[60] Houtkooper RH, Pirinen E, Auwerx J. Sirtuins as regulators of metabolism and healthspan. Nature Reviews Molecular Cell Biology. 2012;13(4):225–238. Epub 2012/03/08. doi: nrm3293 [pii] 10.1038/nrm3293. PubMed PMID: 22395773.

[61] Rajamohan SB, Pillai VB, Gupta M, Sundaresan NR, Birukov KG, Samant S, et al. SIRT1 promotes cell survival under stress by deacetylation-dependent deactivation of poly (ADP-ribose) polymerase 1. Molecular and Cellular Biology. 2009;29(15):4116–4129. Epub 2009/05/28. doi: MCB.00121-09 [pii] 10.1128/MCB.00121-09. PubMed PMID: 19470756. PubMed Central PMCID: PMC2715814.

[62] Bai P, Canto C, Oudart H, Brunyanszki A, Cen Y, Thomas C, et al. PARP-1 inhibition increases mitochondrial metabolism through SIRT1 activation. Cell Metabolism. 2011;13 (4):461–468. Epub 2011/04/05. doi: 10.1016/j.cmet.2011.03.004. PubMed PMID: 21459330. PubMed Central PMCID: PMC3086520.

[63] Berger NA. Oxidant-induced cytotoxicity: a challenge for metabolic modulation. American Journal of Respiratory Cell and Molecular Biology. 1991;4(1):1–3. doi: 10.1165/ajrcmb/4.1.1. PubMed PMID: 1898851.

[64] Lautier D, Lagueux J, Thibodeau J, Menard L, Poirier GG. Molecular and biochemical features of poly (ADP-ribose) metabolism. Molecular and Cellular Biochemistry. 1993;122 (2):171–193. PubMed PMID: 8232248.

[65] Ueda K, Hayaishi O. ADP-ribosylation. Annual Review of Biochemistry. 1985;54:73–100. doi: 10.1146/annurev.bi.54.070185.000445. PubMed PMID: 3927821.

[66] Virag L. PARP-1 and the Shape of Cell Death. In: Bürkle A, editor. Poly(ADP-Ribosyl) ation. New York: Springer US; 2006. pp. 141–152.

[67] Jagtap P, Szabo C. Poly(ADP-ribose) polymerase and the therapeutic effects of its inhibitors. Nature Reviews Drug Discovery. 2005;4(5):421–440. Epub 2005/05/03. doi: 10.1038/nrd1718. PubMed PMID: 15864271.

[68] Malanga M, Althaus FR. The role of poly(ADP-ribose) in the DNA damage signaling network. Biochemistry and Cell Biology. 2005;83(3):354–364. doi: 10.1139/o05-038. PubMed PMID: 15959561.

[69] Elmore S. Apoptosis: a review of programmed cell death. Toxicologic Pathology. 2007;35 (4):495–516. doi: 10.1080/01926230701320337. PubMed PMID: 17562483. PubMed Central PMCID: PMC2117903.

[70] Yu SW, Andrabi SA, Wang H, Kim NS, Poirier GG, Dawson TM, et al. Apoptosis-inducing factor mediates poly(ADP-ribose) (PAR) polymer-induced cell death. Proceedings of the National Academy of Sciences of the United States of America. 2006;103(48):18314–18319. doi: 10.1073/pnas.0606528103. PubMed PMID: 17116881. PubMed Central PMCID: PMC1838748.

[71] Chen M, Zsengeller Z, Xiao CY, Szabo C. Mitochondrial-to-nuclear translocation of apoptosis-inducing factor in cardiac myocytes during oxidant stress: potential role of poly (ADP-ribose) polymerase-1. Cardiovascular Research. 2004;63(4):682–688. doi: 10.1016/j.cardiores.2004.04.018. PubMed PMID: 15306224.

[72] Duriez PJ, Shah GM. Cleavage of poly(ADP-ribose) polymerase: a sensitive parameter to study cell death. Biochemistry and Cell Biology. 1997;75(4):337–349. PubMed PMID: 9493956.

[73] Du L, Zhang X, Han YY, Burke NA, Kochanek PM, Watkins SC, et al. Intra-mitochondrial poly(ADP-ribosylation) contributes to NAD+ depletion and cell death induced by oxidative stress. Journal of Biological Chemistry. 2003;278(20):18426–18433. Epub 2003/03/11. doi: 10.1074/jbc.M301295200M301295200 [pii]. PubMed PMID: 12626504.

[74] Zhang Y, Liu S, Mickanin C, Feng Y, Charlat O, Michaud GA, et al. RNF146 is a poly (ADP-ribose)-directed E3 ligase that regulates axin degradation and Wnt signalling. Nature Cell Biology. 2011;13(5):623–629. Epub 2011/04/12. doi: ncb2222 [pii] 10.1038/ncb2222. PubMed PMID: 21478859.

[75] Zhou ZD, Chan CH, Xiao ZC, Tan EK. Ring finger protein 146/Iduna is a poly(ADP-ribose) polymer binding and PARsylation dependent E3 ubiquitin ligase. Cell Adhesion

and Migration. 2011;5(6):463–471. Epub 2012/01/26. doi: 18356 [pii] 10.4161/cam.5.6.18356. PubMed PMID: 22274711. PubMed Central PMCID: PMC3277779.

[76] Wang Z, Michaud GA, Cheng Z, Zhang Y, Hinds TR, Fan E, et al. Recognition of the iso-ADP-ribose moiety in poly(ADP-ribose) by WWE domains suggests a general mechanism for poly(ADP-ribosyl)ation-dependent ubiquitination. Genes Development. 2012;26 (3):235–240. Epub 2012/01/24. doi: gad.182618.111 [pii] 10.1101/gad.182618.111. PubMed PMID: 22267412; PubMed Central PMCID: PMC3278890.

[77] Dawson VL, editor Symposium S14: stroke: inflammation in the neurovascular unit, ischemic preconditioning. Journal of Neurochemistry, 2004;90 (Suppl. 1): p80.

[78] Andrabi SA, Kang HC, Haince JF, Lee YI, Zhang J, Chi Z, et al. Iduna protects the brain from glutamate excitotoxicity and stroke by interfering with poly(ADP-ribose) polymer-induced cell death. Nature Medicine. 2011;17(6):692–699. Epub 2011/05/24. doi: nm.2387 [pii] 10.1038/nm.2387. PubMed PMID: 21602803.

[79] Kang HC, Lee YI, Shin JH, Andrabi SA, Chi Z, Gagne JP, et al. Iduna is a poly(ADP-ribose) (PAR)-dependent E3 ubiquitin ligase that regulates DNA damage. Proceedings of the National Academy of Sciences of the United States of America. 2011;108(34):14103–14108. Epub 2011/08/10. doi: 1108799108 [pii] 10.1073/pnas.1108799108. PubMed PMID: 21825151; PubMed Central PMCID: PMC3161609.

[80] Jungmichel S, Rosenthal F, Altmeyer M, Lukas J, Hottiger MO, Nielsen ML. Proteome-wide identification of poly(ADP-Ribosyl)ation targets in different genotoxic stress responses. Molecular Cell. 2013;52(2):272–285. doi: 10.1016/j.molcel.2013.08.026. PubMed PMID: 24055347.

[81] Rossi MN, Carbone M, Mostocotto C, Mancone C, Tripodi M, Maione R, et al. Mitochondrial localization of PARP-1 requires interaction with mitofilin and is involved in the maintenance of mitochondrial DNA integrity. Journal of Biological Chemistry. 2009;284 (46):31616–31624. Epub 2009/09/19. doi: M109.025882 [pii] 10.1074/jbc.M109.025882. PubMed PMID: 19762472. PubMed Central PMCID: PMC2797232.

[82] Lapucci A, Pittelli M, Rapizzi E, Felici R, Moroni F, Chiarugi A. Poly(ADP-ribose) polymerase-1 is a nuclear epigenetic regulator of mitochondrial DNA repair and transcription. Molecular Pharmacology. 2011;79(6):932–940. Epub 2011/03/29. doi: mol.110.070110 [pii] 10.1124/mol.110.070110. PubMed PMID: 21441600.

[83] Horvath EM, Szabo C. Poly(ADP-ribose) polymerase as a drug target for cardiovascular disease and cancer: an update. Drug News Perspectives. 2007;20(3):171–181. Epub 2007/05/24. doi: 1092098 [pii] 10.1358/dnp.2007.20.3.1092098. PubMed PMID: 1752 0094.

[84] Pacher P, Szabo C. Role of poly(ADP-ribose) polymerase 1 (PARP-1) in cardiovascular diseases: the therapeutic potential of PARP inhibitors. Cardiovascular Drug Reviews. 2007;25(3):235–260. Epub 2007/10/09. doi: CDR018 [pii] 10.1111/j.1527-3466.2007.00018.x. PubMed PMID: 17919258. PubMed Central PMCID: PMC2225457.

[85] Gao YH, Li CX, Shen SM, Li H, Chen GQ, Wei Q, et al. Hypoxia-inducible factor 1alpha mediates the down-regulation of superoxide dismutase 2 in von Hippel-Lindau deficient renal clear cell carcinoma. Biochemical and Biophysical Research Communications. 2013;435(1):46–51. doi: 10.1016/j.bbrc.2013.04.034. PubMed PMID: 23611775.

[86] Xi H, Gao YH, Han DY, Li QY, Feng LJ, Zhang W, et al. Hypoxia inducible factor-1alpha suppresses peroxiredoxin 3 expression to promote proliferation of CCRCC cells. FEBS Letters. 2014;588(18):3390–3394. doi: 10.1016/j.febslet.2014.07.030. PubMed PMID: 25093297.

[87] Brune B, Zhou J. The role of nitric oxide (NO) in stability regulation of hypoxia inducible factor-1alpha (HIF-1alpha). Current Medicinal Chemistry. 2003;10(10):845–855. PubMed PMID: 12678687.

[88] Ratcliffe PJ, O'Rourke JF, Maxwell PH, Pugh CW. Oxygen sensing, hypoxia-inducible factor-1 and the regulation of mammalian gene expression. The Journal of Experimental Biology. 1998;201(Pt 8):1153–1162. PubMed PMID: 9510527.

[89] Zingarelli B, Cuzzocrea S, Zsengeller Z, Salzman AL, Szabo C. Protection against myocardial ischemia and reperfusion injury by 3-aminobenzamide, an inhibitor of poly (ADP-ribose) synthetase. Cardiovascular Research. 1997;36(2):205–215. Epub 1998/02/17. PubMed PMID: 9463632.

[90] Kovacs K, Toth A, Deres P, Kalai T, Hideg K, Gallyas F, Jr., et al. Critical role of PI3-kinase/Akt activation in the PARP inhibitor induced heart function recovery during ischemia-reperfusion. Biochemical Pharmacology. 2006;71(4):441–452. Epub 2005/12/13. doi: 10.1016/j.bcp.2005.05.036. PubMed PMID: 16337154.

[91] Roesner JP, Mersmann J, Bergt S, Bohnenberg K, Barthuber C, Szabo C, et al. Therapeutic injection of PARP inhibitor INO-1001 preserves cardiac function in porcine myocardial ischemia and reperfusion without reducing infarct size. Shock. 2010;33(5):507–512. Epub 2010/04/17. doi: 10.1097/SHK.0b013e3181c4fb08. PubMed PMID: 20395771.

[92] Desestret V, Riou A, Chauveau F, Cho TH, Devillard E, Marinescu M, et al. In vitro and in vivo models of cerebral ischemia show discrepancy in therapeutic effects of M2 macrophages. PloS One. 2013;8(6):e67063. doi: 10.1371/journal.pone.0067063. PubMed PMID: 23825621. PubMed Central PMCID: PMC3692438.

[93] Pugsley MK. Cardiac Drug Development Guide. Totowa, NJ: Humana Press; 2003. x, 431 p.

[94] Szabo C, Gero D, Hasko G. Anti-Inflammatory and Cytoprotective Effects of Inosine. In: Haskó G, Cronstein BN, Szabó C, editors. Adenosine Receptors: Therapeutic Aspects for Inflammatory and Immune Diseases. Boca Raton, FL: CRC/Taylor & Francis; 2007. pp. 237–256.

[95] Yamada J, Yoshimura S, Yamakawa H, Sawada M, Nakagawa M, Hara S, et al. Cell permeable ROS scavengers, Tiron and Tempol, rescue PC12 cell death caused by pyrogallol or hypoxia/reoxygenation. Neuroscience Research. 2003;45(1):1–8. PubMed PMID: 12507718.

[96] Martinez-Romero R, Canuelo A, Martinez-Lara E, Javier Oliver F, Cardenas S, Siles E. Poly(ADP-ribose) polymerase-1 modulation of in vivo response of brain hypoxia-inducible factor-1 to hypoxia/reoxygenation is mediated by nitric oxide and factor inhibiting HIF. Journal of Neurochemistry. 2009;111(1):150–159. doi: 10.1111/j.1471-4159.2009.06307.x. PubMed PMID: 19656264.

[97] Zhang Y, Zhang X, Park TS, Gidday JM. Cerebral endothelial cell apoptosis after ischemia-reperfusion: role of PARP activation and AIF translocation. Journal of Cerebral Blood Flow and Metabolism: Official Journal of the International Society of Cerebral Blood Flow and Metabolism. 2005;25(7):868–877. doi: 10.1038/sj.jcbfm.9600081. PubMed PMID: 15729291.

[98] Pashevin DO, Nagibin VS, Tumanovska LV, Moibenko AA, Dosenko VE. Proteasome inhibition diminishes the formation of neutrophil extracellular traps and prevents the death of cardiomyocytes in coculture with activated neutrophils during anoxia-reoxygenation. Pathobiology: Journal of Immunopathology, Molecular and Cellular Biology. 2015;82(6):290–298. doi: 10.1159/000440982. PubMed PMID: 26558384.

[99] Tang L, Peng Y, Xu T, Yi X, Liu Y, Luo Y, et al. The effects of quercetin protect cardiomyocytes from A/R injury is related to its capability to increasing expression and activity of PKCepsilon protein. Molecular and Cellular Biochemistry. 2013;382(1–2):145–152. doi: 10.1007/s11010-013-1729-0. PubMed PMID: 23793725.

Chapter 4

Vascular Smooth Muscle as an Oxygen Sensor: Role of Elevation of the $[Na^+]_i/[K^+]_i$

Sergei N. Orlov , Yulia G. Birulina ,
Liudmila V. Smaglii and Svetlana V. Gusakova

Additional information is available at the end of the chapter

http://dx.doi.org/10.5772/65384

Abstract

The article presents a review of data from our own research and data obtained by other authors about the role of intracellular sodium (Na_i^+) and potassium (K_i^+) in transcriptomic changes in vascular smooth muscle cells (VSMC) during hypoxia. It was found that acute hypoxia suppressed $[K^+]_o$ and phenylephrine-induced contractions of aortic rings through voltage-gated as well as by Ca_i^{2+}- and ATP-sensitive K^+ channels; 24-h incubation of VSMC in ischemic conditions resulted in attenuation of ATP content, elevation of $[Na^+]_i$ and loss of $[K^+]_i$. Dissipation of Na^+ and K^+ gradients in low-Na^+, high-K^+ medium completely eliminated increment in Fos, Atf3, Ptgs2 and Per2 mRNAs and sharply diminished augmentation of Klf10, Edn1, Nr4a1 and Hes1 expression evoked by hypoxia. All these data suggest that Na_i^+/K_i^+-mediated signaling contribute to transcriptomic changes in VSMC subjected to sustained hypoxia.

Keywords: smooth muscle cells, hypoxia, intracellular $[Na^+]/[K^+]$ ratio, transcription, contraction

1. Introduction

Maintaining optimal oxygen tension level in cells promotes the metabolic and plastic processes that ensure their functional stability. To date, there are a lot of reports showing the high sensitivity of endothelium-denuded blood vessels to oxygen deficiency (hypoxia) [1–5]. These data allow considering vascular smooth muscle cells (VSMC) as an oxygen sensor involved in modulation of blood vessel tone and gene expression. Previously, using global gene expression profiling, we found that in several cell types including rat aortic VSMC Na^+, K^+-ATPase inhibition by ouabain or K^+-free medium led to the differential expression of dozens of genes whose altered expression was previously detected in cells subjected to hypoxia and ischemia/reperfusion [6, 7]. In view of this finding, we examined the relative impact of canonical hypoxia-inducible factor 1alpha (HIF-1α)-and Na_i^+/K_i^+-mediated signaling on transcriptomic changes evoked by hypoxia and glucose deprivation as well as its possible involvement in regulation of VSMC contraction.

2. Hypoxia affects excitation-contraction and excitation-transcription coupling: role of HIF-1α-mediated signaling

Blood vessels play a key role in the maintenance of a balanced supply of oxygen and nutrition in target tissues under acute and chronic hypoxic conditions. In systemic circulation, acute hypoxic conditions resulted in dilatation of vascular beds via direct actions of attenuated partial oxygen pressure (pO_2) on vascular smooth muscle cells (VSMC) as well as by ATP release from erythrocytes that, in turn, leads to activation of purinergic P2Y receptors and augmented production of nitric oxide by endothelial cells (for comprehensive reviews, see [1–3]).

Figure 1A shows that in the absence of erythrocytes, hypoxia attenuated by 20–30% the contraction of rat aortic strips triggered by agonist of α_1-adrenergic receptors phenylephrine. We found that inhibitory action of hypoxia was partially abolished by 4-aminopyridine (**Figure 1B**) and glibenclamide (**Figure 1C**), thus indicating activation of voltage-gated and ATP-sensitive K^+ channels, respectively. Recently, Gun et al. reported that hypoxic relaxation of mesenteric arteries is suppressed by a selective inhibitor of the large conductance Ca^{2+}-activated K^+ channels (BK_{Ca}) iberiotoxin [4].

Unlike systemic circulation, hypoxia results in augmented contraction of pulmonary arterial smooth muscle cells via inhibition of voltage-gated K^+ channels $K_v1.5$ and $K_v2.1$ and activation of nonselective cation channels TRPC1 (for reviews, see [5, 8]). It was shown that ATP release from erythrocytes triggered by shear stress and activation of cAMP-mediated signaling is sharply decreased in human with primary pulmonary hypertension [9]. To the best of our knowledge, the comparative analysis of hypoxia-induced ATP release from erythrocytes of normotensive and hypertensive patients and implication of purinergic receptors in regulation of vascular tone in systemic and pulmonary circulations have not yet been performed.

In addition, the regulation of vascular tone hypoxia leads to cell type-specific differential expression of hundreds of genes documented in global gene profiling studies [10–16]. It is generally accepted that these transcriptomic changes are mediated by hypoxia-inducible factor 1alpha (HIF-1α) involved in regulation of gene expression via interaction of HIF-1α/HIF-1β heterodimer with hypoxia-response elements (HREs) in promoter/enhancer regions of the target gene's DNA. In normoxia, oxygen-dependent prolyl hydroxylase hydroxylates HIF-1α and induces its proteasomal degradation. In contrast, under hypoxic conditions, HIF-1α is translocated to the nucleus, where it forms HIF-1α/HIF-1β complex [17–20]. The list of HIF-1-sensitive genes includes Hif-1α per se and others related to angiogenesis (vascular endothelial growth factor (Vegf) and its receptor Flt1), vasomotor control (endothelin-1, adrenomedullin,

http://dx.doi.org/10.5772/65384

nitric oxide synthase-2), erythropoiesis and iron metabolism (transferrin, transferrin receptor, erythropoietin, ceruloplasmin), energy metabolism (phosphoenolpyruvate carboxylase, aldose, endolase, phosphoglucokinase-1, -L and -C, lactate dehydrogenase A, tyrosine hydroxylase and plasminogen activator inhibitor-1, glucose transporters Glut1-Glut3), and cell proliferation (Tgfb, Igf1, Igfbp1) [21]. Shimoda and coworkers reported that reduction in voltage-gated K^+ currents following hypoxia was absent in pulmonary arterial smooth muscle cells from heterozygous HIF-1α mice, thus suggesting and implicating this oxygen-sensing machinery in vascular bed-specific contractile responses [22].

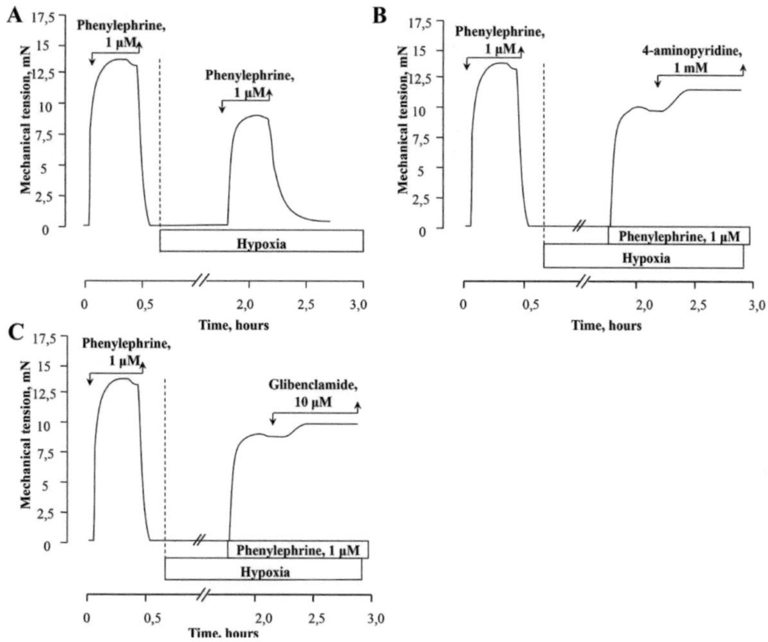

Figure 1. Hypoxia influences on phenylephrine (PE)-induced contraction of ring aortic segments from male Wistar rats. Aortic segments were incubated for 60 min in hypoxic Krebs solution (pO_2 ~ 30 mmHg) and then contacted with phenylephrine (1 μM). Registration of constrictive responses was performed by Myobath-2 Multi-Channel Tissue Bath System. Incubation in hypoxic solution decreased the amplitude of PE-induced constriction in comparison with contraction in normoxic solution (A). Both blocker of voltage-dependent potassium channel 4-aminopyridine (1 mM) (B) and blocker of ATP-dependent potassium channels glibenclamide (10 μM) (C) significantly decreased mechanical tension of aortic segments in comparison with PE-induced contraction in hypoxic solution ($p < 0.05$). *X* axis—time (h), *Y* axis—mechanical tension (mN). The arrows indicate the addition and removal of the respective solutions.

It should be noted that side-by-side with activation of HIF-1α-mediated signaling, attenuation of pO_2 and delivery of cell fuels resulted in decreased intracellular ATP content that, in turn, led to activation of AMP-sensitive protein kinase (AMPK) [23, 24], decline of ion transport ATPase activities and dissipation of electrochemical gradients of K^+, Na^+, Cl^- and Ca^{2+} [25]. Numerous research teams reported that $[Ca^{2+}]_i$ elevation triggers transcriptomic alterations via Ca_i^{2+}-sensitive transcriptional elements [26]. Importantly, along with the increment in $[Ca^{2+}]_i$, even transient ischemia increases $[Na^+]_i$ from 5–8 to 25–40 mM and causes reciprocal changes in $[K^+]_i$ [27]. These data motivate us to propose that Na_i^+/K_i^+-sensitive signaling pathways contribute to cellular responses triggered by sustained hypoxia [6, 28]. Investigations examining this hypothesis are considered below.

3. Intracellular monovalent cations as regulators of gene transcription

In the late 1990s, we observed that elevation of the $[Na^+]_i/[K^+]_i$ ratio protects rat aortic VSMC against apoptosis triggered by serum deprivation and staurosporine addition [29]. To further explore this antiapoptotic pathway, we treated cells with actinomycin D or cycloheximide. Both macromolecular synthesis inhibitors abolished protection against apoptosis by ouabain [30]. Later we employed proteomic technology and detected hundreds of differentially expressed protein spots in VSMC subjected to Na^+, K^+-ATPase inhibition by ouabain and other cardiotonic steroids (CTS) [30]. These data, together with augmented RNA synthesis observed in ouabain-treated VSMC [31], suggest that sharp transcriptomic changes seen in ouabain-treated cells are mediated by immediate response genes (IRG). Indeed, in both RASMC and HeLa cells, ouabain treatment resulted in augmentation of immunoreactive c-Fos and c-Jun by 10-fold and fourfold, respectively [32, 33]. Addition of ouabain induced a fourfold c-Fos mRNA increment accompanied by fivefold increment in $[Na^+]_i$ within 30 min. At the same time, we observed only 10–15% decrease in $[K^+]_i$ [32, 33]. Thus, we can assume that c-Fos expression is more sensitive to increase in $[Na^+]_i$ rather than $[K^+]_i$.

Recent studies have revealed that CTS may affect cells independently of suppression of Na^+, K^+-ATPase. Thus, ouabain induced interaction of α-subunit of the Na^+, K^+-ATPase with the membrane-associated nonreceptor tyrosine kinase Src, activation of Ras/Raf/ERK1,2, phosphatidylinositol 3-kinase (PI(3)K), PI(3)K-dependent protein kinase B, phospholipase C, $[Ca^{2+}]_i$ oscillations and increased production of the reactive oxygen species (for review, see [34–36]). Considering this, we employed K^+-free medium as an alternative approach for Na^+, K^+-ATPase inhibition. To identify Na_i^+,K_i^+-sensitive transcriptomes, both ubiquitous and cell type-specific, we compared the effect of ouabain and K^+-free medium on profiles of gene expression in rat VSMC, human umbilical vein endothelial cells (HUVEC) and the human carcinoma HeLa cell line [26]. Using Affymetrix-based technology, we found that expression of 684, 737 and 1839 transcripts in HeLa, HUVEC and RASMC, respectively, changes up to 60-fold. It is worth noting that there was a strong correlation in cells pretreated with ouabain or K^+-free medium for 3 h. We also found that 80 transcripts of examined Na_i^+/K_i^+-sensitive genes were common for all examined types of cells [26].

We found that genes involved in the regulation of transcription represents a half of ubiquitous Na_i^+,K_i^+-sensitive transcriptome. This amount was ~sevenfold higher than in the total human genome [37]. The group of ubiquitous Na_i^+/K_i^+-sensitive genes, whose expression was increased by more than threefold, included the transcription factor of the steroid-thyroid

http://dx.doi.org/10.5772/65384

hormone-retinoid receptor superfamily Nr4a2, transcriptional regulator of C2H2-type zinc finger protein Egr-1, the basic helix-loop-helix transcription regulator Hes1, members of the superfamily of b-zip transcriptional factors possessing leucine-zipper dimerization motif and basic DNA-binding domain and forming heterodimeric activating protein AP-1 (Fos, FosB, Jun, JunB, Atf3) [26].

4. Evidence for Na_i^+/K_i^+-mediated, Ca_i^{2+}-independent excitation-transcription coupling

Because of the high electrochemical gradient, the opening of calcium channels resulted in rapid elevation of $[Ca^{2+}]_i$ from ~0.1 to 1 μM, its interaction with calmodulin and other $[Ca^{2+}]_i$ sensors, in turn, affects the expression of hundreds of genes, i.e., phenomenon termed excitation-transcription coupling [38]. Increase in $[Ca^{2+}]_i$ affects transcription via several signaling pathways. Thus, $[Ca^{2+}]_i$ elevation induces translocation of kappa-light-chain enhancer of nuclear factor (NFκB) of activated B cells from the cytosol to the nucleus. This process is triggered by activation of Ca^{2+}/calmodulin-sensitive protein kinase (CaMKI, II or III) and phosphorylated IkB kinase that phosphorylates the inhibitor of kB (IkB) [38]. $[Ca^{2+}]_i$ elevation also promotes translocation from cytosol to the nucleus; nuclear factor of activated T cells (NFAT) is evoked by its dephosphorylation by the (Ca^{2+}/calmodulin)-dependent phosphatase calcineurin [39]. In addition, increased cytosolic and nucleoplasmic Ca^{2+} concentrations lead to phosphorylation of cAMP response element-binding protein (CREB) by CaMKII and CaMKIV, respectively. Phosphorylated CREB regulates transcription via their binding to the (Ca^{2+}+cAMP)-response element (CRE) sequences of DNA [40].

Because the c-Fos promoter contains CRE, its augmented expression might be mediated by depolarization of ouabain-treated VSMC and the opening of voltage-gated Ca^{2+} channels. However, unlike high-K^+ medium, c-Fos expression in ouabain-treated cells was not affected by inhibition of L-type Ca^{2+} channels with nicardipine [41]. In additional experiments, we found that augmented c-Fos expression evoked by ouabain was preserved in Ca^{2+}-free medium and in the presence of extracellular (EGTA) and intracellular (BAPTA) Ca^{2+} chelators [30]. To study the role of Ca_i^{2+}-mediated and Na_i^+/K_i^+-independent signaling, we compared transcriptomic changes triggered by elevation of the $[Na^+]_i/[K^+]_i$ ratio in control and Ca^{2+}-depleted cells. Depletion of Ca^{2+} led to prevalent increase in Na_i^+/K_i^+-sensitive genes, both ubiquitous and cell-type specific [26]. For further investigation, we examined ubiquitous Ca_i^{2+}-sensitive genes whose expression is regulated by more than threefold independently of the presence of Ca^{2+} chelators and selected several transcription factors (Fos, Hes1, Nfkbia, Jun), protein phosphatase 1, dual specificity phosphatase Dusp8, interleukin-6, regulatory subunit, type 2 cyclooxygenase COX-2, cyclin L1 [41].

Considering these data, it is important to underline that Ca^{2+} chelators may affect cellular functions independently of Ca^{2+} depletion. Thus, we observed that the addition of EGTA increases permeability of VSMC for Na^+ [41]. It is also known that the affinity of EGTA for Mn^{2+}, Zn^{2+}, Cu^{2+}, Co^{2+}, $Fe^{2+/3+}$ is 10-fold to 10^7-fold higher than for Ca^{2+} [42–44]. These polyvalent cations are important in regulation of metaloenzymes activity and participate in protein-DNA and protein-protein interactions. Moreover, EGTA causes irreversible conformational transition and inactivation of transcriptional adaptor Zn^{2+}-binding domain that affects gene expression [45]. It is worth noting that in the human genome, the C2H2 zinc finger superfamily includes about half of all annotated transcription factors [46]. This implies that this and other chelators have Ca_i^{2+}-independent action on transcriptomic changes evoked by diverse stimuli. Keeping these data in mind, we compared the actions of Ca^{2+} chelators and Na^+, K^+-ATPase inhibitors on transcriptomic changes and concentration of monovalent cations in VSMC [47]. Our results show that transcriptomic changes seen in Ca^{2+}-depleted VSMC are at least partially caused by elevation of the $[Na^+]_i/[K^+]_i$ ratio and activation of Na_i^+/K_i^+-independent signaling pathways. This conclusion is supported by several observations. First, Ca^{2+} depletion led to a ~threefold elevation of $[Na^+]_i$ and a twofold attenuation of $[K^+]_i$. An increment in the $[Na^+]_i/[K^+]_i$ ratio seen in Ca^{2+}-depleted cells was caused by elevation of plasma membrane permeability for monovalent cations. Indeed, Ca^{2+} depletion resulted in almost threefold elevation of the rate of ^{22}Na and ^{86}Rb influx measured in the presence of inhibitors of Na^+, K^+-ATPase and Na^+, K^+, $2Cl^-$ cotransport. Second, the list of genes whose mRNA content was increased in Ca^{2+}-depleted cells by more than fourfold includes a large number of genes whose expression was also attenuated by the Na^+, K^+-ATPase inhibition in K^+-free medium. Third, there was a strong positive correlation in mRNA content of 2071 genes whose expression was changed by more than 1.2-fold in cells subjected to Na^+, K^+-ATPase inhibition in K^+-free medium as well as in Ca^{2+}-depleted cells. Fourth, dissipation of transmembrane gradients of Na^+ and K^+ in high-K^+, low-Na^+ medium abolished the increment in the $[Na^+]_i/[K^+]_i$ ratio as well as sharp elevation of Atf3, Nr4a1 and Erg3 mRNA content triggered by 3-h incubation of VSMC in Ca^{2+}-free, EGTA-containing medium [47]. Thus, novel molecular biological and pharmacological approaches should be developed for precise identification of the relative impact of Ca^{2+}-mediated and Ca^{2+}-independent pathways on transcriptomic changes evoked by elevation of the $[Na^+]_i/[K^+]_i$ ratio.

5. Evidence for implication of $[Na^+]_i/[K^+]_i$-sensitive pathways in transcriptomic changes evoked by hypoxia

The crosstalk between transcriptomic changes and monovalent ion handling was initially supported by comparative analysis of Na_i^+/K_i^+-sensitive genes documented in our investigations [26] and data on genes whose expression in hypoxic conditions was changed in studies performed by other research groups [9, 11, 48–56]. Indeed, among genes whose augmented expression was detected both in vivo and in vitro models of ischemia/reperfusion, we found several ubiquitous Na_i^+/K_i^+-sensitive genes, including transcription factors EGR1, ATF3, NFKBIZ, HES1 as well as type 2 cyclooxygenase, IL6, thioredoxin-interacting protein TXNIP.

http://dx.doi.org/10.5772/65384

Moreover, using IPA-knowledge base data, we observed that ubiquitous Na^+_i,K^+_i-sensitive transcriptomes are highly significantly correlated with differential expression of genes in disorders triggered by kidney, liver and heart ischemia (**Figure 2**). These data allowed us to propose that transcriptomic changes in ischemic tissues are at least partially mediated by a novel Na_i^+, K_i^+-mediated excitation-transcription coupling [26, 27].

To examine this hypothesis, we compared the effect of ouabain and hypoxia on the content of monovalent ions and ATP in VSMC from the rat aorta. We observed that 24-h incubation of VSMC in hypoxia and glucose starvation decreased intracellular ATP content by ~threefold, whereas ouabain attenuated this parameter by <20% (**Figure 3**). Ouabain led to almost 10-fold increase in $[Na^+]_i$ and similar decrease in $[K^+]_i$. Hypoxia also caused threefold increase in $[Na^+]_i$ and twofold decrease in $[K^+]_i$. At the same time, reduction in monovalent cations transmembrane gradients in low-Na^+, high-K^+ medium almost completely eliminated the actions of ouabain and hypoxia on the $[Na^+]_i/]K^+]_i$ ratio [57].

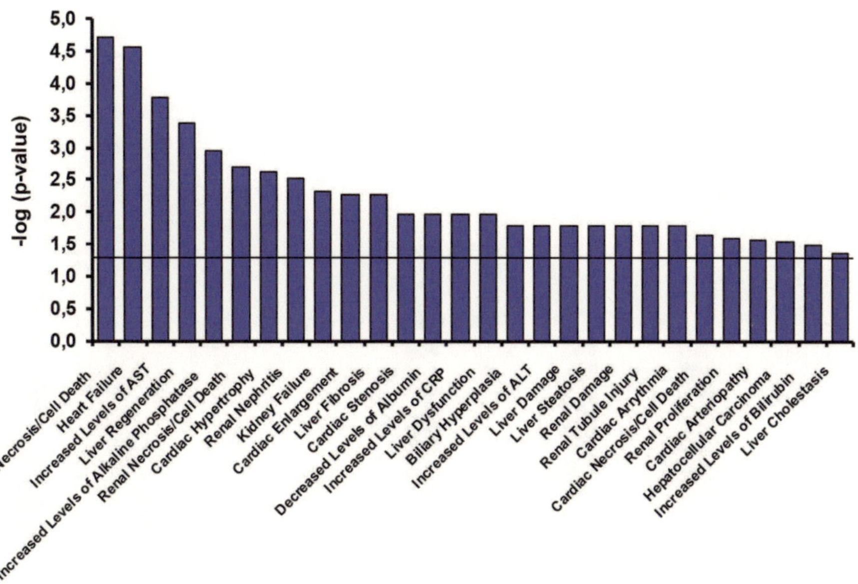

Figure 2. Disorders significantly associated with differential expression of genes whose expression was ubiquitously changed in VSMC from rat aorta, human umbilical vein endothelial cells and HeLa cell line subjected to Na^+,K^+-ATPase inhibition by both ouabain and K^+-free medium. The criteria with a threshold for significance of $p = 0.05$ (or 1.3 when expressed as −log(p-value) are shown as straight line. Adopted with permission from [26].

We then identified the $[Na^+]_i/]K^+]_i$-sensitive transcriptome in rat VSMC. We found that 6-h inhibition of the Na^+, K^+-ATPase with ouabain or in K^+-free medium resulted in differential expression of 6412 transcripts exhibit highly significant ($p < 4 \times 10^{-9}$) and positive ($R^2 > 0.80$) correlation and classified as Ca_i^{2+}-sensitive genes [57]. To continue our studies, we selected genes whose participation in the pathogenesis of hypoxia was shown in previous studies combined with the property of the highest expression increments under sustained Na^+, K^+-

ATPase inhibition. These genes include Fos, Cyp1a1, Klf10, Atf3, Nr4a1, Hes1, Ptgs2 and Per2. Among these genes, Fos, Atf3 and JUN together form dimeric transcription factor AP-1 whose expression increased in all types of cells subjected to hypoxia [58]. Klf10 is a Kruppel-like zinc finger transcription factor family member involved in hypoxia-dependent angiogenesis via COX-1 activation [59]. Ptgs2 encodes an inducible isoform of cyclooxygenase-2 (COX-2) whose role in the pathophysiology of hypoxia is well documented [60]. Nur77 or Nr4a1, also known as nerve growth factor IB, is the nuclear receptor of transcription factors stabilizing HIF-1α which increases its transcriptional activity [61]. Hes1 is the main helix-loop-helix transcription factor that enhances the expression after ischemic renal failure [52]. Clock, Bmal1, Per1, Per2, Cry1 and Cry2 are the positive (Clock and Bmal1) and negative (others) regulators of a transcription-translation feedback loop forming the core circadian oscillator [62]. Cyp1a1 encodes a cytochrome P450 family member and its expression is mediated by HIF-1β [63, 64]. Per2 promotes circadian stabilization of HIF-1α activity that is critical for myocardial adaptation to ischemia. The positive controls for canonical HIF-1α-sensitive genes are endothelin (Edn1) and vascular endothelial growth factor (Vegfa).

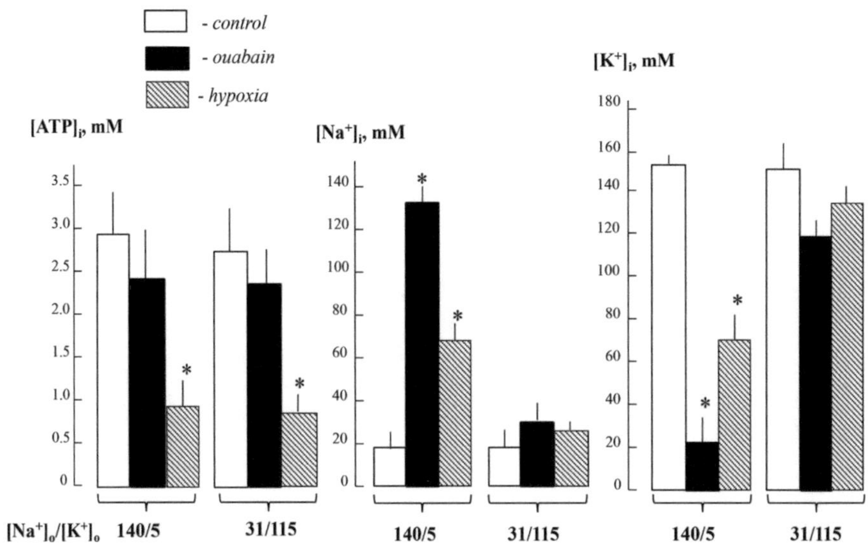

Figure 3. Effect of ouabain and hypoxia on intracellular Na$^+$, K$^+$ and ATP concentrations in VSMC from the rat aorta. Cells were exposed to normal oxygen partial pressure (5% CO_2/air—control) ±3 μM ouabain or exposure to hypoxia (5% CO_2/95% N_2)/glucose deprivation for 24 h in normal high-Na$^+$, low-K$^+$ ([Na$^+$]/[K$^+$] = 140/5) or in low-Na$^+$, high-K$^+$ DMEM-like medium ([Na$^+$]/[K$^+$] = 131/115). Intracellular K$^+$ and Na$^+$ Cl$^-$ content was measured as the steady-state distribution of extra- and intracellular ^{86}Rb and ^{22}Na, respectively. Intracellular ATP content was measured by assaying luciferase-dependent luminescence with ATP bioluminescent assay kit. Means ± S.E. from three independent experiments performed in quadruplicate are shown. *$p < 0.05$ compared to the controls. Adopted with permission from [57].

To assess the role of [Na$^+$]$_i$/[K$^+$]$_i$-dependent and HIF-1α-mediated signaling, we compared expression of the above-listed selected genes in hypoxic conditions and under the action of ouabain in control high-Na$^+$, low-K$^+$ medium and in high-K$^+$, low-Na$^+$ medium with dissipated transmembrane gradients of monovalent cations and after cells transfection with Hif-1a siRNA

[57]. As demonstrated in other cell types [65, 66], hypoxia slightly enhanced Hif-1a mRNA (**Figure 4**) but increased immunoreactive HIF-1α protein content by ~fivefold (**Figure 5**).

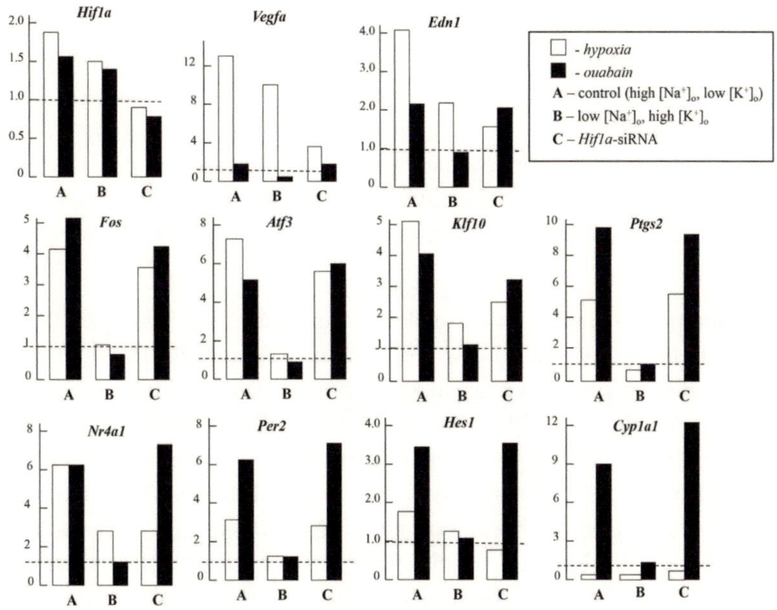

Figure 4. Effect of hypoxia and ouabain on gene expression in VSMC from the rat aorta. Cells were incubated for 24 h under normoxia, hypoxia/glucose deprivation or 3 mM ouabain in control high-Na^+, low-K^+ medium (A, C), or high-K^+, low-Na^+ medium (B). In some experiments, RASMC were transfected with Hif-1α siRNA (C). The content of mRNA in normoxia was taken as 1.00 and shown as broken lines. Adopted with permission from [57].

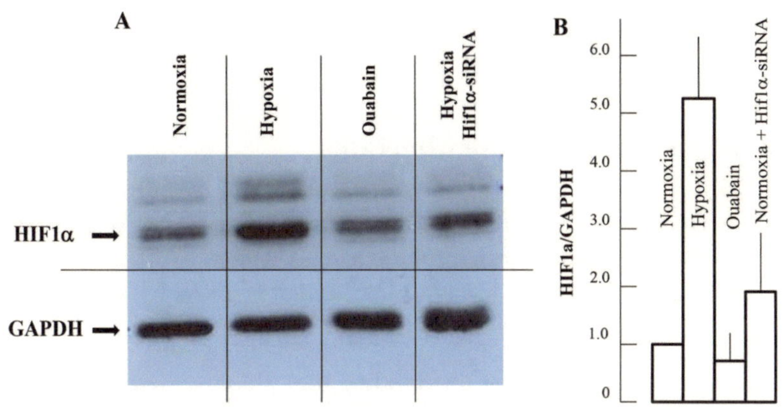

Figure 5. (A). Representative Western blots of GAPDH and HIF-1α in VSMC incubated for 24 h under control conditions (normoxia), hypoxia/glucose deprivation, 3 mM ouabain or hypoxia/glucose deprivation in cells transfected with Hif-1α siRNA. (B). Hypoxia/glucose deprivation and ouabain influence on HIF-1α protein relative content in RASMC. The HIF-1α/GAPDH ratio in control conditions was taken as 1.00. Data obtained in three independent experiments are reported as means ± S.E. Adopted with permission from [57].

Transfection of rat VSMC with Hif-1α siRNA but not with scrambled siRNA led to ~threefold expression reduction in Hif-1a and lowered hypoxia-induced HIF-1a protein gain (**Figure 5**). Pretreatment with ouabain slightly changed HIF-1α protein content (**Figure 5**) and amplified baseline Hif-1a mRNA by ~50% (**Figure 4**). Hypoxia causes fourfold and 12-fold increase in Edn1 and Vegfa mRNA content, respectively, (**Figure 4**), which is consistent with earlier observations [19]. Hypoxia-dependent increase in Edn1 and Vegfa mRNA was attenuated after transfection with Hif-1a siRNA by ~twofold and fourfold, respectively. At the same time, ouabain augmented Edn1 mRNA by 2.5-fold but did not significantly impair Vegfa. Similarly, low-Na^+, high-K^+ medium that is characterized with dissipation of the transmembrane gradients of monovalent cations also did not affect hypoxia-induced expression of Vegfa and reduced Edn1 mRNA by twofold. All these data strongly support the efficacy of Hif1α-siRNA function [57].

In hypoxic conditions, dissipation of monovalent cations transmembrane gradients completely suppressed increments in Fos, Atf3, Ptgs2 and Per2 mRNA and diminished increase in Klf10, Edn1, Nr4a1 and Hes1 expression (**Figure 4**). Hypoxia caused from twofold to sixfold augmentation of Atf3, Fos, Ptgs2, Klf10, Nr4a2, Hes1 and Per2 expression (**Figure 4**). These data 17 are consistent with the observations obtained in other cell types, including human VSMC [67, 68]. Transfection with Hif-1a siRNA led to twofold attenuation of hypoxia-induced increase in Nr4a and Klf10 mRNA without significant influence on expression of Fos, Atf3, Ptgs2 and Per2 evoked by hypoxia. At the same time, hypoxic conditions led to twofold decrease in Cyp1a1 mRNA and attenuated expression of Cyp1a1 obtained from human microvasculature [69]. Ouabain enhanced the expression of all eight tested genes from threefold to 10-fold that were completely abolished in low-Na^+, high-K^+ medium characterized with dissipation of the transmembrane gradients of monovalent cations [57]. However, in ouabain-treated RASMC, the expression of these genes was not affected by transfection with Hif-1a siRNA, but decrease in monovalent cations transmembrane gradient sharply decreased elevation of Edn1, Klf10, Hes1 and Nr4a1 expression seen in hypoxic conditions and completely abolished increase in Atf3, Fos, Ptgs2 and Per2 mRNA (**Figure 4**).

6. Unresolved issues and future directions

Viewed collectively, our results demonstrate a key role of $[Na^+]_i/[K^+]_i$-mediated excitation-transcription coupling in overall transcriptomic changes triggered by sustained ischemia. The molecular organization of sensors for monovalent cation is still unclear in contrast to rapid progress in the identification of Ca_i^{2+} sensors. Initially, such sensors were identified in parvalbumin and calmodulin. These high-affinity binding sites (the so-called EF-hand domains) are formed by a highly conservative linear amino acid sequence consisting of 14 amino acid residues. Further screening of cDNA libraries allowed to identify more than 30 other Ca_i^{2+} [70]. Moreover, high-affinity sensors for Na_i^+ are almost completely saturated at $[Ca^{2+}]_i$ of 1 μM. This allows identifying amino acid residues using ^{45}Ca binding assay. In contrast, molecular sensors for monovalent ion may be presented by 3D protein structures formed with space-separated amino acid residues [27, 71]. Besides this, cellular functions are affected by monovalent cations when they act in the millimolar concentrations that make their detection with radioisotopes more complicate. As it was shown by Ono and coworkers, Na^+ may interact with calpain Ca^{2+}-binding sites at the baseline level of $[Ca^{2+}]_i$ (~100 nM). Thus, calpain functions as Ca_i^{2+}-dependent protease with $K_{0.5}$ of 15 mM for Na^+ [72]. Additional experiments should be performed to examine the role of Ca^{2+}-binding proteins as $[Na^+]_i$ sensors involved in cellular responses evoked by hypoxia.

It is generally accepted that transcription is under the control of proteins interacting with specific response elements within 5′- and 3′-untranslated region (UTR). Considering this, we tried to find Na^+ response element (NaRE) within c-Fos promoter. With the CRE and all other known c-Fos promoter transcription elements, we observed massive accumulation of endogenous c-Fos mRNA and immunoreactive protein in HeLa cells subjected to 6-h inhibition of Na^+, K^+-ATPase, but we did not find any significant increase in luciferase expression in ouabain-treated HeLa cells [33]. Negative results obtained in this study may be explained by the following hypotheses: (i) NaRE is located within the c-Fos 3′-UTR and/or introns. (ii) Elevation of $[Na^+]_i/[K^+]_i$ ratio influences on gene expression through epigenetic modification of regulatory mechanism having a significant impact on various cellular functions, such the DNA, histones or nucleosome remodeling [73]. Importantly, the epigenetic mechanism of gene expression does not contribute to the regulation of L-luc transcription in the plasmid employed in our experiments [33]. (iii) More evidence indicates that gene activation or silencing is under the complex control of three-dimensional (3D) positioning of genetic materials and chromatin in the nuclear space (for review, see [74]). It may be proposed that gene transcription is affected by increased $[Na^+]_i/[K^+]_i$ ratio through changing of the 3D organization of DNA-chromatin complex. These hypotheses will be verified in forthcoming studies.

Some studies have shown that epigenetic modulatory mechanism of histone methylation is a key process that helps cells to adapt to hypoxia [75]. Growing evidence shows that along with the 5′-UTR regulation by transcription factors, gene activation or silencing is controlled by 3D positioning of genetic materials and chromatin in nuclear spaces [74, 76]. The epigenetic regulation of 3D genome organization with considering the $[Na^+]_i/[K^+]_i$ ratio and its role in gene silencing and activation is currently being examined in our laboratory.

Matrix metalloproteinases play an important role in pathophysiology of hypoxic chronic venous disease via their implication in the regulation of migration, proliferation and endothelium-dependent VSMC contraction [77]. We found that sustained elevation of the $[Na^+]_i/[K^+]_i$ ratio resulted in ~fivefold elevation of Mmp28 metalloproteinase expression in rat VSMC [57]. The same procedure resulted in sevenfold elevation of the content of Nccp mRNA encoding natriuretic peptide precursor C [57]. NCCP is proteolytically processed to C-type natriuretic peptide (CNP), i.e., a selective agonist for the B-type natriuretic receptor whose role in cGMP-mediated vasorelaxation is well documented. We noted that in endothelial cells, modest long-term inhibition of the Na^+,K^+-ATPse causes ~sevenfold attenuation of expression of Edn encoding preproendothelin-1 that is proteolytically processed to the most powerful endothelium-derived vasoconstrictor endothelin-1. We also observed ~10-fold elevation of the content of mRNA encoding ubiquitously derived vasodilator adrenomedullin (unpublished results). Do these $[Na^+]_i/[K^+]_i$-mediated transcriptomic changes contribute to the pathophysiology of hypoxic vascular disorders? Does partial dissipation of electrochemical gradients of monovalent cations seen in VSMC subjected to ischemia and glucose deprivation have an impact on the distinct regulation of systemic and pulmonary circulation under hypoxic conditions? We will address these questions to forthcoming studies.

Acknowledgements

This work was supported by Grants from the Russian Foundation for Basic Research #15-04-00101 and the Russian Science Foundation #14-15-00006 and #16-15-10026.

Author details

Sergei N. Orlov[1,2*], Yulia G. Birulina[1], Liudmila V. Smaglii[1] and Svetlana V. Gusakova[1]

*Address all correspondence to: sergei.n.orlov@yandex.ru

1 Siberian State Medical University, Tomsk, Russia

2 MV Lomonosov Moscow State University, Moscow, Russia

References

[1] Ellsworth ML, Ellis CG, Goldman D, Stephenson AH, Dietrich HH, Sprague RS. Erythrocytes: oxygen sensors and modulators of vascular tone. Physiology. 2008; 24: 107–116.

[2] Ralevic V, Dunn WR. Purinergic transmission in blood vessels. Auton Neurosci Basic Clin. 2015; 191: 48–66.

[3] Luneva OG, Sidorenko SV, Maksimov GV, Grygorczyk R, Orlov SN. Erythrocytes as regulators of blood vessel tone. Biochem (Moscow) Suppl Ser A Membr Cell Biol. 2015; 9: 161–171.

[4] Guan Y, Li N, Tian Y-M, Zhang L, Ma H-L, Maslov LN, et al. Chronic intermittent hypobaric hypoxia antagonizes renal vascular hypertension by enhancement of vasorelaxation via activating of BKCa. Life Sci. 2016; 157: 74–81.

[5] Sylvester JT, Shimoda LA, Aaronson PI, Ward JP. Hypoxic pulmonary vasoconstriction. Physiol Rev. 2012; 92: 367–520.

[6] Koltsova SV, Trushina Y, Haloui M, Akimova OA, Tremblay J, Hamet P, Orlov SN. Ubiquitous $[Na^+]_i/[K^+]_i$-sensitive transcriptome in mammalian cells: evidence for Nai+,Ki+-independent excitation-transcription coupling. PLoS One. 2012; 7: e38032.

[7] Taurin S, Seyrantepe V, Orlov SN, Tremblay T-L, Thibaut P, Bennett MR, et al. Proteome analysis and functional expression identify mortalin as an anti-apoptotic gene induced by elevation of $[Na^+]_i/[K^+]_i$ ratio in cultured vascular smooth muscle cells. Circ Res. 2002; 91: 915–922.

[8] Veith C, Schermuly RT, Brandes RP, Weissmann N. Molecular mechanisms of hypoxia-inducible factor-induced pulmonary arterial smooth muscle cell alterations in pulmonary hypertension. J Physiol. 2016; 594: 1167–1177.

[9] Sprague RS, Stephenson AH, Ellsworth ML, Keller C, Lonigro AJ. Impaired release of ATP from red blood cells of humans with primary pulmonary hypertension. Exp Biol Med. 2001; 226: 434–439.

[10] Mazzatti D, Lim F-L, O'Hara A, Wood IS, Trayhurn P. A microarray analysis of the hypoxia-induced modulation of gene expression in human adipocytes. Arch Physiol Biochem. 2012; 118: 112–120.

[11] Lu A, Tang Y, Ran R, Clark JF, Aronow BJ, Sharp FR. Genomics of the periinfarction cortex after focal cerebral ischemia. J Cereb Blood Flow Metab. 2003; 23: 786–810.

[12] Kamphuis W, Dijk F, van Soest S, Bergen AAB. Global gene expression profiling of ischemic preconditioning in the rat retina. Mol Vision. 2007; 13: 1020–1030.

[13] Tang Y, Pacary E, Freret T, Divoux D, Petit E, Schumann-Bard P, Bernaudin M. Effect of hypoxic preconditioning on brain genomic response before and following ischemia in the adult mouse: identification of potential neuroprotective candidate for stroke. Neurobiol Dis. 2006; 21: 18–28.

[14] Ong LL, Oldigs JK, Kaminski A, Gerstmayer B, Piechaczek C, Wagner W, et al. Hypoxic/normoxic preconditioning increases endothelial differentiation potential of human bone marrow CD133+ cells. Tissue End Part C Methods. 2010; 16: 1069–1081.

[15] Manalo DJ, Rowan S, Lavoie T, Natarajan L, Kelly BD, Ye SQ, et al. Transcription regulation of vascular endothelial cell responses to hypoxia by HIF-1. Blood. 2005; 105: 659–669.

[16] Leonard MO, Cottell DC, Godson C, Brady HR, Taylor CT. The role of HIF-1a in transcriptional regulation of the proximal tubular epithelial cell response to hypoxia. J Biol Chem. 2003; 278: 40296–40304.

[17] Forsythe JA, Jiang BH, Iber NV, Agani F, leung SW, Koos RD, Semenza GL. Activation of vascular endothelial growth factor gene transcription by hypoxia-inducible factor 1. Mol Cell Biol. 1996; 16: 4604–4613.

[18] Maxwell PH, Wiesener MS, Chang GW, Clifford SC, Vaux EC, Cockman ME, et al. The tumor suppressor protein VHL targets hypoxia-inducible factor for oxygen-dependent proteolysis. Nature. 1999; 399: 271–275.

[19] Kallio PJ, Pongratz I, Gradin K, McGuire J, Poellinger L. Activation of hypoxia-inducible factor 1a: posttranslational regulation and conformational change by recruitment of the Arnt transcription factor. Proc Natl Acad Sci USA. 1997; 94: 5667–5672.

[20] Semenza GL, Jiang BH, leung SW, Passantino R, Concordet JP, Maire P, Giallongo A. Hypoxia response elements in the aldolase A, enolase 1, and lactate dehydrogenase A gene promoters contain essential binding sites for hypoxia-inducible factor 1. J Biol Chem. 1996; 271: 32529–32537.

[21] Sharp FR, Ran R, Lu A, Tang Y, Strauss KI, Glass T, et al. Hypoxic preconditioning protects against ischemic brain injury. NeuroEx. 2004; 1: 26–35.

[22] Shimoda LA, Manalo DJ, Sham JS, Semenza GL, Sylvester JT. Partial HIF-1a deficiency impairs pulmonary arterial myocyte electrophysiological responses to hypoxia. Am J Physiol Lung Cell Mol Physiol. 2001; 291: L202–L208.

[23] Kahn BB, Alquier T, Carling D, Hardie DG. AMP-activated protein kinase: ancient energy gauge provides clues to modern understanding of metabolism. Cell Metab. 2005; 1: 15–25.

[24] Evans AM, Lewis SA, Ogunbayo OA, Moral-Sanz J. Modulation of the LKB1-AMPK signaling pathways underpins hypoxic pulmonary vasoconstriction and pulmonary hypertension. Adv Exp Med Biol. 2015; 860: 88–99.

[25] Williams RS, Benjamin IJ. Protective responses in the ischemic myocardium. J Clin Invest. 2000; 106: 813–818.

[26] Coulon V, Blanchard J-M. Flux calciques et expression gйnigue. Mйdicine Sciences. 2001; 17: 969–978.

[27] Murphy E, Eisner DA. Regulation of intracellular and mitochondrial sodium in health and disease. Circ Res. 2009; 104: 292–303.

[28] Orlov SN, Hamet P. Salt and gene expression: evidence for Na_i+,K_i+-mediated signaling pathways. Pflugers Arch Eur J Physiol. 2015; 467: 489–498.

[29] Orlov SN, Thorin-Trescases N, Kotelevtsev SV, Tremblay J, Hamet P. Inversion of the intracellular Na^+/K^+ ratio blocks apoptosis in vascular smooth muscle at a site upstream of caspase-3. J Biol Chem. 1999; 274: 16545–16552.

[30] Orlov SN, Taurin S, Thorin-Trescases N, Dulin NO, Tremblay J, Hamet P. Inversion of the intracellular Na^+/K^+ ratio blocks apoptosis in vascular smooth muscle cells by induction of RNA synthesis. Hypertension. 2000; 35: 1062–1068.

[31] Orlov SN, Taurin S, Tremblay J, Hamet P. Inhibition of Na^+,K^+ pump affects nucleic acid synthesis and smooth muscle cell proliferation via elevation of the $[Na^+]_i/[K^+]_i$ ratio: possible implication in vascular remodeling. J Hypertens. 2001; 19: 1559–1565.

[32] Taurin S, Dulin NO, Pchejetski D, Grygorczyk R, Tremblay J, Hamet P, Orlov SN. c-Fos expression in ouabain-treated vascular smooth muscle cells from rat aorta: evidence for an intracellular-sodium-mediated, calcium-independent mechanism. J Physiol. 2002; 543: 835–847.

[33] Haloui M, Taurin S, Akimova OA, Guo D-F, Tremblay J, Dulin NO, et al. Nai+-induced c-Fos expression is not mediated by activation of the 5'-promoter containing known transcriptional elements. FEBS J. 2007; 274: 3257–3267.

[34] Aperia A. New roles for an old Na,K-ATPase emerges as an interesting drug target. J Intern Med. 2007; 261: 44–52.

[35] Schoner W, Scheiner-Bobis G. Endogenous and exogenous cardiac glycosides: their role in hypertension, salt metabolism, and cell growth. Am J Physiol Cell Physiol. 2007; 293: C509–C536.

[36] Liu J, Xie Z. The sodium pump and cardiotonic steroids-induced signal transduction protein kinases and calcium-signaling microdomain in regulation of transporter trafficking. Biochim Biophys Acta. 2010; 1802: 1237–1245.

[37] Tupler R, Perini G, Green MR. Expressing the human genome. Nature. 2001; 409: 832–833.

[38] Santana LF. NFAT-dependent excitation-transcription coupling in heart. Circ Res. 2008; 103: 681–683.

[39] McDonald TF, Pelzer S, Trautwein W, Pelzer DJ. Regulation and modulation of calcium channels in cardiac, skeletal, and smooth muscle cells. Physiol Rev. 1994; 74: 365–512.

[40] Hardingham GE, Chawla S, Johnson CM, Bading H. Distinct functions of nuclear and cytoplasmic calcium in the control of gene expression. Nature. 1997; 385: 260–265.

[41] Orlov SN, Aksentsev SL, Kotelevtsev SV. Extracellular calcium is required for the maintenance of plasma membrane integrity in nucleated cells. Cell Calcium. 2005; 38: 53–57.

[42] Martell AE, Smith RM. Critical stability constants. 1974. New York, Plenum Press.

[43] Bartfai T. Preparation of metal-chelate complexes and the design of steady-state kinetic experiments involving metal nucleotide complexes. Adv Cyclic Nucl Res. 1979; 10: 219–242.

[44] Orlov SN, Grygorczyk R, Kotelevtsev SV. Do we know the absolute values of intracellular free calcium concentration? Cell Calcium. 2003; 34: 511–515.

[45] Matt T, Martinez-Yamout MA, Dyson HJ, Wright PE. The CBP/p300 XAZ1 domain in its native state is not a binding partner of MDM2. Biochem J. 2004; 381: 685–691.

[46] Emerson RO, Thomas JH. Adaptive evolution in zinc finger transcription factors. PLoS Genetics. 2009; 5: e1000325.

[47] Koltsova SV, Tremblay J, Hamet P, Orlov SN. Transcriptomic changes in Ca^{2+}-depleted cells: role of elevated intracellular $[Na^+]/[K^+]$ ratio. Cell Calcium. 2015; 58: 317–324.

[48] Beck H, Semisch M, Culmsee C, Plesnila N, Hatzopoulos AK. Egr-1 regulates expression of the glial scar component phosphacan in astrocytes after experimental stroke. Am J Pathol. 2008; 173: 77–92.

[49] Suzuki S, Tanaka K, Nogawa S, Nagata E, Ito D, Dembo T, Fukuuchi Y. Temporal profile and cellular localization of interleukin-6 protein after focal cerebral ischemia in rats. J Cereb Blood Flow Metab. 1999; 19: 1256–1262.

[50] Yuen PST, Jo S-K, Holly MK, Hu X, Star RA. Ischemic and nephrotoxic acute renal failure are distinguished by their broad transcriptomic responses. Physiol Genomics. 2006; 25: 375–386.

[51] Li HF, Cheng CF, Liao WJ, Lin H, Yang RB. ATF3-mediated epigenetic regulation protects against acute kidney injury. J Am Soc Nephrol. 2010; 21: 1003–1013.

[52] Kobayashi T, Terada Y, Kuwana H, Tanaka H, Okada T, Kuwahara M, et al. Expression and function of the Delta-1/NOtch-2/Hes-1 pathway during experimental acute kidney injury. Kidney Int. 2008; 73: 1240–1250.

[53] Bolli R, Shinmura K, Tang XL, Kodani E, Xuan YT, Guo Y, Dawn B. Discovery of a new function of cyclooxygenase (COX)-2: COX-2 is a cardioprotective protein that alleviates ischemia/reperfusion injury and mediates the late phase of cardioprotection. Cardiovasc Res. 2002; 15: 506–519.

[54] Corss AK, Haddock G, Stock CJ, Allan S, surr J, Bunning BR, et al. ADAMTS-1 and -4 are up-regulated following transient middle cerebral artery occlusion in the rat and their expression is modulated by TNF in cultured astrocytes. Brain Res. 2006; 1088: 19–30.

[55] Cheng O, Ostrowski RP, Wu B, Liu W, Chen C, Zhang JH. Cyclooxygenase-2 mediates hyperbaric oxygen preconditioning in the rat model of transient global cerebral ischemia. Stroke. 2011; 42: 484–490.

[56] Wood IS, Perez de Heredia F, Wang B, Trayhurn P. Cellular hypoxia and adipose tissue dysfunction in obesity. Proc Nutr Soc. 2009; 68: 370–377.

[57] Koltsova SV, Shilov B, Birulina JG, Akimova OA, Haloui M, Kapilevich LV, et al. Transcriptomic changes triggered by hypoxia: evidence for HIF-1a -independent, $[Na^+]_i/[K^+]_i$-mediated excitation-transcription coupling. PLoS One. 2014; 9: e110597.

[58] Cummins EP, Taylor CT. Hypoxia-responsive transcription factors. Pfluger Arch Eur J Physiol. 2005; 450: 363–371.

[59] Yang DH, Hsu CF, Lin CY, Guo JY, Yu WC, Chang VH. Kruppel-like factor 10 upregulates the expression of cyclooxygenase 1 and further modulates angiogenesis in endothelial cell and platelet aggregation in gene-deficient mice. Int J Biochem Cell Biol. 2013; 45: 419–428.

[60] Phillis JW, Horrocks LA, Farooqui AA. Cyclooxygenases, lipoxygenases, and epoxygenases in CNS: their role and involvement in neurological disorders. Brain Res. 2006; 52: 201–243.

[61] Kim B-J, Kim H, Cho E-J, Youn H-D. Nur77 upregulates HIF-a by inhibiting pVHL-mediated degradation. Exp Mol Med. 2008; 40: 71–83.

[62] Hamet P, Tremblay J. Genetics of the sleep-wake cycle and its disorders. Metabolism Clin Exp. 2006; 55: S7–S12.

[63] Koyanagi S, Kuramoto Y, Nakagawa H, Aramaki H, Ohdo S, Soeda S, Shimeno H. A molecular mechanism regulating circadian expression of vascular endothelial growth factor in tumor cells. Cancer Res. 2003; 63: 7277–7283.

[64] Eckle T, Hartmann K, Bonney S, Reithel S, Mittelbronn M, Walker LA, et al. Adora2b-elicited Per2 stabilization promotes a HIF-dependent metabolic switch critical for myocardial adaptation to ischemia. Nature Med. 2012; 18: 774–782.

[65] Ke Q, Costa M. Hypoxia-inducible factor-1 (HIF-1). Mol Pharmacol. 2006; 70: 1469–1480.

[66] Zhang H, Qian DZ, Tan YS, Lee K, Gao P, Ren YR, et al. Digoxin and other cardiac glycosides inhibit HIF-1a synthesis and block tumor growth. Proc Natl Acad Sci USA. 2008; 105: 19579–19586.

[67] Zuloaga KL, Gonzales RJ. Dihydrotestosterone attenuates hypoxia inducible factor-1a and cycloxygenase-2 in cerebral arteries during hypoxia with glucose deprivation. Am J Physiol Heart Circ Physiol. 2011; 301: H1882–H1890.

[68] Camacho M, Rodriguez C, Guadall A, Alcolea S, Orriols M, Escudero J-R, et al. Hypoxia upregulates PGI-synthase and increases PGI2 release in human vascular cells exposed to inflammatory stimuli. J Lipid Res. 2011; 52: 720–731.

[69] Zhang N, Walker MK. Crosstalk between the aryl hydrocarbon receptor and hypoxia on the constitutive expression of cytochrome P4501A1 mRNA. Cardiovasc Toxicol. 2007; 7: 282–290.

[70] Heizmann CW, Hunziker W. Intracellular calcium-binding proteins: more sites than insights. TiBS. 1991; 16: 98–103.

[71] Orlov SN, Hamet P. Intracellular monovalent ions as second messengers. J Membr Biol. 2006; 210: 161–172.

[72] Ono Y, Ojimam K, Torii F, Takaya E, Doi N, Nakagawa K, et al. Skeletal muscle-specific calpain is an intracellular Na^+-dependent protease. J Biol Chem. 2010; 285: 22986–22998.

[73] Graff J, Kim D, Dobbin MM, Tsai L-H. Epigenetic regulation of gene expression in physiological and pathological brain processes. Physiol Rev. 2011; 91: 603–649.

[74] Lanctot C, Cheutin T, Cremer M, Cavalli G, Cremer T. Dynamic genome architecture in the nuclear space: regulation of gene expression in three dimensions. Nature Rev Genet. 2007; 8: 104–115.

[75] Johnson AB, Denko N, Barton MC. Hypoxia induces a novel signature of chromatin modifications and global repression of transcription. Mutat Res. 2008; 640: 174–179.

[76] Gibcus JH, Dekker J. The hierarchy of the 3D genome. Mol Cell. 2013; 49: 773–782.

[77] MacColl E, Khalil RA. Matrix metalloproteinases as regulator of vein structure and function: implications in chronic venous disease. J Pharmacol Exp Ther. 2015; 355: 410–420.

Chapter 5

Hypoxia in Mesenchymal Stem Cell

Wahyu Widowati, Dwi Davidson Rihibiha,
Khie Khiong, M. Aris Widodo,
Sutiman B. Sumitro and Indra Bachtiar

Additional information is available at the end of the chapter

http://dx.doi.org/10.5772/65510

Abstract

Mesenchymal stem cells (MSCs) are non-hematopoietic multipotent stem cells with self-renewal properties and ability to differentiate into a variety of mesenchymal tissues. This chapter overviews effects of hypoxia on MSCs, makes it promising therapy to various diseases. Cultivation of MSCs under hypoxic condition results in variety of outcome that is important to be noted in clinical use. In most studies, hypoxic condition appears to increase proliferation, differentiation, and immune regulatory performance of MSCs without affecting its characteristic. Those benefits are therefore utilized in clinical application. However, there are also studies that report on negative effects of hypoxia in MSCs such as chromosomal instability. Molecular mechanism of MSCs in hypoxic condition is provided for better understanding, which is crucial for further development with better outcome.

Keywords: mesenchymal stem cells, hypoxia

1. Introduction

In these days, stem cell therapy is becoming more believable in treating degenerative diseases compared to conventional medicine. Various diseases such as diabetes, myocardial infarction, spinal cord injury, stroke, and Parkinson's and Alzheimer's diseases have become more prevalent with increasing life expectancy. It has been estimated that in the United States alone, ~128 million individuals would benefit from regenerative stem cell therapy during their lifetime. Mesenchymal stem cells (MSCs) have been highly utilized to treat degenerative diseases among other stem cells. These cells are found in tissues such as bone marrow, adipose tissue, umbilical cord, and dental pulp. Self-renewal and multipotency are the key features of MSCs that make it promising tool. These properties have raised interest on researchers for finding appropriate method to optimize the genetic and environmental factors, which later enhance the biological activities of MSCs.

Many researches have been conducted in the last two decades to study the complex processes in stem cell maintenance. The role of hypoxic conditions (usually 2–9% O_2 concentration) on stem cell biology is very interesting subject due to its beneficial effects. Thus, cultivation of MSCs under hypoxia is currently studied to obtain better understanding, as well as further development to generate better outcome.

2. Mesenchymal stem cell

About 130 years ago, German pathologist Conheim proposed the presence of non-hematopoietic stem cells in the bone marrow that contributes to wound healing in numerous peripheral tissues. Later in the early 1970s, Friedenstein and colleagues demonstrated that the rodent bone marrow had fibroblastoid cells with clonogenic potential *in vitro* [1, 2]. In the study, after the non-adherent cells were removed a few hours later, spindle-like cells, which were morphologically heterogeneous, appeared to attach to the plastic, capable of forming colonies. These cells could also make bone and reconstitute a hematopoietic microenvironment in subcutaneous transplants. Moreover, they could regenerate heterotopic bone tissue in serial transplants, thus indicated their self-renewal potential. Over the years, many studies have investigated these findings and found that these cells were also present in the human bone marrow and could be sub-passaged and differentiated *in vitro* into a variety of the mesenchymal lineages such as osteoblasts, chondrocytes, adipocytes, and myoblasts [3–7]. It has been further renamed as "mesenchymal stem cell" or MSC [4].

MSCs or MSC-like cells are also found in fat, umbilical cord blood, amniotic fluid, placenta, dental pulp, tendons, synovial membrane, and skeletal muscle, yet the complete equivalency of such populations remains unclear [8–16]. Characteristic of MSCs according to The International Society for Cell Therapy [17] consists of (1) adherence to plastic in standard culture conditions; (2) expression of the surface molecules CD73, CD90, and CD105 in the absence of CD34, CD45, HLA-DR, CD14 or CD11b, CD79a, or CD19 surface molecules; and (3) a capacity for differentiation to osteoblasts, adipocytes, and chondroblasts *in vitro*. These criteria were established to standardize human MSC isolation but may not apply uniformly to other species. For instance, marker expression and behavior in murine MSCs were different compared to human MSCs [18]. Certain *in vivo* surface markers may no longer be expressed after Transplantation, although new markers are obtained during expansion. In study done by Jones et al., MSC uniformly expressed HLA-DR (a marker that should not be expressed on MSCs by the above definition) while also expressing CD90 and CD105, adhering to plastic in culture, and differentiating into osteoblasts, adipocytes, and chondroblasts [19]. Indeed, clear definition of MSC-specific characteristics is difficult to apply in both human and animal models.

http://dx.doi.org/10.5772/65510

3. Hypoxia in mesenchymal stem cell

Numerous *in vitro* studies have been conducted in the last two decades to observe the complex processes in stem cell maintenance. However, the role of physiologically hypoxic conditions (usually 2–9% O_2 concentration) on stem cell biology received very little attention. O_2 concentration is an environmental factor that plays a vital role on stem cell fate and function [20]. Stem cells are typically cultured under the ambient O_2 concentration without paying attention to the metabolic milieu of the niche in which they normally grow [21]. The effects of different O_2 levels in MSC culture were first studied in 1958, when Cooper et al. and Zwartouw and Westwood observed that some cells proliferated more rapidly under low O_2 tension levels compared to normal atmospheric levels [22, 23]. MSCs are present in perivascular niches in close association with blood vessels in virtually all tissues [11, 16, 24] and have been compared to pericytes [25]. Even though MSCs are located close to vascular structures, the different tissues where these stem cells are found exhibit low oxygen tensions [26–29]. Therefore, it is possible that maintaining MSCs in an undifferentiated state may require a hypoxic environment, in addition to other factors.

The higher O_2 concentration might cause environmental stress to the *in vitro* cultured MSCs. Recent studies have presented significant evidences regarding the negative outcome under ambient O_2 concentration on MSCs, including early senescence, longer population doubling (PD) time, DNA damage [30, 31], and poor engraftment following transplantation [32, 33]. These have shown the influential effect of O_2 concentration on MSCs biology and raised serious concern over its therapeutic efficiency and biosafety. Thus, the effect of different O_2 concentration on MSCs biology is further discussed based on recent research outcomes.

4. Characteristic of MSCs in hypoxic condition

As described above, MSC immunophenotype is characterized by the expression of CD73, CD90, CD105, CD106, CD146, and MHC class I molecules, and the absence of markers such as CD45 and CD34 or MHC class II molecules [17]. Many studies suggest that hypoxia has no effect on MSCs characteristic, indicated by surface markers. According to one study by Holzwarth et al., there were no significant differences in the expression of cell surface markers after 14 days of culture at 1% when compared to 20% of O_2 [34]. Referring to study carried out by Nekanti et al., WJ-MSCs cultured under both hypoxia and normoxia for 10 passages were positive for CD44, CD73, CD90, CD105, and CD166 and negative for CD34, CD45, and HLA-DR, and there was no significant difference between the two populations [35]. These results are also supported by study carried out by Widowati et al. The surface marker of WJ-MSCs of P4 and P8 both normoxic and hypoxic 5% O_2 were not significantly different. WJ-MSCs were positive for CD105, CD73, and CD90 and negative for CD34, CD45, CD14, CD19, and HLA-II [36].

Morphology changes are also documented in MSCs under hypoxia. Referring to Nekanti et al., WJ-MSC cultured under hypoxia showed a higher amount of large, flattened cells both at early and late passages, compared to normoxic cultures. The enlargement in cell size under hypoxia might be due to a natural response to low oxygen, in which increased surface area would allow for an increase in oxygen diffusion rate [35].

5. MSCs proliferation in hypoxic condition

Capability for self-renewal is a key feature of stem cells. An increased proliferation rate is necessary for more efficient use of stem cells in regenerative therapies. Fehrer et al. demonstrated that bone marrow-derived MSCs (BM-MSCs) cultured in 3% O_2 concentration showed significant increased *in vitro* proliferative lifespan, with ~10 additional population doublings (PDs) (28.5 ± 3.8 PD in 20% O_2 and 37.5 ± 3.4 PD in 3% O_2) before reaching senescence compared to cells cultured in the ambient O_2 environment [31]. In addition, early passaged MSCs cultured in hypoxic conditions also exhibit increased proliferative lifespan along with significant difference in population doubling [30]. Furthermore, it is possible to harvest more than 1×10^9 MSCs from the first five passages cultured in 3% O_2, whereas in ambient condition only 2×10^7 cells can be obtained [30]. Higher *in vitro* expansion rate in hypoxic conditions has also been reported by other researchers [37–39]. Such *in vitro* culture environment also allows to maintain a higher proportion of rapidly self-renewing MSCs for a longer period of time [40]. Other study showed that the increased hypoxic (O_2 2.5%) condition was the best microenvironment for stem cell proliferation compared to normoxic and hypoxic (O_2 5%) for cells at a high passage (P7, P8) [41].

However, various responses of stem cells under hypoxia have been reported [42]. Those differences in cellular responses on hypoxia might be associated with degrees and durations of hypoxia, as well as other cell conditions. Oxygen tension in the stem cell niche for MSCs is suggested to be various from 1 to 7% [43]. A study by Holzwarth et al. showed that rates of MSCs proliferation were reduced after 7 days of culture under hypoxia at 21, 5, 3, and 1% O_2. In their study, only 1.37% of the cells entered the G2/M phase in hypoxic cultures (1% O_2) after 7 days, compared to 2.50% at hyperoxic culture (21% O_2). Reduced O_2 concentrations were therefore confirmed to inhibit cell proliferation as indicated by reduced number of cells in the G2/M phase [34].

6. Chromosomal stability of MSCs in hypoxic condition

Some recent studies have found that human mesenchymal stem cells (hMSCs) retained chromosomal stability following long-term culture *in vitro* [44–46]. Hypoxic environments have shown to increase mutation frequencies in cancer cell lines and trigger genomic rearrangements [47, 48]. It is suggested that oxygen concentration has a major impact on karyotypic aberration. Referring to study of Ueyama et al., chromosomal instability is associated with repeated cell division. A high frequency of chromosomal abnormality breakpoints in common fragile sites (CFSs) was detected by karyotypic analysis (e.g., 2q33, 7q11, 7q36, 8q22.1, 8q24.1,

11p15.1, 19q13) [49]. Generally, chromosomes have fragile sites that are prone to exhibiting gaps and breaks during metaphase [50], in which chromosome rearrangement occurs in cultured cells. Fragile sites are categorized into two main classes, common and rare, according to their frequency in the population [51]. In Ueyama study, several genes involved in regulation of the cell cycle, transcription and cell adhesion, are located in that region with a frequency of 6, 5, and 2%, respectively. In particular, the 11p15.5 domain known as an important tumor suppressor gene region such as tetraspanin 32 (TSPAN32) and tumor-suppressing subtransferable candidate 4 (TSSC4) is present in this region. Alterations in this region have been associated with some neoplasia. It is suggested that the deletion of contiguous genes may induce a multisystem developmental disorder and that these alterations might influence normal functioning and cell survival.

Sex chromosome aneuploidy was also one of the most observed aberrational karyotypes. Frequency of sex chromosome in cultured lymphocytes was significantly higher in females than in males, and that loss of Y chromosomes correlated with age in human bone marrow cells [52, 53]. There are several factors influencing karyotypic stability such as hypoxic culture conditions, donor age, and multiple passages. Karyotypic aberrations increased with passage number and hMSCs undergo spontaneous transformation with tumorigenic potential, especially in later passages under hypoxic culture conditions in hMSCs of elderly donors [49]. Shortly, monitoring of chromosomal stability in culture expanded hMSCs is required prior to exposure to human beings, in order to detect mutations and potentially immortalized clones and to prevent transplant-associated tumor formation.

7. MSCs plasticity in hypoxic condition

The multilineage potential of MSCs is one of the reasons underlying their use in regenerative medicine [54]. Results of MSC differentiation into other lineages diverse according to several studies [34, 55, 56]. Some *in vitro* studies have shown that cultures with low O_2 concentrations stimulated cells to differentiate into adipogenic, osteogenic, or chondrogenic cells. Previous study showed that Rat mesenchymal stem cells (rMSCs) cultured in 5% oxygen produced more bone than cells cultured in 20% O_2 throughout their cultivation time, as indicated by increased markers of osteogenesis, including alkaline phosphatase activity, calcium content, and von Kossa staining. These markers were usually elevated above basal levels when cells were switched from control to low oxygen at first passage and decreased for cells switched from low to control oxygen [57]. Hypoxia appears to exert a potent lipogenic effect independent of PPAR-γ2 maturation pathway [58]. The level of differentiated antigen H-2Dd and the number of G2/S/M phase cells increased evidently under 8% O_2 condition. Also, the proportion of wide, flattened, and epithelial-like cells increased significantly in MSCs. When cultured in adipogenic medium, there was a fivefold to sixfold increase in the number of lipid droplets under hypoxic conditions compared with that in normoxic culture. Oct4 was downregulated under 8% O_2 condition but still expressed after adipocyte differentiation in normoxic culture and treated with hypoxia-mimicking agents, cobalt chloride ($CoCl_2$) and deferoxamine mesylate

(DFX). These findings indicate that hypoxia enhances MSC differentiation and hypoxia and hypoxia-mimicking agents generate different effects on MSC differentiation [59].

Conversely, some others have reported suppressive effects of low O_2 tension levels on the plasticity of MSCs. Differentiation capacity into adipogenic progeny was diminished, and no osteogenic differentiation was detected at 3% oxygen. In turn, MSC that had previously been cultured at 3% oxygen could subsequently be stimulated to successfully differentiate at 20% oxygen [31]. Temporary exposure of MSCs to hypoxia resulted in (i) persistent (up to 14 days postexposure) downregulation of cbfa-1/Runx2, osteocalcin, and type I collagen and (ii) permanent (up to 28 days postexposure) upregulation of osteopontin mRNA expressions [60]. Another study by Widowati et al. showed both nor-WJ-MSCs and hypo-WJ-MSCs differentiated to osteocytes, chondrocytes, and adipocytes, although there was no significant difference among treatments [36]. Study conducted by Georgi et al. showed that molecular fingerprints of human MSCs, primary chondrocytes, and MSC/primary chondrocytes coculture differ when cultured in either normoxic (21% O_2) or hypoxic (2.5% O_2) conditions [61]. In the study, cartilage formation increased in cocultures of MSCs and primary chondrocytes was lost when the cells were cultured under hypoxia which was associated with a decrease in the mRNA expression of the chondrogenic marker SOX9 and FGF-1. This coincided with a significant decrease in lipids. Lipid profiles of normoxic and hypoxic cultures are different. The improved cartilage formation in cocultures of MSCs and chondrocytes may employ soluble factors, including small molecules, lipids, or proteins [62]. Lipids such as phospholipids, cholesterol, and diacylglycerols play significant roles in cellular signaling, membrane integrity, and metabolism [63]. Recent study described that short-term changes in sphingolipid metabolism resulted in long-term effects on the chondrogenic phenotype, and the stimulation of chondrocytes with acylceramidase improves cartilage repair and MSC differentiation [64].

8. Immunomodulatory effects of MSCs in hypoxic condition

One of the key factors of MSC in therapeutics development is their known anti-inflammatory/immunomodulatory properties. Clinical studies showed efficacy of MSC at inhibiting lethal, immune-based condition of graft versus host disease [65–70]. It has been reported that MSCs derived from adipose, bone marrow, and placenta have the capability to recover ischemic injury by increasing vascularization and reducing inflammation in ischemia-injured hindlimb, lung, heart, and brain [71–73]. Thus, these cells have been used in clinical trials to treat ischemic disease [74]. MSCs produce a broad variety of cytokines, chemokines, and growth factors that may potentially be involved in tissue repair. Hypoxia increases the production of several of these factors, although different responses are also noted in few studies. Referring to Chang et al., hypoxic preconditioning enhances the capacity of the secretome obtained from cultured human MSCs to release several of these factors and the therapeutic potential of the cultured MSC secretome in experimental TBI [75].

One of the most studied mechanisms of inflammation-induced MSC activity is treatment with interferon gamma (IFN-γ). This cytokine is usually secreted during inflammatory Th1 immune responses that are associated with autoimmunity mediated by cellular means, such as CD8 T cells and NK cells, which commonly occur in multiple sclerosis, diabetes type 1, and rheumatoid arthritis [76]. Treatment of IFN-γ in MSC has been reported to enhance the immunosuppressive activity through stimulation of the enzyme IDO [77–80]. MSC expression of the tryptophan-catabolizing enzyme indolamine 2,3 deoxygenase (IDO) was markedly upregulated under hypoxia [81]. IDO is critical in immune regulation by MSC through induction of T cell anergy [82] and stimulation of T regulatory cells (T-regs) [83, 84].

Moreover, IFN-γ induced secretion of other inhibitors of inflammation by MSCs, including the complement inhibitor factor H [85], as well as the immunomodulatory molecules TGF-β and HGF [86]. At a functional level, Noone et al. demonstrated that IFN-γ pretreatment of MSC resulted in protection of MSCs from NK-mediated killing via upregulation of prostaglandin E (PGE)-2 synthesis [87]. IFN-γ, along with necrosis factor-alpha (TNF-α), IL-1α, and IL-1β, induces Gal-9 in MSC [88].

Another inflammatory mediator known to induce regenerative activities in MSC is the macrophage-derived cytokine TNF-α. Pretreatment of TNF-α in MSCs provided superior angiogenic activity *in vitro*, as indicated by expression of VEGF, as well as *in vivo* in an animal model of critical limb ischemia, as compared to untreated MSCs [89]. In other study, TNF-α preconditioning increased proliferation, mobilization, and osteogenic differentiation of MSCs and upregulated bone morphogenetic protein-2 (BMP-2) protein level. Osteogenic differentiation of MSC induced by TNF-α was partially inhibited after BMP-2 knockdown by siRNA [90]. Lipopolysaccharide and toll-like receptor (TLR) agonists, as activators of innate immunity, are also responsible for regenerative activity of MSCs by inducing paracrine factors secretion such as VEGF [91]. IFN-γ and TLR also upregulate the glucocorticoids production, which decreases T cells stimulated by radiotherapy in colonic mucosa [92].

Akiyama et al. reported that MSCs induced T cell apoptosis via the Fas/FasL pathway [93]. Telomerase improved immunomodulatory properties of MSCs by upregulating FasL expression [94]. Dental follicle cells and cementoblasts have been reported to trigger apoptosis of ameloblast-lineage cells, as well as Hertwig's epithelial root sheath (HERS)/epithelial rests of Malassez (ERM) cells, via the Fas/FasL pathway during tooth development [95]. FasL regulated the immunomodulatory properties of Human gingiva-derived mesenchymal stem cells (hGMSCs), which is promoted by hypoxia. However, the underlying pathways of such event remain unclear. Further studies regarding the pathways involved in hGMSC-mediated immunomodulation are encouraged.

9. Molecular mechanism of MSCs in hypoxic condition

O_2 concentration in the stem cell niche (usually 2–9% O_2) is considered a driver of cell function [20]. Hypoxia plays a vital role in maintaining homeostasis within the body from the early stage of embryonic development. It facilitates proper embryonic development, maintains stem cell pluripotency, induces differentiation, and regulates the signaling of multiple cascades, including angiogenesis [96]. In hypoxic conditions, these functions are regulated by several transcription factors such as hypoxia-inducible factors (HIFs), prolyl hydroxylases (PHDs), factor-inhibiting HIF-1 (FIH-1), activator protein 1 (AP-1), nuclear factor (NF)-κB, p53, and c-Myc [97]. Although interaction among all of the transcription factors is required for cellular response, HIFs (especially HIF-1) are the key regulators of cellular response to hypoxia [98]. The discovery of HIF-1a by Greg Semenza provided profound insight into the cellular mechanisms that control hypoxic adaptation [99–101].

Generally, under hypoxic conditions, low O_2 level suppresses the prolyl hydroxylation that leads to HIF-1α accumulation and nuclear translocation [102]. After nuclear translocation, it binds with HIF-1β to form the heterodimer. Then, the HIF-1 heterodimer binds to a hypoxia-response element (HRE) in the target genes, associated with coactivators such as CBP/p300, and regulates the transcription (**Figure 1**) of as many as 70 genes involved in metabolism, angiogenesis, invasion/metastasis, and cell fate [103].

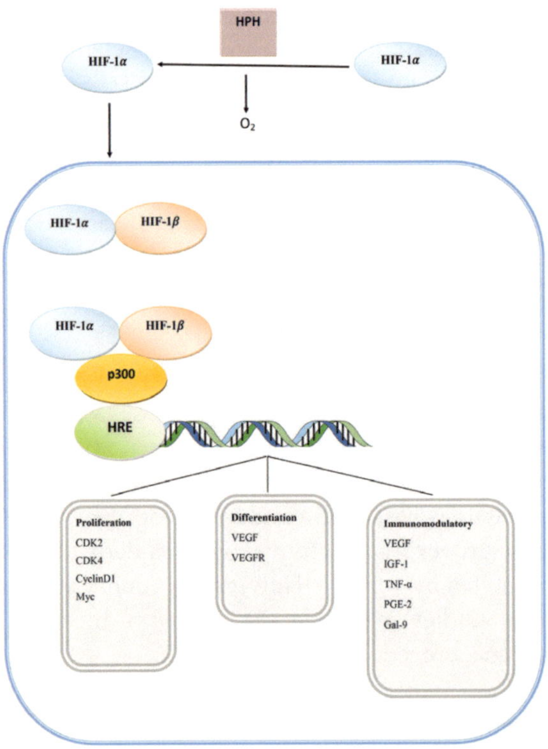

Figure 1. Regulation of hypoxia in MSCs. HIF, hypoxia-inducible factor; HPH, HIF-prolyl hydroxylases; HPE, HIF-prolyl hydroxylases; HRE, hypoxia-response element; CDK, cyclin-dependent kinase; VEGF, vascular endothelial growth factor; VEGFR, vascular endothelial growth factor receptor; IGF, insulin-like growth factor; TNF, tumor necrosis factor; PGE-2, prostaglandin E-2; Gal9, galectin-9. The prolyl hydroxylation process is suppressed due to lack of O_2 that leads HIF-1α accumulation and nuclear translocation after nuclear translocation, and it binds HIF-1β to form the heterodimer. Then, the HIF-1 heterodimer binds HRE in the genes target, associated with coactivators such as CBP/p300, and regulates the transcription of as many as 70 genes involved in proliferation, differentiation, and immunomodulatory.

http://dx.doi.org/10.5772/65510

In 2007, iPSCs were discovered by Shinya Yamanaka and colleagues, and the subsequent identification of the necessary transcriptional programs was required to maintain stem cells in a pluripotent state [104, 105]. The measurement of low partial pressures of oxygen in various stem cell niches raises question whether HIF-1a and iPSCs pathways were converged. It was described initially in Embryonic stem cells (ESCs) [106], hematopoietic stem cells (HSCs) [107], neural stem cells (NSCs) [108], and cancer stem cells (CSCs) [109], which now further expanded to include iPSCs [110]. Remarkably, Yamanaka first reprogrammed fibroblasts to iPSCs using only four transcription factors (Oct4, Sox2, c-Myc, and Klf4) [105] in the same year that Oct4 was shown to be a specific target gene of HIF-2a [111]. The correlation between HIF-2a and Oct4 has been proposed as underlying mechanism of stem cells response to hypoxic conditions in their niche and direct modification of stem cell function by low O_2. HIF-2a expression has recently been investigated in several stem cell lineages, and Oct4 expression is tightly regulated throughout embryogenesis. Loss or even decrease in Oct4 expression leads to differentiation [112]. Oct4 works in concert with Nanog and Sox2 to maintain stem cell identity and repress genes that promote differentiation [113]. The recent identification of HIF-2a upregulation by Oct4 in CSCs and ESCs underscores the importance of this axis in maintaining stemness in both development and disease.

It is known that phosphorylation of protein kinase B (Akt), a downstream gene of phosphatidylinositol 3-kinase (PI3K) signaling pathway, is an important step in signaling pathways that mediate cell proliferation [114, 115]. In PI3K/Akt pathway, a large number of substrates are phosphorylated, including HIF-1 [116]. Referring to study done by Rosová et al., the preculture of MSCs in hypoxia prior to injection activated the PI3K/Akt signaling pathway while maintaining their viability and cell cycle rates [117].

Hypoxia-mediated MSC differentiation by reducing apoptosis via activating the PI3K/Akt/FoxO pathway. Referring to Wang et al., MSCs underwent apoptosis upon induction for chondrogenic differentiation [118]. Apoptosis has been demonstrated as a general phenomenon that occurs during endochondral differentiation of chondrocytes [119]. One study demonstrated that chondrocytes progression to endochondral ossification employed higher FAS receptor and caspase protein as indicators of apoptosis [120]. Other studies showed that both the Wnt/beta-catenin and Indian hedgehog (Ihh) signaling pathways play important roles in endochondral ossification. Beta-catenin is needed at upstream of Ihh signaling for chondrocyte survival and inhibition of apoptosis [121]. The expression of Sox9, col2a1 and aggrecan in prechondrogenic cells 30 and chondrocytes 14 is regulated by PI3K/Akt pathway. It has also been demonstrated that PI3K/Akt regulated col2a1 and aggrecan by modulating Sox9 expression and transcriptional activity in nucleus pulposus cells 31.

Lee et al. [122] showed novel pathway for hypoxia-induced proliferation and migration in human mesenchymal stem cells that employ HIF-1α, FASN, and mTORC1O. Hypoxia treatment stimulates UCB-hMSC proliferation, along with the expression of two lipogenic enzymes: fatty acid synthase (FASN) and stearoyl-CoA desaturase-1 (SCD1). FASN is a key enzyme in UCB-hMSC proliferation and migration. Hypoxia-induced FASN expression was regulated by the HIF-1α/SCAP/SREBP1 pathway. Mammalian target of rapamycin (mTOR) was phosphorylated by hypoxia, whereas inhibition of FASN by cerulenin suppressed hypoxia-induced mTOR phosphorylation, as well as UCB-hMSC proliferation and migration. Hypoxia-induced proliferation and migration are significantly inhibited by raptor small interfering RNA. Hypoxia-induced mTOR also regulates CDK2, CDK4, cyclin D1, cyclin E, and F-actin expression as well as c-myc, p-cofilin, profilin, and Rho GTPase. Moreover, hypoxia-induced FASN stimulates FFA production as well as proliferation and migration. Several studies reported that FAS and FA derivatives inhibited and uncoupled oxidative phosphorylation of various cells [123–125]. Palmitic acid treatment rescues inhibition of mTOR phosphorylation as well as restriction of UCB-hMSC proliferation and migration. Change in cellular metabolite ratios may be another pathway, in addition to the HIF1a/SCAP/SREBP1 pathway, involved in the regulation of lipid metabolism in UCB-hMSCs. Some studies reported that alteration of cellular metabolite ratios, such as NADP/NADPH, by hypoxia has also an important role in the regulation of various stem cell functions such as cell cycle and self-renewal activities [126, 127].

10. Hypoxic MSCs in clinical application

MSCs possess anti-inflammatory/immunomodulatory properties, which are utilized in therapeutics development. Clinical studies on efficacy of MSCs have been shown to inhibit lethal, immune-based condition of graft versus host disease [65–70]. Moreover, MSCs derived from adipose, bone marrow, and placenta have the capability to recover ischemic injury by increasing vascularization and reducing inflammation in ischemia-injured hindlimb, lung, heart, and brain [71–73, 128]. These cells have been used in clinical trials to treat ischemic disease [74], and the safety of MSCs has been evaluated [129, 130]. There are several modified approaches, which have been proposed to improve the effect of MSCs on ischemia-related disease, such as over expression of angiogenesis-related genes such as bFGF on MSCs [131], combination with other cells such as endothelial cells [84], antioxidants such as melatonin [132], serum deprivation [72], and cell spheroids [133].

From isolation to engraftment, the MSCs usually pass through two different phases, consisting of *in vitro* culture condition (from isolation to transplantation) and *in vivo* or physiological condition (before isolation and after transplantation). At present, most of the expansion procedures of MSCs are performed under ambient O_2 concentration, where cells are exposed to 20% O_2, which is ~4–10 times more than the concentration of O_2 in their natural niches [134, 135]. Maintaining genetic stability has been a challenge during *in vitro* expansion of MSCs. Increased rates of aneuploidy, double-stranded DNA breakdown, and faster telomere shortening have been reported for MSCs cultured in ambient condition [30]. According to recent review, major causes behind aneuploidy were defective spindle assembly checkpoint, centrosome amplification, and merotelic attachments [136], which are caused by ROS [137]. ROS also acts in acceleration of telomere shortening and DNA breakdown [138, 139]. Correlation between telomere shortening and aneuploidy in embryonic and hepatocellular carcinoma cells has also been reported in recent studies [140, 141]. The higher ROS production due to the increased mitochondrial respiration during expansion of MSCs in ambient O_2 concentration might be the cause behind genetic instability in them. However, cells undergo anaerobic respiration during hypoxia, which lowers the ROS concentration within the cells. This might reduce the DNA damage, telomere shortening, and aneuploidy which in return may increase the biosafety of stem cell-based therapy.

The ability of stem or progenitor cells to home and engraft into target tissues after transplantation is the key to succeed in clinical application. The degree of homing and engraftment of MSCs in adult recipients is very low [142–144]. Hypoxic culture conditions may also provide a solution for more efficient engraftment. Recently, early passaged mouse BM-MSCs showed better engraftment than late passaged mouse BM-MSCs in *in vivo* model [145]. In other study, hypoxic preconditioned murine MSCs also enhanced skeletal muscle regeneration and improved blood flow and vascular formation compared to normoxic condition [146]. Furthermore, hypoxic conditions cause MSCs to grow faster [30] while maintaining a higher number of rapidly self-renewing cells [40]. Hypoxic environment also upregulated chemokine receptors CXCR4, CXCR7 and CX3CR1 [147, 148], and they may facilitate tissue-specific trafficking of MSCs. Thus, sufficient numbers of MSCs with a higher fraction of rapidly self-renewing cells are suggested, and highly expressed chemokine receptors on their surface can be obtained from the early passages of hypoxic cultures, which could increase the efficiency of damaged tissue-specific migration and engraftment following transplantation.

MSCs cultured under hypoxic conditions also increased in vascular endothelial growth factor receptor 1 (VEGFR1) expression and VEGF- or placental growth factor (PLGF)-dependent migration (Okuyama et al., 2006). Preconditioning with oxygen and combined glucose depletion also increased the survival of stem cell antigen (Sca)-1þ cells via PI3K/Akt-dependent caspase-3 downregulation and thereby increased the engraftment rate [149]. In addition to the increase in migration and survival, MSCs with hypoxic preconditioning have also been shown to enhance revascularization after transplantation for hindlimb ischemia [117]. Therefore, culturing MSCs in hypoxic conditions can also be considered as a solution for tissue-specific engraftment.

Hypoxia-stimulated immune regulation of MSCs has been observed in the situation of allogeneic use of BM-MSCs for stimulation of therapeutic angiogenesis. Recent study showed hypoxia-conditioned BM-MSCs from B6 mice repair limb of Balb/c mice compared to normoxic MSCs. Engraftment in allogeneic recipients increased by decreasing NK cells cytotoxicity and the accumulation of host-derived NK cells when transplanted *in vivo*. These allogeneic hypoxia-treated BM-MSCs increased CD31+ endothelial cells and αSMA+ and desmin + muscle cells, thereby enhancing angiogenesis and restoring muscle structure. Moreover, anti-NK antibodies along with normoxic MSCs enhanced angiogenesis and prevented limb amputation in allogeneic recipients with limb ischemia [150].

Some studies have shown that MSC transplantation contributes to tumor formation *in vivo* [24, 151, 152], whereas Furlani et al. reported that cultured MSCs with spontaneous transformations had no functional effects after intracardiac transplantation [153]. Further studies regarding tumorigenicity and safety of the stem cell-based products are encouraged. However, complexity of cell therapy requires more standards for advanced medicinal products [154]. Thus, especially in the field of regenerative medicine, concrete and specific standards and governmental support systems are necessary to promote their production [154].

11. Perspective of hypoxic MSCs

Hypoxic condition has been confirmed to enhance MSCs proliferation, differentiation, and immune regulatory performance. However, some studies have also reported opposite and negative effects. Different outcomes in each study raise interest in availability of more appropriate methods for cell cultures, which require further study in standardizing the culture of MSCs for use in cell therapy. Optimal conditions for the culture of MSCs have not yet been clearly defined, and it is very crucial to precisely determine the effects of hypoxia on MSCs differentiation, proliferation, and morphology, among other aspects. Moreover, hypoxic MSC-based therapies require a complete understanding of stem cell molecular mechanism. The clarity in stem cell regulation is important for further development such as periodic monitoring of chromosomal stability in culture prior to exposure to human to detect mutations and to prevent transplant-associated tumor formation, and also genetic engineering of physiology of MSCs to acquire better outcome.

12. Conclusion

The growing interest in the potential application of MSCs in regenerative medicine was followed by the several studies measuring the effects of low O_2 levels on the behavior and function of MSCs. Hypoxic condition appears to enhance MSCs proliferation, differentiation, and immune regulatory performance in damaged tissues without affecting its characteristic. However, there are also studies that report on negative effects of hypoxia in MSCs.

Author details

Wahyu Widowati[1*], Dwi Davidson Rihibiha[2], Khie Khiong[2], M. Aris Widodo[3], Sutiman B. Sumitro[4] and Indra Bachtiar[5]

*Address all correspondence to: wahyu_w60@yahoo.com

1 Faculty of Medicine, Maranatha Christian University, Bandung, Indonesia

2 Biomolecular and Biomedical Research Center, Aretha Medika Utama, Bandung, Indonesia

3 Laboratory of Pharmacology, Faculty of Medicine, Brawijaya University, Malang, Indonesia

4 Department of Biology, Faculty of Mathematics and Natural Sciences, Brawijaya University, Malang, Indonesia

5 Stem Cell and Cancer Institute, Jakarta, Indonesia

References

[1] Friedenstein AJ. The development of fibroblast colonies in monolayer cultures of guinea-pig bone marrow and spleen cells. Cell Tissue Kinet. 1970;3:393–403. doi: 10.1111/j.1365-2184.1970.tb00347.x.

[2] Friedenstein AJ. Stromal mechanisms of bone marrow: cloning *in vitro* and retransplantation *in vivo*. Haematol Blood Transfus. 1980;25:19–29. doi:10.1007/978-3-642-67319-1_3.

[3] Bianco P, Robey PG, Simmons PJ. Mesenchymal stem cells: revisiting history, concepts, and assays. Cell Stem Cell. 2008;2:313–319. doi:10.1016/j.stem.2008.03.002.

[4] Caplan AI. Adult mesenchymal stem cells for tissue engineering versus regenerative medicine. J Cell Physiol. 2007;213:341–347. doi:10.1002/jcp.21200.

[5] Kolf CM, Cho E, Tuan RS. Biology of adult mesenchymal stem cells: regulation of niche, self-renewal and differentiation. Arthritis Res Ther. 2007;9:204. doi:10.1186/ar2116.

[6] Pittenger MF, Mackay AM, Beck SC, Jaiswal RK, Douglas R, Mosca JD, et al. Multilineage potential of adult human mesenchymal stem cells. Science. 1999;284:143–147. doi:10.1126/science.284.5411.143.

[7] Prockop DJ. "Stemness" does not explain the repair of many tissues by mesenchymal stem/multipotent stromal cells (MSCs). Clin Pharmacol Ther. 2007;82:241–243. doi: 10.1038/sj.clpt.6100313.

[8] Rogers I, Casper RF. Umbilical cord blood stem cells. Best Pract Res Clin Obstet Gynaecol. 2004;18:893–908. doi:10.1016/j.bpobgyn.2004.06.004.

[9] Bieback K, Kluter H. Mesenchymal stromal cells from umbilical cord blood. Curr Stem Cell Res Ther. 2007;2:310–323.

[10] Xu Y, Malladi P, Wagner DR, Longaker MT. Adipose-derived mesenchymal cells as a potential cell source for skeletal regeneration. Curr Opin Mol Ther. 2005;7:300–305. PMID:16121695.

[11] Shi S, Gronthos S. Perivascular niche of postnatal mesenchymal stem cells in human bone marrow and dental pulp. J Bone Miner Res. 2003;18:696–704. doi:10.1359/jbmr.2003.18.4.696.

[12] Tsai MS, Lee JL, Chang YJ, Hwang SM. Isolation of human multipotent mesenchymal stem cells from second-trimester amniotic fluid using a novel two-stage culture protocol. Hum Reprod. 2004;19:1450–1456. doi:10.1093/humrep/deh279.

[13] Bi Y, Ehirchiou D, Kilts TM, Inkson CA, Embree MC, Sonoyama W, et al. Identification of tendon stem/progenitor cells and the role of the extracellular matrix in their niche. Nat Med. 2007;13:1219–1227. doi:10.1038/nm1630.

[14] Igura K, Zhang X, Takahashi K, Mitsuru A, Yamaguchi S, Takashi TA. Isolation and characterization of mesenchymal progenitor cells from chorionic villi of human placenta. Cytotherapy. 2004;6:543–553. doi:10.1080/14653240410005366-1.

[15] De Bari C, Dell'accio F, Tylzanowski P, Luyten FP. Multipotent mesenchymal stem cells from adult human synovial membrane. Arthritis Rheum. 2001;44:1928–1942. doi: 10.1002/1529-0131(200108)44:8<1928::AID-ART331>3.0.CO;2-P.

[16] Crisan M, Deasy B, Gavina M, Zheng B, Huard J, Lazzari L, et al. Purification and long-term culture of multipotent progenitor cells affiliated with the walls of human blood vessels: myoendothelial cells and pericytes. Methods Cell Biol. 2008;86:295–309. doi: 10.1016/S0091-679X(08)00013-7.

[17] Dominici M, Le Blanc K, Mueller I, Slaper-Cortenbach I, Marini F, Krause D, et al. Minimal criteria for defining multipotent mesenchymal stromal cells: the international society for cellular therapy position statement. Cytotherapy. 2006;8:315–317. doi: 10.1080/14653240600855905.

[18] Peister A, Mellad JA, Larson BL, Hall BM, Gibson LF, Prockop DJ. Adult stem cells from bone marrow (MSCs) isolated from different strains of inbred mice vary in surface epitopes, rates of proliferation, and differentiation potential. Blood. 2004;103:1662–1668. doi:10.1182/blood-2003-09-3070.

[19] Jones EA, Kinsey SE, English A, Jones RA, Straszynski L, Meredith DM, et al. Isolation and characterization of bone marrow multipotential mesenchymal progenitor cells. Arthritis Rheum. 2002;46:3349–3360. doi:10.1002/art.10696.

[20] Simon MC, Keith B. The role of oxygen availability in embryonic development and stem cell function. Nat Rev Mol Cell Biol. 2008;9:285–296. doi:10.1038/nrm2354.

[21] Scadden DT. The stem-cell niche as an entity of action. Nature. 2006;441:1075–1079. doi: 10.1038/nature04957.

[22] Cooper PD, Burt AM, Wilson JN. Critical effect of oxygen tension on rate of growth of animal cells in continuous suspended culture. Nature. 1958;182:1508–1509. doi: 10.1038/1821508b0.

[23] Zwartouw HT, Westwood JC. Factors affecting growth and glycolysis in tissue culture. Br J Exp Pathol. 1958;39:529–539.

[24] Miura M, Miura Y, Padilla-Nash HM, Molinolo AA, Fu B, Patel V, et al. Accumulated chromosomal instability in murine bone marrow mesenchymal stem cells leads to malignant transformation. Stem Cells. 2006;24:1095–1093. doi:10.1634/stemcells. 2005-0403.

[25] Kuhn NZ, Tuan RS. Regulation of stemness and stem cell niche of mesenchymal stem cells: implications in tumorigenesis and metastasis. J Cell Physiol. 2010;222:268–277. doi:10.1002/jcp.21940.

[26] Harrison JS, Rameshwar P, Chang V, Bandari P. Oxygen saturation in the bone marrow of healthy volunteers. Oxygen saturation in the bone marrow of healthy volunteers. Blood. 2002;99:394. PMID:11783438.

[27] Kofoed H, Sjontoft E, Siemssen SO, Olesen HP. Bone marrow circulation after osteotomy. Blood flow, pO2, pCO2, and pressure studied in dogs. Acta Orthop Scand. 1985;56:400–403.

[28] Matsumoto A, Matsumoto S, Sowers AL, Koscielniak JW, Trigg NJ, Kuppusamy P, et al. Absolute oxygen tension (pO(2)) in murine fatty and muscle tissue as determined by EPR. Magn Reson Med. 2005;54:1530–1535. doi:10.1002/mrm.20714.

[29] Pasarica M, Sereda OR, Redman LM, Albarado DC, Hymel DT, Roan LE, et al. Reduced adipose tissue oxygenation in human obesity: evidence for rarefaction, macrophage chemotaxis, and inflammation without an angiogenic response. Diabetes. 2009;58:718–725. doi:10.2337/db08-1098.

[30] Estrada JC, Albo C, Benguria A, Dopazo A, Lopez-Romero P, Carrera-Quintanar L, et al. Culture of human mesenchymal stem cells at low oxygen tension improves growth and genetic stability by activating glycolysis. Cell Death Differ. 2012;19:743–755. doi: 10.1038/cdd.2011.172.

[31] Fehrer C, Brunauer R, Laschober G, Unterluggauer H, Reitinger S, Kloss F, et al. Reduced oxygen tension attenuates differentiation capacity of human mesenchymal stem cells and prolongs their lifespan. Aging Cell. 2007;6:745–757. doi:10.1111/j. 1474-9726.2007.00336.x.

[32] Mohamadnejad M, Pournasr B, Bagheri M, Aghdami N, Shahsavani M, Hosseini LA, et al. Transplantation of allogeneic bone marrow mesenchymal stromal cell-derived hepatocyte-like cells in homozygous familial hypercholesterolemia. Cytotherapy. 2010;12:566–568. doi:10.3109/14653240903511143.

[33] Schachinger V, Erbs S, Elsasser A, Haberbosch W, Hambrecht R, Holschermann H. Intracoronary bone marrow-derived progenitor cells in acute myocardial infarction. N Engl J Med. 2006;355:1210–1221.

[34] Holzwarth C, Vaegler M, Gieseke F, Pfister SM, Handgretinger R, Kerst G, et al. Low physiologic oxygen tensions reduce proliferation and differentia-tion of human multipotent mesenchymal stromal cells. BMC Cell Biol. 2010;11:1–11. doi:10.1186/1471-2121-11-11.

[35] Nekanti U, Dastidar S, Venugopal P, Totey S, Ta M. Increased proliferation and analysis of differential gene expression in human Wharton's jelly-derived mesenchymal stromal cells under hypoxia. Int J Biol Sci. 2010;6:499–512.

[36] Widowati W, Wijaya L, Murti H, Widyastuti H, Agustina D, Laksmitawati DR, et al. Conditioned medium from normoxia (WJMSCs-norCM) and hypoxia-treated WJMSCs (WJMSCs-hypoCM) in inhibiting cancer cell proliferation. BGM. 2015;7:8–17.

[37] Basciano L, Nemos C, Foliguet L, de Isla N, de Carvalho M, Tran N, et al. Long term culture of mesenchymal stem cells in hypoxia promotes a genetic program maintaining their undifferentiated and multipotent status. BMC Cell Biol. 2011;12:1–12. doi: 10.1186/1471-2121-12-12.

[38] Grayson WL, Zhao F, Bunnell B, Ma T. Hypoxia enhances proliferation and tissue formation of human mesenchymal stem cells. Biochem Biophys Res Commun. 2007;358:948–953. doi:10.1016/j.bbrc.2007.05.054.

[39] Weijers EM, Van Den Broek LJ, Waaijman T, Van Hinsbergh VWM, Gibbs S, Koolwijk P. The influence of hypoxia and fibrinogen variants on the expansion and differentiation of adipose tissue-derived mesenchymal stem cells. Tissue Eng Part A. 2011;17:2675–2685. doi:10.1089/ten.tea.2010.0661.

[40] Saller MM, Prall WC, Docheva D, Schönitzer V, Popov T, Anz D, et al. Increased stemness and migration of human mesenchymal stem cells in hypoxia is associated with altered integrin expression. Biochem Biophys Res Commun. 2012;423:379–385. doi:10.1016/j.bbrc.2012.05.134.

[41] Widowati W, Wijaya L, Bachtiar I, Gunanegara RF, Sugeng SU, Irawan YA, et al. Effect of oxygen tension on proliferation and characteristics of Wharton's jelly-derived mesenchymal stem cells. BGM. 2014;6:43–48. doi:10.1016/j.bgm.2014.02.001.

[42] Pattappa G, Thorpe SD, Jegard NC, Heywood HK, de Bruijn JD, Lee DA. Continuous and uninterrupted oxygen tension influences the colony formation and oxidative metabolism of human mesenchymal stem cells. Tissue Eng Part C Methods. 2013;19:68–79. doi:10.1089/ten.TEC.2011.0734.

[43] Yew TL, Chang MC, Hsu YT, He FY, Weng WH, Tsai CC, et al. Efficient expansion of mesenchymal stem cells from mouse bone marrow under hypoxic conditions. J Tissue Eng Regen Med. 2013;7:984–993. doi:10.1002/term.1491.

[44] Rubio D, Garcia-Castro J, Martin MC, de la Fuente R, Cigudosa JC, Lloyd AC, et al. Spontaneous human adult stem cell transformation. Cancer Res. 2005;65:3035–3039. doi:10.1158/0008-5472.CAN-04-4194.

[45] Bernardo ME, Zaffaroni N, Novara F, Cometa AM, Avanzini MA, Moretta A, et al. Human bone marrow derived mesenchymal stem cells do not undergo transformation after long-term *in vitro* culture and do not exhibit telomere maintenance mechanisms. Cancer Res. 2007;67:9142–9149. doi:10.1158/0008-5472.CAN-06-4690.

[46] Zhang ZX, Guan LX, Zhang K, Wang S, Cao PC, Wang YH, et al. Cytogenetic analysis of human bone marrow-derived mesenchymal stem cells passaged *in vitro*. Cell Biol Int. 2007;31:645–648. doi:10.1016/j.cellbi.2006.11.025.

[47] Fischer U, Radermacher J, Mayer J, Mehraein Y, Meese E, et al. Tumor hypoxia: impact on gene amplification in glioblastoma. Int J Oncol. 2008;33:509–515. doi:10.3892/ijo_00000034.

[48] Coquelle A, Toledo F, Stern S, Bieth A, Debatisse M. A new role for hypoxia in tumor progression: induction of fragile site triggering genomic rearrangements and formation of complex DMs and HSRs. Mol Cell. 1998;2:259–265. doi:10.1016/S1097-2765(00)80137-9.

[49] Ueyama H, Horibe T, Hinotsu S, Tanaka T, Inoue T, Urushihara H, et al. Chromosomal variability of human mesenchymal stem cells cultured under hypoxic conditions. J Cell Mol Med. 2012;16:72–82. doi:10.1111/j.1582-4934.2011.01303.x.

[50] Sutherland GR. Chromosomal fragile sites. Genet Anal Biomol Eng. 1991;8:161–166. doi:10.1016/1050-3862(91)90056-W.

[51] Lukusa T, Fryns JP. Human chromosome fragility. Biochim Biophys Acta. 2008;1779:3–16. doi:10.1016/j.bbagrm.2007.10.005.

[52] Nowinski GP, Van Dyke DL, Tilley BC, Jacobsen G, Babu VR, Worsham MJ, et al. The frequency of aneuploidy in cultured lymphocytes is correlated with age and gender but not with reproductive history. Am J Hum Genet. 1990;46:1101–1111. PMCID:PMC1683821.

[53] Pierre RV, Hoagland HC. Age-associated aneuploidy: loss of Y chromosome from human bone marrow cells with aging. Cancer. 1972;30:889–894. doi:10.1002/1097-0142(197210)30:4<889::AID-CNCR2820300405>3.0.CO;2-1.

[54] Baksh D, Song L, Tuan RS. Adult mesenchymal stem cells: characterization, differentiation, and application in cell and gene therapy. J Cell Mol Med. 2004;8:301–316. doi:10.1111/j.1582-4934.2004.tb00320.x.

[55] Hung SP, Ho JH, Shih YR, Lo T, Lee OK. Hypoxia promotes proliferation and osteogenic differentiation potentials of human mesenchymal stem cells. J Orthop Res. 2012;30:260–266.doi:10.1002/jor.21517.

[56] Huang J, Deng F, Wang L, Xiang XR, Zhou WW, Hu N, et al. Hypoxia induces osteogenesis related activities and expression of core binding factor alpha1 in mesenchymal stem cells. Tohoku J Exp Med. 2011;224:7–12. doi:10.1620/tjem.224.7.

[57] Lennon DP, Edmison JM, Caplan AI. Cultivation of rat marrow-derived mesenchymal stem cells in reduced oxygen tension: effects on *in vitro* and *in vivo* osteochondrogenesis. J Cell Physio. 2001;187:345–355. doi:10.1002/jcp.1081.

[58] Fink T, Abildtrup L, Fogd K, Abdallah BM, Kassem M, Ebbesen P, Zachar V. Induction of adipocyte like phenotype in human mesenchymal stem cells by hypoxia. Stem Cells. 2004;22:1346–1355. doi:10.1634/stemcells.2004-0038.

[59] Ren H, Cao Y, Zhao Q, Li J, Zhou C, Liao L, et al. Proliferation and differentiation of bone marrow stromal cells under hypoxic conditions. Biochem Biophys Res Commun. 2006;347:12–21. doi:10.1016/j.bbrc.2006.05.169.

[60] Potier E, Ferreira E, Andriamanalijaona R, Pujol JP, Oudina K, Logeart-Avramoglou D, et al. Hypoxia affects mesenchymal stromal cell osteogenic differentiation

and angiogenic factor expression. Bone. 2007;40:1078–1087. doi:10.1016/j.bone.2006.11.024.

[61] Georgi N, Cillero-Pastor B, Eijkel GB, Periyasamy PC, Kiss A, van Blitterswijk C, et al. Differentiation of mesenchymal stem cells under hypoxia and normoxia: lipid profiles revealed by time-of-flight secondary ion mass spectrometry and multivariate analysis. Anal Chem. 2015;87:3981–3988. doi:10.1021/acs.analchem.5b00114.

[62] Maumus M, Manferdini C, Toupet K, Peyrafitte JA, Ferreira R, Facchini A, et al. Adipose mesenchymal stem cells protect chondrocytes from degeneration associated with osteoarthritis. Stem Cell Res. 2013;11:834–844. doi:10.1016/j.scr.2013.05.008.

[63] Brown AJ. Cholesterol, statins and cancer. Clin Exp Pharmacol Physiol. 2007;34:135–141. doi:10.1111/j.1440-1681.2007.04565.x.

[64] Simonaro CM, Sachot S, Ge Y, He X, Deangelis VA, Eliyahu E, et al. Acid ceramidase maintains the chondrogenic phenotype of expanded primary chondrocytes and improves the chondrogenic differentiation of bone marrow-derived mesenchymal stem cells. PLoS One 2013;8:1–14. doi:10.1371/journal.pone.0062715.

[65] Ringden O, Uzunel M, Rasmusson I, Remberger M, Sundberg B, Lönnies H, Le Blanc K. Mesenchymal stem cells for treatment of therapy resistant graft versus host disease. Transplant. 2006;81:1390–1397. doi:10.1097/01.tp.0000214462.63943.14.

[66] Le Blanc K, Rasmusson I, Sundberg B, Götherström C, Hassan M, Uzunel M, et al. Treatment of severe acute graft versus host disease with third party haploidentical mesenchymal stem cells. Lancet. 2004;363:1439–1441. doi:10.1016/S0140-6736(04)16104-7.

[67] Le Blanc K, Frassoni F, Ball L, Locatelli F, Roelofs H, Lewis I, et al. Mesenchymal stem cells for treatment of steroid-resistant, severe, acute graft versus host disease: a phase II study. Lancet. 2008;371:1579–1586. doi:10.1016/S0140-6736(08)60690-X.

[68] Ning H, Yang F, Jiang M, Hu L, Feng K, Zhang J, et al. The correlation between cotransplantation of mesenchymal stem cells and higher recurrence rate in hematologic malignancy patients: outcome of a pilot clinical study. Leukemia. 2008;22:593–599. doi:10.1038/sj.leu.2405090.

[69] Ball L, Bredius R, Lankester A, Schweizer J, van den Heuvel-Eibrink M, Escher H, et al. Third party mesenchymal stromal cell infusions fail to induce tissue repair despite successful control of severe grade IV acute graft-versus-host disease in a child with juvenile myelo-monocytic leukemia. Leukemia. 2008;22:1256–1257. doi:10.1038/sj.leu.2405013.

[70] Muller I, Kordowich S, Holzwarth C, Isensee G, Lang P, Neunhoeffer F, et al. Application of multipotent mesenchymal stromal cells in pediatric patients following allogeneic stem cell transplantation. Blood Cells Mol Dis. 2008;40:25–32. doi:10.1016/j.bcmd.2007.06.021.

[71] Liu J, Hao H, Xia L, Ti D, Huang H, Dong L, et al. Hypoxia pretreatment of bone marrow mesenchymal stem cells facilitates angiogenesis by improving the function of endothelial cells in diabetic rats with lower ischemia. PLoS One. 2015;10:1–18. doi:10.1371/journal.pone.0126715.

[72] Sun CK, Leu S, Hsu SY, Zhen YY, Chang LT, Tsai CY, et al. Mixed serum-derived and normal adipose-derived mesenchymal stem cells against acute lung ischemia reperfusion injury in rats. Am J Transl Res. 2015;7:209–231.

[73] Zhang GW, Gu TX, Guan XY, Sun XJ, Jiang DQ, Tang R, Qi X, Li XY. Delayed enrichment for c-kit and inducing cardiac differentiation attenuated protective effects of BMSCs transplantation in pig model of acute myocardial ischemia. Cardiovasc Ther. 2015;33:184–192. doi:10.1111/1755-5922.12131.

[74] Bura A, Planat-Benard V, Bourin P, Silvestre JS, Gross F, Grolleau JL, et al. Phase I trial: the use of autologous cultured adipose-derived stroma/stem cells to treat patients with non-revascularizable critical limb ischemia. Cytotherapy. 2014;16:245–257. doi:10.1016/j.jcyt.2013.11.011.

[75] Chang CP, Chio CC, Cheong CU, Chao CM, Cheng BC, Lin MT. Hypoxic preconditioning enhances the therapeutic potential of the secretome from cultured human mesenchymal stem cells in experimental traumatic brain injury. Clin Sci. 2013;124:165–176. doi:10.1042/CS20120226.

[76] Skurkovich B, Skurkovich S. Anti-interferon-gamma antibodies in the treatment of autoimmune diseases. Curr Opin Mol Ther. 2003;5:52–57. PMID:12669471.

[77] Croitoru-Lamoury J, Lamoury FMJ, Caristo M, Suzuki K, Walker D, Takikawa O, et al. Interferon-γ regulates the proliferation and differentiation of mesenchymal stem cells via activation of indoleamine 2,3 dioxygenase (IDO). PLoS One. 2011;6:1–13. doi:10.1371/journal.pone.0014698.

[78] Rong LJ, Chi Y, Yang SG, Chen DD, Chen F, Xu SX, et al. Effects of interferon-γ on biological characteristics and immunomodulatory property of human umbilical cord-derived mesenchymal stem cells. J Exp hematol Chin Assoc Pathophysiol. 2012;20:421–426.

[79] Kang JW, Koo HC, Hwang SY, Kang SK, Ra JC, Lee MH, et al. Immunomodulatory effects of human amniotic membrane-derived mesenchymal stem cells. J Vet Sci. 2012;13:23–31. doi:10.4142/jvs.2012.13.1.23.

[80] Lin W, Oh SKW, Choo ABH, George AJT. Activated T cells modulate immunosuppression by embryonic-and bone marrow-derived mesenchymal stromal cells through a feedback mechanism. Cytotherapy. 2012;14:274–284. doi:10.3109/14653249.2011.635853.

[81] Roemeling-Van Rhijn M, Mensah FKF, Korevaar SS, Leijs MJC, Van Osch GJVM, IJzermans JNM, et al. Effects of hypoxia on the immunomodulatory properties of

adipose tissue-derived mesenchymal stem cells. Front Immunol. 2013;4:1–8. doi:10.3389/fimmu.2013.00203.

[82] English K, Tonlorenzi R, Cossu G, Wood KJ. Mesoangioblasts suppress T cell proliferation through IDO and PGE-2-dependent pathways. Stem Cells Dev. 2013;22:512–523. doi:10.1089/scd.2012.0386.

[83] Engela AU, Baan CC, Peeters AM, Weimar W, Hoogduijn MJ. Interaction between adipose-tissue derived mesenchymal stem cells and regulatory T cells. Cell Transplant. 2013;22:41–54. doi:10.3727/096368912X636984.

[84] Huang CC, Chen DY, Wei HJ, Lin KJ, Wu CT, Lee TY, et al. Hypoxia-induced therapeutic neovascularization in a mouse model of an ischemic limb using cell aggregates composed of HUVECs and cbMSCs. Biomaterials. 2013;34:9441–9550. doi:10.1016/j.biomaterials.2013.09.010.

[85] Tu Z, Li Q, Bu H, Lin F. Mesenchymal stem cells inhibit complement activation by secreting factor H. Stem Cells Dev. 2010;19:1803–1809. doi:10.1089/scd.2009.0418.

[86] Ryan JM, Barry F, Murphy JM, Mahon BP. Interferon-gamma does not break, but promotes the immunosuppressive capacity of adult human mesenchymal stem cells. Clin Exp Immunol. 2007;149:353–363. doi:10.1111/j.1365-2249.2007.03422.x.

[87] Noone C, Kihm A, English K, O'Dea S, Mahon BP. IFN-gamma stimulated human umbilical-tissue derived cells potently suppress NK activation and resist NK mediated cytotoxicity *in vitro*. Stem Cells Dev. 2013;15:3003–3014. doi:10.1089/scd.2013.0028.

[88] Gieseke F, Kruchen A, Tzaribachev N, Bentzien F, Dominici M, Müller I. Proinflammatory stimuli induce galectin-9 in human mesenchymal stromal cells to suppress T-cell proliferation. Eur J Immunol. 2013;43:2741–2749. doi:10.1002/eji.201343335.

[89] Kwon YW, Heo SC, Jeong GO, Yoon JW, Mo WM, Lee MJ, et al. Tumor necrosis factor-α-activated mesenchymal stem cells promote endothelial progenitor cell homing and angiogenesis. Biochim Biophys Acta. 2013;1832:2136–2144. doi:10.1016/j.bbadis.2013.08.002.

[90] Lu Z, Wang G, Dunstan CR, Chen Y, Lu WYR, Davies B, et al. Activation and promotion of adipose stem cells by tumour necrosis factor-alpha preconditioning for bone regeneration. J Cell Physiol. 2013;228:1737–1744. doi:10.1002/jcp.24330.

[91] Grote K, Petri M, Liu C, Jehn P, Spalthoff S, Kokemüller H, et al. Toll-like receptor 2/6-dependent stimulation of mesenchymal stem cells promotes angiogenesis by paracrine factors. Eur Cells Mater. 2013;26:66–79. PMID:24027020.

[92] Bessout R, Sémont A, Demarquay C, Charcosset A, Benderitter M, Mathieu N. Mesenchymal stem cell therapy induces glucocorticoid synthesis in colonic mucosa and suppresses radiation-activated T cells: new insights into MSC immunomodulation. Mucosal Immunol. 2014;7:656–669. doi:10.1038/mi.2013.85.

[93] Akiyama K, Chen C, Wang D, Xu X, Qu C, Yamaza T, et al. Mesenchymal stem cell induced immunoregulation involves FAS-ligand-/FAS-mediated T cell apoptosis. Cell Stem Cell. 2012;10:544–555. doi:10.1016/j.stem.2012.03.007.

[94] Chen C, Akiyama K, Yamaza T, You Y-O, Xu X, Li B, et al. Telomerase governs immunomodulatory properties of mesenchymal stem cells by regulating FAS ligand expression. EMBO Mol Med. 2014;6:322–334. doi:10.1002/emmm.201303000.

[95] Ding, SW. RNA-based antiviral immunity. Nat Rev Immunol. 2010;10:632–644. doi: 10.1038/nri2824.

[96] Lin Q, Kim Y, Alarcon RM, Yun Z. Oxygen and cell fate decisions. Gene Regul Syst Bio. 2008;2:43–51. PMCID:PMC2733087.

[97] Kenneth NS, Rocha S. Regulation of gene expression by hypoxia. Biochem J. 2008;414:19–29. doi:10.1042/BJ20081055.

[98] Stamati K, Mudera V, Cheema U. Evolution of oxygen utilization in multicellular organisms and implications for cell signalling in tissue engineering. J Tissue Eng. 2011;2:1–12. doi:10.1177/2041731411432365.

[99] Semenza GL, Wang GL. A nuclear factor induced by hypoxia via de novo protein synthesis binds to the human erythropoietin gene enhancer at a site required for transcriptional activation. Mol Cell Biol. 1992;12:5447–5454.

[100] Wang GL, Jiang BH, Rue EA, Semenza GL. Hypoxia inducible factor 1 is a basic helix loop helix PAS heterodimer regulated by cellular O2 tension. Proc Natl Acad Sci. 1995;92:5510–5514. PMCID:PMC46495.

[101] Wang GL, Semenza GL. General involvement of hypoxia-inducible factor 1 in transcriptional response to hypoxia. Proc Natl Acad Sci. 1993;90:4304–4308. PMCID: PMC46495.

[102] Weidemann A, Johnson RS. Biology of HIF-1α. Cell Death Differ. 2008;15:621–627. doi: 10.1038/cdd.2008.12.

[103] Brahimi-Horn MC, Pouyssegur J. Oxygen, a source of life and stress. FEBS Lett. 2007;581:3582–3591. doi:10.1016/j.febslet.2007.06.018.

[104] Takahashi K, Tanabe K, Ohnuki M, Narita M, Ichisaka T, Tomoda K, et al. Induction of pluripotent stem cells from adult human fibroblasts by defined factors. Cell. 2007;131:861–872. doi:10.1016/j.cell.2007.11.019.

[105] Takahashi K, Yamanaka S. Induction of pluripotent stem cells from mouse embryonic and adult fibroblast cultures by defined factors. Cell. 2006;126:663–676. doi:10.1016/j.cell.2006.07.024.

[106] Adelman DM, Maltepe E, Simon MC. Multilineage embryonic hematopoiesis requires hypoxic ARNT activity. Genes Dev. 1999;13:2478–2483.

[107] Cipolleschi MG, Dello Sbarba P, Olivotto M. The role of hypoxia in the maintenance of hematopoietic stem cells. Blood. 1993;8:2031–2037. PMID:8104535.

[108] Panchision DM. The role of oxygen in regulating neural stem cells in development and disease. J Cell Physiol. 2009;220:562–568. doi:10.1002/jcp.21812.

[109] Li Z, Bao S, Wu Q, Wang H, Eyler C, Sathornsumetee S, et al. Hypoxia-inducible factors regulate tumorigenic capacity of glioma stem cells. Cancer Cell. 2009;15:501–513. doi: 10.1016/j.ccr.2009.03.018.

[110] Yoshida Y, Takahashi K, Okita K, Ichisaka T, Yamanaka S. Hypoxia enhances the generation of induced pluripotent stem cells. Cell Stem Cell. 2009;5:237–241. doi: 10.1016/j.stem.2009.08.001.

[111] Covello KL, Kehler J, Yu H, Gordan JD, Arsham AM, Hu CJ, et al. HIF-2alpha regulates Oct-4: effects of hypoxia on stem cell function, embryonic development, and tumor growth. Genes Dev. 2006;20:557–570. doi:10.1101/gad.1399906.

[112] Boiani M, Eckardt S, Scholer HR, McLaughlin KJ. Oct4 distribution and level in mouse clones: consequences for pluripotency. Genes. 2002;16:1209–1219. doi:10.1101/gad. 966002.

[113] Boyer LA, Lee TI, Cole MF, Johnstone SE, Levine SS, Zucker JP, et al. Core transcriptional regulatory circuitry in human embryonic stem cells. Cell. 2005;122:947–956. doi: 10.1016/j.cell.2005.08.020.

[114] Borgatti P, Martelli AM, Bellacosa A, Casto R, Massari L, Capitani S, et al. Translocation of AKT/PKB to the nucleus of osteoblast-like MC3T3-E1 cells exposed to proliferative growth factors. FEBS Lett. 2000;477:27–32.

[115] Jung F, Haendeler J, Goebel C, Zeiher AM, Dimmeler S. Growth factor-induced phosphoinositide 3-OH kinase/Akt phosphorylation in smooth muscle cells: induction of cell proliferation and inhibition of cell death. Cardiovasc Res. 2000;48:148–157. doi: 10.1016/S0008-6363(00)00152-8.

[116] Semenza GL. Targeting HIF-1 for cancer therapy. Nat Rev Cancer. 2003;3:721–732. doi: 10.1038/nrc1187.

[117] Rosová I, Dao M, Capoccia B, Link D, Nolta JA. Hypoxic preconditioning results in increased motility and improved therapeutic potential of human mesenchymal stem cells. Stem Cells. 2008;26:2173–2182. doi:10.1634/stemcells.2007-1104.

[118] Wang CY, Chen LL, Kuo PY, Chang JL, Wang YJ, Hung SC. Apoptosis in chondrogenesis of human mesenchymal stem cells: effect of serum and medium supplements. Apoptosis. 2010;15:439–449. doi:10.1007/s10495-009-0431-x.

[119] Cheung JO, Grant ME, Jones CJ, Hoyland JA, Freemont AJ, Hillarby MC. Apoptosis of terminal hypertrophic chondrocytes in an *in vitro* model of endochondral ossification. J Pathol. 2003;201:496–503. doi:10.1002/path.1462.

[120] Aizawa T, Kon T, Einhorn TA, Gerstenfeld LC. Induction of apoptosis in chondrocytes by tumor necrosis factor-alpha. J Orthop Res. 2001;19:785–796. doi:10.1016/S0736-0266(00)00078-4.

[121] Mak KK, Chen MH, Day TF, Chuang PT, Yang Y. Wnt/beta-catenin signaling interacts differentially with Ihh signaling in controlling endochondral bone and synovial joint formation. Development. 2006;133:3695–3707. doi:10.1242/dev.02546.

[122] Lee HJ, Ryu JM, Jung YH, Oh SY, Lee SJ, Han HJ. Novel pathway for hypoxia-induced proliferation and migration in human mesenchymal stem cells: involvement of HIF-1α, FASN, and mTORC1. Stem Cells. 2015;33:2182-2195. doi:10.1002/stem.2020.

[123] Ventura FV, Ruiter JP, Ijlst L, Almeida IT, Wanders RJ. Inhibition of oxidative phosphorylation by palmitoyl-CoA in digitonin permeabilized fibroblasts: implications for long-chain fatty acid beta oxidation disorders. Biochim Biophys Acta. 1995;1272:14–20.

[124] Samartsev VN, Belosludtsev KN, Chezganova SA, Zeldi IP. Effect of ethanol on the palmitate induced uncoupling of oxidative phosphorylation in liver mitochondria. Biochemistry. 2002;67:1240–1247. doi:10.1023/A:1021397220815.

[125] Brustovetskii NN, Dedukhova VN, Egorova MV, Mokhova EN, Skulachev VP. Uncoupling of oxidative phosphorylation by fatty acids and detergents suppressed by ATP/ADP antiporter inhibitors. Biokhimiia. 1991;56:1042–1048.

[126] Cipolleschi MG, Marzi I, Santini R, Fredducci D, Vinci MC, D'Amico M, et al. Hypoxia-resistant profile implies vulnerability of cancer stem cells to physiological agents, which suggests new therapeutic targets. Cell Cycle. 2014;13:268–278. doi:10.4161/cc.27031.

[127] Marzi I, Cipolleschi MG, D'Amico M, Stivarou T, Rovida E, Vinci MC, et al. The involvement of a Nanog, Klf4 and c-Myc transcriptional circuitry in the intertwining between neoplastic progression and reprogramming. Cell Cycle. 2013;12:353–364. doi:10.4161/cc.23200.

[128] Li D, Zhang M, Zhang Q, Wang Y, Song X, Zhang Q. Functional recovery after acute intravenous administration of human umbilical cord mesenchymal stem cells in rats with cerebral ischemia-reperfusion injury. Intractable Rare Dis Res. 2015;4:98–104. doi:10.5582/irdr.2015.01010.

[129] Karussis D, Karageorgiou C, Vaknin-Dembinsky A, Gowda-Kurkalli B, Gomori JM, Kassis I, et al. Safety and immunological effects of mesenchymal stem cell transplantation in patients with multiple sclerosis and amyotrophic lateral sclerosis. Arch Neurol. 2010;67:1187–1194. doi:10.1001/archneurol.2010.248.

[130] Lalu MM, McIntyre L, Pugliese C, Fergusson D, Winston BW, Marshall JC, et al. Safety of cell therapy with mesenchymal stromal cells (safe cell): a systematic review and meta-analysis of clinical trials. PLoS One. 2012;7:1–21. doi:10.1371/journal.pone.0047559.

[131] Zhang JC, Zheng GF, Wu L, Ou Yang LY, Li WX. Bone marrow mesenchymal stem cells overexpressing human basic fibroblast growth factor increase vasculogenesis in ischemic rats. Braz J Med Biol Res. 2014;47:886–894. doi:10.1590/1414-431X20143765.

[132] Yip HK, Chang YC, Wallace CG, Chang LT, Tsai TH, Chen YL, et al. Melatonin treatment improves adipose-derived mesenchymal stem cell therapy for acute lung ischemia-reperfusion injury. J Pineal Res. 2013;54:207–221. doi:10.1111/jpi.12020.

[133] Park IS, Chung PS, Ahn JC. Enhanced angiogenic effect of adipose-derived stromal cell spheroid with low-level light therapy in hind limb ischemia mice. Biomaterials. 2014;35:9280–9289. doi:10.1016/j.biomaterials.2014.07.061.

[134] Antoniou ES, Sund S, Homsi EN, Challenger LF, Rameshwar P. A theoretical simulation of hematopoietic stem cells during oxygen fluctuations: prediction of bone marrow responses during hemorrhagic shock. Shock. 2004;22:415–422.

[135] Chow DC, Wenning LA, Miller WM, Papoutsakis ET. Modeling pO2 distributions in the bone marrow hematopoietic compartment II. Modified Kroghian models. Biophys J. 2001;81:685–696. doi:10.1016/S0006-3495(01)75733-5.

[136] Gordon DJ, Resio B, Pellman D. Causes and consequences of aneuploidy in cancer. Nat Rev Genet. 2012;13:189–203. doi:10.1038/nrg3123.

[137] Wang CY, Liu LN, Zhao ZB. The role of ROS toxicity in spontaneous aneuploidy in cultured cells. Tissue Cell. 2012;45:47–53. doi:10.1016/j.tice.2012.09.004.

[138] Barzilai A, Yamamoto K. DNA damage responses to oxidative stress. DNA Repair (Amst). 2004;3:1109–1115. doi:10.1016/j.dnarep.2004.03.002.

[139] Guachalla LM, Rudolph KL. ROS induced DNA damage and checkpoint responses: influences on aging? Cell Cycle. 2010;9:4058–4060. doi:10.4161/cc.9.20.13577.

[140] Treff NR, Su J, Taylor D, Scott RT. Telomere DNA deficiency is associated with development of human embryonic aneuploidy. PLoS Genetics. 2011;7:1–10. doi:10.1371/journal.pgen.1002161.

[141] Plentz RR, Schlegelberger B, Flemming P, Gebel M, Kreipe H, Manns MP, et al. Telomere shortening correlates with increasing aneuploidy of chromosome 8 in human hepatocellular carcinoma. Hepatology. 2005;42:522–526. doi:10.1002/hep.20847.

[142] LaBarge MA, Blau HM. Biological progression from adult bone marrow to mononucleate muscle stem cell to multinucleate muscle fiber in response to injury. Cell. 2002;111:589–601. doi:10.1016/S0092-8674(02)01078-4.

[143] Ankrum J, Karp JM. Mesenchymal stem cell therapy: two steps forward, one step back. Trends Mol Med. 2010;16:203–209. doi:10.1016/j.molmed.2010.02.005.

[144] Phinney DG, Prockop DJ. Concise review: mesenchymal stem/multipotent stromal cells: the state of trans differentiation and modes of tissue repair—current views. Stem Cells. 2007;25:2896–2902. doi:10.1634/stemcells.2007-0637.

[145] Jin J, Zhao Y, Tan X, Guo C, Yang Z, Miao D. An improved transplantation strategy for mouse mesenchymal stem cells in an acute myocardial infarction model. PLoS One. 2011;6:1–16. doi:10.1371/journal.pone.0021005.

[146] Leroux L, Descamps B, Tojais NF, Seguy B, Oses P, Moreau C, et al. Hypoxia preconditioned mesenchymal stem cells improve vascular and skeletal muscle fiber regeneration after ischemia through a wnt4-dependent pathway. Mol Ther. 2010;18:1545–1552. doi:10.1038/mt.2010.108.

[147] Liu H, Liu S, Li Y, Wang X, Xue W, Ge G, et al. The role of SDF-1-CXCR4/CXCR7 axis in the therapeutic effects of hypoxia-preconditioned mesenchymal stem cells for renal ischemia/reperfusion injury. PLoS One. 2012;7:1–13. doi:10.1371/journal.pone.0034608.

[148] Hung S-C, Pochampally RR, Hsu S-C, Sanchez C, Chen S-C, Spees J, et al. Short-term exposure of multipotent stromal cells to low oxygen increases their expression of CX3CR1 and CXCR4 and their engraftment *in vivo*. PLoS One. 2007;2:1–11. doi:10.1371/journal.pone.0000416.

[149] Lu G, Haider HK, Jiang S, Ashraf M. Sca-1þ stem cell survival and engraftment in the infarcted heart: dual role for preconditioning induced connexin-43. Circulation. 2009;119:2587–2596. doi:10.1161/CIRCULATIONAHA.108.827691.

[150] Huang WH, Chen HL, Huang PH, Yew TL, Lin MW, Lin SJ, et al. Hypoxic mesenchymal stem cells engraft and ameliorate limb ischaemia in allogeneic recipients. Cardiovasc Res. 2014;101:266–276. doi:10.1093/cvr/cvt250.

[151] Guest I, Ilic Z, Ma J, Grant D, Glinsky G, Sell S. Direct and indirect contribution of bone marrow-derived cells to cancer. Int J Cancer. 2010;126:2308–2318. doi:10.1002/ijc.24946.

[152] Tolar J, Nauta AJ, Osborn MJ, Panoskaltsis Mortari A, McElmurry RT, Bell S, et al. Sarcoma derived from cultured mesenchymal stem cells. Stem Cells. 2007;25:371–379. doi:10.1634/stemcells.2005-0620.

[153] Furlani D, Li W, Pittermann E, Klopsch C, Wang L, Knopp A, et al. A transformed cell population derived from cultured mesenchymal stem cells has no functional effect after transplantation into the injured heart. Cell Transplant. 2009;18:319–331. doi:10.3727/096368909788534906.

[154] Tsubouchi M, Matsui S, Banno Y, Kurokawa K, Kawakami K. Overview of the clinical application of regenerative medicine products in Japan. Health Policy. 2008;88:62–72. doi:10.1016/j.healthpol.2008.02.011.

Chapter 6

Cardiovascular Adaptation to High-Altitude Hypoxia

Jun Ke, Lei Wang and Daliao Xiao

Additional information is available at the end of the chapter

http://dx.doi.org/10.5772/65354

Abstract

High-altitude exposure has been well recognized as a hypoxia exposure that significantly affects cardiovascular function. However, the pathophysiologic adaptation of cardiovascular system to high-altitude hypoxia (HAH) varies remarkably. It may depend on the exposed time and oxygen partial pressure in the altitude place. In short-term HAH, cardiovascular adaptation is mainly characterized by functional alteration, including cardiac functional adjustments, pulmonary vascular constriction, transient pulmonary hypertension, and changes in cerebral blood flow (CBF). These changes may be explained mainly by ventilatory acclimatization and variation of autonomic nervous activity. In long-term HAH, cardiovascular adaptation is mainly characterized by both functional and structural alterations. These changes include right ventricle (RV) hypertrophy, persistent pulmonary hypertension, lower CBF and reduced uteroplacental and fetal volumetric blood flows.

Keywords: high altitude, hypoxia, cardiovascular adaptation, compensatory and pathologic adaptation

1. Introduction

High-altitude environment exerts a unique challenge to human life, which is chiefly characterized by lower partial pressure of O_2 (PO_2) relative to sea level at the same latitudes. The conventional definition of high-altitude hypoxia (HAH) is that arterial blood O_2 saturation (SaO_2) in body measurably begins to fall at altitudes >2500 m [1]. It is one of the hypoxemic types, which is due to a decrease in the amount of breathable oxygen caused by the low atmospheric pressure of high altitudes, and in turn low maximal oxygen uptake (VO_2 max), and the arterial partial pressure of O_2 (PaO_2) in the body [2]. Reduced oxygen availability at high altitude is associated with significant changes in cardiovascular function and increased the risk of cardiovascular disease. Human body has both short-term and long-term adaptations to altitude that allow it to partially compensate for the lowered amount of oxygen in the atmosphere [3]. In this chapter we present the physiologic and pathologic adaptation of cardiovascular system to short-term and long-term HAH and its underlying mechanisms.

2. Cardiovascular adaptation to high-altitude hypoxia

2.1. Cardiovascular adaptation to short-term high-altitude hypoxia and the underlying mechanisms

With ascent to high altitude, there is a nonlinear decrease in barometric pressure and a reduction in ambient partial pressure of oxygen (PO_2), and, subsequently a decrease in the PO_2 at every point along the oxygen transport cascade from inspired air to the alveolar space, arterial blood, the tissues, and venous blood. The higher the elevation attained, the greater the drop in PO_2 in the human body. These declines in oxygen tensions trigger a variety of physiologic responses in the cardiovascular system over a period of minutes to weeks after the initial altitude hypoxia exposure that enable the individual adapt to or compensate for the hypoxic environment.

At high altitude, in the short term, the low PO_2 of inspired air will typically concomitantly reduce SaO_2, so a compensatory adjustment may immediately take place to meet the large and consistent O_2 demand of the aerobic metabolism of tissues and cells. Initial lack of oxygen is sensed by the carotid bodies, which causes an increase in the breathing rate. Then the cardiovascular functions are changed in response to the short-term HAH.

2.1.1. Cardiac system

The main cardiac response to short-term HAH is the adjustment of cardiac function, which includes the changes in heart rate (HR) and cardiac output, left ventricular ejection fraction (LVEF), both ventricular systolic and diastolic function, and arterial blood pressure (ABP). At high altitude, an initial response is that the heart beats faster. Cardiac contractility and submaximal cardiac output also increase acutely during the first few days at altitude. This acute increase in cardiac output may largely be explained by the increased heart rate and may be offset by reduced stroke volume. For example, an earlier study demonstrated that acutely breathing an inspired fraction of O_2 of 0.12 caused 22% increase in cardiac output accompanied with 18% increase in heart rate and unchanged stroke volume, so the oxygen delivery to the tissues remained unchanged [4]. In addition, an evaluation of ventricular functions by Doppler echocardiography with tissue Doppler imaging (TDI) in volunteers exposed to acutely short-term (90 min) HAH reported that short-term HAH significantly increased HR, LVEF, isovolumic contraction wave velocity (ICV), acceleration (ICA), and systolic ejection wave velocity at the mitral annulus, indicating enhanced left ventricular systolic function. However, there was no change in right ventricular area shortening fraction, tricuspid annular plane systolic excursion (TAPSE), ICV, and ICA at the tricuspid annulus, demonstrating preserved right ventricular systolic function. Furthermore, increase in isovolumic relaxation time (IRT) at both annuli indicated altered diastolic function of both ventricles [5].

In response to a short-term high-altitude exposure, blood pressure is likely increased to a variable extent in many individuals. The changes in blood pressure may be dependent on individual conditions, the absolute altitude of exposure, and the duration of stay at altitude. A recent study has reported that after acute exposure to 3700 m, diastolic blood pressure and mean arterial blood pressure rose gradually and continually in healthy male young adults [6]. Further analysis showed that higher blood pressure accompanied poor sleeping quality and higher incidence of acute mountain sickness. In addition, systolic blood pressure also significantly increased after high-altitude exercise [6]. Significant rise in systolic and diastolic blood pressure in the initial phase of exposure to altitude was also reported in other studies [7, 8].

There are several possible mechanisms involved in short-term HAH-mediated cardiac dysfunction. One of the important mechanisms is the changes of autonomic nervous system including parasympathetic nervous system and sympathetic nervous system (SNS). A functional approach to assess the role of parasympathetic nerves by muscarinic blockade reported that tachycardia after 8 hours of exposure to hypoxia can be prevented by muscarinic blockade, which indicated that a muscarinic effect was involved in the tachycardia after short-term HAH [9]. Acute exposure to high altitude induced a statistically significant increase in heart rate associated with a shift of sympathovagal balance towards more sympathetic and less parasympathetic activity, which suggests a depression of autonomic functions and a relative increase in sympathetic activity at higher hypoxic levels [10]. These adaptations consist of significantly increased sympathetic activation as evidenced by heightened circulating catecholamine levels (such as norepinephrine) [11–14]. Mazzeo et al. reported a different catecholamine response between acute and chronic high-altitude exposure [13]. In response to acute exposure to 4300 m (4 hours), the arterial plasma epinephrine levels but not norepinephrine levels were significantly increased. However, both epinephrine and norepinephrine concentrations were increased after 21 days of chronic exposure [13]. These findings provide evidence for a differential adaptive response between sympathetic neural activity and that of the adrenal medulla during high-altitude exposure.

The increase in sympathetic tone may be a natural response by acute nonadapted subjects to counteract the effects of hypoxia. Indeed, short-term altitude exposure can directly or indirectly affect the vascular tone of systemic resistance vessels and enhances ventilation and sympathetic activity through the activation of peripheral chemoreceptors [15]. The peripheral chemoreceptors mainly include carotid bodies and aortic chemoreceptor, which are served as hypoxia sensors in the arterial walls. Carotid bodies act as sensitive monitors of arterial O_2 tension (PaO_2), whereas aortic chemoreceptors mainly monitor arterial O_2 content (CaO_2). So, carotid bodies evoke stronger respiratory responses than aortic chemoreceptors [16]. A study in humans exposed to hypoxia demonstrated that carotid bodies are chiefly responsible for ventilatory and vascular response, whereas aortic chemoreceptors mainly mediated the tachycardic response [17]. Another study indicated that hyperventilation induced by hypoxic stimulation of carotid bodies decreased vagal traffic to the heart through Hering-Breuer reflex, which plays an important indirect role in tachycardic response to hypoxia [18]. Meanwhile, hypoxic stimulation of carotid bodies also directly activated SNS to accelerate HR through increasing circulating catecholamine [19]. In addition, hypoxic activation of peripheral chemoreceptors was addressed to reset the baroreflex control of both HR and sympathetic nervous system (SNS) activity to higher levels, so that HR and sympathetic vasoconstriction were increased, which were independent of breathing rate and tidal volume [20].

2.1.2. Pulmonary vascular system

Pulmonary circulation is the important portion of the cardiovascular system responsible for the gas exchange. Short-term HAH can immediately trigger hypoxic pulmonary vasoconstriction

(HPV), which, in conjunction with increased cardiac output, leads to an enhanced pulmonary vascular resistance and a rise in pulmonary artery pressure. An investigation reported that human pulmonary vascular tone rose rapidly to reach a maximum within 5 min and was then maintained for the duration of the altitude exposure. This acute hypoxic pulmonary vasoconstriction (HPV) was reversed to baseline values within 5 min after breathing oxygen [21]. HPV is intrinsic to the pulmonary vascular smooth cells and independent of the endothelium, as demonstrated in experiments with endothelium-denuded pulmonary arteries (PAs) [22]. In short-term HAH, it was confirmed that small resistance pulmonary arteries (<200 μm) were highly sensitive to the alveolar O_2 tension. There is a functional "O_2-sensing unit" in the pulmonary artery smooth muscle cell (PASMC) mitochondria, which can detect falls in alveolar O_2, leading to produce a mediator to modulate the function of effector proteins. During hypoxia, the production of the mediator is low, which causes the inhibition of specific O_2-sensitive K^+ channels resulting in depolarization of PASMCs and activation of voltage-gated L-type Ca^{2+} channels. Ca^{2+} influx is thereby increased and cytosolic Ca^{2+} elevated, resulting in activation of the PASMCs' contractile machinery and development of HPV [23]. Given the fact that there is a lack of voltage-gated L-type Ca^{2+} channels in endothelium, it is most likely that HPV is endothelium-independent and intrinsic to pulmonary smooth muscle cells. However, endothelium-dependent and -independent mechanisms could modulate this response. Hypoxia may enhance pulmonary artery resistance through endothelin (ET) and sympathetic stimulation, whereas HPV may be attenuated by increased release of NO, hyperventilation improving alveolar PO_2, and respiratory alkalosis [24].

High-altitude pulmonary edema (HAPE) is not an uncommon form of acute altitude illness that occurs in otherwise healthy mountaineers at altitudes typically above 2500 m. The initial cause of HAPE is a shortage of oxygen caused by the lower air pressure at high altitudes. The mechanisms underlying this oxygen shortage-induced HAPE are poorly understood, but one of the critical mechanisms is an excessive rise in pulmonary vascular resistance or hypoxic pulmonary vasoconstriction leading to increased microvascular pressures. This enhanced hydrostatic stress causes dynamic changes in the permeability of the alveolar capillary barrier and induces a high-permeability noninflammatory lung edema. Previous report indicated that decreased nitric oxide release and enhanced endothelin levels following acute high-altitude exposure may be the major determinants of exaggerated hypoxic pulmonary vasoconstriction in HAPE-susceptible individuals [25]. In addition, other hypoxia-mediated changes of sympathetic nervous activity, endothelial function, and altered levels of other vasoactive mediators such as endothelin and angiotensin II may also contribute additionally to HAPE susceptibility. Although higher pulmonary arterial pressure is associated with the development of HAPE, pulmonary hypertension may not in itself be sufficient to explain the development of high-altitude pulmonary edema. Development of pulmonary hypertension can occur in the absence of HAPE in humans at high altitude.

2.1.3. Cerebrovascular system

The brain is the most oxygen-dependent organ in the body. In response to acute exposure to high altitude, cerebral blood flow (CBF) rises significantly to ensure an adequate supply of O_2 to meet the brain tissues' large and consistent demand [26–28]. The mechanisms underlying the regulation of CBF during short-term HAH are complex and depend partly on the degree of hypoxia per se and on the partial pressures of arterial oxygen (PaO_2) and arterial carbon dioxide ($PaCO_2$) [29]. Upon ascent to high altitude, a severe drop in PaO_2 (to <40–45 mmHg) induces a cerebral vasodilation, which suggests that altitude-mediated reduced PaO_2 may act as a cerebral vasodilator. However, the fall in $PaCO_2$ following hyperventilation caused by hypoxic-induced activation of peripheral chemoreceptor also produces cerebral vasoconstriction. Therefore, the changes in CBF at high altitude are highly related to the balance of PaO_2/$PaCO_2$ in the circulation. Indeed, it has been demonstrated that the low PaO_2-to-$PaCO_2$ ratio explains 40% of the increase in brain blood flow upon arrival at high altitude (5050 m) [26]. The increased CBF is mainly due to heightened hypoxic-induced dilatation in the cerebral circulation prior to ventilatory adjustments [26]. A number of mechanisms are proposed to contribute to the cerebral vasodilation. One of the mechanisms is that hypoxia may increase adenosine and nitric oxide level, which causes an increase in arterial diameter [27]. In addition, the cerebral dilatation can be also regulated through other factors (such as hypoxia inducible factor). Furthermore, the fact that acute altitude exposure-mediated increased CBF and cerebral vasodilation can be reversed by supplemental oxygen suggests a direct hypoxic effect. With increasing altitude, increased CBF is believed to be one compensatory mechanism serving to maintain normal oxygen flux to the brain in the face of arterial hypoxemia. However, the profound hypoxemia experienced by climbers at extreme altitude (>5500 m) is known to be related with cerebral dysfunction. Previous investigation has shown that hypoxia-mediated cerebral vascular dysfunction and cerebral edema is one of the major cause of deaths over 8000 m on Everest [30].

High-altitude cerebral edema (HACE) is a medical condition in which the brain swells with fluid because of ascending to a high altitude. It occurs when the body fails to acclimatize while ascending to a high altitude. HACE can be prevented by ascending to heights slowly to allow the body more time to acclimatize. The major cause of HACE is oxygen deprivation. It is most often a complication of acute mountain sickness or high-altitude pulmonary edema. The current leading theory of its pathophysiology is that HACE is likely a result of vasogenic edema [31]. High-altitude hypoxia increases vascular permeability, which passes through the vasogenic endothelium in the brain. The leaking may be caused by increased pressure, or it may be caused by inflammation that makes the endothelium vulnerable to leaking. It has been reported that activation of vascular endothelial growth factor (VEGF) by hypoxia-inducible factor may be one of the major causes leading to overperfusion of microvascular beds, endothelial leakage, and hence edema [31]. In addition, high-altitude hypoxia can alter cerebral vasodilation coupled with a possible impairment of the autoregulation of cerebral blood flow and disruption of the integrity of the blood brain barrier possibly by hypoxia-mediated release of certain neuromodulators such as VEGF and calcitonin gene-related peptide (CGRP). Furthermore, the increased sympathetic nervous activity at high altitude may also play a role in the development of cerebral edema.

2.2. Cardiovascular adaptation to long-term HAH and the underlying mechanisms

Acute short-term exposure to high altitude has been recognized as a type of cardiovascular stress, and results in an immediate increase in heart rate, cardiac output, and a transient rise in the blood pressure but without significant changes in the ejection fraction. However, long-term exposure to high altitude or people who reside at high altitude show compensate change in cardiovascular system that has allowed them to adapt to high-altitude chronic hypoxia.

2.2.1. *Cardiac system*

In long-term HAH, the changes in cardiac function are different from those in acute short-term HAH. Similar to the short-term HAH, heart rate and arterial blood pressure may remain increased, but stroke volume is decreased and the cardiac output returns to baseline after a longer hypoxic exposure [4]. In long-term HAH, the heart must preserve adequate contractile function in spite of lowered oxygen tension in the cardiac circulation. Suarez et al. had conducted studies in young men during acclimation to a simulated altitude in a chamber for 40 days and their results showed that left ventricular systolic function indices including ejection fraction, ratio of peak systolic pressure to end systolic volume, and mean normalized systolic ejection rate at rest and exercise, were sustained in all subjects at high altitude despite reduced preload, pulmonary hypertension and severe hypoxemia, which means remarkably preserved contractility and excellent tolerance of the normal myocardium to long-term HAH [32]. Another study also demonstrated that cardiac contractility remained normal during exposure to altitude-induced hypoxia with preservation of LV ejection fraction and LV percent fractional shortening [33].

Cardiac adaptation to long-term HAH is characterized by a variety of functional adjustments to maintain homeostasis with minimum expenditure of energy. Such adjustments may help to protect the heart from development of ischemic heart disease. An epidemiological study reported that men residing at high altitude resulted in protection against death from ischemic heart disease [34]. The epidemiological observations on the cardioprotective effect of high altitude were confirmed in various experimental models [35–37]. It has been reported that the hearts of animals adapted to long-term HAH develop better functional recovery following ischemia and produce smaller cardiac infarction. In addition, it has also been reported that adaptation to HAH could protect the heart against ischemia-induced arrhythmias [38]. However, the cardioprotective effect of adaptation to HAH is age-dependent. For example, a recent experiment with rats at stimulated altitude of 5000 m from 7-week-old to their entire lifetime [39] showed that cardiac tolerance to acute hypoxia was significantly increased in up to 18 months-old rats, but it was lost in senescent rats (25 months-old). Similarly, people living at high altitude in the Andeans lost their adaptation and have higher incidence of pulmonary hypertension in their aged life.

The mechanisms underlying cardiac functional changes in response to long-term HAH remain far from being understood. However, recent studies in animals and man have highlighted the role of both sympathetic and parasympathetic nervous system in cardiac adaptation following long-term HAH. The role of the parasympathetic system in regulation of heart rate has been examined in humans from the response to muscarinic blockade. A study in human after exposing to an altitude of 5260 m for 9 weeks found that muscarinic blockade increased HR both at rest and during exercise, which suggested that enhanced parasympathetic activity involves in the altered HR during long-term HAH [40]. Meanwhile, another study in animals reported that the muscarinic receptor density in animals native to high altitude was significantly higher than in those living at low altitude. After 5 weeks of relocation to sea level the muscarinic receptor density concomitantly declined to the level in sea level animals [41]. In addition, similar to the short-term HAH, the sympathetic nervous system also plays a key role in the regulation of HR and cardiac function during long-term HAH, but the pattern is different from those in short-term HAH. Previous studies in long-term HAH subjects reported that plasma norepinephrine level increased more significantly than epinephrine levels [13, 14, 42, 43]. Although the resting heart rate remains increased, the maximal heart rate (the heart rate at maximal exercise) is reduced at long-term HAH. In view of the evidence of elevated systemic catecholamine levels after long-term HAH, the lower maximal heart rate suggests a change in adrenergic receptor density. Indeed, several studies in animals have shown the change in adrenergic receptor density in response to long-term HAH. For example, a study in rats exposed to 21 days of hypobaric hypoxia found that there was a significant reduction in β-adrenergic receptor density [44]. Another study in rats following 21 days of exposure to a simulated altitude of 5500 m also reported a downregulation of α- and β-adrenergic receptor density in ventricular tissues [45]. Furthermore, studies in humans using isoprenaline as an indirect measure of density of β-adrenergic receptors demonstrated a downregulation of β-adrenergic receptors at high altitude [46]. It has been reported that prolonged HAH exposure could also alter peripheral and central adrenergic receptor expression, leading to changes in cardiac function [47, 48]. Taken together, sustained long-term HAH exposure causes progressive enhancement of both sympathetic and parasympathetic activity, resulting in alteration of cardiovascular function.

In addition to cardiac functional adaptation, cardiac structural adaptation also occurs following long-term HAH exposure. One of the changes in response to sustained HAH is development of right ventricle (RV) hypertrophy. Long-term high altitude-induced RV hypertrophy is a beneficial adaptation that helps to counteract the increased afterload caused by persistent pulmonary hypertension and maintain a normal cardiac output [49]. During the compensated phase of hypertrophy, a study using an isolated preparation of the RV working heart demonstrated that mechanical performance was almost doubled compared with the control group, while the index of contractility remained unchanged, which means that the elevated ventricular performance is merely the result of the increased muscle mass. Meantime, the markedly improved ability of the RV maintaining cardiac output against increased pulmonary resistance was observed [49]. Hypertrophic RV is associated with significant changes of cardiac protein profiling [50]. Experimental results in rats exposed to intermittent high-altitude hypoxia have shown that the concentration of collagenous and noncollagenous proteins was significantly increased both in hypertrophic RV and nonhypertrophic LV [51]. Cardiac enlargement may be the result of both an increase in the number of individual cell elements (hyperplasia) and an increase in their volume (hypertrophy).

2.2.2. Pulmonary vascular system

The most common effect of long-term sustained HAH exposure is the development of pulmonary hypertension. Previous studies have reported a prevalence of high-altitude pulmonary hypertension between 5% and 18% of the population living at high altitude [52]. High-altitude pulmonary hypertension is characterized by increased pulmonary vascular resistance secondary to hypoxia-induced pulmonary vasoconstriction and vascular remodeling. The pulmonary vascular adaptations involve all elements of the vessel wall and include endothelial dysfunction, extension of smooth muscle into previously nonmuscular vessels and adventitial thickening. Long-term high-altitude-induced pulmonary hypertension was not completely reversed by oxygen breathing, suggesting that pulmonary arteries structural remodeling plays a pivotal role in pulmonary hypertension during long-term HAH [53]. Pulmonary arteries (PAs) remodeling involves cellular hypertrophy and hyperplasia in all three structural layers of PAs, namely adventitia, media, and intima. In addition, long-term HAH also causes other structural changes, such as the migration of medial smooth muscle cells (SMCs) into the intima, fibroblast proliferation and increased collagen deposition in the adventitia, more extracellular matrix proteins secreted by endothelial cells, and the appearance of SM-like cells in previously nonmuscularized vessels of the alveolar wall. All these changes eventually result in a reduction of the vascular lumen diameter and an increase in pulmonary vascular resistance [54].

The molecular mechanisms underlying the pathogenesis of high altitude-induced pulmonary hypertension are not fully understood, but several hypoxia-mediated signaling pathways are thought to play a key role. In the pulmonary vasculature, some membrane-bound receptors and signaling proteins are sensitive to hypoxia and play important role in the vascular medial proliferation. For example, a recent study in a sheep model of in utero high-altitude long-term hypoxia exposure demonstrated pulmonary vascular remodeling similar to that seen in other animal models of pulmonary hypertension [55]. The results indicated that pulmonary arteries of long-term HAH-exposed fetuses exhibited medial wall thickening and distal muscularization associated with an increased epidermal growth factor receptor (EGFR) protein expression in the pulmonary arteries. Furthermore, it has been demonstrated that the proliferation of fetal ovine pulmonary vascular smooth muscle cell was attenuated by inhibition of EGFR with a specific EGFR protein tyrosine kinase inhibitor [55]. These findings suggest that EGFR plays a role in fetal ovine pulmonary vascular remodeling following long-term HAH and that inhibition of EGFR signaling may reverse high altitude-induced pulmonary vascular remodeling. Similar to EGFR, platelet-activating factor (PAF) and PAF receptor have also been implicated in the pathogenesis of long-term HAH-induced pulmonary remodeling and hypertension in different animal models [56, 57]. In those studies, high PAF and PAF receptor expression levels in the pulmonary arteries have been reported in the long-term hypoxia-exposed animals [56, 57]. Furthermore, PAF receptor antagonists attenuated hypoxia-induced pulmonary hypertension and pulmonary vascular remodeling [56], suggesting that PAF receptor-mediated signaling also plays a key role in pulmonary vascular remodeling.

Accumulating evidence indicates that intrinsic changes in the ionic balance and calcium homeostasis of pulmonary arterial smooth muscle cells (PASMCs) caused by long-term hypoxia have a profound effect on PA remodeling. The membrane depolarization of PASMCs following the hypoxic inhibition of O_2 sensitive K^+ channels activated Ca^{2+} influx and elevated cytoplasmic ionized Ca^{2+} via voltage-gated Ca^{2+} channels. Changes in the transport of K^+ and Ca^{2+} through their respective ion channels modulate these processes by affecting cell volume, membrane potential, gene transcription, apoptosis, and cell-cycle progression. The adaptation of these ion channels at high altitude appears to involve in pulmonary arteries remodeling [58].

Although PASMCs are the major components of arteries that actively involve long-term HAH-mediated sustained vasoconstriction and enhanced medial hypertrophy, endothelial cells, on

http://dx.doi.org/10.5772/65354

the other hand, can sense humoral and hemodynamic changes incurred by high-altitude hypoxia, triggering their production of vasoactive and mitogenic factors that then affect PASMCs' function and growth [54, 59, 60]. Endothelin (ET)-1 is an important mediator of hypoxia-induced pulmonary vasoconstriction and vascular remodeling [61]. Chronic hypoxia increases ET-1 gene transcription and peptide synthesis in cultured endothelial cells. ET-1 and its receptors are selectively upregulated in patients with primary pulmonary hypertension and in humans exposed to high altitude [61]. Rats exposed to chronic hypoxia exhibit increased pulmonary artery pressure associated with an increase in ET-1 peptide levels. Moreover, hypoxic pulmonary vascular remodeling can be prevented and reversed by administration of ET receptor antagonist [61], suggesting a key role of ET-1 and its receptor-mediated signaling in chronic hypoxia-induced pulmonary hypertension and vascular remodeling.

2.2.3. *Cerebrovascular system*

Upon ascent to high altitude, cerebral blood flow (CBF) rises substantially. However, as HAH-exposed time is increased, the increased CBF will return to near sea level values within 1–3 weeks, which displays clear time-dependent changes during acclimatization. In general, high-altitude native residents have lower CBF values compared to sea level natives. The major mechanism underlying the reduction in CBF of high-altitude residents is the reported elevation in hematocrit and consequently increased arterial oxygen content (CaO_2), suggesting an inverse relationship between CBF and CaO_2. There are at least four reflex mechanisms that regulate CBF: (1) hypoxic ventilator response; (2) hypercapnic ventilatory response; (3) hypoxic cerebral vasodilation; and (4) hypocapnic cerebral vasoconstriction [62]. On initial arrival at high altitude, hypobaric hypoxia changes the mediators of CBF because of a decrease in arterial oxygen tension, which is an independent mediator of cerebral arteriolar dilatation. In addition, hypoxemia can trigger hyperventilation associated decrease in arterial carbon dioxide tension, which will cause cerebral arterial constriction because of an associated increase in periarteriolar pH. Therefore, over a few days period at a constant altitude, the influence of the arterial oxygen tension-induced threshold for cerebral vasodilation is attenuated and the degree of hypocapnia is enhanced. Furthermore, during a prolonged stay at altitude, the hematocrit also increases, resulting in an increased arterial oxygen content at an unchanged oxygen tension. This change will tend to decrease CBF. Therefore, cerebral hemodynamics during acclimatization to altitude is the result of these homeostatic mechanisms. In addition to these reflex responses, CBF is also regulated by some other hypoxia-induced changes. For example, high-altitude hypoxia-induced changes of cerebral capillary density, hypoxia-induced factor (HIF), nitric oxide, endothelin-1, reactive oxygen species (ROS), and neurotransmitters may be responsible for the falling CBF during long-term HAH [29].

2.2.4. *Uteroplacental vascular system*

Pregnancy is associated with a significant increase in uterine blood flow that optimizes the delivery of oxygen and nutrients to the developing fetus. The greater fall in uteroplacental vascular resistance preferentially directs blood flow to this vascular bed, raising the uterine blood flow from 20–50 ml/min in the nonpregnant state to 450–800 ml/min in the near-term pregnant stage [63]. The adaptations in the uterine circulation to pregnancy are complex and are mainly achieved through the remodeling of uterine vasculature, enhanced vasodilator response, blunted vasoconstrictor response, and reduced pressure-dependent myogenic reactivity. At sea level pregnant uterine artery diameter doubles due to the vascular growth and remodeling as well as due to alterations in vasoreactivity, and changes in the active and passive properties of the uterine artery vascular wall. The molecular mechanisms prompting uterine vascular growth and enlargement of the vascular diameter are not fully understood. However, one of the major mechanisms underlying pregnancy-mediated decreased uterine vascular resistance may be regulated through hormonal stimuli. It has been reported that estradiol is likely a key player because of its angiogenic properties and stimulatory effects on nitric oxide-mediated vasodilation [64]. Estrogen receptors (ERs) have been identified in uterine artery vascular smooth muscle and their expressions are significantly increased in pregnant uterine arteries as compared with nonpregnant uterine arteries [65]. The pregnancy-associated increased ER expression may directly upregulate vascular endothelial growth factor (VEGF), MAP kinase, and eNOS expression and their activities, leading to promote uterine vascular growth and vasodilation [65]. The decreased uterine vascular resistance can also be regulated by contractile agonists or related proteins. For example, pregnancy decreases PKC activity but increases ERK kinase activity in uterine arteries, leading to decrease in uterine artery contractility [66, 67]. In addition, myogenic tone and distensibility are additional factors that can alter uterine arterial intraluminal diameter and uterine vascular resistance. It has been reported that pregnancy significantly downregulates pressure-dependent myogenic tone and increases the pressure-dependent passive uterine arterial diameter. The reduced myogenic tone is mediated by an increase in the inhibitory effect of ERK and a decrease in the PKC signal pathway [68].

High-altitude hypoxia has profound effects on uteroplacental circulation including altered uteroplacental and fetal volumetric blood flows, resulting in fetal intrauterine growth restriction. It has been demonstrated that high-altitude hypoxia decreases the pregnancy-associated rise in uterine blood flow [69]. Reduced uterine blood flow and inadequate perfusion of the placenta have been attributed to the increased incidence of preeclampsia and fetal intrauterine growth restriction [1]. One of the mechanisms that contributes to the decreased uterine blood flow may be a significant inhibition of pregnancy-associated increase in uterine vascular growth. It has been reported that there is only half as much pregnancy-mediated increase in uterine arterial DNA synthesis in chronic hypoxic vs. normoxic animals [70]. The proliferative response to serum stimulation in cultured uterine arterial smooth muscle cells is also attenuated by hypoxia exposure [70]. In addition, high-altitude hypoxia also can alter pregnancy-associated responses to contractile proteins and vasodilator-mediated signaling pathways. Experimental studies in sheep, that experienced long-term high-altitude exposure during pregnancy, showed significant increase in the pressure-dependent myogenic tone of resistance-sized uterine arteries by suppressing the ERK1/2 activity and increasing the PKC signaling pathway [65]. Furthermore, high-altitude hypoxia exposure selectively downregulated estrogen-α receptor expression in uterine arteries of pregnant animals and inhibited the steroid hormone-mediated adaptation of ERK1/2 and PKC signaling pathways to cause an increase in the myogenic tone of uterine arteries in pregnancy [65]. These observations provide a novel molecular mechanism underlying high altitude-induced decrease in uterine blood flow by inhibition of estrogen/receptor-mediated signaling in pregnancy. The large-conductance Ca^{2+}-activated K^+ (BKca) is abundantly expressed in vascular smooth muscle cells. Previous studies have suggested that BKca channel is involved in the regulation of uterine circulation and the increase in uterine blood flow during pregnancy [71]. The BKca channel in vascular smooth muscle is a major effector in response to hypoxia. Studies in pregnant sheep model of long-term high-altitude (3801 m) exposure provide novel evidence that long-term high-altitude hypoxia during pregnancy adversely affects the uterine circulation via downregulating BKca channel function in uterine vasculatures [72]. High-altitude hypoxia during gestation significantly inhibited pregnancy-associated upregulation of BKca channel activity and attenuated BKca channel current density in pregnant uterine arteries [72]. This was mediated by a selective downregulation of BKca channel β1 subunit expression in the uterine arteries. In accordance, high-altitude hypoxia impaired the role of the BKca channel in regulating pressure-induced myogenic tone of uterine arteries that was enhanced in pregnant animals acclimatized to high altitude. These results suggest that selectively targeting BKca channel may be another key mechanism in the maladaptation of uteroplacental circulation caused by high-altitude hypoxia, which may contribute to the decreased uterine blood flow and fetal intrauterine growth restriction associated with maternal hypoxia. The molecular mechanisms underlying high-altitude hypoxia-mediated alteration of targeting gene expression in pregnant uterine arteries are not completely understood. However, recent studies suggest that epigenetic mechanism plays an important role in regulation of gene expression in adaptation to high altitude [73]. The results showed that chronic hypoxia increased estrogen receptor α subunit (ER-α) promoter DNA methylation at both specific protein-1 and upstream stimulatory factor binding sites, decreased specificity protein-1 and upstream stimulatory factor binding to the promoter, and suppressed ER-α expression in uterine arteries of pregnant animals [73]. Furthermore, the studies provide novel evidence that hypoxia-mediated DNA methylation plays a causal role in ER-α gene repression and ablation of estrogen-mediated adaptation of uterine arterial BKca channel activity, resulting in increased uterine arterial myogenic tone in pregnancy [73].

There are significant differences in uterine arterial adaptation to pregnancy between the long- and short-resident high-altitude populations. The weight of the babies born to Tibetan residents at high altitude is more than that of those born to Han women living at the same altitude, which is associated with a higher uterine flow velocity and larger uterine arterial diameters [1]. The uterine arterial diameters in Andean pregnant women are also most doubling increased at high altitude whereas there are about half as much increase in European pregnant women [74]. As a result, Andean pregnant women have much higher uterine blood flows and birth weights of their babies than Europeans at high altitude. However, the values are the same at low altitude in both Andean and European women, which suggests a much higher protective effect of Andean ancestry at high altitude. The questions why long-resident high-altitude populations (such as Tibetan and Andean women) have higher resistant to the adverse effects of high-altitude hypoxia than the short-resident populations (such as Han and European women) are not fully understood. However, recent reports suggest that genetic background may play a key role in the altitude-related changes in birth weight and uterine blood flow [1].

3. Conclusion

The adaptation of the cardiovascular system to altitude is variable, depending on individual predisposition, the actual elevation, the rate of ascent, and the duration of exposure. In acute short-term exposure to HAH, the initial response is increasing sympathetic activity and hyperventilation resulting in increases in systemic vascular resistance, blood pressure, heart rate, and cardiac output. Pulmonary vasoconstriction leads to pulmonary hypertension. However, in response to acute HAH, cerebral blood flow (CBF) rises significantly to ensure an adequate supply of O_2 to meet the brain tissues' large and consistent demand. The sympathetic excitation results from acute HAH, partly through chemoreceptor reflexes and partly through altered baroreceptor function. In long-term HAH exposure or resident at high altitude, cardiovascular system progresses a compensatory adaptation. The cardiovascular system may promote adaptational changes in cardiovascular structure, remodeling, and functional proteins through different molecular mechanisms including epigenetic regulatory and/or genetic factor-mediated mechanisms. However, cardiovasculatures may progress a pathologic adaptation and develop a maladaptation syndrome known as high-altitude pulmonary edema, cerebral edema, chronic mountain sickness, pulmonary hypertension, heart failure, and fetal intrauterine growth restriction. In conclusion, cardiovascular system progresses a compensatory and pathologic adaptation to HAH. Understanding those adaptation processes will help us to reduce the development of adverse changes and simultaneously preserve the beneficial signs of the process of adaptation.

Author details

Jun Ke[1,2], Lei Wang[1,3] and Daliao Xiao[1*]

*Address all correspondence to: Dxiao@llu.edu

1 Center for Perinatal Biology, Department of Basic Science, Loma Linda University School of Medicine, Loma Linda, California, USA

2 Guangdong Cardiovascular Institute, Guangdong General Hospital, Guangdong Academy of Medical Science, Guangzhou, Guangdong, China

3 Department of Traditional Chinese Medicine, People's Hospital of Shanghai Putuo District, Shanghai, China

References

[1] Moore LG, Charles SM, Julian CG. Humans at high altitude: hypoxia and fetal growth. Respir Physiol Neurobiol 2011;178:181–190. DOI: 10.1016/j.resp.2011.04.017.

[2] Naeije R. Physiological adaptation of the cardiovascular system to high altitude. Prog Cardiovasc Dis 2010;52:456–466. DOI: 10.1016/j.pcad.2010.03.004.

[3] Wagner PD. Reduced maximal cardiac output at altitude—mechanisms and significance. Respir Physiol 2000;120:1–11. DOI: 10.1016/S0034-5687(99)00101-2.

[4] Klausen K. Cardiac output in man in rest and work during and after acclimatization to 3,800 m. J Appl Physiol 1966;21:609–616.

[5] Huez S, Retailleau K, Unger P, Pavelescu A, Vachiery JL, Derumeaux G, et al. Right and left ventricular adaptation to hypoxia: a tissue Doppler imaging study. Am J Physiol Heart Circ Physiol 2005;289:H1391–H1398. DOI: 10.1152/ajpheart.00332.2005.

[6] Liu Y, Zhang JH, Gao XB, Wu XJ, Yu J, Chen JF, et al. Correlation between blood pressure changes and AMS, sleeping quality and exercise upon high-altitude exposure in young Chinese men. Mil Med Res 2014;1:19. DOI: 10.1186/2054-9369-1-19.

[7] Rhodes HL, Chesterman K, Chan CW, Collins P, Kewley E, Pattinson KT, Myers S, Imray CH, Wright AD. Systemic blood pressure, arterial stiffness and pulse waveform analysis at altitude. JR Army Med Corps 2011;157:110–113. DOI: 10.1136/jramc-157-01-18.

[8] D'Este D, Mantovan R, Martino A, D'Este F, Artusi L, Allibardi P, Franceschi M, Zerio C, Pascotto P. The behavior of the arterial pressure at rest and under exertion in normotensive and hypertensive subjects exposed to acute hypoxia at a median altitude. G Ital Cardiol 1991;21:643–649.

[9] Clar C, Dorrington KL, Fatemian M, Robbins PA. Effects of 8 h of isocapnic hypoxia with and without muscarinic blockade on ventilation and heart rate in humans. Exp Physiol 2001;86:529–538.

[10] Princi T, Zupet P, Finderle Z, Accardo A. Linear and nonlinear assessment of heart rate variability in nonacclimatized middleaged subjects at different hypoxic levels. Biomed Sci Instrum 2008;44:380–385.

[11] Bogaard HJ, Hopkins SR, Yamaya Y, Niizeki K, Ziegler MG, Wagner PD. Role of the autonomic nervous system in the reduced maximal cardiac output at altitude. J Appl Physiol 2002;93:271–279. DOI: 10.1152/japplphysiol.00323.2001.

[12] Kotchen TA, Hogan RP, Boyd AF, Li TK, Sing HC, Mason JW. Reini, noradrenaline and adrenaline responses to simulated altitude. Clin Sci (Colch) 1973;44:243–251.

[13] Mazzeo RS, Bender PR, Brooks GA, Butterfield GE, Groves BM, Sutton JR, et al. Arterial catecholamine responses during exercise with acute and chronic high-altitude exposure. Am J Physiol 1991;261:E419–E424.

[14] Mazzeo RS, Child A, Butterfield GE, Mawson JT, Zamudio S, Moore LG. Catecholamine response during 12 days of high-altitude exposure (4, 300 m) in women. J Appl Physiol 1998;84(4):1151–1157.

[15] Bartsch P, Gibbs JS. Effect of altitude on the heart and the lungs. Circulation 2007;116:2191–2202. DOI: 10.1161/CIRCULATIONAHA.106.650796.

[16] Lahiri S, Mulligan E, Nishino T, Mokashi A, Davies RO. Relative responses of aortic body and carotid body chemoreceptors to carboxyhemoglobinemia. J Appl Physiol Respir Environ Exerc Physiol 1981;50:580–586.

[17] Niewinski P, Janczak D, Rucinski A, Tubek S, Engelman ZJ, Jazwiec P, et al. Dissociation between blood pressure and heart rate response to hypoxia after bilateral carotid body removal in men with systolic heart failure. Exp Physiol 2014;99:552–561. DOI: 10.1113/expphysiol.2013.075580.

[18] Kato H, Menon AS, Slutsky AS. Mechanisms mediating the heart rate response to hypoxemia. Circulation 1988;77:407–414.

[19] Hanada A, Sander M, Gonzalez-Alonso J. Human skeletal muscle sympathetic nerve activity, heart rate and limb haemodynamics with reduced blood oxygenation and exercise. J Physiol 2003;551:635–647. DOI: 10.1113/jphysiol.2003.044024.

[20] Halliwill JR, Morgan BJ, Charkoudian N. Peripheral chemoreflex and baroreflex interactions in cardiovascular regulation in humans. J Physiol 2003;552:295–302. DOI: 10.1113/jphysiol.2003.050708.

[21] Talbot NP, Balanos GM, Dorrington KL, Robbins PA. Two temporal components within the human pulmonary vascular response to approximately 2 h of isocapnic hypoxia. J Appl Physiol 2005;98:1125–1139.

[22] Olschewski A, Weir EK. Hypoxic pulmonary vasoconstriction and hypertension. In: Peacock A, Rubin LJ, Eds, Pulmonary Diseases and Their Treatment. London, UK: Arnold; 2004:33–44.

[23] Platoshyn O, Golovina VA, Bailey CL, Limsuwan A, Krick S, Juhaszova M, et al. Sustained membrane depolarization and pulmonary artery smooth muscle cell proliferation. Am J Physiol Cell Physiol 2000;279:C1540–C1549.

[24] Bartsch P, Mairbaurl H, Maggiorini M, Swenson E. Physiological aspects of high-altitude pulmonary edema. J Appl Physiol 2005;98:1101–1110. DOI: 10.1152/japplphysiol.01167.2004.

[25] Swenson ER, Bartsch P. High-altitude pulmonary edema. Compr Physiol 2012;2:2753–2773. DOI: 10.1002/cphy.c100029.

[26] Lucas SJ, Burgess KR, Thomas KN, Donnelly J, Peebles KC, Lucas RA, et al. Alterations in cerebral blood flow and cerebrovascular reactivity during 14 days at 5050 m. J Physiol 2011;589:741–753. DOI: 10.1113/jphysiol.2010.192534.

[27] Wilson MH, Edsell ME, Davagnanam I, Hirani SP, Martin DS, Levett DZ, et al. Cerebral artery dilatation maintains cerebral oxygenation at extreme altitude and in acute hypoxia—an ultrasound and MRI study. J Cereb Blood Flow Metab 2011;31:2019–2029. DOI: 10.1038/jcbfm.2011.81.

[28] Subudhi AW, Fan JL, Evero O, Bourdillon N, Kayser B, Julian CG, et al. AltitudeOmics: effect of ascent and acclimatization to 5260 m on regional cerebral oxygen delivery. Exp Physiol 2014;99:772–781. DOI: 10.1113/expphysiol.2013.075184.

[29] Ainslie PN, Ogoh S. Regulation of cerebral blood flow during chronic hypoxia: a matter of balance. Exp Physiol 2010;95:251–262. DOI: 10.1113/expphysiol.2008.045575.

[30] Firth PG, Zheng H, Windsor JS, Sutherland AI, Imray CH, Moore GW, Semple JL, Roach RC, Salisbury RA. Mortality on Mount Everest, 1921 to 2006: descriptive study. BMJ 2008;337:a2654. DOI: 10.1136/bmj.a2654.

[31] Hackett PH, Roach RC. High altitude cerebral edema. High Alt Med Biol 2004;5:136–146. DOI: 10.1089/1527029041352054.

[32] Suarez J, Alexander JK, Houston CS. Enhanced left ventricular systolic performance at high altitude during Operation Everest II. Am J Cardiol 1987;60:137–142.

[33] Boussuges A, Molenat F, Burnet H, Cauchy E, Gardette B, Sainty JM, et al. Operation Everest III (Comex '97): modifications of cardiac function secondary to altitude-induced hypoxia. An echocardiographic and Doppler study. Am J Respir Crit Care Med 2000;161:264–270. DOI: 10.1164/ajrccm.161.1.9902096.

[34] Mortimer Jr EA, Monson RR, McMahon B. Reduction in mortality from coronary heart disease in men residing at high altitude. N Engl J Med 1977;296:581–585.

[35] Turek, Z, Kubat K, Ringnalda BEM. Experimental myocardial infarction in rats acclimated to simulated high altitude. Basic Res Cardiol 1980;75:544–553.

[36] Neckar J, Szarszoi O, Koten L, Papousek F, Ostadal B, Grover GJ, Kolar F. Effects of mitochondrial KATP modulators on cardioprotection induced by chronic high altitude hypoxia in rats. Cardiovasc Res 2002:55:567–575. DOI: 10.1016/S0008-6363(02)00456-X.

[37] Tajima M, Katayose D, Bessho M, Isoyama S. Acute ischaemic preconditioning and chronic hypoxia independently increase myocardial tolerance to ischaemia. Cardiovasc Res 1994:28:312–319.

[38] Asemu G, Papousek F, Ostadal B, Kolar F. Adaptation to high altitude hypoxia protects the rat heart against ischemia-induced arrhythmias. Involvement of mitochondrial K (ATP) channel. J Mol Cell Cardiol 1999:31:1821–1831.

[39] La Padula P, Costa LE. Effect of sustained hypobaric hypoxia during maturation and aging on rat myocardium. I. Mechanical activity. J Appl Physiol 2005;98(6):2363–2369. DOI: 10.1152/japplphysiol.00988.2004.

[40] Boushel R, Calbet JA, Radegran G, Sondergaard H, Wagner PD, Saltin B. Parasympathetic neural activity accounts for the lowering of exercise heart rate at high altitude. Circulation 2001;104:1785–1791.

[41] Leon-Velarde F, Richalet JP, Chavez JC, Kacimi R, Rivera-Chira M, Palacios JA, et al. Hypoxia- and normoxia-induced reversibility of autonomic control in Andean guinea pig heart. J Appl Physiol 1996;81:2229–2234.

[42] Calbet JA. Chronic hypoxia increases blood pressure and noradrenaline spillover in healthy humans. J Physiol 2003;551:379–386. DOI: 10.1113/jphysiol.2003.045112.

[43] Mazzeo RS, Brooks GA, Butterfield GE, Podolin DA, Wolfel EE, Reeves JT. Acclimatization to high altitude increase muscle sympathetic activity both at rest and during exercise. Am J Physiol 1995;269:R201-R207.

[44] Kacimi R, Richalet JP, Corsin A, Abousahl I, Crozatier B. Hypoxia-induced downregulation of beta-adrenergic receptors in rat heart. J Appl Physiol 1992;73:1377–1382.

[45] Leon-Velarde F, Bourin MC, Germack R, Mohammadi K, Crozatier B, Richalet JP. Differential alterations in cardiac adrenergic signaling in chronic hypoxia or norepinephrine infusion. Am J Physiol Regul Integr Comp Physiol 2001;280:R274-R281.

[46] Richalet JP, Larmignat P, Rathat C, Keromes A, Baud P, Lhoste F. Decreased cardiac response to isoproterenol infusion in acute and chronic hypoxia. J Appl Physiol 1988;65:1957–1961.

[47] Fischetti F, Fabris B, Zaccaria M, Biagi A, Calci M, Candido R, et al. Effects of prolonged high-altitude exposure on peripheral adrenergic receptors in young healthy volunteers. Eur J Appl Physiol 2000;82:439–445.

[48] Gavras I, Manolis AJ, Gavras H. The alpha2-adrenergic receptors in hypertension and heart failure: experimental and clinical studies. J Hypertens 2001;19:2115–2124.

[49] Kolar F, Ostadal B. Right ventricular function in rats with hypoxic pulmonary hypertension. Pflugers Arch 1991;419:121–126.

[50] Ostadal B, Kolar F. Cardiac adaptation to chronic high-altitude hypoxia: beneficial and adverse effects. Respir Physiol Neurobiol 2007;158:224–236. DOI: 10.1016/j.resp.2007.03.005.

[51] Ostadal B, Mirejovska E, Hurych J, Pelouch V, Prochazka J. Effect of intermittent high altitude hypoxia on the synthesis of collagenous and non-collagenous proteins of the right and left ventricular myocardium. Cardiovasc Res 1978;12:303–308.

[52] Xu XQ, Jing ZC. High-altitude pulmonary hypertension. Eur Respir Rev 2009;18:13–17. DOI: 10.1183/09059180.00011104.

[53] Groves BM, Reeves JT, Sutton JR, Wagner PD, Cymerman A, Malconian MK, et al. Operation Everest II: elevated high-altitude pulmonary resistance unresponsive to oxygen. J Appl Physiol 1987;63:521–530.

[54] Stenmark KR, Fagan KA, Frid MG. Hypoxia-induced pulmonary vascular remodelling: cellular and molecular mechanisms. Circ Res 2006;99:675–691. DOI: 10.1161/01.RES.0000243584.45145.3f.

[55] Sheng L, Zhou W, Hislop AA, Ibe BO, Longo LD, Raj JU. Role of epidermal growth factor receptor in ovine fetal pulmonary vascular remodelling following exposure to high altitude long-term hypoxia. High Alt Med Biol 2009;10:365–372. DOI: 10.1089/ham.2008.1034.

[56] Ono S, Westcott JY, Voelkel NF. PAF antagonists inhibit pulmonary vascular remodelling induced by hypobaric hypoxia in rats. J Appl Physiol 1992;73:1084–1092.

[57] Bixby CE, Ibe BO, Abdallah MF, Zhou W, Hislop AA, Longo LD, Raj JU. Role of platelet-activating factor in pulmonary vascular remodeling associated with chronic high altitude hypoxia in ovine fetal lambs. Am J Physiol Lung Cell Mol Physiol 2007;293:L1475–L1482. DOI: 10.1152/ajplung.00089.2007.

[58] Remillard CV, Yuan JX. High altitude pulmonary hypertension: role of K+ and Ca2+ channels. High Alt Med Biol 2005;6:133–146. DOI: 10.1089/ham.2005.6.133.

[59] Gerasimovskaya EV, Davie NJ, Ahmad S, Tucker DA, White CW, Stenmark KR. Extracellular adenosine triphosphate: a potential regulator of vasa vasorum neovascularization in hypoxia-induced pulmonary vascular remodeling. Chest 2005;128:608s–610s. DOI: 10.1378/chest.128.6_suppl.608S.

[60] Emery CJ. Vascular remodelling in the lung. Eur Respir J 1994;7(2):217–219. DOI: 10.1183/09031936.94.07020217.

[61] Chen YF, Oparil S. Endothelin and pulmonary hypertension. J Cardiovasc Pharmacol 2000;35:S49–S53.

[62] Ainslie PN, Subudhi AW. Cerebral blood flow at high altitude. High Alt Med Biol 2014;15 (2):133–140. DOI: 10.1089/ham.2013.1138.

[63] Palmer SK, Zamudio S, Coffin C, Parker S, Stamm E, Moore LG. Quantitative estimation of human uterine artery blood flow and pelvic blood flow redistribution in pregnancy. Obstet Gynecol 1992;80:1000–1006.

[64] Burton GJ, Woods AW, Jauniaux E, Kingdom JC. Rheological and physiological consequences of conversion of the maternal spiral arteries for uteroplacental blood flow during human pregnancy. Placenta 2009;30:473–482. DOI: 10.1016/j.placenta.2009.02.009.

[65] Chang K, Xiao D, Huang X, Xue Z, Yang S, Longo LD, Zhang L. Chronic hypoxia inhibits sex steroid hormone-mediated attenuation of ovine uterine arterial myogenic tone in pregnancy. Hypertension 2010;56:750–757. DOI: 10.1161/HYPERTENSIONAHA. 110.155812.

[66] Xiao D, Zhang L. ERK MAP kinases regulate smooth muscle contraction in ovine uterine artery: effect of pregnancy. Am J Physiol Heart Circ Physiol 2002;282:H292–H300.

[67] Chang K, Xiao D, Huang X, Longo LD, Zhang L. Chronic hypoxia increases pressure-dependent myogenic tone of the uterine artery in pregnant sheep: role of ERK/PKC pathway. Am J Physiol Heart Circ Physiol 2009;296:H1840–H1849. DOI: 10.1152/ajpheart.00090.2009.

[68] Xiao D, Buchholz JN, Zhang L. Pregnancy attenuates uterine artery pressure-dependent vascular tone: role of PKC/ERK pathway. Am J Physiol Heart Circ Physiol 2006;290: H2337–H2343. DOI: 10.1152/ajpheart.01238.2005.

[69] Julian CG, Galan HL, Wilson MJ, Desilva W, Cioffi-Ragan D, Schwartz J, Moore LG. Lower uterine artery blood flow and higher endothelin relative to nitric oxide metabolite levels are associated with reductions in birth weight at high altitude. Am J Physiol Regul Integr Comp Physiol 2008;295:R906–R915. DOI: 10.1152/ajpregu.00164.2008.

[70] Rockwell LC, Dempsey EC, Moore LG. Chronic hypoxia diminishes the proliferative response of Guinea pig uterine artery vascular smooth muscle cells in vitro. High Alt Med Biol 2006;7:237–244. DOI: 10.1089/ham.2006.7. 237.

[71] Rosenfold CR, Toy T, DeSpain K, Cox BE. Large-conductance Ca2+ dependent K+ channels regulate basal uteroplacental blood flow in ovine pregnancy. J Soc Gynecol Investig 2005;12:402–408. DOI: 10.1016/j.jsgi. 2005.04.009.

[72] Hu XQ, Xiao D, Zhu R, Huang X, Yang S, Wilson SM, Zhang L. Chronic hypoxia suppresses pregnancy-induced upregulation of large-conductance Ca2+-activated K+ channel activity in uterine arteries. Hypertension 2012;60:214–222. DOI: 10.1161/HYPERTENSIONAHA.112.196097.

[73] Chen M, Xiao D, Hu XQ, Dasgupta C, Yang S, Zhang L. Hypoxia represses ER-alpha expression and inhibits estrogen-induced regulation of Ca2+-activated K+ channel activity and myogenic tone in ovine uterine arteries: causal role of DNA methylation. Hypertension 2015;66:44–51. DOI: 10.1161/HYPERTENSIONAHA.115.05299.

[74] Wilson MJ, Lopez M, Vargas M, Julian C, Tellez W, Rodriguez A, Bigham A, Armaza JF, Niermeyer S, Shriver M, Vargas E, Moore LG. Greater uterine artery blood flow during pregnancy in multigeneration (Andean) than shorter-term (European) high-altitude residents. Am J Physiol Regul Integr Comp Physiol 2007;293:R1313–R1324. DOI: 10.1152/ajpregu.00806.2006.

Chapter 7

Arterial Oxygen Saturation During Ascent to 5010 m: Heart Rate and AMS Scores

Christopher B. Wolff, Annabel H. Nickol and David J. Collier

Additional information is available at the end of the chapter

http://dx.doi.org/10.5772/66088

Abstract

The hypothesis here is that tissues exposed to the hypoxia of altitude have increased blood flow so that the rate of arrival of oxygen is as rapid as normal. If the ascent is too rapid, the system starts to fail. The study involves an ascent to high altitude (5010 m) during which 59 subjects recorded their resting arterial oxygen saturation (SaO_2), heart rate (HR) and Lake Louise acute mountain sickness (AMS) scores, twice daily. During the major ascent SaO_2 fell progressively. In 42 subjects, HR increased in a highly significant, negative, relationship to SaO_2. In 10 subjects heart rate (HR) remained unchanged. Three subjects showed extreme HR variability. Data were incomplete in four subjects. For nine of the subjects, showing the progressive HR versus SaO_2 correlation during ascent, the sequence terminated with a lower HR than would be expected from the correlation so far. Individual AMS scores showed no correlation with SaO_2 but averaged values from 19 of the subjects from each 'one night' stopover; showed a strong, negative, correlation. Average stopover HR values correlated negatively with the average SaO_2 values. Cardiac output (CO) is likely to have increased during ascent as HR increased, since there is a progressive relationship between HR and cardiac output (CO). Hence, despite the progressive fall in SaO_2, tissue oxygen delivery (DO_2) would have remained close to normal in the 42 subjects who showed the significant HR: SaO_2 relationship.

Keywords: high altitude, SaO_2, heart rate, acute mountain sickness, oxygen delivery

1. Introduction

During ascent to high altitude, the fractional concentration of oxygen in the atmospheric gas is unchanged but overall barometric pressure falls. This means that there are less oxygen molecules per unit volume, so the activity, or oxygen partial pressure, falls. Breathing will only compensate for this, with a closer approach to normal concentration of oxygen in the blood (known as 'content,' CaO_2), if it is increased. Initially, lowered oxygen in the lung and hence in the blood causes blood flow to the brain to increase, washing out carbon dioxide (CO_2) from the brain environment. The increase in blood flow allows the rate of arrival of oxygen at the brain to normalize, the higher flow compensating for the lower CaO_2. So the rate of arrival of oxygen (oxygen delivery, DO_2) is sustained at or near the normal rate—three times the rate of cerebral oxygen consumption cerebral metabolic rate for oxygen, $CMRO_2$ [1]. However, the lower CO_2 in the brain, and resulting alkalinity, inhibits breathing via the central chemoreceptor, counteracting the stimulating effect of low oxygen at the peripheral arterial chemoreceptor. There is therefore an initial pause in ventilatory stimulation. Over 2–5 days, for a subject remaining at the same altitude, brain inhibition is removed as acidity is corrected. This restores the central chemoreceptor level of respiratory stimulus (removal of inhibition). So now the ventilatory stimulus from the peripheral arterial chemoreceptor activity stimulates ventilation, with improvement in the arterial oxygen level [1]. Since these effects are operating at the same time as subjects ascend, with environmental oxygen falling progressively, arterial oxygen content (CaO_2) and oxygen saturation (SaO_2) usually fall progressively during ascent.

Since individual breathing responses (known as ventilatory responses) vary between individuals the progressive drop in CaO_2 also varies between individuals. Most of the oxygen in the blood is carried on hemoglobin in the red cells and low CaO_2 is paralleled by lower arterial oxygen saturation of the hemoglobin (SaO_2). With little change in hemoglobin concentration (Hb) during ascent, SaO_2 therefore provides a guide to CaO_2 change. If there was no change in cardiac output (CO) the rate of oxygen delivery to the tissues ($DO_2 = CO \times CaO_2$) would fall in proportion to the fall in SaO_2. Here we are interested in the possibility that there may be compensatory increases in CO helping to sustain a more normal DO_2. During ascent, the use of a pulse oximeter provides SaO_2 and also gives the heart rate (HR). Cardiac output is equal to stroke volume (SV) times HR, that is, $CO = HR \times SV$. With only modest changes in SV during ascent HR changes can therefore act as a surrogate for CO changes. Increases in HR as SaO_2 falls during ascent would suggest that CO increases too. Increases in CO as SaO_2/CaO_2 fall will mean that there is compensatory response helping to maintain DO_2. It is therefore important to see whether there is a significant HR increase in relation to falling SaO_2 and to see whether this occurs in all or some subjects. Increases in heart rate can therefore be used as an indirect indicator of any cardiac output increase mitigating DO_2 reduction.

In a recent high-altitude study [2], undertaken in South America, eight normal subjects acclimatized to moderately high altitude during an initial 5-day sojourn at Cusco (3324 m). This was followed by two brief ascents to around 5000 m over a 4-week period. The preliminary acclimatization and brief ascents meant the subjects were likely to be less stressed by their hypoxic exposure than occurs with progressive ascents from sea level. Total time at high

http://dx.doi.org/10.5772/66088

altitude was 28 days, the largest proportion at Cusco. SaO_2 and HR were recorded twice daily. For seven of the subjects, there was a highly significant relationship between HR and SaO_2, with the highest HR accompanying the lowest SaO_2 value. The remaining subject sustained near normal SaO_2 and HR. HR × SaO_2 (assumed to give a value changing in relation to DO_2) remained near constant throughout the trek in all subjects. Since HR × SaO_2 will have a similar trend to CO × CaO_2, DO_2 will have been well sustained despite the varying degrees of hypoxia. Despite apparently relatively good DO_2 maintenance, for these subjects, individual mean acute mountain sickness (AMS) scores correlated significantly with mean SaO_2 values both at rest and with mild exercise (30 cm step up over 2 min).

In a second high-altitude study, undertaken by 14 schoolboys and their teacher, an ascent was made to Annapurna base camp (4130 m) [3]. There was no preliminary acclimatization and, due to shortage of stopover sites, the final two ascent stages were large. The subjects each recorded SaO_2 and HR soon after arrival at each new altitude both at rest and with mild exercise. Not all subjects showed individually significant HR versus SaO_2 changes, but the overview across subjects (mean values at each altitude) was highly significant both for rest and exercise. Of interest was the fact that, for exercise, HR × SaO_2, otherwise constant, showed a large fall for the last ascent stage and base camp. Anecdotally, most subjects suffered considerable AMS symptoms during the 1 day stop at base camp. A plot of the mean values of HR versus SaO_2 for exercise shows a highly significant trend (**Figure 1**), but the HR value for base camp gives a point lower than expected from the rest of the values trend for HR versus SaO_2. This may well represent a failure of DO_2 compensation.

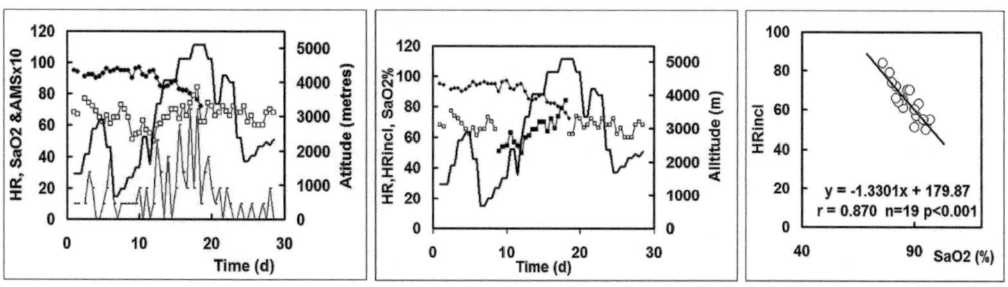

Figure 1. Data from this subject (15) illustrates rising HR during ascent. On the left HR (open squares), SaO_2 (filled circles) and AMS × 10 scores (mini flags) are shown (left hand axis) with altitude (right hand axis, continuous line). The middle plot shows the ascending values of HR as filled squares and omits the AMS scores. The plot on the right shows the ascending HR values plotted against SaO_2—slope significant at the $p < 0.001$ level.

1.1. Reasons why DO_2 control is important

Surprisingly, oxygen combines extreme toxicity with capability to provide energy more efficiently than other biochemical means utilized by other species. The ready conversion of oxygen to dangerous free radicals is largely prevented in our cells by the specific energy-generating biochemical sequences, especially featuring the Krebs cycle. There is an optimum rate at which oxygen flows to a particular tissue and this bears a constant relationship to the rate at which oxygen is utilized (VO_2). Hence, we have values for DO_2/VO_2 which are normally sustained at values specific to the tissue: for the brain 3:1, for heart 1.6:1 and at exercise rates below competitive levels skeletal muscle sustains a ratio 1.5:1 [4]. Maintaining these DO_2 values not only provides sufficient oxygen but also avoids an excess, which would endanger toxicity. Inadequacy of oxygen supply can endanger life following surgery partly from a tendency for an oxygen debt to develop during an operation. This results from reduced arterial pressure since some of the arterial volume escapes into veins relaxed by the anesthesia. The reduced pressure lowers cardiac output so that DO_2 falls, hence development of an oxygen debt [5].

Cerebral arterial blood flow and metabolic rate obtained by Severinghaus et al. [6] were further examined and showed that cerebral oxygen delivery was sustained after ascent to 3100 m, over the next 5 days. There was an initial fall in SaO_2 and compensatory rise in cerebral blood flow. The acclimatization process allowed the initially lowest SaO_2 to improve over the 5 days at altitude [7, 8].

2. Methods

Fifty-nine normal subjects undertook the trek to Kanchenjunga base camp (altitude 5010 m) from Kathmandu (1345 m). The first leg by plane took them to Tumlingtar (470 m) and then they made an initial partial ascent to 2900 m. There was then a descent to 675 m by the 7th day. From there, the rest of the trek (the main ascent) took around 14 days (a conservative ascent profile of just over 300 m per day). Parties of 7–11 subjects set off from Kathmandu separated by a few days. Each group was accompanied by porters and cooks who went ahead each day to prepare the next stopover site. Porters and yaks carried most of the research equipment for other studies and much of the individual luggage, largely housed in individual 60 L barrels. This meant that each subject carried a low-weight 'day pack.' Each subject measured their arterial saturation (SaO_2) and heart rate (HR) using a (Nonin, model 9500, Nonin Medical Inc. MIN, USA) oximeter. The evening measurement was made after at least 5 min rest, seated in the mess tent prior to supper. Readings were made after around 1 min to allow stability. A second measurement of SaO_2 and HR was made in the morning at each stopover site. Again, each measurement was made after at least 5 min rest in the mess tent prior to breakfast. At both morning and evening sessions, each subject filled in individual 'altitude sickness scores' for each of five symptom complexes (head, guts, tired, dizzy, sleep). Each category belongs to the mode of acute mountain sickness (AMS) assessment known as the Lake Louise consensus AMS scoring system [9]. The numerical system requires scores of 0–3 for each category. The AMS score is the total of the values entered in each category. For each category, zero represents no effect and for three, the symptom in the category is severe. Hence, the total possible range, theoretically, for a given score is from 0 to 15. A subject is deemed to be sick, however, with AMS with scores above 3.

3. Results

AMS scores showed no obvious trends during the major ascent for any individual, whereas SaO_2 fell during ascent in all cases (where the data had been recorded—a few subjects omitted variable amounts of data). The heart rate, however, showed an obvious progressively increasing trend in 42 individuals. For 10 subjects, there was no HR change during ascent.

Figure 1 shows a particularly clear example of increasing HR and decreasing SaO_2 for one individual during the major ascent. The AMS score is included in the left-hand panel and omitted in the middle panel, where the square HR symbol during ascent is filled in, to emphasis the progressively increasing HR. In the right-hand panel, HR from the ascent is plotted against SaO_2, showing the highly significant trend in this subject. For the 42 subjects showing increasing HR during ascent and falling SaO_2, individual least squares regression plots (HR versus SaO_2) give significance levels (p values). The degree of the HR versus SaO_2 relationship significance is shown for each subject in **Table 1**, according to the subject's identification number. Nineteen subjects (32%) showed significance at the 0.001 level; 17 (29%) at the 0.01 level and for 6 subjects (10%) significance level was only 0.05. The status for each of the remaining subjects is also shown: four subjects with poor data (very few recorded points or none at all), three subjects with apparently random data (labeled 'variability') and the ten subjects in whom HR was effectively unchanged. **Figure 2** shows HR, SaO_2, AMS score and altitude against time for three of the subjects in whom there was an unchanging HR. The first stopped recording prior to reaching base camp, the second stopped recording at base camp and the third continued, at least HR recording, even during descent.

Significance	Subject No.	Total	Percent
<0.001	1,3,6,8,20,25,26,27,30,32,34,36,40,48, 51,54,55,56,57	19	32
<0.01	4,16,17,21,22,23,24,31,33,35,39,43,45,46,47,50,52	17	29
<0.05	14,28,49,53,58,59	6	10
Ns			29
Poor data	2,5,13,29	4	
Variability	12,18,11	3	
Constant HR	7,9,10,15,19,37,38,41,42,44	10	

Table 1. Listing of all subjects according to (a) whether they showed a significant relationship between HR and SaO_2 during ascent in the upper part of the table ($p < 0.001$, $p < 0.01$ and $p < 0.05$) and (b) those without a significant relationship (poor data, variability or a constant HR).

In the face of any clear individual indication of progress of AMS scores during ascent, it was important to see whether the expected general tendency held good. Mean values for AMS scores and for HR and SaO_2 were calculated for 19 subjects (numbers 1–19) at each altitude. Mean AMS increased progressively with increasing altitude and was significantly related to SaO_2 (**Figure 3**, middle panel). This simply confirms the trend expected with ascent to altitude.

Mean arterial oxygen saturation at each one-night stopover fell progressively during ascent (**Figure 3**, left panel, $SaO_2\% = -0.0043 \times$ altitude (m) + 102.24; $R^2 = 0.972$) though there was considerable variation for the mean values at each stopover site. The error bars show the maximum and minimum individual values.

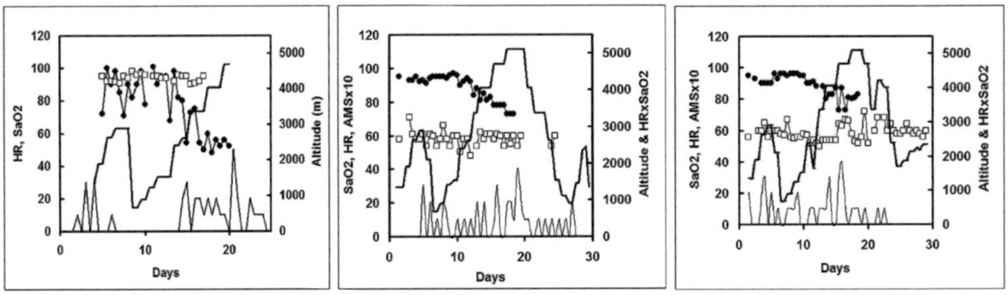

Figure 2. Plots against time of HR (open squares), SaO_2 (filled circles), AMS score (mini-flag) and altitude (continuous line) against time. Each is an example of data from a subject in whom HR remained near constant (subjects, 15, 44 and 38).

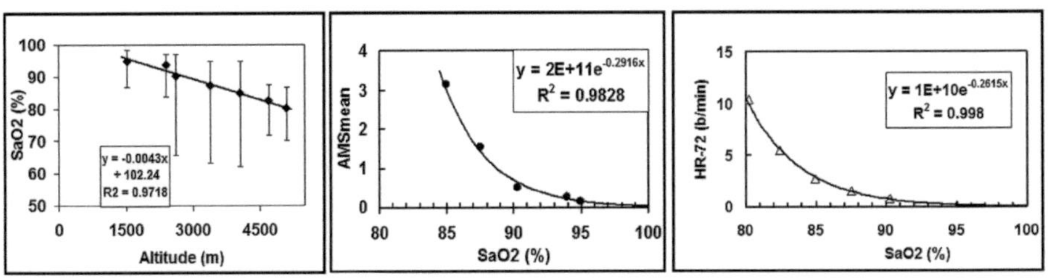

Figure 3. Mean values at each altitude of, $SaO_2\%$, AMS score and HR. The left panel shows SaO_2 against altitude with maximum and minimum values as 'error bars.' The middle panel shows mean AMS score against SaO_2 for one-night stopovers during the major ascent. The right-hand panel shows mean (HR - 72) plotted against $SaO_2\%$ above the first two stopovers of the major ascent. The points are from the lowest altitudes were probably from subjects who were not fully rested).

For mean HR (minus 72 as an assumed normal at sea level), values at each stopover site show a smooth relationship to SaO_2 for altitudes above 2400 m (**Figure 3**, right-hand panel). The higher mean HR at lower SaO_2 is consistent with the tendency for an increasing heart rate during ascent, found for most individuals.

Most subjects in the present study ($n = 42$, 71%) showed the significant HR: SaO_2 relationship. The trend relative to SaO_2 was sustained in 33 subjects; however, for nine subjects (numbered: 20, 25, 48, 50, 52, 53, 55, 56 and 57), the trend ended at the lowest SaO_2 with a lower HR than predicted by the trend to date. **Figure 4** shows an example (subject 25). HR (open rectangles) changes in the figure during base camp to larger open circles, where the points are obviously lower than expected from the trend during ascent. Although anecdotal, it may be no coincidence that the AMS scores are at their maximum at the same time.

Most subjects in the present study (n = 42, 71%) showed the significant HR: SaO_2 relationship. The trend relative to SaO_2 was sustained in 33 subjects; however, for nine subjects (numbered: 20, 25, 48, 50, 52, 53, 55, 56 and 57), the trend ended at the lowest SaO_2 with a lower HR than predicted by the trend to date. **Figure 4** shows an example (subject 25). HR (open rectangles) change in the figure during base camp to larger open circles, where the points are obviously lower than expected from the trend during ascent. Although anecdotal, it may be no coincidence that the AMS scores are at their maximum at the same time.

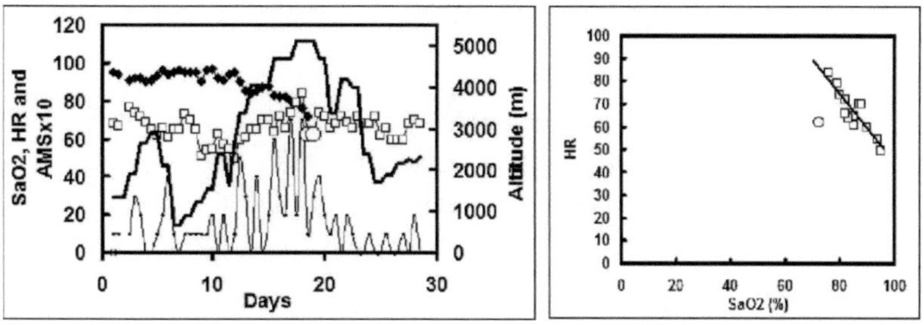

Figure 4. Example of late fall in HR. For subject 25, there was a steady rise in HR (left figure, open squares) during ascent (the period 9–18 days—from 1235 m to base camp at 5100 m). The next two values of HR after reaching base camp (large open circles) were significantly reduced. SaO_2 (filled diamonds) had fallen as usual during ascent. On the left, altitude is shown as a continuous line and AMS score (×10) shows as a thin jagged line. The plot on the right shows HR during the ascent plotted against SaO_2. The open circle represents the one of the two lower HR values for which SaO_2 was recorded. The lowered HR is thought to reflect impaired compensation for hypoxia.

4. Discussion

This HR, SaO_2 and AMS data, collected during a high-altitude trek to Kanchenjunga base camp in 1998, has shown important variations in individual responses. These differences raise questions concerning physiological mechanisms, such as the reason why a significant proportion of subjects (10 out of a total of 59 or 52 if we exclude 3 with inadequate data and variability—see **Table 1**) maintained a constant resting HR, despite falling SaO_2 during ascent. In contrast, in most subjects (42), HR increased in relation to falling SaO_2. Despite inspection of the individual time-based plots of AMS scores, there seemed no help there with its prediction, though there was, of course, the overall upward trend in the average AMS scores during ascent, accompanying lowered SaO_2 (**Figure 3**, middle panel).

A highly significant difference in vulnerability to acute mountain sickness (AMS) has been shown to be related to differences in the type of ACE gene (angiotensin-converting enzyme) carried by the subject. It is part of the renin-angiotensin system, which regulates blood pressure and the balance of fluids and salts in the body. Those with so-called 'double insertion' of the ACE gene experience far less trouble with high-altitude ascent than do those with 'double deletion.' Subjects with the mixed 'insertion/deletion' properties are intermediate [10]. It seems likely that good compensation with maintained DO_2 will be the background reason for the altitude advantage of those with double insertion ACE gene but this, of course, would need detailed examination in a major study. It is also possible that the subjects who sustained a constant heart rate with progressive lowering of SaO_2 belong to the double deletion group. Specific measurement would be required in the study to answer this question. There seems no known difference in responses to hypoxic exposure between men and women.

The significant inverse correlation between HR and SaO_2 in 42 subjects is consistent with the DO_2 priority of body tissues, illustrated for skeletal muscle [11], the brain [7, 8] and heart [4] and demonstrated for the whole body [12] in subjects breathing 12% oxygen—resting DO_2 for each individual was the same on 12% oxygen as on air, despite variations in SaO_2 in each individual on 12% oxygen.

It has been pointed out that HR usually increases as CO increases, but there may not have been complete DO_2 compensation in those who increased their HR during ascent. It is possible that the CO increase falls short of sustaining normal DO_2. Again, it would be useful to know whether the compensation indicated by the HR increase with falling SaO_2 is actually complete.

The depression of HR below that expected from the trend, usually found when it occurs, close to or actually at base camp was most likely to reflect inadequate DO_2. If this did represent a significant fall in DO_2 such subjects could be more vulnerable to AMS. For the subject, illustrated AMS scores were already increasing. It would be helpful in confirmation or refutation of assertions about HR if CO (in preference to HR) could be measured during ascent. Suitable portable equipment is awaited though none is at present on the horizon.

4.1. The value of the study

It is hoped that the illustration here of a variety of different features of the responses of individuals to the hypoxic environment of altitude will help guide future investigation and throw light on mechanisms responsible for AMS.

The study reported here is consistent with the ability of the body to sustain normal and adequate rates of oxygen delivery to the tissues. This has been shown to be limited by the severity of the hypoxic exposure with variation between subjects as to whether the limit is reached, the level of SaO_2 at which it happens, and the fact that a significant proportion of subjects do not make the compensatory adjustments seen in the majority.

The novelty of this study is the new insight that the heart rate increase is a reflection of increased cardiac output sustaining a compensatory rate of oxygen delivery to the tissues. When the heart rate fails to increase as expected from results to date it may be a clue that compensation is failing.

Acknowledgements

Thanks are due to Medical Expeditions (Altitude Education and Research Charity). This work was facilitated by the NIHRB Biomedical Research Unit in Cardiovascular Disease at Barts.

http://dx.doi.org/10.5772/66088

Author details

Christopher B. Wolff[1*], Annabel H. Nickol[2] and David J. Collier[1]

*Address all correspondence to: chriswolff@doctors.org.uk

1 William Harvey Heart Centre, Barts and the London School of Medicine and Dentistry, Queen Mary University of London, London, UK

2 Oxford Centre, for Respiratory Medicine, Churchill Hospital, Oxford, UK

References

[1] Wolff CB. Physiological processes during respiratory acclimatization to low inspired oxygen. In: Mountains: Geology, Topography and Environmental Concern. Goncalves AJB and Vieria AAB, Nova publishers, Hauppauge, New York 2014, Ch. 11.

[2] Brierley G, Parks T, Wolff CB. The relationship of acute mountain sickness to arterial oxygen saturation at altitudes of 3324 to 5176 m. Adv Exp Med Biol. 2012;737:207–212.

[3] Holdsworth L and Wolff CB. Oxygen delivery deficit in exercise with rapid ascent to high altitude. Adv Exp Med Biol. 2013;765:95–99.

[4] Wolff CB Normal cardiac output, oxygen delivery and oxygen extraction. Adv Exp Med Biol. 2007;599:169–182.

[5] Shoemaker WC, Appel PL, Kram HB. Role of oxygen debt in the development of organ failure, sepsis and death in high-risk surgical patients, Chest. 1992;102:208–215.

[6] Severinghaus JW, Chiodi H, Eger EI, Brandstater B, Hornbein TF. Cerebral blood flow in man at high altitude. Circ Res. 1966;19:274–282.

[7] Wolff CB. Cerebral blood flow and oxygen delivery at high altitude. High Altd Med Biol. 2000;1(1):33–38.

[8] Wolff CB, Barry P, Collier DJ. Cardiovascular and respiratory adjustments at altitude sustain cerebral oxygen delivery – Severinghaus revisited. Comp Bioch and Physiol Part A. 2002;132:221–229.

[9] Hackett PH and Oeltz O. The Lake Louis Consensus on the definition and quantification of altitude illness. In: Hypoxia and Mountain Medicine, edited by Sutton JR, Coates G and Houston CS. Burlington: Queen City Printers, 1992, pp 327–330.

[10] Montgomery HE, Marshall RM, Hemingway H Myerson S, Clarkson P, Dollery C et al. Human gene for physical performance. Nature (London). 1998;393:221–222

[11] Wolff CB. Cardiac output, oxygen consumption and muscle oxygen delivery in submaximal exercise: normal and low O_2 states. Adv Exp Med Biol. 2003;510:279–284.

[12] Bell M, Thake CD, Wolff CB. Effect of Inspiration of 12% O_2 (balance N_2) on cardiac output, respiration, oxygen saturation and oxygen delivery. Adv Exp Med Biol. 2011;915:327–332.

Chapter 8

Hypoxia-Induced Molecular and Cellular Changes in the Congenitally Diseased Heart: Mechanisms and Strategies of Intervention

Dominga Iacobazzi, Massimo Caputo and
Mohamed T Ghorbel

Additional information is available at the end of the chapter

http://dx.doi.org/10.5772/66038

Abstract

Tissue hypoxia plays a critical role in the pathobiology of congenital heart diseases, especially with regard to cyanotic patients. Here, we describe the cellular and molecular mechanisms induced by hypoxia in the diseased heart, with particular attention to the metabolic and functional changes that underlie the hypoxia-induced right ventricle remodelling. The role of reactive oxygen species in transcriptomic changes, DNA damage, contractile dysfunction and extracellular matrix remodelling will be addressed. Furthermore, the reoxygenation injury, which occurs when oxygen is reintroduced upon initiation of cardiopulmonary bypass, will be discussed. This allows a better understanding of the risks associated with the reoxygenation injury in children undergoing open-heart surgery and helps to improve strategies of intervention for myocardial protection.

Keywords: hypoxia, congenital heart disease, cyanosis, reoxygenation injury, cardiovascular disease

1. Hypoxia in cardiovascular disease and congenital heart disease

The term hypoxia refers to a condition where the tissues are not adequately oxygenated, usually due to interrupted coronary blood flow or a reduction in arterial blood oxygen partial pressure [1]. With the heart being a highly oxidative organ, relying on high oxygen consumption for the work of its contractile machinery, it appears obvious that cardiac cells are very sensitive to oxygen deprivation [2]. Heart hypoxia, which originates as a result of disproportion between the amount of oxygen supplied to the cardiac cell and the amount required by the cell, plays a critical role in the pathobiology of several cardiovascular diseases [3]. These include myocardial infarction, coronary artery diseases, heart failure secondary to pulmonary disease and congenital heart diseases [1, 4, 5]. In patients with coronary artery diseases and myocardial infarction, hypoxia is usually due to the formation of an atherosclerotic plaque in the wall of coronary arteries, which reduces the perfusion of myocardial tissue [6]. In addition, a rupture of the plaque might result in complete arterial occlusion, leading to the death of the ischemic tissue [6]. The increased O_2 consumption caused by pressure overload and reduced O_2 delivery, due to impaired coronary blood flow, are the main causes of hypoxia in patients suffering from heart failure secondary to pulmonary hypertension [7].

The scenario looks different when shifting the focus to myocardial hypoxia in paediatric patients with congenital heart diseases (CHDs). Diseases affecting the heart, in fact, have usually a different pathophysiology in children compared to adult population [8]. Furthermore, as a result of the different pathophysiological function of the defective heart, the paediatric and adult patients are differently susceptible to stress insults, although there is still disagreement on whether the vulnerability of immature heart is less or more than for adult heart [9–12].

Congenital heart diseases include a wide spectrum of anomalies of the cardiac architecture, and they are usually classified based on the anatomical and pathophysiological nature of the defect. The main anomalies involve atrioventricular junctions and valves [i.e. atrial septal defect (ASD), ventricular septal defect (VSD), atrioventricular septal defect (AVSD)], the ventricular outflow tracts [like in tetralogy of Fallot (TOF)] or can consist of univentricular hearts [like single ventricle (SV)] [13].

More often, congenital heart defects are simply classified as cyanotic and acyanotic, depending on whether or not the defect affects the amount of oxygen in the body. In cyanotic heart defects, as consequence of a mixture between oxygenated and de-oxygenated blood, less oxygen-rich blood reaches the different tissues of the body, resulting in a bluish skin, lips and nail bed colour. This category includes defects such as TOF, transposition of the great vessels or truncus arteriosus. On the other hand, non-cyanotic CHD patients do not experience a lack in blood oxygen supply; therefore, they rarely develop the bluish colour, except for few occasion, when the baby needs more oxygen, such as when crying and feeding. Atrial and/or ventricular septal defects or coarctation of the aorta are examples of acyanotic CHDs [14, 15].

Several studies have shown that, among CHDs, cyanotic patients are much more prone to develop a severe chronic hypoxia state, compared to the acyanotic ones, as the lack of oxygen exposes the cardiac tissue to an increase in free oxygen radicals [16, 17]. Therefore, when considering the treatment of these patients, the oxidative stress problem has to be taken into account, in addition to the other anomalies that characterize these defects. Nevertheless, care must be taken also for the treatment of acyanotic patients, to prevent the hypoxia that might develop in a later stage.

2. Mechanism underlying the hypoxia response in Congenital Heart Disease

2.1. Depletion of antioxidant defences

The exposure of a defective heart to chronic hypoxia induces molecular and cellular changes that affect the myocardial function and metabolism. One of the most typical sign of a heart-developing chronic hypoxia is the unbalance between the level of reactive oxygen species (ROS) and the antioxidant defence system. ROS are physiologically produced during cell metabolic and energetic reactions [18]. Nevertheless, the body is endowed with antioxidant enzymes such as catalase, glutathione peroxidase, and superoxide dismutase and vitamins (retinoic acid, alpha-tocopherol, ascorbic acid) that can counteract this physiological production [19]. Even in case of excessive free radical production, the body responds to restore harmony balance [20]. However, under chronic hypoxia, a downregulation of antioxidant defences occurs, making the cells vulnerable to oxidant damage. Two different studies analysing the oxidant status of paediatric patients with CHDs revealed that the oxidative stress index, given by the ratio between pro-oxidants and antioxidants factors, was higher in the plasma of cyanotic children compared to the controls [16, 17]. No difference was found between acyanotic and control groups, thus confirming that the anatomical defect dictates the hypoxic level and the oxidative status [16, 17].

2.2. Hypoxia-induced metabolic and functional changes: the basis of right ventricle remodelling

Metabolic markers of oxidative stress, such as 8-isoprostane, were shown to be high in cyanotic patients' heart as revealed by our study evaluating the transcriptomic analysis of patients with tetralogy of Fallot (TOF) [21]. In a different study, we performed a genome-wide investigation to determine the global gene expression profiles associated with chronic hypoxia in the heart of patients with TOF, undergoing corrective cardiac surgery. The data revealed that 795 genes were differently expressed in cyanotic versus acyanotic hearts. In particular, genes associated with the contractility machinery function and MAPK signalling, involved in cell survival and antioxidant defence, were downregulated, whereas growth, remodelling and apoptosis-related genes were upregulated in the cyanotic group compared to the acyanotic one [22].

The altered gene expression triggered by the rise in reactive oxygen species is mostly responsible for the cellular and molecular changes that affect the myocardial function and metabolism, thus predisposing the heart to hypertrophy and failure. The hypoxia-induced downregulation of the sodium-calcium (Na^+–Ca^{2+}) exchanger (NCX1) in cyanotic patients decreases myocyte calcium handling capacity, leading to mechanical dysfunction [22]. In addition, ROS can induce oxidative modification of the sarcoplasmic membrane channels: the ryanodine receptor2 (RyR2) becomes abnormally activated while sarcoplasmic reticulum Ca^{2+}-ATPase (SERCA) is inhibited, causing an abnormal Ca^{2+} transient between cytosol and sarcoplasmic reticulum that contributes to the cardiomyocytes contractile dysfunction [23, 24]. ROS accumulation has also a detrimental effect on mitochondrial function by sustaining mitochondrial permeability transition pore (mPTP) opening and mitochondrial membrane depolarization. As a result, mitochondrial respiration is inhibited with less ATP production. The insufficient energy production also arises from the switch from an aerobic metabolism to a high glycolytic metabolic profile. Protein kinase D (PDK), which inhibits pyruvate dehydrogenase during glucose oxidation, is a key factor in the deficient energy supply [25, 26]. Another aspect of redox imbalance is the extracellular matrix (ECM) modification deriving from the matrix metalloproteinases (MMP) activation, which leads to heart remodelling and fibrosis [27].

Within the complex architecture of the heart, the right ventricle (RV) seems to be the most susceptible structure to be affected by the above-mentioned hypoxia-induced changes. The different morphology and metabolism between the left and the right ventricle can in part explain the different susceptibility [28]. Furthermore, the anatomy of most of the CHD exposes the right ventricle to higher stresses, making it more prone to fail than the left counterpart [24]. One of the main insults to which the RV is subjected is the pressure overload that can derive from pulmonary artery hypertension (PAH) or RV outflow obstruction, with both events leading to right ventricular hypertrophy (RVH) and eventually to right ventricular failure.

2.3. HIF-1alpha mediated angiogenic response

One of the key features of chronic hypoxia is the activation of the HIF-1alpha (HIF-1α) signalling, an essential regulator of the angiogenic response. The mechanisms by which HIF-1α is triggered are relatively well-understood: under hypoxia, HIF1-alpha degradation is prevented by the hydroxylation of specific protein residues, and therefore, its translocation to the nucleus promotes the transcriptions of pro-angiogenic genes like vascular endothelial growth factor (VEGF), platelet-derived endothelial cell growth factor/thymidine phosphorylase (PD-ECGF/TP) and erythropoietin (EPO) [29–31].

The role of HIF-1α in adult ischemic heart disease and pressure overload heart failure has been widely demonstrated by different research groups [6, 30, 32]. However, only few studies have investigated its involvement in the pathogenesis of congenital heart disease [6, 33, 34].

An important increase in HIF-1α and related pro-angiogenic genes and proteins have been reported in ventricular biopsies from children with cyanotic congenital heart disease, compared with acyanotic or control groups [22, 35]. In addition, mRNA level of HIF-1α as well as that of two of its representative target genes, VEGF and EPO, were found to be upregulated in blood samples of newborns with cyanosis and persistent pulmonary hypertension, therefore representing early markers of generalized hypoxia [36]. If the HIF-1α/VEGF-induced collateral vessel formation in hypoxemic myocardium is essential to compensate the lack of oxygen supply in cyanotic hearts, especially in cases of coarctation of aorta, an abnormal vessel formation can become a source of morbidity, due to arteriovenous malformations [34]. However, a correlation between VEGF increase and abnormal vessel formation has not yet been found [37]. Nevertheless, increased activation of HIF-1α/VEGF signalling might be detrimental in newborn with persistent pulmonary hypertension, as these patients normally present an overexpression of VEGF receptor 1 (VEGFR1), which accounts for the vasoconstrictor effect of VEGF [38].

Further mechanisms, independent from HIF-1α might account for the hypoxia-induced VEGF production in CHDs. As hypoxia is often associated with tissue damage and apoptosis, cytokines or other mediators (IL-10, TNF-α, TGF-β, etc.) might as well initiate the cascade that leads to VEGF production [31].

2.4. Hypoxia-induced DNA damage

The induction of p53 pathway, as a result of the ROS accumulation triggered by hypoxia, is one of the primary event that initiates the apoptotic cascade that occurs in hypoxic states. The activation of p53 leads to an altered expression of the pro-apoptotic gene Bcl-2, which, in turn, causes the DNA damage [39]. It has been shown that the extent of DNA damage depends on the anatomical anomaly and to the grade of cyanosis, with persistent cyanotic patients being more prone to DNA damage. In particular, children with TOF and with septal defects associated with great vessel anomaly displayed a significantly increased DNA damage compared to the ones with isolated septal defects [39, 40]. These data support the evidence that DNA damage can represent a marker of oxidative stress in CHDs as well as the common biochemical modifications and the oxidant status index.

2.5. miRNA involvement in myocardial adaptation to chronic hypoxia

Among the tissue and circulating biomarkers, microRNAs (miRNAs) have emerged as important tools to assess the hypoxic status of a variety of organs. Briefly, miRNAs are small (19–24 nucleotides) non-coding single-stranded RNAs that form complementary pair with specific target mRNAs to negatively regulate these mRNAs' expression via translational repression or degradation [41]. It has been documented that a hypoxic environment can alter the miRNA profile and their regulation of related pathways, especially with regard to apoptosis/proliferation functions [42]. Furthermore, intensive studies in cardiovascular field have shown how the heart pathophysiology is tightly regulated by miRNAs expression and function [43]. Several miRNAs (i.e. miR-208a, miR21, mi-R29) are involved in myocardial development, and their dysregulation has been linked to cardiac remodelling and hypertrophy; miR-145 upregulation was found in smooth muscle cells of vessels from both a murine model and patients with pulmonary arterial hypertension, whereas plasma upregulation of a huge number of miRNAs (miR-1, miR-133a, miT-499, miR-208) has been reported in patients with acute ischemia and, therefore, hypoxic myocardium [44–48]. Experimental studies performed on cardiac cells further validate the finding that miRNAs expression is modulated with hypoxic stimuli: 145 microRNAs were found to be differently expressed in a study conducted on the human cardiac cell cultured under hypoxia compared the normoxia [49]. Among these, miR-146b was shown to play an important role in the adaptation of cardiomyocytes to chronic hypoxia and its inhibition augmented hypoxia-induced cardiomyocyte apoptosis [50].

A wide array of miRNAs have been reported to be dysregulated in children with CHDs, most of which are crucial in RV development and are specifically linked to a particular defect [24]. In addition, the hypoxic state of some CHDs further affects the miRNA profile of the heart. A recent study by Huang and colleagues shed a light on miRNA-184 as a possible player involved in the mechanism leading to cyanotic CHDs [51]. miRNA-184 expression was, in fact, markedly decreased in myocardial samples from cyanotic CHDs patients, compared to controls and its suppression *in vitro* was also associated with decreased proliferation and induction of apoptosis, through a mechanism that likely involves the activation of Caspase-3 and -9 by the oxidised miRNA-184 [51]. In another study aimed to evaluate the involvement of miRNAs in the hypoxic response of cardiomyocytes, the expression of miR-138 in myocardial samples of cyanotic patients with TOF was almost twofold miR-138 expression in acyanotic group (VSD) patients [52]. This finding suggests that miR-138 might be used to discriminate TOF from other subtypes of CHDs and further supports the evidence that miRNAs can shed a light on the knowledge of the aetiology of different CHDs and be predictive of the clinical outcome/management of these diseases.

3. Reoxygenation and reperfusion injuries

After a hypoxic event or status of the heart, it is crucial to intervene to re-establish a normal oxygen level. In most cases, the intervention involves heart surgery with cardiopulmonary bypass (CPB) and cardioplegic arrest (CA). During such heart surgery, the standard protocol involves the administration of high level of oxygen upon initiation of CPB and before CA. This causes what is commonly referred to as reoxygenation injury [53]. Following the establishment of CPB, the heart is stopped (ischemic period) to carry out the corrective surgery. When the ischemic heart is reperfused at the end of intervention, a reperfusion injury occurs. The severity of this reperfusion injury depends on the severity of the ischemic period and may be linked to delayed post-operative recovery [54].

It has been widely reported that free oxygen radical formation plays an important role in the development of ischemia-reperfusion injury in the heart as well as in various organs. In the reperfused heart, this oxidant formation derives form a series of interacting pathways in cardiac myocytes and endothelial cells, which involve also leukocyte chemotaxis and inflammation. The white blood cells are, in fact, another great source of ROS: when activated by the binding to the hypoxic endothelium, they produce chemotactic substances and oxygen radicals, which are the main responsible for cellular damage [55]. In addition, nitric oxide (NO) production is greatly increased in post-ischemic hearts, thus impairing vascular reactivity [56].

It has been demonstrated that the damage resulting from the reperfusion event is more severe in hypoxic (low oxygen supply), compared to ischemic (low coronary flow) hearts [57]. When comparing the effects of reperfusion, respectively, in ischemic and hypoxic hearts, Samaja et al. found that the myocardial depression, the energy demand, and the associated O_2 free radicals were higher in the hypoxic rat hearts than the ischemic ones. Furthermore, the hearts subjected to chronic hypoxia are even more prone to the reoxygenation injury than the hearts that have experienced acute hypoxic events. The compensatory changes that occur in chronic lack of oxygen may account for the higher predisposition to generate larger amounts of oxygen radicals with the reintroduction of high levels of oxygen [58].

With many CHDs being characterized by a chronic hypoxic status, the subset of cyanotic children is obviously at a higher risk than the acyanotic CHDs population [59]. Clinical studies have shown that, despite similar cross-clamp times during open heart surgery, cyanotic children have worse clinical outcome and more reoxygenation injury, measured by troponin I release, compared with acyanotic children [11]. The major problem arises from the oxygen reintroduction during the cardiopulmonary bypass (CPB), which is a necessary procedure for the surgical management of CHDs [55]. As the chronic hypoxia produces long-term changes in the myocardial metabolism and function, the sudden oxygen reintroduction further exacerbates these effects. The impaired contractility due to hypoxia-induced calcium overload and the loss of high energy phosphates are examples of the pathological events amplified by the reoxygenation [59, 60]. In addition, the depletion of endogenous antioxidants that characterize chronic cyanosis cannot counteract the oxygen radical-mediated injury when oxygen is reintroduced [61]. On the contrary, minimal changes in the antioxidant reserve capacity were reported before and after the CPB in acyanotic infants, suggesting that, in the absence of hypoxia, a small amount of oxygen free radicals are produced [62].

The effect of reoxygenation injury due to CPB in corrective heart surgery in cyanotic children has further been proven by a significant change in the myocardial gene expression profile [21]. In particular, a wide genome expression array study found 32 significantly downregulated and three upregulated genes in cyanotic heart biopsies taken before and after hyperoxic CPB. Among the upregulated genes after reoxygenation, MOSC1, a factor involved in superoxide generation [63], showed a great increase at a mRNA level, thus suggesting its possible involvement in the increase in CPB-induced oxidative stress. On the other hand, the downregulation of the taurine transporter (TAUT) and the consequent depletion of the documented cardioprotective taurine [64] may in part explain some aspects of the myocardial injury, such as the mitochondrial and myofibers dysfunction. In addition, 8-isoprostane, a reliable marker of oxidative stress, was increased after CPB, and this correlated with the downregulation of keys genetic pathways related to myocardial function and to the reduction in antioxidant defenses [21]. It, therefore, appears obvious that the maintenance of endogenous antioxidants during hypoxia is a crucial determinant of tissue recovery on reoxygenation.

It has been suggested that HIF-α might as well stand as target for cardioprotection upon reoxygenation, by inhibiting mitochondrial oxidative metabolism and therefore reducing the generation of ROS under hypoxia-reoxygenation [6].

MicroRNA expression also appears to be affected by the reoxygenation event. In a study by Bolkier et al., the plasma levels of some cardiac-associated miRNA were dramatically increased after surgery of children undergoing open-heart surgery for CHDs. The increase in the selected miRNAs (microRNA-208a, -208b and -499) correlated with higher troponin levels and delayed hospital discharge [65]. This evidence further justifies the use of circulating miRNAs as biomarkers not only for the diagnosis but also for prognosis and prediction of surgical clinical outcome. In addition, through two different approaches—overexpression and inhibition—miRNAs might represent a suitable target to therapeutically treat those defect characterized by an altered expression of their level.

4. Strategies of surgical intervention

In order to reduce the risk associated with reoxygenation injury in children undergoing open-heart surgery, different interventional strategies have been explored. One of the strategies proposed to avoid this injury is the "controlled reoxygenation", achieved by using a partial pressure of oxygen in arterial blood (PaO_2) similar to the patient's preoperative oxygen saturation when starting CPB [66].

Before its adoption in current clinical practices, several experimental studies on animal models have provided the evidence that the biochemical and the functional status of the cyanotic heart are improved by delaying reoxygenation upon cardiopulmonary bypass. Morita and colleagues set up an *in vivo* experimental animal model where immature piglet hearts were subjected to hypoxemia followed by uncontrolled reoxygenation at high oxygen tension (400 mmHg) or controlled oxygenation at ambient tension (40 mmHg) followed by a raising in the tension to 100 mmHg first and 400 mmHg later. The authors found that lipid peroxidation was reduced while antioxidant reserve capacity preserved in the controlled-reoxygenation group, with this outcome correlating with improved ventricular contractility and functional recovery [67]. In addition, using a modified cold blood cardioplegia, enriched with potassium, the calcium influx was limited and the impaired contractility restored upon reoxygenation [66]. Similar results were obtained in another animal study where controlled normoxic reoxygenation showed a better outcome than abrupt oxygen reintroduction at high pressure. Furthermore, the effect of leukodepletion was examined in this study, in order to verify whether the removal of an important source of ROS, the white blood cells, would minimize the reoxygenation injury. The depletion of leukocytes from the blood-reduced oxygen free radical formation and preserved ventricular contractility at similar extent to the one achieved by controlled reoxygenation [55].

The beneficial effect of controlling the rate of re-introduction of molecular oxygen was also evident in adult patients. Lower lipid peroxidation and preserved antioxidant levels were observed in patients receiving normoxic reoxygenation, compared to the hyperoxic ones, although no significant difference between the two groups was found in the cardiac performance after CBP, likely because this was measured at one low time point of the Starling fraction curve [68]. The controlled-reoxygenation procedure has subsequently been adopted in the operations of cyanotic infants undergoing cardiac surgery, obtaining similar results to the ones seen in the acute experimental model [58].

Subsequent studies have further confirmed these findings and stressed the importance of controlled reoxygenation on starting CPB in cyanotic patients. In two randomized controlled trials including cyanotic children receiving CBP, we showed that the reduced myocardial injury in the controlled normoxic group was accompanied by a reduction in cerebral and hepatic injury, assessed by S100 and άGT measurement, which are markers of neuron and hepatocytes damage, respectively [69, 70]. In a different study, we have also analysed the effect of the two reoxygenation approaches on the myocardial gene expression profile of cyanotic paediatric patients undergoing corrective heart surgery. Results showed that the controlled reoxygenation reduced the transcriptomic alteration observed following hyperoxic CPB. The most differentially expressed genes, mainly downregulated, were related to remodelling and metabolic processes, suggesting that the hearts subjected to hyperoxic reoxygenation had lower adaptation and remodelling capacity than the ones with controlled reoxygenation CBP [21].

Another approach of intervention, in the management of CPB, has involved the effect of whole body temperature during the paediatric cardiac surgery.

Although standard CPB procedures have always been conducted by cooling down the body temperature to 28° (hypothermic CPB), in order to reduce the metabolic rate and oxygen consumption, and therefore to protect organs from ischemic injury, recent evidences have demonstrated that normothermic (35°–37°) CPB is associated with lower inflammatory response and organ injury, both in adult and children [71–73].

In addition, we have shown that normothermic CPB in paediatric patients is also associated with reduced oxidative stress, assessed by troponin I and Isoprostane-8 release, compared with hypothermic CPB, while the inflammatory response has similar levels in the two groups [74].

Other researches have also investigated the effect of the temperature of cardioplegia during paediatric CPB. Warm blood cardioplegia, for long time adopted only in adult heart surgery, has proved to be safe and effective compared to standard cold CPB, with even better hydric balance and hemodynamic stability [75]. Once again, the pre-existent hypoxic status affects the biochemical and clinical outcome of the cardioplegic technique used. We have also shown that while for acyanotic patients the cardioplegic technique is not critical, for cyanotic patients, the use of cold blood cardioplegia with terminal warm blood cardioplegic reperfusion ("hot shot") improves the metabolic and functional recovery. The hot shot cardioplegia resulted in higher reperfusion ATP, ATP/ADP and glutamate levels than acyanotic patients, suggesting that this technique is advantageous only in stressed hearts [76]. Furthermore, the study shows that even if the blood cardioplegia is kept at cold temperature, this still offers a higher myocardial protection, compared to the crystalloid cardioplegia, confirming previous experimental and clinical results [77–79].

Besides CPB strategies, a pharmacological approach could be used as an interventional strategy for perioperative cardioprotection of hypoxic hearts. Experimental studies have shown that the selective inhibition of the enzyme phosphodiesterase-5 (PDE-5) can offer myocardial protection in infant hearts by improving myocardial function and reducing infarct size during reperfusion. However, no direct evidence between this protective effect and the hypoxia-induced injury was shown [80].

As for its established role in hypoxia, HIF-1α has also been investigated as a target for hypoxia-induced myocardial injury in reperfusion. By stabilizing its active form, through the compound dimethyloxyglycine (DMOG), a novel HIF-1α stabilizer, Zhang et al. showed that the progression of hypoxia-induced right ventricle remodelling was significantly reduced in a murine model of chronic hypoxia, most likely as a result of the induction of genes related to adaptive processes [81].

Furthermore, as previously mentioned, miRNAs are being extensively investigated as potential therapeutic tools in the management of CHDs. However, despite the fact that the road ahead looks promising and appealing, some obstacles, like the stability, the off-target effects and the immunogenicity of the delivery vehicles, still need to be overcome before getting miRNA-based therapeutics into clinical practice.

5. Conclusion

In conclusion, important steps ahead have been made in the knowledge of the mechanisms by which hypoxia takes part to the onset of congenital heart diseases, especially with regard to cyanotic patients. Likewise, significant advances have been made in the strategies of intervention involving open-heart surgery of children with these defects; in order to reduce the injury induced by CPB reoxygenation. Hopefully, the further understanding of the signalling pathways and the mechanism underlying the pathophysiology of hypoxia and hypoxia-induced reoxygenation injury in each kind of defect will result in the development of even better therapeutic strategies and in the design of specific interventions, particularly for the high-risk population.

Author details

Dominga Iacobazzi, Massimo Caputo and Mohamed T Ghorbel*

*Address all correspondence to: m.ghorbel@bristol.ac.uk

University of Bristol, School of Clinical Sciences, Bristol Heart Institute, Bristol, UK

References

[1] Essop MF. Cardiac metabolic adaptations in response to chronic hypoxia. J Physiol. 2007;584(Pt 3):715–26.

[2] Braunwald E. 50th anniversary historical article. Myocardial oxygen consumption: the quest for its determinants and some clinical fallout. J Am Coll Cardiol. 1999;34(5):1365–8.

[3] Ostadal B, Ostadalova I, Dhalla NS. Development of cardiac sensitivity to oxygen deficiency: comparative and ontogenetic aspects. Physiol Rev. 1999;79(3):635–59.

[4] Budev MM, Arroliga AC, Wiedemann HP, Matthay RA. Cor pulmonale: an overview. Semin Respir Crit Care Med. 2003;24(3):233–44.

[5] Grifka RG. Cyanotic congenital heart disease with increased pulmonary blood flow. Pediatr Clin North Am. 1999;46(2):405–25.

[6] Semenza GL. Hypoxia-inducible factor 1 and cardiovascular disease. Annu Rev Physiol. 2014;76:39–56.

[7] Shohet RV, Garcia JA. Keeping the engine primed: HIF factors as key regulators of cardiac metabolism and angiogenesis during ischemia. J Mol Med (Berl). 2007;85(12):1309–15.

[8] Roche SL, Redington AN. The failing right ventricle in congenital heart disease. Can J Cardiol. 2013;29(7):768–78.

[9] Starnes JW, Bowles DK, Seiler KS. Myocardial injury after hypoxia in immature, adult and aged rats. Aging (Milano). 1997;9(4):268–76.

[10] Jonas RA. Myocardial protection for neonates and infants. Thorac Cardiovasc Surg. 1998;46(Suppl. 2):288–91.

[11] Imura H, Caputo M, Parry A, Pawade A, Angelini GD, Suleiman MS. Age-dependent and hypoxia-related differences in myocardial protection during pediatric open heart surgery. Circulation. 2001;103(11):1551–6.

[12] Lopaschuk GD, Spafford MA. Differences in myocardial ischemic tolerance between 1- and 7-day-old rabbits. Can J Physiol Pharmacol. 1992;70(10):1315–23.

[13] Houyel L, Khoshnood B, Anderson RH, Lelong N, Thieulin AC, Goffinet F, et al. Population-based evaluation of a suggested anatomic and clinical classification of congenital heart defects based on the International Paediatric and Congenital Cardiac Code. Orphanet J Rare Dis. 2011;6:64.

[14] Fraser CD, Carberry KE. Congenital heart disease. In: Townsend CM Jr, Beauchamp RD, Evers BM, Mattox KL, eds. *Sabiston Textbook of Surgery*. 19th ed. Philadelphia, PA: Elsevier Saunders; 2012:chap 59.

[15] Webb GD, Smallhorn JF, Therrien J, Redington AN. Congenital heart disease. In: Mann DL, Zipes DP, Libby P, Bonow RO, *Braunwald E, eds. Braunwald's Heart Disease: A Textbook of Cardiovascular Medicine*. 10th ed. Philadelphia, PA: Elsevier Saunders; 2015:chap 62.

[16] Rokicki W, Strzalkowski A, Klapcinska B, Danch A, Sobczak A. Antioxidant status in newborns and infants suffering from congenital heart defects. Wiad Lek. 2003;56(7–8):337–40.

[17] Ercan S, Cakmak A, Kosecik M, Erel O. The oxidative state of children with cyanotic and acyanotic congenital heart disease. Anadolu Kardiyol Derg. 2009;9(6):486–90.

[18] Scandalios JG. The rise of ROS. Trends Biochem Sci. 2002;27(9):483–6.

[19] Birben E, Sahiner UM, Sackesen C, Erzurum S, Kalayci O. Oxidative stress and antioxidant defense. World Allergy Organ J. 2012;5(1):9–19.

[20] Espinosa-Diez C, Miguel V, Mennerich D, Kietzmann T, Sanchez-Perez P, Cadenas S, et al. Antioxidant responses and cellular adjustments to oxidative stress. Redox Biol. 2015;6:183–97.

[21] Ghorbel MT, Mokhtari A, Sheikh M, Angelini GD, Caputo M. Controlled reoxygenation cardiopulmonary bypass is associated with reduced transcriptomic changes in cyanotic tetralogy of Fallot patients undergoing surgery. Physiol Genomics. 2012;44(22):1098–106.

[22] Ghorbel MT, Cherif M, Jenkins E, Mokhtari A, Kenny D, Angelini GD, et al. Transcriptomic analysis of patients with tetralogy of Fallot reveals the effect of chronic hypoxia on myocardial gene expression. J Thorac Cardiovasc Surg. 2010;140(2):337–45.e26.

[23] Sharma K, Kass DA. Heart failure with preserved ejection fraction: mechanisms, clinical features, and therapies. Circ Res. 2014;115(1):79–96.

[24] Iacobazzi D, Suleiman MS, Ghorbel M, George SJ, Caputo M, Tulloh RM. Cellular and molecular basis of RV hypertrophy in congenital heart disease. Heart. 2016;102(1):12–7.

[25] Piao L, Sidhu VK, Fang YH, Ryan JJ, Parikh KS, Hong Z, et al. FOXO1-mediated upregulation of pyruvate dehydrogenase kinase-4 (PDK4) decreases glucose oxidation and impairs right ventricular function in pulmonary hypertension: therapeutic benefits of dichloroacetate. J Mol Med (Berl). 2013;91(3):333–46.

[26] Ryan JJ, Archer SL. The right ventricle in pulmonary arterial hypertension: disorders of metabolism, angiogenesis and adrenergic signaling in right ventricular failure. Circ Res. 2014;115(1):176–88.

[27] Qipshidze N, Tyagi N, Metreveli N, Lominadze D, Tyagi SC. Autophagy mechanism of right ventricular remodeling in murine model of pulmonary artery constriction. Am J Physiol Heart Circ Physiol. 2012;302(3):H688–96.

[28] Friedberg MK, Redington AN. Right versus left ventricular failure: differences, similarities, and interactions. Circulation. 2014;129(9):1033–44.

[29] Jaakkola P, Mole DR, Tian YM, Wilson MI, Gielbert J, Gaskell SJ, et al. Targeting of HIF-alpha to the von Hippel-Lindau ubiquitylation complex by O2-regulated prolyl hydroxylation. Science. 2001;292(5516):468–72.

[30] Semenza GL. O2-regulated gene expression: transcriptional control of cardiorespiratory physiology by HIF-1. J Appl Physiol (1985). 2004;96(3):1173–7; discussion 0-2.

[31] Felmeden DC, Blann AD, Lip GY. Angiogenesis: basic pathophysiology and implications for disease. Eur Heart J. 2003;24(7):586–603.

[32] Holscher M, Silter M, Krull S, von Ahlen M, Hesse A, Schwartz P, et al. Cardiomyocyte-specific prolyl-4-hydroxylase domain 2 knock out protects from acute myocardial ischemic injury. J Biol Chem. 2011;286(13):11185–94.

[33] Himeno W, Akagi T, Furui J, Maeno Y, Ishii M, Kosai K, et al. Increased angiogenic growth factor in cyanotic congenital heart disease. Pediatr Cardiol. 2003;24(2):127–32.

[34] El-Melegy NT, Mohamed NA. Angiogenic biomarkers in children with congenital heart disease: possible implications. Ital J Pediatr. 2010;36:32.

[35] Qing M, Gorlach A, Schumacher K, Woltje M, Vazquez-Jimenez JF, Hess J, et al. The hypoxia-inducible factor HIF-1 promotes intramyocardial expression of VEGF in infants with congenital cardiac defects. Basic Res Cardiol. 2007;102(3):224–32.

[36] Lemus-Varela ML, Flores-Soto ME, Cervantes-Munguia R, Torres-Mendoza BM, Gudino-Cabrera G, Chaparro-Huerta V, et al. Expression of HIF-1 alpha, VEGF and EPO in peripheral blood from patients with two cardiac abnormalities associated with hypoxia. Clin Biochem. 2010;43(3):234–9.

[37] Ootaki Y, Yamaguchi M, Yoshimura N, Oka S, Yoshida M, Hasegawa T. Vascular endothelial growth factor in children with congenital heart disease. Ann Thorac Surg. 2003;75(5):1523–6.

[38] Nadeau S, Baribeau J, Janvier A, Perreault T. Changes in expression of vascular endothelial growth factor and its receptors in neonatal hypoxia-induced pulmonary hypertension. Pediatr Res. 2005;58(2):199–205.

[39] Vidya G, Suma HY, Vishnu Bhat B, Parkash Chand, Ramachandra Rao K. Hypoxia induced DNA damage in children with isolated septal defect and septal defect with great vessel anomaly of heart. J Clin Diagn Res. 2014;8(4):SC01–3.

[40] Srujana K, Begum SS, Rao KN, Devi GS, Jyothy A, Prasad MH. Application of the comet assay for assessment of oxidative DNA damage in circulating lymphocytes of Tetralogy of Fallot patients. Mutat Res. 2010;688(1–2):62–5.

[41] Bartel DP. MicroRNAs: genomics, biogenesis, mechanism, and function. Cell. 2004;116(2):281–97.

[42] Kulshreshtha R, Ferracin M, Wojcik SE, Garzon R, Alder H, Agosto-Perez FJ, et al. A microRNA signature of hypoxia. Mol Cell Biol. 2007;27(5):1859–67.

[43] Condorelli G, Latronico MV, Cavarretta E. microRNAs in cardiovascular diseases: current knowledge and the road ahead. J Am Coll Cardiol. 2014;63(21):2177–87.

[44] Thum T, Gross C, Fiedler J, Fischer T, Kissler S, Bussen M, et al. MicroRNA-21 contributes to myocardial disease by stimulating MAP kinase signalling in fibroblasts. Nature. 2008;456(7224):980–4.

[45] van Rooij E, Sutherland LB, Thatcher JE, DiMaio JM, Naseem RH, Marshall WS, et al. Dysregulation of microRNAs after myocardial infarction reveals a role of miR-29 in cardiac fibrosis. Proc Natl Acad Sci U S A. 2008;105(35):13027–32.

[46] Caruso P, Dempsie Y, Stevens HC, McDonald RA, Long L, Lu R, et al. A role for miR-145 in pulmonary arterial hypertension: evidence from mouse models and patient samples. Circ Res. 2012;111(3):290–300.

[47] Wang GK, Zhu JQ, Zhang JT, Li Q, Li Y, He J, et al. Circulating microRNA: a novel potential biomarker for early diagnosis of acute myocardial infarction in humans. Eur Heart J. 2010;31(6):659–66.

[48] Cheng Y, Tan N, Yang J, Liu X, Cao X, He P, et al. A translational study of circulating cell-free microRNA-1 in acute myocardial infarction. Clin Sci (Lond). 2010;119(2):87–95.

[49] Chen YT, Liew OW, Richards AM. MicroRNA expression profiles of human left ventricle derived cardiac cells in normoxic and hypoxic conditions. Genom Data. 2015;5:59–60.

[50] Li JW, He SY, Feng ZZ, Zhao L, Jia WK, Liu P, et al. MicroRNA-146b inhibition augments hypoxia-induced cardiomyocyte apoptosis. Mol Med Rep. 2015;12(5):6903–10.

[51] Huang J, Li X, Li H, Su Z, Wang J, Zhang H. Down-regulation of microRNA-184 contributes to the development of cyanotic congenital heart diseases. Int J Clin Exp Pathol. 2015;8(11):14221–7.

[52] He S, Liu P, Jian Z, Li J, Zhu Y, Feng Z, et al. miR-138 protects cardiomyocytes from hypoxia-induced apoptosis via MLK3/JNK/c-jun pathway. Biochem Biophys Res Commun. 2013;441(4):763–9.

[53] Tan S, Yokoyama Y, Wang Z, Zhou F, Nielsen V, Murdoch AD, et al. Hypoxia-reoxygenation is as damaging as ischemia-reperfusion in the rat liver. Crit Care Med. 1998;26(6):1089–95.

[54] Ferrari R, Alfieri O, Curello S, Ceconi C, Cargnoni A, Marzollo P, et al. Occurrence of oxidative stress during reperfusion of the human heart. Circulation. 1990;81(1):201–11.

[55] Allen BS, Ilbawi MN. Hypoxia, reoxygenation and the role of systemic leukodepletion in pediatric heart surgery. Perfusion. 2001;16(Suppl):19–29.

[56] Zweier JL, Talukder MA. The role of oxidants and free radicals in reperfusion injury. Cardiovasc Res. 2006;70(2):181–90.

[57] Samaja M, Motterlini R, Santoro F, Dell' Antonio G, Corno A. Oxidative injury in reoxygenated and reperfused hearts. Free Radic Biol Med. 1994;16(2):255–62.

[58] Allen BS, Rahman S, Ilbawi MN, Kronon M, Bolling KS, Halldorsson AO, et al. Detrimental effects of cardiopulmonary bypass in cyanotic infants: preventing the reoxygenation injury. Ann Thorac Surg. 1997;64(5):1381–7; discussion 7-8.

[59] Corno AF, Milano G, Samaja M, Tozzi P, von Segesser LK. Chronic hypoxia: a model for cyanotic congenital heart defects. J Thorac Cardiovasc Surg. 2002;124(1):105–12.

[60] Najm HK, Wallen WJ, Belanger MP, Williams WG, Coles JG, Van Arsdell GS, et al. Does the degree of cyanosis affect myocardial adenosine triphosphate levels and function in children undergoing surgical procedures for congenital heart disease? J Thorac Cardiovasc Surg. 2000;119(3):515–24.

[61] Teoh KH, Mickle DA, Weisel RD, Li RK, Tumiati LC, Coles JG, et al. Effect of oxygen tension and cardiovascular operations on the myocardial antioxidant enzyme activities in patients with tetralogy of Fallot and aorta-coronary bypass. J Thorac Cardiovasc Surg. 1992;104(1):159–64.

[62] Bolling KS, Halldorsson A, Allen BS, Rahman S, Wang T, Kronon M, et al. Prevention of the hypoxic reoxygenation injury with the use of a leukocyte-depleting filter. J Thorac Cardiovasc Surg. 1997;113(6):1081–9; discussion 9-90.

[63] Morita K, Ihnken K, Buckberg GD, Sherman MP, Young HH. Studies of hypoxemic/reoxygenation injury: without aortic clamping. IX. Importance of avoiding perioperative hyperoxemia in the setting of previous cyanosis. J Thorac Cardiovasc Surg. 1995;110(4 Pt 2):1235–44.

[64] Ito T, Kimura Y, Uozumi Y, Takai M, Muraoka S, Matsuda T, et al. Taurine depletion caused by knocking out the taurine transporter gene leads to cardiomyopathy with cardiac atrophy. J Mol Cell Cardiol. 2008;44(5):927–37.

[65] Bolkier Y, Nevo-Caspi Y, Salem Y, Vardi A, Mishali D, Paret G. Micro-RNA-208a, -208b, and -499 as biomarkers for myocardial damage after cardiac surgery in children. Pediatr Crit Care Med. 2016;17(4):e193–7.

[66] Ihnken K, Morita K, Buckberg GD. Delayed cardioplegic reoxygenation reduces reoxygenation injury in cyanotic immature hearts. Ann Thorac Surg. 1998;66(1):177–82.

[67] Morita K, Ihnken K, Buckberg GD. Studies of hypoxemic/reoxygenation injury: with aortic clamping. XII. Delay of cardiac reoxygenation damage in the presence of cyanosis: a new concept of controlled cardiac reoxygenation. J Thorac Cardiovasc Surg. 1995;110(4 Pt 2):1265–73.

[68] Ihnken K, Winkler A, Schlensak C, Sarai K, Neidhart G, Unkelbach U, et al. Normoxic cardiopulmonary bypass reduces oxidative myocardial damage and nitric oxide during cardiac operations in the adult. J Thorac Cardiovasc Surg. 1998;116(2):327–34.

[69] Caputo M, Mokhtari A, Rogers CA, Panayiotou N, Chen Q, Ghorbel MT, et al. The effects of normoxic versus hyperoxic cardiopulmonary bypass on oxidative stress and inflammatory response in cyanotic pediatric patients undergoing open cardiac surgery: a randomized controlled trial. J Thorac Cardiovasc Surg. 2009;138(1):206–14.

[70] Caputo M, Mokhtari A, Miceli A, Ghorbel MT, Angelini GD, Parry AJ, et al. Controlled reoxygenation during cardiopulmonary bypass decreases markers of organ damage, inflammation, and oxidative stress in single-ventricle patients undergoing pediatric heart surgery. J Thorac Cardiovasc Surg. 2014;148(3):792–801, e8; discussion 0-1.

[71] Birdi I, Caputo M, Underwood M, Angelini GD, Bryan AJ. Influence of normothermic systemic perfusion temperature on cold myocardial protection during coronary artery bypass surgery. Cardiovasc Surg. 1999;7(3):369–74.

[72] Birdi I, Regragui I, Izzat MB, Bryan AJ, Angelini GD. Influence of normothermic systemic perfusion during coronary artery bypass operations: a randomized prospective study. J Thorac Cardiovasc Surg. 1997;114(3):475–81.

[73] Ohata T, Sawa Y, Kadoba K, Taniguchi K, Ichikawa H, Masai T, et al. Normothermia has beneficial effects in cardiopulmonary bypass attenuating inflammatory reactions. ASAIO J. 1995;41(3):M288–91.

[74] Caputo M, Bays S, Rogers CA, Pawade A, Parry AJ, Suleiman S, et al. Randomized comparison between normothermic and hypothermic cardiopulmonary bypass in pediatric open-heart surgery. Ann Thorac Surg. 2005;80(3):982–8.

[75] Durandy Y, Hulin S. Intermittent warm blood cardioplegia in the surgical treatment of congenital heart disease: clinical experience with 1400 cases. J Thorac Cardiovasc Surg. 2007;133(1):241–6.

[76] Modi P, Suleiman MS, Reeves B, Pawade A, Parry AJ, Angelini GD, et al. Myocardial metabolic changes during pediatric cardiac surgery: a randomized study of 3 cardioplegic techniques. J Thorac Cardiovasc Surg. 2004;128(1):67–75.

[77] Bolling K, Kronon M, Allen BS, Wang T, Ramon S, Feinberg H. Myocardial protection in normal and hypoxically stressed neonatal hearts: the superiority of blood versus crystalloid cardioplegia. J Thorac Cardiovasc Surg. 1997;113(6):994–1003; discussion 1003-5.

[78] del Nido PJ, Mickle DA, Wilson GJ, Benson LN, Weisel RD, Coles JG, et al. Inadequate myocardial protection with cold cardioplegic arrest during repair of tetralogy of Fallot. J Thorac Cardiovasc Surg. 1988;95(2):223–9.

[79] Modi P, Imura H, Caputo M, Pawade A, Parry A, Angelini GD, et al. Cardiopulmonary bypass-induced myocardial reoxygenation injury in pediatric patients with cyanosis. J Thorac Cardiovasc Surg. 2002;124(5):1035–6.

[80] Bremer YA, Salloum F, Ockaili R, Chou E, Moskowitz WB, Kukreja RC. Sildenafil citrate (viagra) induces cardioprotective effects after ischemia/reperfusion injury in infant rabbits. Pediatr Res. 2005;57(1):22–7.

[81] Zhang S, Ma K, Liu Y, Pan X, Chen Q, Qi L, et al. Stabilization of hypoxia-inducible factor by DMOG inhibits development of chronic hypoxia-induced right ventricular remodeling. J Cardiovasc Pharmacol. 2016;67(1):68–75.

Chapter 9

Adaptations to Chronic Hypoxia Combined with Erythropoietin Deficiency in Cerebral and Cardiac Tissues

Raja El Hasnaoui-Saadani

Additional information is available at the end of the chapter

http://dx.doi.org/10.5772/66974

Abstract

Chronic anemia-induced hypoxia triggers regulatory pathways that mediate long-term adaptive cardiac and cerebral changes, particularly at the transcriptional level. These adaptative mechanisms include a regulated cerebral blood flow and cardiac output, angiogenesis and cytoprotection triggered by hypoxia-inducible factor 1 alpha (HIF-1α), vascular endothelial growth factor (VEGF), neuronal nitric oxide synthase (nNOS) and Epo pathways. All these compensatory mechanisms aim to optimize oxygen delivery and to protect the brain and heart from hypoxic injury. We reviewed the effects of chronic hypobaric hypoxia as well as chronic anemia in the heart and brain, and we compared for the first time the effects of chronic hypobaric hypoxia combined with a severe lack of Epo (chronic anemia) in these vital organs. Functional cardiac adaptations such as cardiac hypertrophy, increased cardiac output as well as angiogenesis occurred along with the activation of HIF1α/VEGF and Epo/EpoR pathways under chronic anemia or hypoxia. Similarly, cerebrovascular adaptations take place through the same molecular mechanisms under chronic hypoxia or anemia. However, when both arterial pressure and content of oxygen are decreased, the cerebral and cardiac adaptative mechanisms showed their limitations. In addition, cerebral and cardiac cell injuries may have occurred following the combined effect of chronic anemia and hypoxia. By emphasizing the anemia and hypoxia-induced cerebral and myocardial adaptations, this review highlighted the crucial role of Epo in its non-erythropoietic functions such as angiogenesis and neuroprotection. Indeed, a better understanding of these protective mechanisms is of great clinical importance to the development of new therapeutic strategies for the management of ischemic heart and brain.

Keywords: chronic hypoxia, chronic anemia, angiogenesis, cardiac function, cerebral blood flow, oxygen homeostasis, neuroprotection, HIF-1-VEGF-Epo

1. Introduction

Inadequate level of oxygen like in chronic hypoxia or anemia is especially detrimental for cerebral and heart tissues. Indeed, hypoxia plays an important role in the pathogenesis of cerebral and myocardial ischemia, and chronic heart and lung diseases [1]. That is why specific mechanisms at a systemic, cellular and molecular level take place to maintain the oxygen homeostasis. It is important to clearly distinguish the differences between hypoxia and anemia. Hypoxia is a reduction of arterial pressure of oxygen (PaO_2), while anemia is a reduction of arterial content of oxygen (CaO_2) as it occurs during a decrease in hemoglobin concentration. This review focus mainly on chronic hypobaric hypoxia that occurs at high altitude and chronic anemia is referred to our model of transgenic mice that presents a constitutive erythropoietin deficiency. Furthermore, emphasis is placed on effects of chronic hypoxia and anemia in the cerebral and cardiac tissues. The discussion is mostly based on animal studies unless otherwise indicated, even though similarities of adaptative mechanisms are shown by human studies [2, 3].

Chronic hypoxia promotes angiogenesis by modulating the transcriptional regulator hypoxia-inducible factor 1 alpha (HIF-1α), which in turn triggers the upregulation of the erythropoietin [4], a major factor of acclimatization to hypoxia. HIF-1α is a master regulator of the hypoxic response and its proangiogenic activities include regulation of vascular endothelial growth factor (VEGF), but also Epo and its receptors (EpoR) [1, 5]. Erythropoietin primarily regulates red blood cell formation, and Epo serum levels are increased under hypoxic stress (e.g., anemia and altitude) [6]. However, several non-hematopoietic functions of Epo and its receptors have been exposed by experimental studies using genetically modified mice [7]. It is of great clinical importance that Epo has been shown to have protective functions in many different tissues. Indeed, these studies using recombinant human EPO (rHuEPO) suggested new therapeutic indications of Epo for the management of ischemic injuries of several tissues such as myocardium and brain [8–10].

Epo-induced angiogenesis may lead to an improvement in brain perfusion since Epo protects vascular bed integrity and stimulates angiogenesis [11–14] by acting indirectly on endothelial cells via activation of VEGF/VEGF receptor system, which is the most important regulator of endothelial growth and angiogenesis. Furthermore, Epo may have a positive effect on cerebral vasculature in addition to the cerebral blood flow (CBF) through alteration in nitric oxide (NO) production, which mainly derived from arginine and catalyzed by endothelial nitric oxide synthase (eNOS) [15]. Therefore, it seems that cellular protection and angiogenesis in heart and brain tissues are the dual role of erythropoietin and VEGF. These both cytokines are triggered by HIF-1α to maintain an adequate cellular oxygen supply and protect the brain and heart against hypoxic and or anemic injuries.

Our model of erythropoietin-SV40 T antigen (Epo-TAg^h) transgenic mice has a targeted disruption in the 5′ untranslated region of the Epo gene that dramatically reduces its expression. The homozygous animals are thus severely and chronically anemic [16, 17]. Therefore, these transgenic anemic mice provided us an interesting model to study the adaptive mechanisms to chronic anemia and hypoxia, especially in vital organs, such as brain and heart. The present

http://dx.doi.org/10.5772/66974

review aims to give a brief synthesis of adaptations to chronic hypoxia in the brain and heart tissues, in absence of Epo. The first part will briefly describe the similarities of the signaling process of hypoxia-induced angiogenesis, as well as the other mechanisms that take place to protect the brain and heart against anemic and hypoxic injuries. The second part will focus on these adaptations in response to chronic anemia due to Epo deficiency (in comparison with adaptations induced by hypoxia). The third part will mainly describe the effect of both constraints (anemia and hypoxia) in cerebral and cardiac tissues.

2. Adaptations to chronic hypoxia in cerebral and cardiac tissues

2.1. Brain under chronic hypoxia

In the central nervous system, cerebrovascular and energy metabolism adaptations occur under hypoxic conditions in order to preserve an adequate tissue oxygen supply needed to support an optimal neuronal function. An acute hypoxic exposure triggers both a CBF and glucose consumption increases [18]. The stabilization of HIF-1α rapidly up regulates the vasodilatory enzyme inducible nitric oxide synthase (iNOS) [19]. NO, the enzymatic product of iNOS, relaxes vascular smooth muscle cells, providing a short-term increase in blood flow. Thus, an increase in cerebral NO following a rise in NOS isoforms expression is most probably responsible for the rise in CBF [20–23]. With longer hypoxic exposure, polycythemia and cerebral angiogenesis take place to enhance cerebral oxygenation, while cerebral NO level returns to basal value [23, 24]. Indeed, in a chronic hypoxic challenge to the central nervous system, the cerebral cortex is known to undergo a significant cerebrovascular remodeling, in order to preserve tissue oxygen and energy supply [24–29]. These microvascular changes occur relatively late compared to the physiological adaptations [30]. In the rat brain, the capillary density almost doubles, and the average intercapillary distance decreases from about 50 to about 40 μm [31]. Also, by 3 weeks of adaptation, the initial hypoxic-induced increased flow returns to baseline by 5 days [22], concomitantly there is an increasing hematocrit, glucose consumption is slightly elevated by about 15% [32–34] and tissue oxygen tension is restored [35, 36]. Finally, it is well accepted that blood flow alterations serve acute changes in oxygen delivery, while persistent changes are due to capillary density adjustments.

Molecular mechanisms underlying hypoxia-induced capillary increases are now well documented and involve specifically HIF-1α/VEGF pathway [23, 26, 33, 37, 38]. The HIF pathway regulates a host of pro-angiogenic genes, including VEGF, angiopoietin-1, angiopoietin-2 (Ang-2) and many others [39, 40]. HIF-regulated pro-angiogenic factors execute the HIF-specific angiogenic program by increasing vascular permeability (most probably through interaction with NO [41]), endothelial cell proliferation, sprouting, migration, adhesion and tube formation. In rats, HIF-1α is detected in the brain, in all cell types, shortly after the onset of hypoxia and persists for at least 2 weeks, until cerebral angiogenesis is completed within 3 weeks of exposure to hypoxia [23, 29, 35]. Brain angiogenesis also requires additional pro-angiogenic factors such as Ang-2. Ang-2, which is not constitutively expressed under normoxic conditions, is upregulated in rat and mouse endothelial cells following hypoxia [28, 38]. Ang-2 induction during hypoxia is known to occur independently of HIF-1 and is due to cyclooxygenase-2 (COX-2) enzyme activity [42, 43]. More recent results also demonstrated that the hypoxic capillary response in aged mice was preserved after 3 weeks of hypoxia despite a significant delay in the response during the first week of exposure to hypoxia [25].

2.2. Heart under chronic hypoxia

In humans, the most characteristic and important cardiovascular response to hypoxia is pulmonary vasoconstriction, which reduces the caliber of pulmonary vessels and raises vascular resistance in a region of low alveolar PO_2. However, severe hypoxia has a direct deleterious effect on cardiac function. Hypoxic pulmonary vasoconstriction can cause chronic pulmonary hypertension. Myocardial contractility and maximum output are diminished during conditions of reduced oxygen supply. While maximum oxygen consumption is reduced in chronic hypoxia, cardiac output (CO) remains normal at rest, owing primarily to an increased red blood cell mass [44, 45].

In our animal model, we showed that all parameters of cardiac function were preserved when comparing wild-type (WT) mice under normoxic and chronic hypoxic conditions. Indeed, systolic blood pressure was not affected by 14-day hypoxia at 4500 m, and hypoxic wild-type mice did not develop pulmonary hypertension. Moreover, there was no cardiac hypertrophy at variance with what was shown in rats or humans in similar hypoxic conditions [46]. Moreover, cardiac output was not affected by chronic hypoxia alone and oxygen delivery was maintained. In addition, hypoxic wild-type mice responded by increasing plasma Epo and blood hemoglobin, resulting in a rise in oxygen-carrying capacity [47].

Furthermore, many reports now stated that heart could be an additional Epo productive tissue [48, 49]. Hoch et al. first showed an Epo gene and protein expression in cardiac progenitor cells [50]. Through specific binding to its receptor EpoR, Epo triggers intracellular signaling events that depend on the activation of Jak2 tyrosine kinase [51]. The exploration of these pathways revealed that Epo is also an angiogenic as well as an anti-apoptotic factor as described respectively in the brain [52] and the heart [47, 50, 53, 54]. As previously described [55], chronic hypoxia led to the activation of HIF-1α/VEGF pathway in the heart of adult wild-type mice most probably responsible for their enhanced myocardial angiogenesis. Also we demonstrated the activation of cardioprotective pathways, involving HIF-1α and Epo, as suggested by the increase of EpoR expression and P-STAT-5/STAT-5 ratio [47]. Furthermore, we could not exclude a cardiac metabolic gene remodeling since temporal changes in glucose metabolic genes in response to moderate hypobaric hypoxia [56] have been demonstrated.

However, these adaptive responses contribute to maintain an adequate tissue oxygen supply for the preservation of cardiac function and to protect the heart against hypoxic insults.

3. Adaptations to chronic Epo deficiency in cerebral and cardiac tissues

Anemia is defined as a lack of oxygen-carrying red blood cells which also results in a lack of oxygen delivery to tissue. The physiological and molecular responses to tissue hypoxia are increasingly understood while the effects of anemia are still poorly documented [57]. Our model of erythropoietin-SV40 T antigen (Epo-TAg^h) transgenic mice presents a severe reduction of Epo expression that induces chronic anemia [16, 17]. The first studies demonstrated that Epo-Tag^h mice could survive in chronic hypoxia (14 days at 4500 m), in part through an increase in ventilation and probably a higher cardiac output as suggested by a significant cardiac hypertrophy [58–60]. Hence, it was of interest of our team to compare the physiological and cellular responses to chronic anemia (low Hb) and chronic hypoxia (low P_aO_2) in cerebral and cardiac tissues. Indeed, the objectives of our studies were to determine if chronic anemic mice developed compensatory mechanisms in the brain and heart (vascular remodeling, adaptative function, pathways involving HIF-1α) to offset the decrease in hemoglobin concentration.

3.1. Brain under chronic anemia

Low O_2 environment is the principal regulator of HIF activity. The HIF pathway mediates the primary cellular responses to low O_2, which promotes both short- and long-term adaptation to hypoxia as already described in the previous paragraph. In this regard, we considered that anemia-induced cerebral hypoxia involved the same hypoxic molecules. It has already been described that anemia increases cerebral hypoxic genes expression such as HIF, VEGF and nNOS which are involved in O_2 homeostasis [61]. Indeed, studies on severe hemodilution using NOS-deficient mice showed an increased expression of HIF and nNOS proteins in the brain as well as an increased whole body HIF activity [57, 61–64]. Many other molecules, including Epo, VEGF and iNOS have also been shown to be upregulated in the anemic brain [61, 65]. Thus, it seems that during anemia, HIF-1α has the potential to regulate cerebral cellular responses under both hypoxic and normoxic conditions [23, 47, 57, 64, 65].

Then, we focused on potential mediators of the increase in CBF associated with both hypoxia and anemia. Indeed, local production of NO by endothelial NOS (eNOS), and nNOS mediates CBF under a number of physiological conditions, including anemia and hypoxia [24, 61, 63, 64]. Relatively specific inhibition of nNOS has been demonstrated to impair the increase in CBF associated with acute anemia [61] and hypoxia [66–68], implicating nNOS as an important mediator of CBF in both cases [63, 64]. In our studies, we also found an increase in nNOS, while iNOS and eNOS were unchanged but no corresponding change in cerebral NO concentration. The stabilization of HIF-1α, as already described in the brain in acute [61, 69] and chronic anemia [23], promote VEGF-induced angiogenesis as shown in normoxic Epo-TAg^h mice with a rise in the capillary/fiber ratio, thus optimizing oxygen diffusion as previously described in the brain [24]. Erythropoietin also plays an important role in angiogenesis through upregulation of VEGF in ischemic rats [11]. Indeed, Wang et al. showed that neural progenitor cells treated with Epo were able to produce VEGF and consequently to promote angiogenesis through the upregulation of VEGFR2 expression in cerebral endothelial cells [70].

Our work provided novel physiological data about cerebral adaptations to chronic anemia. Indeed, we evidenced that Epo deficiency activated cerebral hypoxic mechanisms through HIF activation that promote angiogenesis [23]. In addition, the JAK/STAT signaling pathway mediated by the Epo/EpoR complex seems to be activated by chronic anemia [23, 47] and could promote neuroprotection and cell proliferation [71]. Furthermore, more recent results showed that nNOS is specifically protective during anemia [57]. All these responses were probably able to minimize brain damage that could be induced by chronic anemia. Finally, the mechanisms responsible for matching capillary density to tissue oxygen levels are not unique to environmental hypoxic stimuli. Rather, these processes appear to be responsible for maintaining the oxygen availability through local blood flow in order to optimize the neuronal function.

3.2. Heart under chronic anemia

The classic physiological cardiovascular responses to anemia include an increased CO, a redistribution of blood flow and a decrease of hemoglobin-oxygen affinity. Two mechanisms are most probably responsible for the increased CO during anemia: reduced blood viscosity and increased sympathetic stimulation of the cardiovascular effectors. Blood viscosity affects both preload and afterload, two of the major determinants of the CO, whereas sympathetic stimulation primarily increases heart rate and contractility [72]. If cardiac function is normal, the increase in venous return or left ventricular preload will be the most important determinant of the increased CO during normovolemic anemia [72]. It is also known that anemia induces right and left ventricular hypertrophy [59, 73, 74] and increases CO, offsetting the fall in arterial oxygen content to maintain oxygen delivery. Our data confirmed the increase in CO by an increase in the stroke volume associated with a left ventricular dilatation as expected by Olivetti et al. [74]. Taken together, these data suggest that the enhancement in CO could be explained by both an increase in preload and autonomous nervous system stimulation. Indeed, our data showed an increase in myocardial function parameters in normoxic anemic mice. However, although the CO was increased in Epo-Tag^{h} mice, oxygen delivery remained lower than in controls. This could induce the stabilization of the transcription factor HIF-1α as already described in the brain in both models of acute and chronic anemia [61, 69]. This stabilization promotes VEGF-induced angiogenesis as shown in normoxic Epo-TAg^{h} mice with a rise in the capillaries/fibers ratio, thus optimizing oxygen diffusion as described in the brain [24]. This increase in capillary density could allow the development of cardiac hypertrophy without myocardial dysfunction, as previously described in rats in a model of anemia induced by iron-deficient diet [74]. Furthermore, we could not exclude that increased expression of nNOS also contributed to these adaptive cardiovascular responses in chronic anemic mice. Indeed, acute anemia resulted in an increase in CO and a reduced stroke volume in WT anemic mice while in contrast, CO and stroke volume responses were severely attenuated in anemic nNOS$^{-/-}$ mice [57]. In addition, a model of *Hif1a*$^{+/-}$ hemizigous mice revealed impaired increases in hematocrit, right ventricular mass and right ventricular pressure, allowing us to speculate that increased HIF-1α may have participated in these physiological responses to anemia in our model [75].

4. Effects of chronic anemia and hypoxia on cerebral and cardiac tissues

As previously explained, plethora of studies are available to describe cerebral and cardiac adaptations and their underlying molecular mechanisms in response to chronic hypoxia or anemia separately. Our group investigated for the first time, the effects of chronic hypobaric hypoxia combined with chronic anemia in the heart and brain of the transgenic Epo-TAg^h mice. So far, the few studies from other groups that also use transgenic mice overexpressing Epo (Tg6 and Tg21) display results that are complementary to our data but also more detailed. Indeed, these studies also describe the pathways involved in the ventilatory responses to hypoxia and aim to clarify the role of Epo in respiratory acclimatization to hypoxia at physiological, cellular and molecular levels. Even though, we were not able to find other animal studies combining the effects of both chronic hypoxia and anemia on cardiac or cerebral tissues, comparing studies at a multidisciplinary level may provide new approaches and therapies for diseases associated with hypoxia.

4.1. Brain under chronic hypoxia and anemia

In the brain, both Epo and its receptor are upregulated during ischaemia/hypoxia [76, 77] and Epo administration considerably inhibits apoptosis after middle cerebral artery occlusion [78]. Apart from its positive effects in acute ischaemic brain damage, Epo is a potent stimulator of the hypoxic ventilatory response (HVR) by interacting with respiratory centers in the brainstem [79]. Indeed, the blockade of Epo's activity in the brainstem of adult C57Bl6 mice by intracisternal injections of the soluble Epo receptor (sEpoR) induced a reduction of the basal minute ventilation, but it did not affect the central chemosensitivity [80, 81]. In contrast, recent study using transgenic mice Tg6 (that present a human Epo gene overexpression in brain and circulation; Tg21: Epo overexpression in brain) suggested that Epo blunts the HVR through an interaction with central and peripheral respiratory chemocenters [81]. In our model, acute hypoxic ventilatory response was increased after chronic hypoxia in wild-type mice but remained unchanged in Epo-TAg^h mice, confirming that adequate erythropoietin level is necessary to obtain an appropriate HVR and a significant ventilatory acclimatization to hypoxia. Surprisingly, both constraints (chronic hypoxia and anemia) did not trigger a synergic effect in any studied parameters except a high cerebral NO level that could suggest an improved brain perfusion. Finally, the response to chronic hypoxia was divergent in the brain of wild-type and anemic mice. Indeed, these adaptation processes including angiogenesis and neuroprotection were globally altered in Epo-TAg^h mice exposed to chronic hypoxia.

Taken together, all these data suggest that Epo/EpoR pathways activation is necessary to initiate neuroprotection mechanisms as well as cerebral angiogenesis under hypoxia but also might help to better understand respiratory disorders at high altitude.

4.2. Heart under chronic hypoxia and anemia

Independently, chronic anemia and chronic hypoxia increased the expression of HIF-1α, VEGF and Epo, cytokines that are involved in both angiogenesis and cardioprotection through specific signaling pathways acting to compensate oxygen transport deficiency. Recent studies also involved these same cytokines in the cardiovascular responses as well as increased cardiac output observed in acute anemia [57, 75]. Our data showed a decrease in left ventricular hypertrophy and functional left ventricular adaptation as well as a reduced oxygen delivery in the heart of hypoxic Epo-TAg^h mice. Results from other groups showed that Tg6 mice did not develop pulmonary hypertension in normoxia or after exposure to chronic hypoxia (10% O_2 for 3 weeks) [82] suggesting an important role of Epo in functional adaptation of the heart to chronic hypoxia. Similarly to what occurred in the brain, we did not observe a synergic effect of these combined constraints on the expression of the hypoxic genes in the heart of chronically hypoxic Epo-TAg^h mice suggesting that adaptive responses to both constraints are already maximal. However, the increased P-STAT-5/STAT-5 ratio is concordant with a direct protective effect of Epo on cardiomyocytes and endothelial cells as well as stimulation of angiogenesis in the ischaemic heart [83]. Capillary density was unchanged in spite of the fall in HIF-1α/VEGF pathway probably because the initiation of the capillarization with acute hypoxia necessitates VEGF, while its maintenance in chronic hypoxia involves other factors such as angiopoietins [38, 43].

Taken together, our results suggest that adaptative mechanisms that take place with chronic anemia are somewhat similar to those in response to 14 days of hypoxia. However, when both constraints are applied, these mechanisms failed to maintain an adequate cardiac adaptation with a secondary decrease in body oxygen supply, despite the activation of cardioprotective pathways.

5. Perspectives and significance

In this review, a proposal is made that chronic anemia-induced hypoxia triggers regulatory pathways that mediate long-term adaptive cardiac and cerebral changes, particularly at the transcriptional level. These adaptative mechanisms include a regulated increase in cerebral blood flow, cardiac output, angiogenesis and cytoprotection triggered by HIF-1α, VEGF and Epo pathways. All these compensatory mechanisms aim to optimize oxygen delivery and to protect the brain and heart from hypoxic injury to allow acclimatization. However, when both arterial pressure and content of oxygen are decreased, the cerebral and cardiac adaptative mechanisms showed their limitations. We could not exclude that cerebral and cardiac cell injuries occurred following the combined effect of chronic anemia and hypoxia as well as of the NO toxicity. **Figure 1** summarizes the cerebral and cardiac plasticity induced by chronic anemia and/or hypoxia. Data shown in this figure are all based on animal studies. Moreover, a recent review of our group includes also ventilatory [60], muscular [84, 85] and rheologic [86] adaptations in this model of mice. Finally, investigating the molecular mechanisms of O_2 homeostasis represents a mean of gaining new insights to the hypoxia-induced cerebral and myocardial injuries. But it is of great clinical importance to study extensively these non-erythropoietic functions of Epo to contribute to the development of new therapeutic strategies for the management of brain and heart ischemia.

Figure 1 summarizes the physiological adaptations to chronic hypoxia and anemia in the heart and brain of our model of Epo-TAg^h mice. The green color represents the responses of normoxic anemic mice. The blue color represents the responses of hypoxic control mice. The red color represents the responses of hypoxic anemic mice. The arrows represent an increase or decrease of the response, while the '=' symbol means no change between normoxia and hypoxia. PaO_2 is arterial pressure of oxygen, CaO_2 is arterial content of oxygen, PiO_2 is inspired pressure of oxygen and TO_2 is transport of oxygen.

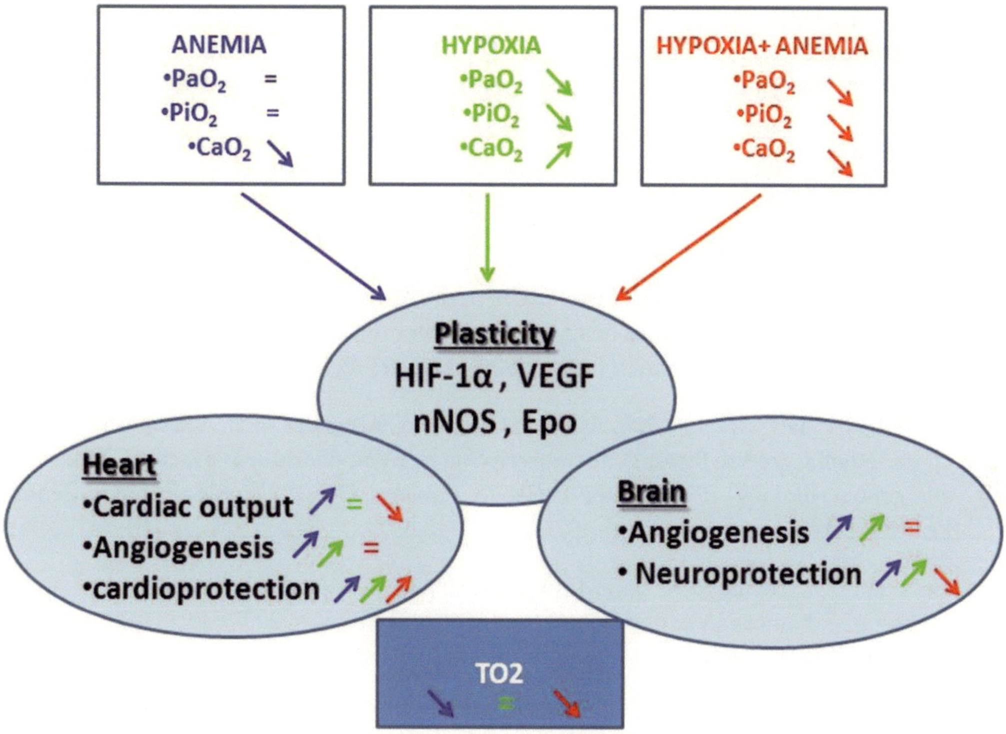

Figure 1. Cerebral and cardiac plasticity induced by chronic anemia and/or hypoxia in Epo-Tag^h mice.

Grants

All the original articles of our group cited in this review were supported by "Agence Nationale de la Recherche" n°ANR-08-GENOPAT-029.

Author details

Raja El Hasnaoui-Saadani

Address all correspondence to: rajaelhasnaoui@hotmail.com

Research center-College of Medicine- Princess Nourah bint Abdulrahmane University, Riyadh, Saudi Arabia

References

[1] Semenza GL. Vascular responses to hypoxia and ischemia. Arteriosclerosis, thrombosis, and vascular biology. 2010 Apr;30(4):648–52. PubMed PMID: 19729615. Pubmed Central PMCID: 2841694.

[2] Ehrenreich H, Hasselblatt M, Dembowski C, Cepek L, Lewczuk P, Stiefel M, et al. Erythropoietin therapy for acute stroke is both safe and beneficial. Molecular medicine. 2002 Aug;8(8):495–505. PubMed PMID: 12435860. Pubmed Central PMCID: 2040012.

[3] Ehrenreich H, Weissenborn K, Prange H, Schneider D, Weimar C, Wartenberg K, et al. Recombinant human erythropoietin in the treatment of acute ischemic stroke. Stroke; a journal of cerebral circulation. 2009 Dec;40(12):e647–56. PubMed PMID: 19834012.

[4] Cohen R, Shainberg A, Hochhauser E, Cheporko Y, Tobar A, Birk E, et al. UTP reduces infarct size and improves mice heart function after myocardial infarct via P2Y2 receptor. Biochemical pharmacology. 2011 Nov 1;82(9):1126–33. PubMed PMID: 21839729.

[5] Forsythe JA, Jiang BH, Iyer NV, Agani F, Leung SW, Koos RD, et al. Activation of vascular endothelial growth factor gene transcription by hypoxia-inducible factor 1. Molecular and cellular biology. 1996 Sep;16(9):4604-13. PubMed PMID: 8756616. Pubmed Central PMCID: 231459.

[6] Gassmann M, Heinicke K, Soliz J, Ogunshola OO. Non-erythroid functions of erythropoietin. Advances in experimental medicine and biology. 2003;543:323–30. PubMed PMID: 14713131.

[7] Vogel J, Gassmann M. Erythropoietic and non-erythropoietic functions of erythropoietin in mouse models. The journal of physiology. 2011 Mar 15;589(Pt 6):1259–64. PubMed PMID: 21282290. Pubmed Central PMCID: 3082089.

[8] Wu H, Lee SH, Gao J, Liu X, Iruela-Arispe ML. Inactivation of erythropoietin leads to defects in cardiac morphogenesis. Development. 1999 Aug;126(16):3597–605. PubMed PMID: 10409505.

[9] Liu C, Shen K, Liu Z, Noguchi CT. Regulated human erythropoietin receptor expression in mouse brain. The journal of biological chemistry. 1997 Dec 19;272(51):32395–400. PubMed PMID: 9405448.

[10] Chen ZY, Warin R, Noguchi CT. Erythropoietin and normal brain development: receptor expression determines multi-tissue response. Neuro-degenerative diseases. 2006;3(1–2):68–75. PubMed PMID: 16909040.

[11] Wang L, Zhang Z, Wang Y, Zhang R, Chopp M. Treatment of stroke with erythropoietin enhances neurogenesis and angiogenesis and improves neurological function in rats. Stroke; a journal of cerebral circulation. 2004 Jul;35(7):1732–7. PubMed PMID: 15178821.

[12] Ribatti D, Vacca A, Roccaro AM, Crivellato E, Presta M. Erythropoietin as an angiogenic factor. European journal of clinical investigation. 2003 Oct;33(10):891–6. PubMed PMID: 14511361.

[13] Marti HH, Bernaudin M, Petit E, Bauer C. Neuroprotection and angiogenesis: dual role of erythropoietin in brain ischemia. News in physiological sciences: an international journal

of physiology produced jointly by the International Union of Physiological Sciences and the American Physiological Society. 2000 Oct;15:225–9. PubMed PMID: 11390915.

[14] Jaquet K, Krause K, Tawakol-Khodai M, Geidel S, Kuck KH. Erythropoietin and VEGF exhibit equal angiogenic potential. Microvascular research. 2002 Sep;64(2):326–33. PubMed PMID: 12204656.

[15] Xiong Y, Mahmood A, Meng Y, Zhang Y, Qu C, Schallert T, et al. Delayed administration of erythropoietin reducing hippocampal cell loss, enhancing angiogenesis and neurogenesis, and improving functional outcome following traumatic brain injury in rats: comparison of treatment with single and triple dose. Journal of neurosurgery. 2010 Sep;113(3):598–608. PubMed PMID: 19817538. Pubmed Central PMCID: 2898921.

[16] Maxwell PH, Osmond MK, Pugh CW, Heryet A, Nicholls LG, Tan CC, et al. Identification of the renal erythropoietin-producing cells using transgenic mice. Kidney international. 1993 Nov;44(5):1149–62. PubMed PMID: 8264149.

[17] Binley K, Askham Z, Iqball S, Spearman H, Martin L, de Alwis M, et al. Long-term reversal of chronic anemia using a hypoxia-regulated erythropoietin gene therapy. Blood. 2002 Oct 1;100(7):2406–13. PubMed PMID: 12239150.

[18] Xu K, Lamanna JC. Chronic hypoxia and the cerebral circulation. Journal of applied physiology. 2006 Feb;100(2):725–30. PubMed PMID: 16421279.

[19] Yin JH, Yang DI, Ku G, Hsu CY. iNOS expression inhibits hypoxia-inducible factor-1 activity. Biochemical and biophysical research communications. 2000 Dec 9;279(1):30–4. PubMed PMID: 11112413.

[20] Hudetz AG, Shen H, Kampine JP. Nitric oxide from neuronal NOS plays critical role in cerebral capillary flow response to hypoxia. The American journal of physiology. 1998 Mar;274(3 Pt 2):H982-9. PubMed PMID: 9530212.

[21] LaManna JC, McCracken KA, Strohl KP. Changes in regional cerebral blood flow and sucrose space after 3-4 weeks of hypobaric hypoxia (0.5 ATM). Advances in experimental medicine and biology. 1989;248:471–7. PubMed PMID: 2506740.

[22] LaManna JC. Rat brain adaptation to chronic hypobaric hypoxia. Advances in experimental medicine and biology. 1992;317:107–14. PubMed PMID: 1288116.

[23] El Hasnaoui-Saadani R, Pichon A, Marchant D, Olivier P, Launay T, Quidu P, et al. Cerebral adaptations to chronic anemia in a model of erythropoietin-deficient mice exposed to hypoxia. American journal of physiology regulatory, integrative and comparative physiology. 2009 Mar;296(3):R801–11. PubMed PMID: 19109375.

[24] LaManna JC, Chavez JC, Pichiule P. Structural and functional adaptation to hypoxia in the rat brain. The Journal of experimental biology. 2004 Aug;207(Pt 18):3163–9. PubMed PMID: 15299038.

[25] Benderro GF, Sun X, Kuang Y, Lamanna JC. Decreased VEGF expression and microvascular density, but increased HIF-1 and 2alpha accumulation and EPO expression in chronic moderate hyperoxia in the mouse brain. Brain research. 2012 Aug 30;1471:46–55. PubMed PMID: 22820296. Pubmed Central PMCID: 3454487.

[26] Boero JA, Ascher J, Arregui A, Rovainen C, Woolsey TA. Increased brain capillaries in chronic hypoxia. Journal of applied physiology. 1999 Apr;86(4):1211–9. PubMed PMID: 10194205.

[27] Dore-Duffy P, LaManna JC. Physiologic angiodynamics in the brain. Antioxidants & redox signaling. 2007 Sep;9(9):1363–71. PubMed PMID: 17627476.

[28] Ward NL, Moore E, Noon K, Spassil N, Keenan E, Ivanco TL, et al. Cerebral angiogenic factors, angiogenesis, and physiological response to chronic hypoxia differ among four commonly used mouse strains. Journal of applied physiology. 2007 May;102(5):1927–35. PubMed PMID: 17234796.

[29] Pichiule P, Agani F, Chavez JC, Xu K, LaManna JC. HIF-1 alpha and VEGF expression after transient global cerebral ischemia. Advances in experimental medicine and biology. 2003;530:611–7. PubMed PMID: 14562758.

[30] Xu K, Puchowicz MA, LaManna JC. Renormalization of regional brain blood flow during prolonged mild hypoxic exposure in rats. Brain research. 2004 Nov 19;1027(1-2):188–91. PubMed PMID: 15494170.

[31] Lauro KL, LaManna JC. Adequacy of cerebral vascular remodeling following three weeks of hypobaric hypoxia. Examined by an integrated composite analytical model. Advances in experimental medicine and biology. 1997;411:369–76. PubMed PMID: 9269451.

[32] Pelligrino DA, LaManna JC, Duckrow RB, Bryan RM, Jr., Harik SI. Hyperglycemia and blood-brain barrier glucose transport. Journal of cerebral blood flow and metabolism: official journal of the International Society of Cerebral Blood Flow and Metabolism. 1992 Nov;12(6):887–99. PubMed PMID: 1400643.

[33] Harik SI, Hritz MA, LaManna JC. Hypoxia-induced brain angiogenesis in the adult rat. The journal of physiology. 1995 Jun 1;485 (Pt 2):525–30. PubMed PMID: 7545234. Pubmed Central PMCID: 1158011.

[34] Harik SI, Lust WD, Jones SC, Lauro KL, Pundik S, LaManna JC. Brain glucose metabolism in hypobaric hypoxia. Journal of applied physiology. 1995 Jul;79(1):136–40. PubMed PMID: 7559210.

[35] Chavez JC, Agani F, Pichiule P, LaManna JC. Expression of hypoxia-inducible factor-1alpha in the brain of rats during chronic hypoxia. Journal of applied physiology. 2000 Nov;89(5):1937–42. PubMed PMID: 11053346.

[36] Dunn JF, Grinberg O, Roche M, Nwaigwe CI, Hou HG, Swartz HM. Noninvasive assessment of cerebral oxygenation during acclimation to hypobaric hypoxia. Journal of cerebral

blood flow and metabolism: official journal of the International Society of Cerebral Blood Flow and Metabolism. 2000 Dec;20(12):1632–5. PubMed PMID: 11129779.

[37] Mironov V, Hritz MA, LaManna JC, Hudetz AG, Harik SI. Architectural alterations in rat cerebral microvessels after hypobaric hypoxia. Brain research. 1994 Oct 10;660(1):73–80. PubMed PMID: 7828003.

[38] Pichiule P, LaManna JC. Angiopoietin-2 and rat brain capillary remodeling during adaptation and deadaptation to prolonged mild hypoxia. Journal of applied physiology. 2002 Sep;93(3):1131–9. PubMed PMID: 12183511.

[39] Krock BL, Skuli N, Simon MC. Hypoxia-induced angiogenesis: good and evil. Genes & cancer. 2011 Dec;2(12):1117–33. PubMed PMID: 22866203. Pubmed Central PMCID: 3411127.

[40] Fong GH. Mechanisms of adaptive angiogenesis to tissue hypoxia. Angiogenesis. 2008;11(2):121–40. PubMed PMID: 18327686.

[41] Agani FH, Puchowicz M, Chavez JC, Pichiule P, LaManna J. Role of nitric oxide in the regulation of HIF-1alpha expression during hypoxia. American journal of physiology cell physiology. 2002 Jul;283(1):C178–86. PubMed PMID: 12055086.

[42] Kanaan A, Farahani R, Douglas RM, Lamanna JC, Haddad GG. Effect of chronic continuous or intermittent hypoxia and reoxygenation on cerebral capillary density and myelination. American journal of physiology regulatory, integrative and comparative physiology. 2006 Apr;290(4):R1105–14. PubMed PMID: 16322350.

[43] Pichiule P, Chavez JC, LaManna JC. Hypoxic regulation of angiopoietin-2 expression in endothelial cells. The journal of biological chemistry. 2004 Mar 26;279(13):12171–80. PubMed PMID: 14702352.

[44] Banchero N. Cardiovascular responses to chronic hypoxia. Annual review of physiology. 1987;49:465–76. PubMed PMID: 3551810.

[45] Pierson DJ. Pathophysiology and clinical effects of chronic hypoxia. Respiratory care. 2000 Jan;45(1):39–51; discussion-3. PubMed PMID: 10771781.

[46] Leon-Velarde F, Villafuerte FC, Richalet JP. Chronic mountain sickness and the heart. Progress in cardiovascular diseases. 2010 May–Jun;52(6):540–9. PubMed PMID: 20417348.

[47] El Hasnaoui-Saadani R, Marchant D, Pichon A, Escoubet B, Pezet M, Hilfiker-Kleiner D, et al. Epo deficiency alters cardiac adaptation to chronic hypoxia. Respiratory physiology & neurobiology. 2013 Apr 1;186(2):146–54. PubMed PMID: 23333855.

[48] Bin-Jaliah I, Ammar HI, Mikhailidis DP, Dallak MA, Al-Hashem FH, Haidara MA, et al. Cardiac adaptive responses after hypoxia in an experimental model. Angiology. 2010 Feb;61(2):145–56. PubMed PMID: 19939823.

[49] Cai Z, Semenza GL. Phosphatidylinositol-3-kinase signaling is required for erythropoietin-mediated acute protection against myocardial ischemia/reperfusion injury. Circulation. 2004 May 4;109(17):2050–3. PubMed PMID: 15117842.

[50] Hoch M, Fischer P, Stapel B, Missol-Kolka E, Sekkali B, Scherr M, et al. Erythropoietin preserves the endothelial differentiation capacity of cardiac progenitor cells and reduces heart failure during anticancer therapies. Cell stem cell. 2011 Aug 5;9(2):131–43. PubMed PMID: 21816364.

[51] Koury MJ, Bondurant MC. The molecular mechanism of erythropoietin action. European journal of biochemistry/FEBS. 1992 Dec 15;210(3):649–63. PubMed PMID: 1483451.

[52] Digicaylioglu M, Lipton SA. Erythropoietin-mediated neuroprotection involves cross-talk between Jak2 and NF-kappaB signalling cascades. Nature. 2001 Aug 9;412(6847):641–7. PubMed PMID: 11493922.

[53] Kertesz N, Wu J, Chen TH, Sucov HM, Wu H. The role of erythropoietin in regulating angiogenesis. Developmental biology. 2004 Dec 1;276(1):101–10. PubMed PMID: 15531367.

[54] Marzo F, Lavorgna A, Coluzzi G, Santucci E, Tarantino F, Rio T, et al. Erythropoietin in heart and vessels: focus on transcription and signalling pathways. Journal of thrombosis and thrombolysis. 2008 Dec;26(3):183–7. PubMed PMID: 18338108.

[55] Ray PS, Estrada-Hernandez T, Sasaki H, Zhu L, Maulik N. Early effects of hypoxia/reoxygenation on VEGF, ang-1, ang-2 and their receptors in the rat myocardium: implications for myocardial angiogenesis. Molecular and cellular biochemistry. 2000 Oct;213(1–2):145–53. PubMed PMID: 11129953.

[56] Sharma S, Taegtmeyer H, Adrogue J, Razeghi P, Sen S, Ngumbela K, et al. Dynamic changes of gene expression in hypoxia-induced right ventricular hypertrophy. American journal of physiology heart and circulatory physiology. 2004 Mar;286(3):H1185–92. PubMed PMID: 14630626.

[57] Tsui AK, Marsden PA, Mazer CD, Adamson SL, Henkelman RM, Ho JJ, et al. Priming of hypoxia-inducible factor by neuronal nitric oxide synthase is essential for adaptive responses to severe anemia. Proceedings of the National Academy of Sciences of the United States of America. 2011 Oct 18;108(42):17544–9. PubMed PMID: 21976486. Pubmed Central PMCID: 3198321.

[58] Macarlupu JL, Buvry A, Morel OE, Leon-Velarde F, Richalet JP, Favret F. Time course of ventilatory acclimatisation to hypoxia in a model of anemic transgenic mice. Respiratory physiology & neurobiology. 2006 Aug;153(1):14–22. PubMed PMID: 16330260.

[59] Macarlupu JL, Buvry A, Morel OE, Leon-Velarde F, Richalet JP, Favret F. Characterisation of the ventilatory response to hypoxia in a model of transgenic anemic mice. Respiratory physiology & neurobiology. 2006 Jan 25;150(1):19–26. PubMed PMID: 15878311.

[60] Voituron N, Jeton F, Cholley Y, Hasnaoui-Saadani RE, Marchant D, Quidu P, et al. Catalyzing role of erythropoietin on the nitric oxide central pathway during the ventilatory responses to hypoxia. Physiological reports. 2014 Feb 1;2(2):e00223. PubMed PMID: 24744892. Pubmed Central PMCID: 3966246.

[61] McLaren AT, Marsden PA, Mazer CD, Baker AJ, Stewart DJ, Tsui AK, et al. Increased expression of HIF-1alpha, nNOS, and VEGF in the cerebral cortex of anemic rats. American journal of physiology Regulatory, integrative and comparative physiology. 2007 Jan;292(1):R403–14. PubMed PMID: 16973934.

[62] Hare GM, Mazer CD, Hutchison JS, McLaren AT, Liu E, Rassouli A, et al. Severe hemodilutional anemia increases cerebral tissue injury following acute neurotrauma. Journal of applied physiology. 2007 Sep;103(3):1021–9. PubMed PMID: 17556499.

[63] Hare GM, Mazer CD, Mak W, Gorczynski RM, Hum KM, Kim SY, et al. Hemodilutional anemia is associated with increased cerebral neuronal nitric oxide synthase gene expression. Journal of applied physiology. 2003 May;94(5):2058–67. PubMed PMID: 12533500.

[64] Hare GM, Tsui AK, McLaren AT, Ragoonanan TE, Yu J, Mazer CD. Anemia and cerebral outcomes: many questions, fewer answers. Anesthesia and analgesia. 2008 Oct;107(4):1356–70. PubMed PMID: 18806052.

[65] Tsui AK, Marsden PA, Mazer CD, Sled JG, Lee KM, Henkelman RM, et al. Differential HIF and NOS responses to acute anemia: defining organ-specific hemoglobin thresholds for tissue hypoxia. American journal of physiology Regulatory, integrative and comparative physiology. 2014 Jul 1;307(1):R13–25. PubMed PMID: 24760996.

[66] Pearce WJ. Mechanisms of hypoxic cerebral vasodilatation. Pharmacology & therapeutics. 1995 Jan;65(1):75–91. PubMed PMID: 7716183.

[67] Serrano J, Encinas JM, Salas E, Fernandez AP, Castro-Blanco S, Fernandez-Vizarra P, et al. Hypobaric hypoxia modifies constitutive nitric oxide synthase activity and protein nitration in the rat cerebellum. Brain research. 2003 Jun 20;976(1):109–19. PubMed PMID: 12763628.

[68] Serrano J, Encinas JM, Fernandez AP, Rodrigo J, Martinez A. Effects of acute hypobaric hypoxia on the nitric oxide system of the rat cerebral cortex: Protective role of nitric oxide inhibitors. Neuroscience. 2006 Oct 27;142(3):799–808. PubMed PMID: 16952423.

[69] Rakusan K, Cicutti N, Kolar F. Effect of anemia on cardiac function, microvascular structure, and capillary hematocrit in rat hearts. American journal of physiology Heart and circulatory physiology. 2001 Mar;280(3):H1407–14. PubMed PMID: 11179091.

[70] Wang L, Chopp M, Gregg SR, Zhang RL, Teng H, Jiang A, et al. Neural progenitor cells treated with EPO induce angiogenesis through the production of VEGF. Journal of cerebral blood flow and metabolism: official journal of the International Society of Cerebral Blood Flow and Metabolism. 2008 Jul;28(7):1361–8. PubMed PMID: 18414495. Pubmed Central PMCID: 3971950.

[71] Lopez TV, Lappin TR, Maxwell P, Shi Z, Lopez-Marure R, Aguilar C, et al. Autocrine/paracrine erythropoietin signalling promotes JAK/STAT-dependent proliferation of human cervical cancer cells. International journal of cancer. 2011 Dec 1;129(11):2566–76. PubMed PMID: 21442620.

[72] Hebert PC, Van der Linden P, Biro G, Hu LQ. Physiologic aspects of anemia. Critical care clinics. 2004 Apr;20(2):187–212. PubMed PMID: 15135460.

[73] Naito Y, Tsujino T, Matsumoto M, Sakoda T, Ohyanagi M, Masuyama T. Adaptive response of the heart to long-term anemia induced by iron deficiency. American journal of physiology heart and circulatory physiology. 2009 Mar;296(3):H585–93. PubMed PMID: 19136608.

[74] Olivetti G, Lagrasta C, Quaini F, Ricci R, Moccia G, Capasso JM, et al. Capillary growth in anemia-induced ventricular wall remodeling in the rat heart. Circulation research. 1989 Nov;65(5):1182–92. PubMed PMID: 2529998.

[75] Yu AY, Shimoda LA, Iyer NV, Huso DL, Sun X, McWilliams R, et al. Impaired physiological responses to chronic hypoxia in mice partially deficient for hypoxia-inducible factor 1alpha. The journal of clinical investigation. 1999 Mar;103(5):691–6. PubMed PMID: 10074486. Pubmed Central PMCID: 408131.

[76] Sakanaka M, Wen TC, Matsuda S, Masuda S, Morishita E, Nagao M, et al. In vivo evidence that erythropoietin protects neurons from ischemic damage. Proceedings of the national academy of sciences of the United States of America. 1998 Apr 14;95(8):4635–40. PubMed PMID: 9539790. Pubmed Central PMCID: 22542.

[77] Siren AL, Knerlich F, Poser W, Gleiter CH, Bruck W, Ehrenreich H. Erythropoietin and erythropoietin receptor in human ischemic/hypoxic brain. Acta neuropathologica. 2001 Mar;101(3):271–6. PubMed PMID: 11307627.

[78] Siren AL, Fratelli M, Brines M, Goemans C, Casagrande S, Lewczuk P, et al. Erythropoietin prevents neuronal apoptosis after cerebral ischemia and metabolic stress. Proceedings of the National Academy of Sciences of the United States of America. 2001 Mar 27;98(7):4044–9. PubMed PMID: 11259643. Pubmed Central PMCID: 31176.

[79] Soliz J, Joseph V, Soulage C, Becskei C, Vogel J, Pequignot JM, et al. Erythropoietin regulates hypoxic ventilation in mice by interacting with brainstem and carotid bodies. The journal of physiology. 2005 Oct 15;568(Pt 2):559–71. PubMed PMID: 16051624. Pubmed Central PMCID: 1474739.

[80] Soliz J, Gassmann M, Joseph V. Soluble erythropoietin receptor is present in the mouse brain and is required for the ventilatory acclimatization to hypoxia. The journal of physiology. 2007 Aug 15;583(Pt 1):329–36. PubMed PMID: 17584830. Pubmed Central PMCID: 2277219.

[81] Soliz J, Soulage C, Hermann DM, Gassmann M. Acute and chronic exposure to hypoxia alters ventilatory pattern but not minute ventilation of mice overexpressing erythropoietin. American journal of physiology regulatory, integrative and comparative physiology. 2007 Oct;293(4):R1702–10. PubMed PMID: 17652365.

[82] Weissmann N, Manz D, Buchspies D, Keller S, Mehling T, Voswinckel R, et al. Congenital erythropoietin over-expression causes "anti-pulmonary hypertensive" structural and functional changes in mice, both in normoxia and hypoxia. Thrombosis and haemostasis. 2005 Sep;94(3):630–8. PubMed PMID: 16268482.

[83] Ruifrok WP, de Boer RA, Westenbrink BD, van Veldhuisen DJ, van Gilst WH. Erythropoietin in cardiac disease: new features of an old drug. European journal of pharmacology. 2008 May 13;585(2–3):270–7. PubMed PMID: 18407263.

[84] Hagstrom L, Agbulut O, El-Hasnaoui-Saadani R, Marchant D, Favret F, Richalet JP, et al. Epo is relevant neither for microvascular formation nor for the new formation and maintenance of mice skeletal muscle fibres in both normoxia and hypoxia. Journal of biomedicine & biotechnology. 2010;2010:137817. PubMed PMID: 20414335. Pubmed Central PMCID: 2855079.

[85] Hagstrom L, Canon F, Agbulut O, Marchant D, Serrurier B, Richalet JP, et al. Skeletal muscle intrinsic functional properties are preserved in a model of erythropoietin deficient mice exposed to hypoxia. Pflugers archiv: European journal of physiology. 2010 Apr;459(5):713–23. PubMed PMID: 20119684.

[86] Pichon A, Lamarre Y, Voituron N, Marchant D, Vilar J, Richalet JP, et al. Red blood cell deformability is very slightly decreased in erythropoietin deficient mice. Clinical hemorheology and microcirculation. 2014;56(1):41–6. PubMed PMID: 23302595.

Chapter 10

Hypothermia in Stroke Therapy: Systemic versus Local Application

Mitchell Huber, Hong Lian Duan, Ankush Chandra,
Fengwu Li, Longfei Wu, Longfei Guan,
Xiaokun Geng and Yuchuan Ding

Additional information is available at the end of the chapter

http://dx.doi.org/10.5772/65899

Abstract

Presently, there are no effective, widely applicable therapies for ischemic stroke. There is strong clinical evidence for the neuroprotective benefits of hypothermia, and surface-cooling methods have been utilized for decades in the treatment of cerebral ischemia during cardiac arrest, but complications with hypothermia induction have hindered its clinical acceptance in ischemic stroke therapy. Recently, the microcatheter-based local endovascular infusion (LEVI) of cold saline directly to the infarct site has been proposed as a solution to the drawbacks of surface cooling. The safety and efficacy of LEVI in rat models have been established, and implementation in larger animals has been similarly encouraging. A recent pilot study even established the safety of LEVI in humans. This review seeks to outline the major research on LEVI, discusses the mechanisms that mediate its superior neuroprotection over surface and systemic cooling, and identifies areas that warrant further investigation. While LEVI features improvements on surface cooling, its core mechanisms of neuroprotection are still largely shared with therapeutic hypothermia in general. As such, the mechanisms of hypothermia-based neuroprotection are discussed as well.

Keywords: local endovascular infusion, therapeutic hypothermia, ischemic stroke therapy, neuroprotection, microcatheter

1. Introduction

Ischemic stroke is the leading cause of death and disability worldwide, yet effective treatment is limited. Despite considerable research efforts, intravenous (IV) thrombolysis with recombinant tissue plasminogen activator (rt-PA) within the first 4.5 h of symptom onset remains the only proven acute therapy for ischemic stroke [1]. Outside of the treatment window, rt-PA fails to be an option, and given that only 25.4% of stroke patients arrive to the hospital within 3 h of symptom onset, a significant minority of patients are even eligible to receive rt-PA [2]. Thus, alternative treatment strategies for ischemic stroke are urgently needed. Although over a thousand drugs and nonpharmacological strategies have been tested for neuroprotective ability in acute stroke as of 2003, none have proven effective and applicable enough for widespread clinical acceptance [3]. However, hypothermia has prevailed as a promising therapeutic option for stroke patients. In fact, hypothermia is the only neuroprotective approach found thus far whose efficacy has been experimentally demonstrated in a randomized controlled clinical trial [4]. The neuroprotective benefits of hypothermia have been utilized for decades in the treatment of global cerebral ischemia following cardiac arrest and for hypoxic-ischemic encephalopathy in newborns, but its use in stroke therapy has garnered attention only in recent years [4, 5].

Hypothermia has been consistently shown to reduce infarct volumes and improve functional outcomes in animal models of focal cerebral ischemia. In a meta-analysis, the use of hypothermia in animal models of ischemic stroke was shown to reduce infarct volumes by 44% on average [6]. Given the robust neuroprotective effects of therapeutic hypothermia (TH) in animal models of temporary artery occlusion, studies are being conducted at an increasing rate to empirically establish hypothermia as a high-yield front-line stroke therapy.

1.1. Degrees of hypothermia

Therapeutic hypothermia is defined as the deliberate reduction of core body temperature for therapeutic benefit [7]. While there is no exact consensus on the optimal degree of cooling, several studies have found cooling at 33°C to be most effective [7–10]. The vast majority of investigations on the topic feature a mild to moderate degree of cooling, with very few venturing into moderate-deep to deep hypothermia (**Table 1**). In fact, temperature depressions to such an extent have been reported to primarily provide negative consequences [9]. For this review, therapeutic hypothermia refers to mild-moderate hypothermia, unless otherwise specified.

Degree of hypothermia	Mild	Moderate	Moderate-deep	Deep
Body temperature (°C)	35.9–34	33.9–32	31.9–30	<30

Table 1. Terms for degrees of hypothermia by body temperature.

2. Systemic hypothermia

The majority of studies on the induction of TH in acute ischemic stroke therapy have applied whole-body cooling. Therapeutic cerebral hypothermia can be most easily established by either surface cooling or systemic endovascular infusion cold saline [11, 12]. In clinical stroke cases, surface and endovascular cooling have both been used for successful whole-body hypothermia induction and maintenance.

The sentinel study on therapeutic hypothermia exclusively considered "surface cooling," cooling with ice packs or air-circulating cooling blankets/mattresses. This study demonstrated improved survival outcomes in cardiac arrest patients with therapeutic hypothermia [5, 12]. The Cooling for Acute Ischemic Brain Damage (COOL AID) study additionally showed that moderate therapeutic hypothermia (target temperature 32°C by surface cooling) in patients with acute ischemic stroke is feasible and can be accomplished safely by surface cooling [13]. Surface-cooling methods are easy to use and permit early treatment initiation, which makes them an attractive option. However, there are numerous logistical problems associated with surface cooling that outweigh its benefit.

Systemic endovascular infusion methods reduce body temperature invasively using intravenously placed cooling catheters or intravenous cold infusions of isotonic saline into a major systemic blood vessel. The safety of endovascular cooling in patients with acute ischemic stroke was assessed in both the COOL AID II study [14] and the Intravascular Cooling in the Treatment of Stroke (ICTuS) study [15]. The approach was shown in both cases to reduce body temperature more rapidly than surface cooling could accomplish, and since a temperature probe is embedded in the catheter, precise temperature monitoring and regulation was far superior to surface-cooling methods. The disadvantages of systemic endovascular hypothermia induction stem from its invasive nature; the method carries a much higher risk of deep venous thrombosis (DVT), bacteremia, and sepsis than surface cooling [16, 17]. Additionally, the Intravascular Cooling in the Treatment of Stroke-Longer tPA Window (ICTuS-L) study results showed a statistically significant increase in the occurrence of pneumonias in patients receiving systemic endovascular TH [18].

Unfortunately, whole-body cooling by either method creates a number of serious complications. Chiefly, whole-body cooling frequently causes shivering and dermal vasoconstriction, which can complicate effective progression to optimal cooling ranges; whole-body cooling frequently requires 3–7 h to reach target temperatures [19]. Shivering also raises intracranial pressure (ICP) and requires the use of several pharmacological agents to inhibit these effects along with skin warming to address physical discomfort [20, 21]. Another side effect of whole-body cooling is the risk of shear-induced platelet aggregation, which can develop as blood viscosity increases at low temperatures [22]. Even a minor amount of coagulation can cause a blockage of the microcirculation of the brain and heart, which ironically creates the exact problem that hypothermia attempts to treat [21]. Furthermore, whole-body cooling increases the likelihood of ventricular fibrillations, bradycardia, reduced cardiac output, hemostatic or hemorrhagic changes, decreased urine output, and metabolic dysfunction [14, 23, 24]. With this extensive list of severe complications, a more graceful therapeutic modality is urgently needed.

3. Hypothermia via local endovascular infusion

Recently, the selective induction of hypothermia into the ischemic region using an endovascular microcatheter has garnered attention as a novel strategy to optimize the neuroprotective benefits of therapeutic hypothermia with the myriad of comorbidities accompanying full-body cooling. In contrast to other cooling methods, which require hypothermia to slowly spread into the ischemic region, local endovascular infusion (LEVI) reduces infarct temperatures effectively by perfusing ice-cold saline directly to the ischemic region. This allows for more rapid achievement of target temperatures and permits greater specificity of hypothermia while avoiding the side effects of systemic cooling. During these procedures, an infusion microcatheter, guided to the site of the lesion via the guide catheter over a microguidewire, is advanced distally to the site of occlusion, and cold saline is perfused [25] for a variable length of time, usually from 5 to 30 min. The logistics of actually performing LEVI in humans are relatively simple, as this is a normal part of performing endovascular interventions for many neuroendovascular surgeons [26]. Therefore, it is expected that this new therapy could easily be added to an angiography suite [27].

LEVI has been tested in animal models of stroke both before and after reperfusion. Pre-reperfusion flushing was first proposed by Ding et al. [28], when the technique was used in a transient middle cerebral artery occlusion (MCAO) rat model. The study produced a 65% reduction in infarct volumes and 61% reduction in leukocyte infiltration when resolution of a 2-h middle cerebral artery occlusion was preceded by LEVI (23°C saline infused at 2 mL/min for 3–4 min) [28]. Pre-reperfusion LEVI has since been shown to reduce infarct volumes by 75 [29] to 90% [30] and significantly conserve motor function both hours and weeks after stroke [29, 30]. Post-reperfusion LEVI has also been considered in some studies, in which a catheter was introduced into the internal carotid artery after blood flow to the ischemic territory had been reestablished [31, 32]. Significant improvements in both infarct volume and functional recovery were observed in every post-reperfusion LEVI trial tested, but these improvements were not as pronounced as those from pre-reperfusion LEVI.

Although the majority of current experimental data on LEVI in stroke are based on rat models, a few large animal studies that have been conducted are equally encouraging. A recent investigation using swine showed that LEVI significantly reduced infarct volumes following 4–4.5-h MCAO (the longest delay of hypothermia in any LEVI large animal study) [33]. The credibility [34], safety, and efficacy of LEVI in Rhesus monkeys were also confirmed, as infusion of cold-lactated Ringer's solution was used to achieve statistically significant degrees of peri-infarct cooling without apparent vasogenic edema or other comorbidities [35]. Additionally, the safety and feasibility of LEVI was recently verified in humans [36]. In nine human patients with partially or completely treated cerebrovascular diseases undergoing diagnostic cerebral angiogram, 7°C LEVI at ~33 mL/min for 10–13 min was able to reduce jugular venous blood temperature (a proxy for brain temperature) by 0.84°C while reducing rectal temperature by 0.15°C and having no significant effects on vital signs. LEVI was also recently implemented in patients actively undergoing ischemic stroke (within 8 h of symptom onset), which confirmed the safety and feasibility of the procedure [25]. The neuroprotective efficacy of LEVI, however, remains to be established in a clinical setting.

Despite recent milestones in LEVI testing, several systematic obstacles have hindered widespread acceptance. Chief among these obstacles is heterogeneity of experimental designs. Since TH is only widely used for cardiac arrest, the majority of studies utilize a global ischemia model, which has been found to unfaithfully simulate the physiological conditions of

http://dx.doi.org/10.5772/65899

focal ischemia [37]. Hypothermia-based investigations also vary in animal model, animal age, duration of ischemia, duration of hypothermia, depth of hypothermia, method of hypothermia induction, and rate of cooling, all of which have consistently been shown to play critical roles in the efficacy of TH treatments. Additionally, current animal models have failed to adequately simulate the reaction of a human to such an intervention. While the majority of LEVI studies have used rat models, rats have been widely criticized for their poor translatability to clinical practice [38]. There even exists heterogeneity among the species; rats of similar strains from different suppliers have been found to show variations in response to ischemia [12]. Given that stroke accounts for 9% of deaths worldwide and ~25% of stroke survivors are permanently disabled [39], such a promising therapy is in serious need of further exploration.

3.1. Benefits of LEVI over systemic infusion

LEVI is an optimized version of general TH. As such, its mechanisms of neuroprotection are predominately the same as those of full-body cooling. However, LEVI retains a few unique features that make it considerably more effective than global cooling. These features are summarized in the present section.

3.1.1. Maximized rate of cooling

Although there is no consensus on the exact treatment window for therapeutic hypothermia, it would be difficult to dispute the time-sensitive nature of hypothermia induction [31, 40]. While one author found that TH is ineffective after 45 min of ischemia [41] and most others have found neuroprotective efficacy when induction follows 2–3 h of ischemia [30, 42], there is a strong consensus that this efficacy diminishes over the course of hours. Considering that surface-cooling methods frequently take 3–7 h to reach target temperatures [19], it would be impossible for any stroke patient to fall within an optimal treatment window. By contrast, LEVI can establish target temperatures in a matter of minutes [36]; in a 300-g localized cerebral infarct, LEVI attained target temperatures 30 times faster than classic surface cooling and 10–20 times faster than systemic infusion of cold saline into the inferior vena cava [27]. The time saved by using LEVI translates to superior degrees of neuroprotection and an improved quality of life for ischemic stroke patients.

3.1.2. Metabolite washout and attenuated hyper- or hypoperfusion

One mechanism by which ischemic stroke damages the brain is through postischemic hyperperfusion. Under ischemic conditions, brain cells are forced to conduct anaerobic respiration, the byproducts of which (lactate, prostaglandins, and carbon dioxide) are vasodilatory at elevated levels [43]. In the absence of adequate perfusion, these vasodilatory metabolites accumulate in the ischemic region and trigger an excessive vasodilation once perfusion is restored. Literature on postischemic hyperperfusion has been discrepant, but suggests that the phenomenon is associated with larger infarcts and early death [44, 45]. This "luxury reperfusion" has been implicated in post-reperfusion edema formation, the primary cause of death within 1 month of ischemic stroke [45, 46]. While hypothermia prevents intracranial-pressure elevations by itself, LEVI provides an additional protective mechanism by washing out vasodilatory metabolites built up during the ischemic period, which minimizes the extent of hyperperfusion-related injury [29, 47]. As evidence of this mechanism, fast warm (37°C)-saline LEVI has been shown to significantly reduce infarct volumes and improve functional recoveries compared to systemic infusion of warm saline [28].

Pre-reperfusion flushing also significantly reduces leukocyte infiltration and ICAM-1 expression in the peri-infarct vasculature [28, 48], leading to improved postischemic perfusion. Luan et al. showed that LEVI was able to reduce cerebral poststroke ICAM-1 expression and leukocyte infiltration to a significantly greater degree than that of local warm-saline infusion or systemic cold-saline infusion were able to [48]. Other studies have reported similar reductions in ICAM-1 expression and infiltration/activation of PMN leukocytes and microglia [49]. These data imply that the neuroprotective advantages of LEVI over systemic infusion rely partially on its metabolite-washout ability and subsequent improved perfusion.

3.1.3. Drug delivery into ischemic territory through LEVI

In addition to the hypothermia-associated benefits of cold-saline infusion, LEVI allows for coadministration of neuroprotective drugs directly into the ischemic region along with hypothermic fluids, which maximizes local drug concentrations while minimizing systemic drug concentrations, thereby circumventing dose-dependent systemic side effects [50]. Preliminary studies using LEVI with neuroprotective drugs have shown exceptional promise; a 2012 study by Song et al. found that LEVI of a magnesium sulfate solution at 15°C caused a 65% reduction in infarct volumes compared to a 48% reduction from LEVI alone [51]. Similar results were found following LEVI of a 20% human albumin solution cooled to 0°C [52]. Normothermic local infusion of drugs has shown potential as well, as LEVI of erythropoietin at room temperature reduced infarct volumes by 21% (significant compared to control), decreased apoptosis in the ischemic core and penumbra, and significantly preserved neurological scores [53].

LEVI can also aid in drug permeation into the brain parenchyma. Blood-brain barrier (BBB) impermeability has been described as the most important factor limiting the growth of neurotherapeutic drugs [54] and remains a challenging issue today. However, BBB breakdown is a natural product of cerebral ischemia, which allows for the perfusion of drugs into the brain parenchyma that would otherwise be prevented from reaching their target [50]. When coupled with LEVI-based drug administration, BBB breakdown can be capitalized on to provide benefits for stroke therapy. This hypothesis was confirmed experimentally in a 2007 study by Woitzik et al. in which microcatheter-based infusion of MK-801 (an NMDA receptor antagonist) into the ischemic region resulted in 30% smaller infarct volumes at 24 h after infusion than when MK-801 was infused systemically [50]. MK-801 has shown significant neuroprotective potential, but has not attained clinical acceptance due to significant side effects when administered at high enough doses to be effective when infused systemically [55], a problem nullified by LEVI-based administration. While LEVI with neuroprotective drugs has never been tested in a clinical setting, it is possible that the combination could open the door for the use of neuroprotective pharmacotherapies that would otherwise be prohibited from reaching target tissues [50, 56].

http://dx.doi.org/10.5772/65899

4. Mechanisms underlying hypothermia-induced neuroprotection

In addition to LEVI-specific neuroprotective mechanisms, LEVI benefits from neuroprotective mechanisms of therapeutic hypothermia in general. These mechanisms exhibit significant redundancy, as they affect multiple steps in several parallel pathways of hypoxia-induced brain injury. Hypothermia primarily exerts its neuroprotective effects by slowing essential metabolic processes while preserving life, which subsequently attenuates pathways involved in excitotoxicity, free radical production, inflammation, edema, and apoptosis [12, 37, 57, 58]. However, a common theme in literature on the topic is consensus on effects and uncertainty of mechanisms. While virtually every paper finds TH administration to be neuroprotective, there is very little agreement on how this works. This is due, in part, to the correlative goal of most studies. The majority of work on the topic identifies alterations in the levels of one indicator or another when TH is implemented, but fails to elucidate exactly where TH exerts its neuroprotective effects. While this is valuable information, without a causative component, these studies always leave the door open for the participation of a third variable. In light of frequently conflicting findings, this section features few concrete lessons from the literature. Rather, we attempt to discuss the pathways that TH acts on, and consider the most likely points at which TH exerts its neuroprotective effects.

4.1. Metabolic crisis

The primary culprit of ischemia-induced brain damage is oxygen-supply cessation, which initiates a cascade of secondary problems. In the absence of oxygen, neurons are unable to generate high-energy metabolites, which prohibit effective maintenance of ion gradients. Ion-gradient breakdown leads to involuntary depolarization, which allows for excessive glutamate release. This wave of glutamate then stimulates NMDA and AMPA receptors, which results in increased intracellular calcium levels and ultimately leads to excitotoxicity, a phenomenon characterized by mitochondrial membrane depolarization, caspase activation, production of reactive oxygen and nitrogen species, and apoptosis [37, 59]. In addition to excitotoxicity, ion-gradient breakdown causes Na^+ to build up in brain cells and in particular astrocytes. This establishes an osmotic gradient favoring the movement of water into astrocytes (and to a lesser extent, all other brain cells), thereby creating cytotoxic edema [60]. The edema increases intracranial pressure and ultimately exacerbates brain damage (**Figure 1**).

Hypothermia combats this cascade at several points (**Figure 1**). Reduced brain temperatures have been shown to lower cerebral metabolic rate by 5% for every 1°C reduction in body temperature, allowing for prolonged maintenance of ion gradients (preventing excitotoxicity) and minimized need to conduct anaerobic respiration, thereby diminishing the extent of reperfusion injury [58]. In patients with traumatic brain injury who received therapeutic hypothermia to 32–33°C, cerebral oxygen consumption was reduced to 27% after 24 h of hypothermia [61]. Hypothermia has also been shown to reduce the production of glycolytic intermediates by an average of 30% and tricarboxylic acid (TCA) cycle intermediates by 30–70% [62]. Alternatively, ratios of phosphocreatinine:inorganic phosphate and adenosine triphosphate (ATP):inorganic phosphate seem to increase slightly during transient hypothermia, implying that the real energy conservation mechanism at play is one of the slowing energy-consuming reactions, rather than slowing glycolytic flux [62]. Hypothermia has also been routinely reported to improve ATP recovery after reperfusion [37]; mild hypothermia has led to a 10–20% increase in the rate of metabolic recovery in the first 10–25 min after reperfusion compared to normothermic animals [63], a finding echoed in other studies [62, 64]. It is possible, then, that the primary energy conservation mechanism that underlies TH is that of accelerated energy recovery after reperfusion rather than energy preservation during hypoxia. However, while metabolic depression during hypothermia has been well documented as a phenomenon, its underlying mechanism is still poorly understood. Thus, the points at which hypothermia exerts its neuroprotective effects are unclear, and whether its main mechanism of neuroprotection involves cellular respiration at all remains to be elucidated.

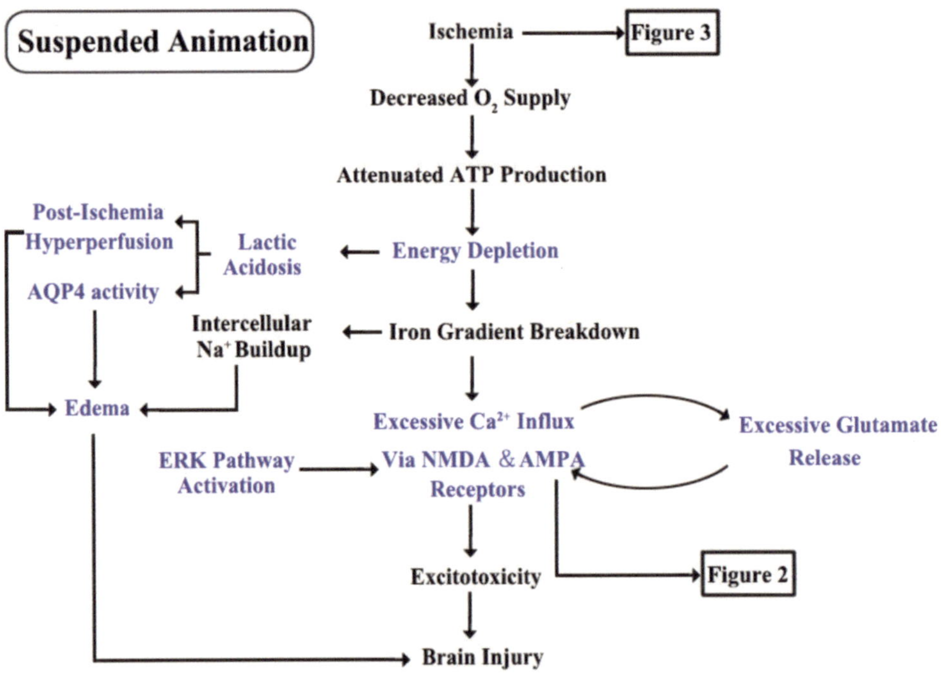

Figure 1. The figure describes the pathogenesis of stroke as it relates to ischemia-induced metabolic crisis. The points at which hypothermia exerts its neuroprotective effects remain largely unclear. Studies have shown that TH attenuates a multitude of steps in the cascade of ischemia-induced brain damage compared to stroke without hypothermia, but whether the observed attenuations are direct effects of TH or byproducts of upstream attenuations has yet to be elucidated. As such, blue font indicates steps discussed in the present review that hypothermia has been shown to attenuate. Black font indicates steps that we have not discussed in the present review, but does not necessarily indicate that these steps are unaffected by hypothermia.

Hypothermia has also been shown to prevent anoxic depolarization. In an aged rat model, mild hypothermia was shown to completely inhibit the efflux of excitatory amino acids (glutamate and aspartate) while significantly increasing the release of the inhibitory amino acid taurine [65]. While no mechanism has been firmly tied to this phenomenon, several have been speculated. TH has been reported to prevent activation of protein kinase C (PKC) and calcium-calmodulin kinase II during ischemia, both of which are associated with neurotransmitter release [65]. Therapeutic cooling also attenuates ischemia-induced downregulation of the GluR2 (glutamate receptor 2) CA1 subunit, which is responsible for limiting Ca^{2+} influx through AMPA receptors in a global cerebral ischemia model [66]. It is also possible that this facet of hypothermic neuroprotection is accomplished by the preservation of ion gradients due to metabolic downregulation. However, some reports have suggested that hypothermia simply delays anoxic depolarization rather than preventing it [67]. In light of conflicting research on the topic, it is likely that multiple mechanisms are at play, culminating in the robust excitation prevention associated with therapeutic hypothermia.

Hypothermia has also been found to combat cytotoxic edema after ischemic stroke (**Figure 1**). This edema is largely mediated by aquaporin 4 (AQP4), which is expressed in the glial-limiting membranes, ependyma, and pericapillary foot processes of astrocytes [68]. In mice, AQP4 knockout has been associated with reduced infarct sizes, decreased brain water content, and improved neurological and survival outcomes [60]. While the brain naturally downregulates AQP4 expression following hypoxia [60], hypothermia has been shown to augment this downregulation [60, 69, 70]. It is possible that this downregulation is a downstream effect of TH. In experimental models, AQP4 levels in astrocyte cell membranes were increased by increased lactic acid concentration, but AQP4 mRNA levels were unchanged, which implies that the observed increases in membrane-bound AQP4 came as the result of redistribution or posttranslational modification, rather than increased expression [71]. Several other mechanisms have also been proposed for this upregulation [72]; thus, the specifics of ischemia-induced aquaporin modulation have still yet to be fully elucidated.

At the molecular level, several studies have implicated immediate induction of early gene expression (miRNAs) and cellular stress response (heat-shock proteins, HSPs) activation in hypothermia-induced neuroprotection. Hypothermia has been shown to suppress transcription of some pro-inflammatory molecules (interleukin (IL)-1β and osteopontin) and enhance transcription of anti-inflammatory substances (HSP70) [73]. The duration of post-reperfusion hypothermia seems to play a role in the modulation of transcriptional rate, as the expression of numerous genes differs when hypothermia is sustained for 8 h compared to 4 h. One such gene is early growth response-1 (Egr-1), which is an early regulator of other pro-inflammatory mediators (IL-1β MCK-1, and MIP-2) [73]. This is consistent with other reports on the topic, which suggests that Egr-1 is the key component modulated by TH. However, information regarding early cellular response to ischemia and hypothermia has largely been conflicting, leaving the specifics of its involvement unclear [38] and inconsistent [31, 32].

While there exists a general consensus that TH is neuroprotective, the precise mechanisms of this effect are still very much theoretical. Additionally, if TH attenuated metabolic crisis alone, it would not be able to accomplish such a robust degree of neuroprotection [74]. It comes as no surprise, then, that suspended animation is just the appetizer in the multicourse meal that is TH-mediated neuroprotection.

4.2. Inflammation and blood-brain barrier breakdown

In stroke therapy, the restoration of blood flow is of chief concern. Surprisingly, however, recanalization is not exclusively beneficial. Reperfusion often initiates a detrimental cascade, collectively termed ischemia/reperfusion injury, which can be disastrous; in some animal models, reperfusion after an extended period of ischemia caused larger infarct volumes than if the occlusion had been left permanently [45]. Reperfusion injury is a complex, multifaceted injury cascade initiated by sterile inflammation from anoxic tissue damage, and propagated by both the innate and adaptive immune systems and complement system [75, 76].

Mechanistically, ischemia/reperfusion injury is initiated by the aberrant Ca^{2+} influx characteristic of ischemic stroke, which activates phospholipases and eventually results in the production of pro-inflammatory mediators from microglia, including proteases, leukotrienes, IL-1β IL-6, NO, and tumor necrosis factor (TNF)-a [77]. These mediators contribute to post-reperfusion insult directly, by increasing vascular permeability, and indirectly, by increasing endothelial ICAM-1 expression and serving as potent chemotactic agents for polymorphonuclear leukocytes, both of which increase leukocyte extravasation into the brain parenchyma [46, 78]. The pro-inflammatory transcription factor nuclear factor kappa B (NF-κB) is likely the cause of this upregulation, as it is responsible for inducing the expression of IL-1β IL-6, TNF-α, and ICAM-1 [78]. In addition to recruiting leukocytes to the infarct site, IL-1β and TNF-α have also been found to increase the production of matrix metalloproteinases (MMPs) [79]. MMP-2 and MMP-9 have been shown to contribute to vasogenic edema by degrading extracellular matrix components during ischemic stroke, and MMP-9 knockout mice experience reduced infarct volumes and less severe motor deficits than wild-type mice [79]. The effect of MMPs ultimately perpetuates the development of inflammation and edema, which further encourages leukocyte extravasation. Once leukocytes enter the brain tissue, they produce ROS and pro-inflammatory factors of their own, thereby creating a viscous cycle of brain injury, inflammation, and blood-brain barrier (BBB) breakdown (**Figure 2**).

A common effect of reperfusion injury mechanisms is BBB disruption. Reperfusion activates matrix-degrading proteases within hours, which makes the vessels particularly leaky and allows for migration of albumin and other blood proteins into the brain parenchyma within 4–6 h of BBB disruption [72]. Water osmotically follows these proteins, thereby creating vasogenic edema, which may increase brain water content by more than 100% in poorly perfused regions [72, 80]. Vasogenic edema is the primary cause of death within the first month of an ischemic stroke [46], as it increases intracranial pressure (ICP) and compresses cerebrovasculature within the inflexible confines of the skull, causing further ischemia and eventually brain herniation [56].

Therapeutic hypothermia is able to confer anti-inflammatory neuroprotection by reducing the secretion of pro-inflammatory cytokines (IL-1β TNF-α, and IL-6) and inflammatory mediators (reactive oxygen and nitrogen species, E-selectin, and HMGB1) [81]. TH can also prevent leukocyte extravasation into neural tissue directly by reducing the endothelial expression of ICAM-1 [27, 48]. ICAM-1 is constitutively expressed by endothelial cells at very low levels, but the expression is precipitously increased following endothelial damage when it functions as an attachment point for the CD11/CD18 integrin of leukocytes (preceding extravasation

http://dx.doi.org/10.5772/65899

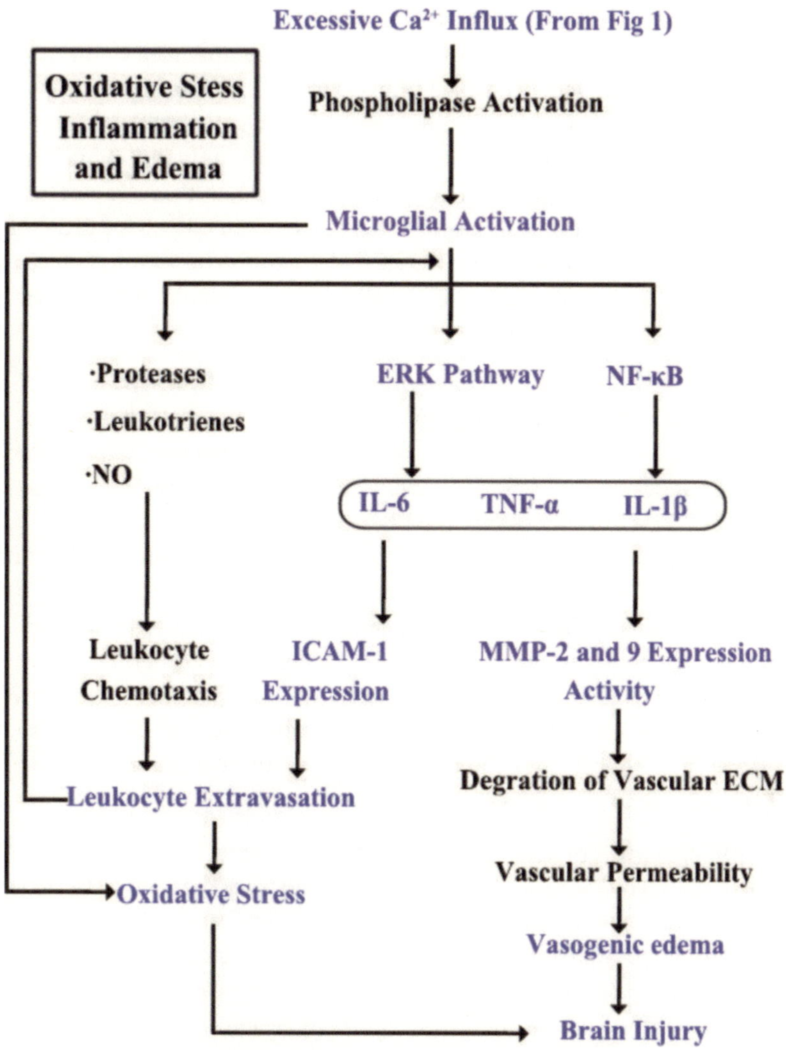

Figure 2. The figure describes the pathogenesis of stroke as it relates to ischemia-induced oxidative stress, inflammation, and edema. It is not known exactly where hypothermia exerts its neuroprotective effects. Studies have shown that TH attenuates a multitude of steps in the cascade of ischemia-induced brain damage compared to stroke without hypothermia, but whether the observed attenuations are direct effects of TH or byproducts of upstream attenuations has yet to be elucidated. As such, blue font indicates steps discussed in the present review that hypothermia has been shown to attenuate. Black font indicates steps that we have not discussed in the present review, but does not necessarily indicate that these steps are unaffected by hypothermia.

into damaged tissue) [82]. ICAM-1 knockout mice are resistant to cerebral ischemic injury [83], and antagonization of CD11/CD18 has been shown to substantially reduce leukocyte infiltration and subsequent cerebral edema (**Figure 2**) [82].

These effects seem to be associated with the inhibition of the extracellular signal-regulated kinase (ERK) pathway (**Figure 2**). ERK plays a significant role in the regulation of cell survival signals, and in the brain it is involved in responses to stress stimuli, including glutamate receptor stimulation and oxidative stress [84, 85]. ERK has been shown to contribute to NO and TNF-α secretion, and inhibition of the pathway prevents the release of excitotoxic amino acids following focal ischemia [86]. Transient hypothermia has been shown to reduce microglial activation, which translated to reduced phosphorylation (activation) of ERK and decreased IL-6 and TNF-α secretion [84]. However, induction of hypothermia in conjunction with U0216 (an ERK inhibitor) provided equal functional recovery to rats that did not receive U0216, implying that poststroke functional recovery progresses independently of ERK signaling [87]. Hypothermia has also been shown to reduce ICAM-1 expression in microglia in correlation with the ERK pathway, as administration of TH led to decreases in the activation of ERK as well as the inhibition of ICAM-1 expression [84].

Hypothermia-associated decreases in the expression of ICAM-1, IL-1β and TNF-α may also be due to attenuation of the NF-κB pathway (**Figure 2**). Therapeutic hypothermia has been shown to increase the expression of HSP70 in ischemic brains (but not in non-ischemic brains), and reports have suggested that HSP70 stabilizes NF-κB, thereby preventing its phosphorylation (activation) [73]. However, other NF-κB-associated proteins contribute as well. This pathway is puzzling, as the mechanism of NF-κB suppression varies depending on the type of ischemia. In models of focal ischemia, hypothermia suppresses NF-κB activity by inhibiting the activity of NF-κB kinase (IKK), a protein essential for degradation of the NF-κB inhibitor (IκB). In models of global ischemia, nuclear NF-κB levels in hypothermic subjects were still below normothermic levels, but IKK and IκB levels were unchanged [78]. These results are surprising, but emphasize the complexity of stroke pathogenesis and TH-associated neuroprotection. Moreover, regardless of the precise mechanism, therapeutic hypothermia seems to serve a beneficial role in NF-κB-associated neuroprotection.

Hypothermia can also prevent BBB breakdown directly. Nagel et al. recently found that TH increased functional recovery and reduced MMP-2 and -9 activities to the same degree as normothermic application of the MMP inhibitor minocycline, and that the application of TH in conjunction with minocycline was only marginally more effective than either by itself [88]. In addition to decreasing MMP activity, minocycline has been shown to decrease MMP production at the transcriptional level, and this report suggested that TH functions in the same way [88]. Other groups have found similar results, and this TH-induced MMP downregulation indeed translated to smaller infarct volumes and improved functional recovery [79, 89]. These data consistently show that TH is a powerful downregulator of MMP expression and activity, and that the modulation of MMP function leads to marked improvements in big-picture end goals of stroke therapy (decreased infarct volume, increased functional recovery, etc.) (**Figure 2**).

4.3. Apoptosis

Following the initial ischemia-induced insults (hours to days), long-term brain damage (days to weeks) is greatly influenced by cellular proapoptotic mechanisms. Hypothermia has been shown to affect several aspects of apoptotic cell death in both the intrinsic (intracellular-mediated) and extrinsic (receptor-mediated) cell death pathways, and ultimately prevent apoptosis after experimental stroke (**Figure 3**) [37].

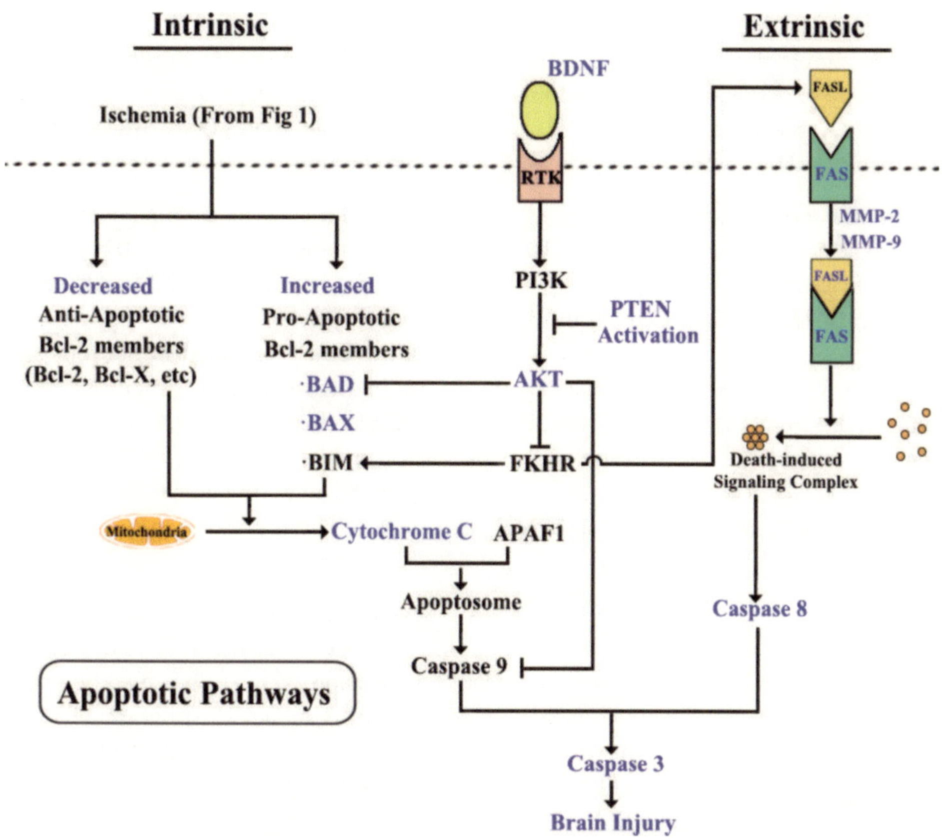

Figure 3. The figure describes the pathogenesis of stroke as it pertains to apoptotic pathways. It is not known exactly where hypothermia exerts its neuroprotective effects. Studies have shown that TH attenuates a multitude of steps in the cascade of ischemia-induced brain damage compared to stroke without hypothermia, but whether the observed attenuations are direct effects of TH or byproducts of upstream attenuations has yet to be elucidated. As such, blue font indicates steps discussed in the present review that hypothermia has been shown to attenuate. Black font indicates steps that we have not discussed in the present review, but does not necessarily indicate that these steps are unaffected by hypothermia. BDNF, brain-derived neurotropic factor; MMP, matrix metalloproteinase; RKT, receptor tyrosine kinase; PI3K, phosphoinositide-3 kinase; PTEN, phosphatase and tensin homologue; FKHR, forkhead transcription factor; APAF1, apoptotic protease-activating factor 1.

The extrinsic apoptotic pathway is initiated by ligand binding to cell death receptors; the best studied being the FAS-ligand (FASL) and its receptor, FAS. When FASL interacts with FAS, it triggers the intercellular assembly of death-induced-signaling complexes (DISCs), which leads to caspase 8 activation. Activated caspase 8 then triggers a caspase activation cascade resulting in the stimulation of apoptosis-inducing proteins such as caspase 3, thereby mediating cell death (**Figure 3**).

Hypothermia affects this pathway at multiple levels (**Figure 3**). Cooling has been shown to suppress the expression of caspase 8, caspase 3, FAS, and FASL [90]. Additionally, there is evidence that the FAS-FASL complex must be cleaved from the cell membrane by MMPs before becoming active [91]. TH has been shown to reduce levels of both MMPs and soluble

FASL in cooled rat brains [91], so is possible that the reduction in levels of these downstream effectors is simply the byproduct of inhibiting the FAS-FASL cleavage. While there are little available data to this end, the fact remains that, by one mechanism or another, hypothermia significantly reduces the production of a number of extrinsic apoptotic pathway intermediates, which translates to the preservation of penumbral tissue.

The intrinsic apoptotic pathway is triggered by intracellular cell stress signals including hypoxia, DNA damage, and cellular detachment from the extracellular matrix. These signals initiate apoptosis by disrupting the balance between proapoptotic Bcl-2 family members (BID, BAX, BAD, etc.) and anti-apoptotic Bcl-2 members (Bcl-2, Bcl-x, etc.) by a variety of mechanisms. Bcl-2 and Bcl-xL have both been found to be upregulated in neurons surviving hypoxia, while proapoptotic Bcl-2 members are highly expressed in neurons that will eventually die from hypoxic damage [37]. The imbalance between pro- and anti-apoptotic Bcl-2 members leads to the liberation of cytochrome C from the mitochondrial intermembrane space into the cytosol where it couples with APAF1 to form an apoptosome. The apoptosome activates caspase 9, which triggers a caspase activation cascade resulting in the activation of caspase 3 and apoptosis (**Figure 3**).

Hypothermia exerts its neuroprotective effects at several points along the intrinsic apoptotic pathway (**Figure 3**). TH has been found to inhibit BAX overexpression 4 h after 30 min of partial ischemia while having no effect on Bcl-2 expression [92]. TH has also been shown to diminish cytochrome C release without modifying BAX or Bcl-2 expression. This study did not observe caspase activity, which implied that TH endowed neuroprotection functions independently of caspases [93]. Interestingly, the same group found that hypothermia increased Bcl-2 expression in a global ischemia model [94], which underlines the importance of designing studies specific to local cooling in focal ischemia models. Additionally, mild hypothermia has been found to decrease cytochrome C translocation 5 h after reperfusion while leaving levels of caspase 9 and caspase 3 unchanged [74]. The conflicting nature of these findings leaves the point at which TH exerts its protective effects in question, but emphasizes the intricacy of TH-mediated neuroprotection.

Some of the anti-apoptotic effects of TH are mediated through the anti-apoptotic factor Akt/protein kinase B (**Figure 3**). Hypothermia attenuates decreases in Akt dephosphorylation (inactivation) after hypoxia [90]. In response to growth factors including BDNF (brain-derived neurotropic factor), membrane receptor tyrosine kinases activate PI3 kinase, which activates Akt via phosphorylation (p-Akt), thereby allowing it to phosphorylate (inhibit) numerous proapoptotic factors, including BAD, caspase 9, and forkhead transcription factor (FKHR) [90, 95]. Under normal physiological conditions, these proteins are phosphorylated by Akt, and their dephosphorylation can have severe repercussions. Dephosphorylation of BAD allows it to migrate into the mitochondria where it triggers the release of cytochrome C [91]. Dephosphorylated FKHR functions as a transcription factor to encourage overexpression of FASL and BIM [90]. Activation of caspase 9 activates a caspase cascade that results in apoptosis.

In normothermia, poststroke p-Akt levels fluctuate constantly; Zhao et al. found that, in normothermic rats, p-Akt levels decreased 30 min after stroke, increased at 1.5 and 5h, decreased at 9 and 24h, and increased again at 48h. Moderate hypothermia was found to stabilize these fluctuations at every time point except 24h, which translated to reduced infarct volumes and improved functional recovery up to 2 months after hypoxia. Interestingly, the reduction in infarct volumes was considerably less pronounced when TH was administered in conjunction with the PI3K inhibitor LY294002, although infarcts were still substantially smaller than in control animals [90]. It is very likely that this pathway provides a significant portion of TH-mediated neuroprotection. In line with this premise, mild hypothermia has also been found to inhibit the expression of caspase-3 and Fas after resolution of focal ischemia, which also translated to significantly decreased infarct volumes [96]. Hypothermia has also been shown to augment BDNF expression during cerebral ischemia [97], as well as attenuate the decrease in the Akt activity after stroke [90], so it is also possible that the effects of hypothermia on Akt activity are mediated at the level of BDNF.

While direct enhancement of the Akt pathway likely constitutes a portion of TH-mediated neuroprotection, cerebral cooling intervenes at other steps in the pathway as well. The PI3K/Akt pathway is inhibited by phosphatase and tensin homologue (PTEN), which de-phosphorylates upstream activators of Akt. PTEN is inhibited by phosphorylation (p-PTEN), and p-PTEN levels seem to play a crucial role in TH-mediated neuroprotection. Hypothermia has been found to stabilize p-PTEN levels more effectively than levels of p-Akt and other PI3K/Akt pathway participants (p-PDK1, p-GSK3β p-FKHR) [37]. A recent investigation from Lee et al. found that TH administered 15 min before reperfusion led to massive decreases in infarct volume while TH administered 15 min after reperfusion only had modest infarct reductions. Interestingly, while early and late TH had nearly identical effects on levels of p-Akt and other proteins, only early TH maintained high levels of p-PTEN [98]. Additionally, independent of hypothermia, PTEN inhibition was recently shown to confer a 75% reduction in infarct volume in rat models [95]. PTEN clearly plays a critical part in the story of neuroprotection, and should not be neglected in future investigations on the topic.

4.4. Long-term neuroprotection

There is compelling clinical evidence of neuroprotection with prolonged moderate cerebral hypothermia initiated within a few hours after hypoxia-ischemia and continued through the resolution of ischemia in term infants and adults [99–101]. The mechanisms underlying the neuroprotection are currently under investigation. Volser et al. showed that during the post-ischemic phase, the brain naturally activates restorative mechanisms to counteract the effects of the ischemic insult even without the induction of hypothermia [102]. This study, among others put forth the idea of long-term neuroprotection following an ischemic event in the brain. A study by Feng et al. went a step further and found that acute brain insult led to stimulation of neural stem cell proliferation, particularly in the subventricular and hippocampal subgranular zone, corroborating long-term neuroprotection [103]. However, evident from the lasting symptoms of acute ischemia, the brain is unable to completely regenerate and recover from the injury on its own. Thus, there is a dire need for the development of effective regenerative techniques and therapies to maximize patient recovery. This is where LEVI and hypothermia can be used to further the recovery of the brain.

Over the past decade, researchers have proposed the following mechanisms of long-term neuroprotection: neurogenesis, angiogenesis, gliogenesis, preservation of the integrity of neural networks, and inhibition of apoptosis [55]. These mechanisms will be discussed in detail below.

4.4.1. Neurogenesis

Contrary to prior belief, neurogenesis is a common event observed in the brain and while it is primarily limited to two neurogenic areas of the brain, the dentate gyrus of the hippocampus and the subventricular zone of the lateral ventricles, this process plays an important role in maintaining normal brain function [104, 105]. Two potential mechanisms can be attributed to neurogenesis: enhanced differentiation of neuroprogenitor cells into neurons and preferential differentiation of neuroprogenitor cells toward neurogenesis over gliogenesis.

The formation of new neural cells from neural progenitor cells has been identified as a major contributor to new populations of neurons, and TH seems to encourage this formation. An *in vivo* study by Silasi et al. found that when forebrain ischemia was induced in adult rodents, mild hypothermia following the ischemic event led to significantly increased neurogenesis in the dentate gyrus when compared to control groups with no hypothermia induction following an ischemic event [106]. Moreover, a very recent study in a neonatal hypoxic-ischemic injury mouse model showed that hypothermia provided partial protection for neural stem and progenitor cells (NSPCs) in the dentate gyrus subgranular zone, which may facilitate the recovery of function after injury and does not impair the proliferation of NSPCs during recovery [107]. This TH-mediated neurogenesis is thought to confer a more robust, long-term conservation of brain function than would be seen in normoxic stroke patients.

Preferential differentiation of neuroprogenitor cells into neurons also plays a major role in neuroprotection. Interestingly, an *in vivo* study found that cooling of rat brains to 33°C under hypoxic conditions led to an inhibition of hypoxia-induced apoptosis of proliferating neural stem cells and an increase in preferential maturation of neural progenitor cells into neural cells in the striatum [108]. Moreover, an *in vitro* study by Saito et al. found that moderate hypothermia to 32°C prevented apoptosis, preserved the naivety of neural stem cells, and led to lower expression of GFAP in neural stem cell culture, indicating less glial differentiation [109].

On the other hand, a study from early 2016 found that in aged rats, hypothermia induced by H_2S gas for 24 h after resolution of an MCAO only provided temporary therapeutic benefit and did not correlate with enhanced neurogenesis in the subventricular zone or infarcted area [110]. However, the duration of hypothermia induction in this study was shorter than the duration of hypothermia used in most clinical trials (24–48 h) and thus led to suboptimal hypothermia which is reflected in the temporary therapeutic effects [110]. Additionally, the use of hydrogen sulfide to induce hypothermia may not be representative of the conventional hypothermia-inducing agents used in other animal studies. H_2S is a weak and reversible inhibitor of oxidative phosphorylation, thus causing a suspended animation state with hypothermia [111]. It is quite possible that the mechanism of induction of hypothermia by H_2S may have interfered with various long-term protective mechanisms observed in other studies and in clinic using conventional hypothermia techniques.

4.4.2. *Angiogenesis*

Angiogenesis is a normal yet important biological process that is highly regulated and leads to the formation of new blood vessels during development, wound repair, and reproduction [111]. A study on rats by Xie et al. found that mild hypothermia enhanced angiogenesis in focal cerebral ischemia by increasing microvessel diameter, number of vascular branch points, and overall vessel surface area [112]. This was found to be a brain-derived neurotrophic factor (BDNF)-dependent process. Moreover, another study using a rat MCAO model showed that the injection of BDNF fused with a collagen-binding domain (CBD-BDNF) into the lateral ventricle specifically bound to collagen of the ventricular ependyma and consequently led to neural regeneration, angiogenesis, and reduced cell death [113]. This study further confirms the pro-angiogenic activity of BDNF in ischemic conditions. Vascular endothelial growth factor (VEGF) upregulation has also been found to correlate with acute cerebral ischemia [114, 115]. A very recent prospective cohort study observed increased brain perfusion over the first month in term-asphyxiated newborn babies treated with hypothermia during the first few days of life. This increase in brain perfusion came as a result of increased angiogenesis, which was found to be associated with VEGF expression in the injured brain of asphyxiated newborns treated with hypothermia [116]. VEGF has been consistently shown to increase angiogenesis, which translates to increased functional recovery in the months following an ischemic stroke [117–119].

4.4.3. *Gliogenesis*

While gliogenesis refers to the development of microglia, oligodendrocytes, and astrocytes in the brain, intriguingly, oligodendrocytes have been found to have a similar susceptibility to neurons for cell death. Early studies found that combined deprivation of oxygen and glucose led to selective death of mature oligodendrocytes over other glial cells *in vitro* [120–122]. *In vivo* studies have shown that cerebral white matter, specifically oligodendrocytes and astrocytes, are highly vulnerable to focal ischemia [123]. However, *in vitro* studies have shown that hypothermia increases the number of oligodendrocyte precursors in primary neural and glial cultures from mouse brains and maintains a cell population of oligodendrocyte progenitors in a less well-differentiated state [124]. Recent studies have found that susceptible oligodendrocyte progenitors and mature oligodendrocytes exposed to hypoxia could be protected by deep hypothermia [125]. Another study demonstrated that hypothermia promoted the differentiation and maturation of oligodendrocyte precursor cells (OPCs), and indicated that OPC death was significantly suppressed by hypothermia *in vitro*, alluding to the fact that hypothermia is protective of oligodendrogliogenesis [126]. More recent studies in fetal sheep have shown that cerebral ischemia is associated with significant loss in total numbers of oligodendrocytes, decreased myelin basic protein expression, and increased microglial activation [127, 128]. However, another study in fetal sheep countered these results by showing that delayed cerebral hypothermia partially protects white matter after global cerebral ischemia by stimulating oligodendrocyte proliferation, reducing microglial induction, and restoring the amount and pattern of expression of myelin basic protein, once again confirming the neuroprotective role of hypothermia toward oligodendrogenesis [129, 130]. Moreover, researchers have found that hypothermia attenuates demyelination, trauma-induced oligodendrocyte cell death, and overall circuit dysfunction [131, 132]. While a study in preterm fetal sheep found that TH was correlated with an overall reduction in the hypoxia-induced death of immature oligodendrocytes, hypothermia did not prevent the hypoxia-induced inhibition of oligodendrocyte proliferation in the periventricular white matter zone [133, 134]. Most importantly, a recent study in rats found that hypothermia reduced the extent of hypoxia-ischemia damage in axons and increased oligodendrocyte lineage proliferation, which was reflected in the increase in myelination of axons and decreases apoptosis and pre-oligodendrocyte lineage accumulation [134]. While an ischemic environment has been shown to be detrimental to oligodendrogenesis and oligodendrocyte survival, hypothermia has been shown to rescue these processes *in vivo* and *in vitro*, as discussed above.

Since astrocytes are the largest population of cells present in the ischemic core during the subacute to chronic period of stroke, astrogliogenesis is often considered to be therapeutic following insult to the brain [131, 135, 136]. However, we still lack much information and need more investigation in this area. Most of the current literature suggests astrogliogenesis as detrimental to the brain rather than neuroprotective. As we know, activated astrocytes form the glial scar in the brain following insult or injury [112, 137]. This brings about doubt on whether astrogliogenesis is therapeutic and may actually impede the postischemic healing process by forming a glial scar that could hinder neurite growth and synaptogenesis, and lead to leakage of proapoptotic factors from astrocyte gap junctions within the glial scar [138]. Moreover, a very recent study found that in mice, hypoxia diminished the protective function of astrocytes and activated them to initiate astrogliosis in the ischemic region [139]. In fact, many studies have shown that decreased astrogliosis correlates with decreased infarct size [140]. Intriguingly, a study conducted by Xiong et al. showed that postischemic hypothermia in rats for 24 h rescued hippocampal neurons by decreasing astrocyte activation and inflammatory cytokine release [141]. Such studies truly call into question the role of astrogliogenesis in neuroprotection. More investigation needs to be done in this area to better understand the role of astrogliogenesis in neuroprotection under hypothermic conditions.

4.4.4. Preservation of the integrity of neural networks

Neural networks are functional units representing the high complexity and processivity of the brain and thus repair and preservation of this circuitry is the key for recovery from brain injury. Some of the key processes involved in neural network maintenance are axonal and neurite growth, synaptogenesis, and maintenance of neuronal architecture. Studies have found that hypothermia of the brain by 17°C enhanced neurite and axonal outgrowth in brain slices [142, 143]. A recent study on spinal cord injury rat models found that regional hypothermia promoted neurite, axonal, and nerve fiber growth to the point that hind limb function was recovered in these rats, which emphasizes the plasticity and extent of recovery via hypothermia that the central nervous system is capable of [144]. However, deep hypothermia (20°C) followed by subsequent rewarming did not change the stability of dendritic spines or the presynaptic boutons in mouse somatosensory cortex [145]. Moreover, a gene profiling study on rat model of traumatic brain injury found that mild hypothermia had significant effects on gene expression for synapse organization and biogenesis; an analysis of the hippocampal gene expression profiles of these rats found that 133 genes showed statistically significant changes in expression compared to injured rat in normoxic conditions. Of the 133, 57 genes were upregulated and were responsible for synaptic organization and biogenesis [146]. An *in vitro* study showed that hypothermia to 33°C following *in* vitro ischemia decreased the neuronal actin polymerization that reduced spine calcium kinetics, disrupted detrimental cell signaling, and protected the neurons against damage [147]. While hypoxic conditions caused changes in F-actin architecture of dendritic spines, hypothermia decreased the actin modifications in dendritic spines preventing the neuronal death [148]. All of these studies support the notion of spine and synaptogenesis preservation by hypothermia treatment.

In a functional study on ischemic gerbils treated with moderate postischemic hypothermia, the untreated (normothermic) groups experienced a 95% reduction in CA1 cells, while cell counts in the TH group were equivalent to that of sham animals. Additionally, postischemic hypothermia preserved the electrophysiological properties of CA1 neurons, which reflects the functional preservation of neural networks [149]. Moreover, mice subjected to ischemia followed by hypothermia treatment showed neuroprotection against ischemia-induced long-term potentiation (LTP) impairment as well as synaptic plasticity [150]. While there are encouraging studies on mechanisms of neural network preservation by hypothermia treatment, further research is needed to better understand how neuronal networks are preserved in the ischemic and penumbra regions in response to hypothermia.

5. Future research directions

Between 1935 and 2010, cancer, heart disease, and stroke have consistently been in the top five causes of death in the United States [151]. While all three are complex, multifaceted diseases, stroke differs from cancer and heart disease in one critical way; a highly effective, easily administered, cost-effective therapy has already been devised. The main factor hindering significant progress on stroke therapy is not a lack of ideas, but rather a lack of research moving hypothermia toward clinical acceptance. Since TH is still predominately discussed in the context of cardiac arrest, the majority of studies on TH feature a global ischemia (cardiac arrest) model, which cannot always be extrapolated to studies on focal cerebral ischemia. Several papers in the present review alone have arrived at a finding using a global ischemia model that is directly opposed by results from a model of focal ischemia or vice versa [37, 93, 94]. In focal ischemia models, there is significant heterogeneity in experimental methods. Studies on TH in focal cerebral ischemia frequently differ in animal model, animal age, duration of ischemia, duration of hypothermia, depth of hypothermia, method of hypothermia induction, and rate of cooling, all of which have consistently been shown to play critical roles in the efficacy of TH treatments. It is also important to note that the vast majority of investigations on neuroprotective efficacy have used transient occlusion models, which produce much more uniform and encouraging results than those using a permanent occlusion model [37]. This is problematic, considering that an estimated 50% of ischemic stroke patients display vessel occlusion 3–4 days after symptom onset, which is considered a relatively permanent occlusion [152]. This heterogeneity is likely a large source of conflicting findings, and surely prevents investigators from coming to an agreement on TH mechanisms. Another issue with present research is the goal of hypotheses. While there have been innumerable studies on the mechanisms of hypothermia-mediated neuroprotection, these reports are usually correlative rather than causative, which makes it difficult to derive any concrete, widely applicable mechanisms from the literature. This overall lack of research has hindered publicization of the procedure; given that LEVI was only developed in 2002, many groups are simply unaware that such a procedure has been proposed. For instance, a highly cited 2012 review on the topic discussed numerous problems with global cooling, but failed to mention LEVI to any extent despite the fact that the procedure remedies every problem highlighted in the paper [58]. However, as the body of research on LEVI grows, so too will its clinical acceptance.

Overall, the picture of therapeutic hypothermia-mediated neuroprotection is favorable and encouraging. TH consistently decreases infarct volumes and facilitates short- and long-term preservation of function to an unprecedented degree. Although there is little widespread consensus as to how this is accomplished, a review of the literature is scarce with detrimental effects of TH. While many questions remain to be answered before TH can be consistently implemented in humans, such a promising therapy to such a ubiquitously disastrous disease warrants a significant time investment going forward.

Acknowledgements

This work was partially supported by the American Heart Association Grant-in-Aid (14GRNT20460246), Merit Review Award (I01RX-001964-01) from the US Department of Veterans Affairs Rehabilitation R&D Service, the National Natural Science Foundation of China (81501141), and the Beijing New-Star Plan of Science and Technology (xx2016061).

Author details

Mitchell Huber[1#], Hong Lian Duan[2#], Ankush Chandra[1], Fengwu Li[2], Longfei Wu[3], Longfei Guan[2], Xiaokun Geng[1,2*] and Yuchuan Ding[1,2]

*Address all correspondence to: xgeng@ccmu.edu.cn

1 Department of Neurological Surgery, Wayne State University School of Medicine, Detroit, MI, USA

2 Institute of Neuroscience, Beijing Luhe Hospital, Capital Medical University, Beijing, China

3 China-America Institute of Neuroscience, Xuanwu Hospital, Capital Medical University, Beijing, China

# These authors contributed equally for this work

References

[1] The National Institute of Neurological Disorders and Stroke rt-PA Stroke Study Group Tissue plasminogen activator for acute ischemic stroke. N Engl J Med, 1995. **333**(24): p. 1581–1588.

[2] Demaerschalk, B.M., et al., Scientific rationale for the inclusion and exclusion criteria for intravenous alteplase in acute ischemic stroke: a statement for healthcare professionals from the American Heart Association/American Stroke Association. Stroke, 2016. **47**(2): p. 581–641.

[3] O'Collins, V.E., et al., 1,026 experimental treatments in acute stroke. Ann Neurol, 2006. **59**(3): p. 467–477.

[4] Bernard, S.A., Gray, T.W., and Buist, M.D., Treatment of comatose survivors of out-of-hospital cardiac arrest with induced hypothermia. ACC Curr J Rev, 2002. **11**(4): p. 82–83.

[5] The Hypothermia After Cardiac Arrest Study Group Mild therapeutic hypothermia to improve the neurologic outcome after cardiac arrest. N Engl J Med, 2002. **346**(8): p. 549–556.

[6] van der Worp, H.B., et al., Hypothermia in animal models of acute ischaemic stroke: a systematic review and meta-analysis. Brain, 2007. **130**(12): p. 3063–3074.

[7] Hemmen, T.M. and Lyden, P.D., Hypothermia after acute ischemic stroke.J Neurotrauma, 2009. **26**(3): p. 5.

[8] Kollmar, R., et al., Different degrees of hypothermia after experimental stroke - Short- and long-term outcome. Stroke, 2007. **38**(5): p. 1585–1589.

[9] Gunn, A.J. and Thoresen, M., Animal studies of neonatal hypothermic neuroprotection have translated well in to practice. Resuscitation, 2015. **97**: p. 88–90.

[10] Gunn, A.J. and Bennet, L., Timing still key to treating hypoxic ischaemic brain injury. The Lancet Neurology. 2016. **15**(2): p. 126–127.

[11] Christian, E., et al., A review of selective hypothermia in the management of traumatic brain injury. Neurosurg Focus, 2008. **25**(4): p. 8.

[12] Ginsberg, M.D., et al., Therapeutic modulation of brain temperature: relevance to ischemic brain injury. Cerebrovasc Brain Metab Rev, 1992. **4**(3): p. 189–225.

[13] Krieger, D.W., et al., Cooling for acute ischemic brain damage (cool aid): an open pilot study of induced hypothermia in acute ischemic stroke. Stroke, 2001. **32**(8): p. 1847–1854.

[14] De Georgia, M.A., et al., Cooling for acute ischemic brain damage (COOL AID): a feasibility trial of endovascular cooling. Neurology, 2004. **63**(2): p. 312–317.

[15] Lyden, P.D., et al., Intravascular cooling in the treatment of stroke (ICTuS): early clinical experience. J Stroke Cerebrovasc Dis, 2005. **14**(3): p. 107–114.

[16] Pichon, N., et al., Efficacy of and tolerance to mild induced hypothermia after out-of-hospital cardiac arrest using an endovascular cooling system. Crit Care, 2007. **11**(3): p. R71.

[17] Simosa, H.F., et al., Increased risk of deep venous thrombosis with endovascular cooling in patients with traumatic head injury. Am Surg, 2007. **73**(5): p. 461–464.

[18] Hemmen, T.M., et al., Intravenous thrombolysis plus hypothermia for acute treatment of ischemic stroke (ICTuS-L): final results. Stroke, 2010. **41**(10): p. 2265–2270.

[19] Kammersgaard, L.P., et al., Feasibility and safety of inducing modest hypothermia in awake patients with acute stroke through surface cooling: a case-control study: The Copenhagen stroke study. Stroke, 2000. **31**(9): p. 2251–2256.

[20] Jeon, S.B., et al., Critical care for patients with massive ischemic stroke. J Stroke, 2014. **16**(3): p. 146–160.

[21] Polderman, K.H., Mechanisms of action, physiological effects, and complications of hypothermia. Crit Care Med, 2009. **37**(7 Suppl): p. S186–202.

[22] Zhang, J.N., et al., Effects of low temperature on shear-induced platelet aggregation and activation. J Trauma, 2004. **57**(2): p. 216–223.

[23] Connolly, J.E., Boyd, R.J., and Calvin, J.W., The protective effect of hypothermia in cerebral ischemia-experimental and clinical application by selective brain cooling in the human. Surgery, 1962. **52**(1): p. 15–24.

[24] Parkins, W.M., Jensen, J.M., and Vars, H.M., Brain cooling in the prevention of brain damage during periods of circulatory occlusion in dogs. AnnSurg, 1954. **140**(3): p. 284–289.

[25] Chen, J., et al., Endovascular hypothermia in acute ischemic stroke: pilot study of selective intra-arterial cold saline infusion. Stroke, 2016. **47**(7): p. 1933–1935.

[26] Ringer, A.J. and Tomsick, T.A., Developments in endovascular therapy for acute ischemic stroke. Neurol Res, 2002. **24(Suppl 1)**: p. S43–46.

[27] Ding, Y., Justin, C., Research progress of hypothermia: selective intra-arterial infusion and regional brain cooling in acute stroke therapy. Exp Stroke, 2012.

[28] Ding, Y., et al., Prereperfusion saline infusion into ischemic territory reduces inflammatory injury after transient middle cerebral artery occlusion in rats. Stroke, 2002. **33**(10): p. 2492–2498.

[29] Ding, Y., et al., Prereperfusion flushing of ischemic territory: a therapeutic study in which histological and behavioral assessments were used to measure ischemia-reperfusion injury in rats with stroke. J Neurosurg, 2002. **96**(2): p. 310–319.

[30] Ding, Y., et al., Local saline infusion into ischemic territory induces regional brain cooling and neuroprotection in rats with transient middle cerebral artery occlusion. Neurosurgery, 2004. **54**(4): p. 956–964; discussion 964-5.

[31] Ji, Y., et al., Therapeutic time window of hypothermia is broader than cerebral artery flushing in carotid saline infusion after transient focal ischemic stroke in rats. Neurol Res, 2012. **34**(7): p. 657–663.

[32] Ji, Y.-B., et al., Interrupted intracarotid artery cold saline infusion as an alternative method for neuroprotection after ischemic stroke. Neurosurg Focus, 2012. **33**(1): p. E10.

[33] Mattingly, T.K., et al., Catheter based selective hypothermia reduces stroke volume during focal cerebral ischemia in swine. J Neurointerv Surg, 2016. **8**(4): p. 418–422.

[34] Zhao, B., et al., A more consistent intraluminal rhesus monkey model of ischemic stroke. Neural Regener Res, 2014. **9**(23): p. 2087–2094.

[35] Wang, B., et. Al., Local cerebral hypothermia induced by selective infusion of cold lactated ringer's: a feasibility study in rhesus monkeys. 2016. Neurological Research. 38(6): p. 545 - 552.

[36] Choi, J.H., et al., Selective brain cooling with endovascular intracarotid infusion of cold saline: a pilot feasibility study.Am J Neuroradiol, 2010. **31**(5): p. 928–934.

[37] Zhao, H., Steinberg, G.K., and Sapolsky, R.M., General versus specific actions of mild-moderate hypothermia in attenuating cerebral ischemic damage. J Cereb Blood Flow Metab, 2007. **27**(12): p. 1879–1894.

[38] van der Worp, H.B., et al., Can animal models of disease reliably inform human studies? PLoS Med., 2010. **7**(3): p. e1000245.

[39] Esposito, E., et al., In cold blood: intraarteral cold infusions for selective brain cooling in stroke. J Cereb Blood Flow Metab, 2014. **34**(5): p. 743–752.

[40] Roelfsema, V., et al., Window of opportunity of cerebral hypothermia for postischemic white matter injury in the near-term fetal sheep. J Cereb Blood Flow Metab, 2004. **24**(8): p. 877–886.

[41] Markarian, G.Z., et al., Mild hypothermia: therapeutic window after experimental cerebral ischemia. Neurosurgery, 1996. **38**(3): p. 542–550; discussion 551.

[42] Li, J., et al., Long-term neuroprotection induced by regional brain cooling with saline infusion into ischemic territory in rats: a behavioral analysis. Neurol Res, 2004. **26**(6): p. 677–683.

[43] Lassen, N.A., The luxury-perfusion syndrome and its possible relation to acute metabolic acidosis localised within the brain.Lancet, 1966. **288**(7473): p. 1113–1115.

[44] Heiss, W.D., et al., Repeat positron emission tomographic studies in transient middle cerebral artery occlusion in cats: residual perfusion and efficacy of postischemic reperfusion. J Cereb Blood Flow Metab, 1997. **17**(4): p. 388–400.

[45] Pan, J., et al., Reperfusion injury following cerebral ischemia: pathophysiology, MR imaging, and potential therapies. Neuroradiology, 2007. **49**(2): p. 93–102.

[46] Hsu, C.Y., et al., Arachidonic acid and its metabolites in cerebral ischemia. Ann N Y Acad Sci, 1989. **559**: p. 282–295.

[47] Chen, J., et al., The effect of a microcatheter-based selective intra-arterial hypothermia on hemodynamic changes following transient cerebral ischemia. Neurol Res, 2015. **37**(3): p. 263–268.

[48] Luan, X.D., et al., Regional brain cooling induced by vascular saline infusion into ischemic territory reduces brain inflammation in stroke. Acta Neuropathol, 2004. **107**(3): p. 227–234.

[49] Toyoda, T., et al., Intraischemic hypothermia attenuates neutrophil infiltration in the rat neocortex after focal ischemia-reperfusion injury. Neurosurgery, 1996. **39**(6): p. 1200–1205.

[50] Woitzik, J. and Schilling, L., A new method for superselective middle cerebral artery infusion in the rat. J Neurosurg, 2007. **106**(5): p. 872–878.

[51] Song, W., et al., Intra-carotid cold magnesium sulfate infusion induces selective cerebral hypothermia and neuroprotection in rats with transient middle cerebral artery occlusion. Neurol Sci, 2013. **34**(4): p. 479–486.

[52] Chen, J., et al., Enhanced neuroprotection by local intra-arterial infusion of human albumin solution and local hypothermia. Stroke, 2013. **44**(1): p. 260–262.

[53] Dang, S., et al., Neuroprotection by local intra-arterial infusion of erythropoietin after focal cerebral ischemia in rats. Neurol Res, 2011. **33**(5): p. 520–528.

[54] Pardridge, W.M., The blood-brain barrier: bottleneck in brain drug development. NeuroRx, 2005. **2**(1): p. 3–14.

[55] Lyden, P.D. and Lonzo, L., Combination therapy protects ischemic brain in rats. A glutamate antagonist plus a gamma-aminobutyric acid agonist. Stroke, 1994. **25**(1): p. 189–196.

[56] Huang, Z.G., et al., Biphasic opening of the blood-brain barrier following transient focal ischemia: effects of hypothermia. Can J Neurol Sci, 1999. **26**(4): p. 298–304.

[57] Polderman, K.H., Application of therapeutic hypothermia in the intensive care unit. Opportunities and pitfalls of a promising treatment modality-Part 2: Practical aspects and side effects. Intensive Care Med, 2004. **30**(5): p. 757–769.

[58] Yenari, M.A. and Han, H.S., Neuroprotective mechanisms of hypothermia in brain ischaemia. Nat Rev Neurosci, 2012. **13**(4): p. 267–278.

[59] Dong, X.-X., Wang, Y., and Qin, Z.-H., Molecular mechanisms of excitotoxicity and their relevance to pathogenesis of neurodegenerative diseases. Acta Pharmacol Sin, 2009. **30**(4): p. 379–387.

[60] Previch, L.M., L.; Wright, J.; Singh, S.; Geng, X.; Ding, Y., Progress in AQP research and new developments in therapeutic approaches to ischemic and hemorrhagic stroke. Int J Mol Sci, 2016. **17**(7).

[61] Yenari, M., et al., Metabolic downregulation: a key to successful neuroprotection? Stroke, 2008. **39**(10): p. 2910–2917.

[62] Erecinska, M., Thoresen, M., and Silver, I.A., Effects of hypothermia on energy metabolism in Mammalian central nervous system. J Cereb Blood Flow Metab, 2003. **23**(5): p. 513–530.

[63] Kimura, T., et al., Effect of mild hypothermia on energy state recovery following transient forebrain ischemia in the gerbil. Exp Brain Res, 2002. **145**(1): p. 83–90.

[64] Shimizu, H., et al., Effect of brain, body, and magnet bore temperatures on energy metabolism during global cerebral ischemia and reperfusion monitored by magnetic resonance spectroscopy in rats. Magn Reson Med, 1997. **37**(6): p. 833–839.

[65] Ooboshi, H., et al., Hypothermia inhibits ischemia-induced efflux of amino acids and neuronal damage in the hippocampus of aged rats. Brain Res, 2000. **884**(1–2): p. 23–30.

[66] Colbourne, F., et al., Hypothermia rescues hippocampal CA1 neurons and attenuates down-regulation of the AMPA receptor GluR2 subunit after forebrain ischemia. Proc Natl Acad Sci USA, 2003. **100**(5): p. 2906–2910.

[67] Kristian, T., Katsura, K., and Siesjo, B.K., The influence of moderate hypothermia on cellular calcium uptake in complete ischaemia: implications for the excitotoxic hypothesis. Acta Physiol Scand, 1992. **146**(4): p. 531–532.

[68] Papadopoulos, M.C., et al., Aquaporin-4 facilitates reabsorption of excess fluid in vasogenic brain edema. FASEB J, 2004. **18**(9): p. 1291-+.

[69] Zhao, H., et al., Molecular mechanisms of therapeutic hypothermia on neurological function in a swine model of cardiopulmonary resuscitation. Resuscitation, 2012. **83**(7): p. 913–920.

[70] Kurisu, K., et al., Transarterial regional brain hypothermia inhibits acute aquaporin-4 surge and sequential microvascular events in ischemia/reperfusion injury. Neurosurgery, 2016. **79**(1): p. 125–134.

[71] Morishima, T., et al., Lactic acid increases aquaporin 4 expression on the cell membrane of cultured rat astrocytes. Neurosci Res, 2008. **61**(1): p. 18–26.

[72] Vella, J., et al., The central role of aquaporins in the pathophysiology of ischemic stroke. Front Cell Neurosci, 2015. **9**: p. 108.

[73] Shintani, Y., Terao, Y., and Ohta, H., Molecular mechanisms underlying hypothermia-induced neuroprotection. Stroke Res Treat, 2010. **2011**: p. 809874.

[74] Xu, L., et al., Mild hypothermia reduces apoptosis of mouse neurons in vitro early in the cascade. J Cereb Blood Flow Metab, 2002. **22**(1): p. 21–28.

[75] Nour, M., Scalzo, F., and Liebeskind, D.S., Ischemia-reperfusion injury in stroke. Interv Neurol, 2013. **1**(3–4): p. 185–199.

[76] Eltzschig, H.K. and Eckle, T., Ischemia and reperfusion-from mechanism to translation. Nat Med, 2011. **17**(11): p. 1391–1401.

[77] Kim, J.Y., Kawabori, M., and Yenari, M.A., Innate inflammatory responses in stroke: mechanisms and potential therapeutic targets. Curr Med Chem, 2014. **21**(18): p. 2076–2097.

[78] Yenari, M.A. and Han, H.S., Influence of hypothermia on post-ischemic inflammation: role of nuclear factor kappa B (NFkappaB). Neurochem Int, 2006. **49**(2): p. 164–169.

[79] Truettner, J.S., Alonso, O.F., and Dalton Dietrich, W., Influence of therapeutic hypothermia on matrix metalloproteinase activity after traumatic brain injury in rats. Journal of cerebral blood flow and metabolism, 2005. **25**: p. 1516.

[80] Kahles, T. and Brandes, R.P., NADPH oxidases as therapeutic targets in ischemic stroke. Cell Mol Life Sci, 2012. **69**(14): p. 2345–2363.

[81] Ceulemans, A.-G., et al., The dual role of the neuroinflammatory response after ischemic stroke: modulatory effects of hypothermia. J Neuroinflamm, 2010. **7**: p. 74.

[82] Yenari, M.A., et al., Hu23F2G, an antibody recognizing the leukocyte CD11/CD18 integrin, reduces injury in a rabbit model of transient focal cerebral ischemia. Exp Neurol, 1998. **153**(2): p. 223–233.

[83] Connolly, E.S., Jr., et al., Cerebral protection in homozygous null ICAM-1 mice after middle cerebral artery occlusion. Role of neutrophil adhesion in the pathogenesis of stroke. J Clin Invest, 1996. **97**(1): p. 209–216.

[84] Schmitt, K.R., Hypothermia suppresses inflammation via ERK signaling pathway in stimulated microglial cells. Journal of neuroimmunology, 2007. **189**: p. 16.

[85] Aikawa, R., et al., Oxidative stress activates extracellular signal-regulated kinases through Src and Ras in cultured cardiac myocytes of neonatal rats. J Clin Invest, 1997. **100**(7): p. 1813–1821.

[86] Alessandrini, A., et al., MEK1 protein kinase inhibition protects against damage resulting from focal cerebral ischemia. Proc Natl Acad Sci U S A, 1999. **96**(22): p. 12866–12869.

[87] D'Cruz, B.J., et al., Hypothermia and ERK activation after cardiac arrest. Brain research, 2005. **1064**: p. 118.

[88] Nagel, S., Minocycline and hypothermia for reperfusion injury after focal cerebral ischemia in the rat: effects on BBB breakdown and MMP expression in the acute and subacute phase. Brain research, 2008. **1188**: p. 206.

[89] Burk, J., et al., Protection of cerebral microvasculature after moderate hypothermia following experimental focal cerebral ischemia in mice. Brain Res, 2008. **1226**: p. 248–255.

[90] Zhao, H., et al., Akt contributes to neuroprotection by hypothermia against cerebral ischemia in rats. J Neurosci, 2005. **25**(42): p. 9794–9806.

[91] Liu, L., et al., FasL shedding is reduced by hypothermia in experimental stroke. J. Neurochem, 2008. **106**(2): p. 541–550.

[92] Eberspacher, E., et al., The effect of hypothermia on the expression of the apoptosis-regulating protein Bax after incomplete cerebral ischemia and reperfusion in rats. J Neurosurg Anesthesiol, 2003. **15**(3): p. 200–208.

[93] Yenari, M.A., Mild hypothermia attenuates cytochrome c release but does not alter Bcl-2 expression or caspase activation after experimental stroke. 2002. **22**: p. 38.

[94] Zhang, Z., et al., Mild hypothermia increases Bcl-2 protein expression following global cerebral ischemia. Brain research. Molecular brain research, 2001. **95**: p. 85.

[95] Shi, G.D., et al., PTEN deletion prevents ischemic brain injury by activating the mTOR signaling pathway. Biochem Biophys Res Commun, 2011. **404**(4): p. 941–945.

[96] Phanithi, P.B., et al., Mild hypothermia mitigates post-ischemic neuronal death following focal cerebral ischemia in rat brain: immunohistochemical study of Fas, caspase-3 and TUNEL. Neuropathology, 2000. **20**(4): p. 273–282.

[97] Vosler, P.S., et al., Delayed hypothermia preferentially increases expression of brain-derived neurotrophic factor exon III in rat hippocampus after asphyxial cardiac arrest. Brain research. Molecular brain research, 2005. **135**: p. 29.

[98] Lee, S.M., et al., The protective effect of early hypothermia on PTEN phosphorylation correlates with free radical inhibition in rat stroke. J Cereb Blood Flow Metab, 2009. **29**(9): p. 1589–1600.

[99] Gunn, A.J. and Gluckman, P.D., Head cooling for neonatal encephalopathy: the state of the art. Clin Obstet Gynecol, 2007. **50**(3): p. 636–651.

[100] Hoehn, T., et al., Therapeutic hypothermia in neonates. Review of current clinical data, ILCOR recommendations and suggestions for implementation in neonatal intensive care units. Resuscitation, 2008. **78**(1): p. 7–12.

[101] Shah, P.S., Hypothermia: a systematic review and meta-analysis of clinical trials. Semin Fetal Neonatal Med, 2010. **15**(5): p. 238–246.

[102] Kernie, S.G. and Parent, J.M., Forebrain neurogenesis after focal Ischemic and traumatic brain injury. Neurobiol Dis, 2010. **37**(2): p. 267–274.

[103] Feng, J.F., et al., Effect of therapeutic mild hypothermia on the genomics of the hippocampus after moderate traumatic brain injury in rats. Neurosurgery, 2010. **67**(3): p. 730–742.

[104] Gage, F.H., Mammalian neural stem cells. Science, 2000. **287**(5457): p. 1433–1438.

[105] Ming, G.L. and Song, H., Adult neurogenesis in the mammalian brain: significant answers and significant questions. Neuron, 2011. **70**(4): p. 687–702.

[106] Silasi, G. and Colbourne, F., Therapeutic hypothermia influences cell genesis and survival in the rat hippocampus following global ischemia. J Cereb Blood Flow Metab, 2011. **31**(8): p. 1725–1735.

[107] Kwak, M., et al., Effects of neonatal hypoxic-ischemic injury and hypothermic neuroprotection on neural progenitor cells in the mouse hippocampus. Dev Neurosci, 2015. **37**(4–5): p. 428–439.

[108] Xiong, M., et al., Post-ischemic hypothermia promotes generation of neural cells and reduces apoptosis by Bcl-2 in the striatum of neonatal rat brain. Neurochem Int, 2011. **58**(6): p. 625–633.

[109] Saito, K., et al., Moderate low temperature preserves the stemness of neural stem cells and suppresses apoptosis of the cells via activation of the cold-inducible RNA binding protein. Brain Res, 2010. **1358**: p. 20–29.

[110] Sandu, R.E., et al., Twenty-four hours hypothermia has temporary efficacy in reducing brain infarction and inflammation in aged rats. Neurobiol Aging, 2016. **38**: p. 127–140.

[111] Otrock, Z.K., et al., Understanding the biology of angiogenesis: Review of the most important molecular mechanisms. Blood Cells Mol Dis, 2007. **39**(2): p. 212–220.

[112] Hawthorne, A.L., et al., The unusual response of serotonergic neurons after CNS Injury: lack of axonal dieback and enhanced sprouting within the inhibitory environment of the glial scar. J Neurosci, 2011. **31**(15): p. 5605–5616.

[113] Guan, J., et al., Neuronal regeneration and protection by collagen-binding BDNF in the rat middle cerebral artery occlusion model. Biomaterials, 2012. **33**(5): p. 1386–1395.

[114] Wang, Y., et al., VEGF overexpression induces post-ischaemic neuroprotection, but facilitates haemodynamic steal phenomena. Brain, 2005. **128**(Pt 1): p. 52–63.

[115] Margaritescu, O., Pirici, D., and Margaritescu, C., VEGF expression in human brain tissue after acute ischemic stroke. Rom J Morphol Embryol, 2011. **52**(4): p. 1283–1292.

[116] Shaikh, H., et al., Increased brain perfusion persists over the first month of life in term asphyxiated newborns treated with hypothermia: does it reflect activated angiogenesis? Transl Stroke Res, 2015. **6**(3): p. 224–233.

[117] Dzietko, M., et al., Delayed VEGF treatment enhances angiogenesis and recovery after neonatal focal rodent stroke. Transl Stroke Res, 2013. **4**(2): p. 189–200.

[118] Sun, Y., et al., VEGF-induced neuroprotection, neurogenesis, and angiogenesis after focal cerebral ischemia. J Clin Invest, 2003. **111**(12): p. 1843–1851.

[119] Lee, H.J., et al., Human neural stem cells over-expressing VEGF provide neuroprotection, angiogenesis and functional recovery in mouse stroke model. PLoS One, 2007. **2**(1): p. e156.

[120] McDonald, J.W., et al., Oligodendrocytes from forebrain are highly vulnerable to AMPA/kainate receptor-mediated excitotoxicity. Nat Med, 1998. **4**(3): p. 291–297.

[121] Lyons, S.A. and Kettenmann, H., Oligodendrocytes and microglia are selectively vulnerable to combined hypoxia and hypoglycemia injury in vitro. J Cereb Blood Flow Metab, 1998. **18**(5): p. 521–530.

[122] Yoshioka, A., et al., Non-N-methyl-D-aspartate glutamate receptors mediate oxygen–glucose deprivation-induced oligodendroglial injury. Brain Res, 2000. **854**(1–2): p. 207–215.

[123] Pantoni, L., Garcia, J.H., and Gutierrez, J.A., Cerebral white matter is highly vulnerable to ischemia. Stroke, 1996. **27**(9): p. 1641–1647.

[124] Imada, S., et al., Hypothermia-induced increase of oligodendrocyte precursor cells: Possible involvement of plasmalemmal voltage-dependent anion channel 1. J Neurosci Res, 2010. **88**(16): p. 3457–3466.

[125] Agematsu, K., et al., Effects of preoperative hypoxia on white matter injury associated with cardiopulmonary bypass in a rodent hypoxic and brain slice model. Pediatr Res, 2014. **75**(5): p. 618–625.

[126] Xiong, M., et al., Effects of hypothermia on oligodendrocyte precursor cell proliferation, differentiation and maturation following hypoxia ischemia in vivo and in vitro. Exp Neurol, 2013. **247**: p. 720–729.

[127] Davidson, J.O., et al., Non-additive effects of delayed connexin hemichannel blockade and hypothermia after cerebral ischemia in near-term fetal sheep. J Cereb Blood Flow Metab, 2015. **35**(12): p. 2052–2061.

[128] Davidson, J.O., et al., Connexin hemichannel blockade improves outcomes in a model of fetal ischemia. Ann Neurol, 2012. **71**(1): p. 121–132.

[129] Davidson, J.O., et al., Extending the duration of hypothermia does not further improve white matter protection after ischemia in term-equivalent fetal sheep. Sci Rep, 2016. **6**: p. 25178.

[130] Davidson, J.O., et al., How long is too long for cerebral cooling after ischemia in fetal sheep? J Cereb Blood Flow Metab, 2015. **35**(5): p. 751–758.

[131] Lotocki, G., et al., Oligodendrocyte vulnerability following traumatic brain injury in rats: effect of moderate hypothermia. Ther Hypothermia Temp Manag, 2011. **1**(1): p. 43–51.

[132] Lotocki, G., et al., Oligodendrocyte vulnerability following traumatic brain injury in rats. Neurosci Lett, 2011. **499**(3): p. 143–148.

[133] Bennet, L., The effect of cerebral hypothermia on white and grey matter injury induced by severe hypoxia in preterm fetal sheep. Journal of Physiology, 2007. **578**: p. 506.

[134] Xiong, M., et al., Short-term effects of hypothermia on axonal injury, preoligodendrocyte accumulation and oligodendrocyte myelination after hypoxia-ischemia in the hippocampus of immature rat brain. Dev Neurosci, 2013. **35**(1): p. 17–27.

[135] Font, M.A., Arboix, A., and Krupinski, J., Angiogenesis, neurogenesis and neuroplasticity in ischemic stroke. Curr Cardiol Rev, 2010. **6**(3): p. 238–244.

[136] Gopurappilly, R., Stem cells in stroke repair: current success & future prospects. CNS & Neurological disorders drug targets, 2011. **10**: p. 756.

[137] Trendelenburg, G. and Dirnagl, U., Neuroprotective role of astrocytes in cerebral ischemia: focus on ischemic preconditioning, Glia, 2005. **50**: p. 320.

[138] Lin, J.H., et al., Gap-junction-mediated propagation and amplification of cell injury. Nat Neurosci, 1998. **1**(6): p. 494–500.

[139] Agematsu, K., et al., Hypoxia diminishes the protective function of white-matter astrocytes in the developing brain. J Thorac Cardiovasc Surg, 2016. **151**(1): p. 265–272 e1-3.

[140] Zhao, Y. and Rempe, D.A., Targeting astrocytes for stroke therapy. Neurotherapeutics, 2010. **7**(4): p. 439–451.

[141] Xiong, M., et al., Post-ischemic hypothermia for 24h in P7 rats rescues hippocampal neuron: association with decreased astrocyte activation and inflammatory cytokine expression. Brain Res Bull, 2009. **79**(6): p. 351–357.

[142] Schmitt, K.R.L., et al., Hypothermia-induced neurite outgrowth is mediated by tumor necrosis factor-alpha. Brain Pathol, 2010. **20**(4): p. 771–779.

[143] Schmitt, K.R., S100B modulates IL-6 release and cytotoxicity from hypothermic brain cells and inhibits hypothermia-induced axonal outgrowth. Neuroscience research, 2007. **59**: p. 173.

[144] Xu, X., et al., Beneficial effects of local profound hypothermia and the possible mechanism after experimental spinal cord injury in rats. J Spinal Cord Med, 2016. **39**(2): p. 220–228.

[145] Xie, Y., Chen, S., and Murphy, T., Dendritic spines and pre-synaptic boutons are stable despite local deep hypothermic challenge and re-warming in vivo. PLoS One, 2012. **7**(5): p. e36305.

[146] Feng, J.-F., et al., Effect of therapeutic mild hypothermia on the genomics of the hippocampus after moderate traumatic brain injury in rats. Neurosurgery, 2010. **67**(3): p. 730–742.

[147] Gisselsson, L.L., Matus, A., and Wieloch, T., Actin redistribution underlies the sparing effect of mild hypothermia on dendritic spine morphology after in vitro ischemia. J Cereb Blood Flow Metab, 2005. **25**(10): p. 1346–1355.

[148] Muniz, J., et al., Neuroprotective effects of hypothermia on synaptic actin cytoskeletal changes induced by perinatal asphyxia. Brain Res, 2014. **1563**: p. 81–90.

[149] Dong, H., et al., Electrophysiological properties of CA1 neurons protected by postischemic hypothermia in gerbils. Stroke, 2001. **32**(3): p. 788–795.

[150] Dietz, R.M., et al., Therapeutic hypothermia protects against ischemia-induced impairment of synaptic plasticity following juvenile cardiac arrest in sex-dependent manner. Neuroscience, 2016. **325**: p. 132–141.

http://dx.doi.org/10.5772/65899

[151] Hoyert, D.L., 75 years of mortality in the United States, 1935–2010. NCHS Data Brief, 2012(88): p. 1–8.

[152] Kassem-Moussa, H. and Graffagnino, C., Nonocclusion and spontaneous recanalization rates in acute ischemic stroke: a review of cerebral angiography studies. Arch Neurol, 2002. **59**(12): p. 1870–1873.

Chapter 11

Hypoxia and Pulmonary Hypertension

Nicoletta Charolidi and Veronica A. Carroll

Additional information is available at the end of the chapter

http://dx.doi.org/10.5772/67151

Abstract

Vasoconstriction in response to low oxygen tension (hypoxia) in pulmonary arteries is an important physiological adaptation to reroute blood flow to areas of higher oxygenation for effective gaseous exchange. However, chronic hypoxia is a common feature of lung disease, such as chronic obstructive pulmonary disease (COPD). Hypoxic stress triggers cellular phenotypic alterations including increased proliferation and migration of vascular smooth muscle cells (VSMCs), as well as synthesis of extracellular matrix (ECM) proteins that remodel lung vasculature. Remodelling of vessels increases the risk of pulmonary hypertension (PH)—elevated pulmonary arterial pressure—and eventually right heart failure. This chapter will summarise the major pathways and mechanisms involved in hypoxia-driven pulmonary hypertension (PH).

Keywords: hypoxia, pulmonary hypertension, HIF-1α, HIF-2α, mTOR, VHL

1. Introduction

The main function of the cardiovascular system is to circulate and deliver oxygen to metabolically active tissues of the body. At physiologically normal oxygen levels, the pulmonary vasculature of healthy individuals is highly distensible, allowing the cardiac output to adjust to levels of activity. In varying degrees of oxygen availability, as in different altitudes, adaptive cardiovascular responses are employed. In acute hypoxia (short, transient reduction in oxygen tension), the pulmonary vascular bed constricts rapidly [1]. When oxygen levels are restored, it dilates again in a swift and reversible manner. With a sustained hypoxic exposure (hours to days), the response is different. There is a loss of pulmonary distensibility, increased arterial pressure, tachycardia and increased workload for the right cardiac ventricle. In return to normoxic conditions, there is, at least in the short term, a limited reversibility of these effects. The Operation Everest II study [2] demonstrated this phenomenon by monitoring the pulmonary vascular pressure of healthy individuals who were exposed to progressive partially pressured oxygen over a period of a few weeks. However, for high-altitude populations, such as the Tibetans, this is not the case. Due to natural selection and adaptation over many thousands of years living under low oxygen conditions, Tibetans have altered oxygen-sensing mechanisms and pulmonary vascular resistance to sustained hypoxia (discussed later in this chapter) [3].

Healthy, native sea-level dwellers, who move to high altitude, develop high pulmonary arterial pressure, but with time, in the majority of cases, it stabilises and becomes well tolerated [4]. By contrast, people with pre-existing lung pathologies, such as chronic obstructive pulmonary disease (COPD), cystic fibrosis, idiopathic pulmonary fibrosis, bronchiectasis or restrictive chest wall abnormalities, are at risk of developing pulmonary hypertension (PH). Chronic PH lowers quality of life and decreases life expectancy for the affected individuals [5–8].

The pathophysiology of hypoxia-associated PH is characterised by extensive vascular remodelling that leads to arterial narrowing rather than reversible vessel vasoconstriction (**Figure 1**). Processes that take place include endothelial cell dysfunction, muscularisation of normally non-muscular arteries, phenotypic switching and proliferation of vascular smooth muscle cells (VSMCs), increased extracellular matrix deposition and erythrocytosis [7, 9, 10]. In this chapter, recent developments in mechanistic aspects underlying hypoxia-induced pathophysiological changes in PH will be briefly summarised.

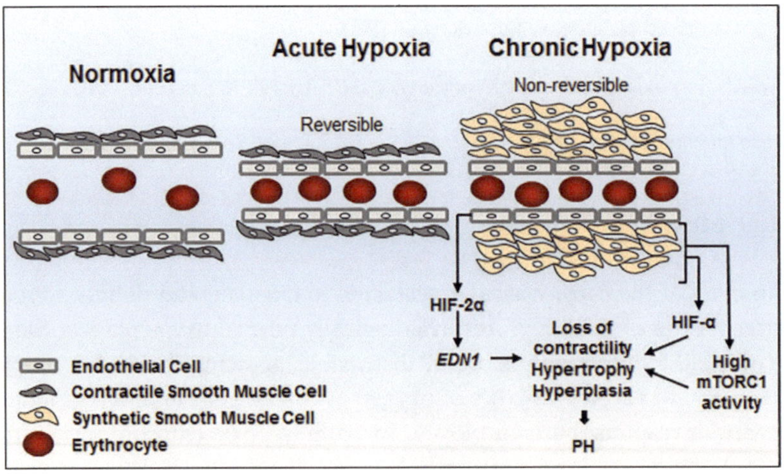

Figure 1. Schematic representation of pulmonary arterial responses to normoxia, acute hypoxia and chronic hypoxia. With acute and chronic hypoxia, the pulmonary artery undergoes vasoconstriction. In the case of acute hypoxia, the artery can reversibly dilate. But in chronic hypoxia, the artery undergoes nonreversible vascular remodelling characterised by intimal thickening due to VSMC dedifferentiation (loss of contractility, hypertrophy and hyperplasia). Additionally, there is distal muscularisation of non-muscular vessels, a settled-in endothelial cell dysfunction and erythrocytosis. Activation of HIF-1α and HIF-2α as well as over-activation of mTORC1 contributes to VSMC dedifferentiation and the establishment of hypoxic PH. Abbreviations: HIF-1α, hypoxia-inducible factor 1α; HIF-2α, hypoxia-inducible factor 2α; mTORC1, mechanistic target of rapamycin complex 1; PH, pulmonary hypertension.

http://dx.doi.org/10.5772/67151

2. Role of endothelial cell dysfunction

Endothelial cells in pulmonary vessels first sense hypoxic stress. Having a role in maintaining homeostasis, endothelial cells contribute to reducing the vascular tone in order for vasoconstriction to take place and regulate vessel adaptation to increased blood flow [11]. In healthy individuals, the endothelium is responsible for the balanced expression of vasoactive mediators that have either vasodilator ability, such as nitric oxide (NO) and prostacyclin (PGI_2), or vasoconstrictive properties, such as endothelin-1 (ET-1) [11–14]. ET-1 is released abluminally and triggers vasoconstriction through binding to its VSMC receptors ET_A and ET_B [15]. However, when ET-1 binds to its endothelial ET_B receptor, it can induce vasodilation through NO and PGI_2 recruitment [15], while this route also serves for ET-1 clearance from the lung [16].

In pathological PH, as in COPD, endothelial cell dysfunction is one of the major contributing factors for the progression of the condition. It has been found that endothelial NO synthase (eNOS), the enzyme responsible for NO production, as well as prostacyclin synthase, the enzyme responsible for PGI_2 production, is markedly diminished in patients with COPD [12, 17]. Furthermore, ET-1 has been reported to have an increased expression in the lungs of patients with PH and is a therapeutic target [14]. ET-1, as well as being a potent vasoconstrictor, is also a VSMC mitogen, acting through smooth muscle ET_A and ET_B receptors [15]. So in effect, during hypoxic endothelial dysregulation, the pathogenic excess of ET-1 maintains vessel constriction and VSMC proliferation.

3. Phenotypic switching of vascular smooth muscle cells

In hypoxia, the highly plastic VSMCs switch from a contractile to a synthetic phenotype, which is characterised by increased proliferation and extracellular matrix deposition [18]. Differentiated smooth muscle cells express a repertoire of contractile proteins, signalling molecules and receptors for their primary function of vessel contraction. These contractile VSMCs have little capacity for proliferation, protein synthesis or migration [18]. However, pulmonary VSMCs, under chronic hypoxic stimulation, switch to a synthetic state exhibiting hypertrophy, hyperplasia, loss of contractility and migration, contributing to the enlargement of the arterial intimal layer (**Figure 1**) and in the muscularisation of non-muscular pulmonary vessels [9]. Additionally, there is a deposition of collagen and elastic fibres. In extreme cases, the excessive VSMC proliferation can progress from vascular lesions to calcification. These phenomena seem to correlate with the degree of PH extent and COPD severity [19–21].

The endothelial dysfunction that takes place in PH may also contribute to the dedifferentiation and proliferation of VSMCs [22]. Specifically, dysregulated endothelial cells can cause alterations in AKT signalling in VSMCs, which in turn triggers their phenotypic switch [23]. This pathway is also affected by aberrant regulation of the mechanistic target of rapamycin (mTOR) pathway (discussed later in this chapter).

4. Hypoxia and pulmonary hypertension

The major cellular oxygen-sensing mechanism implicated in hypoxia-induced pulmonary hypertension is the hypoxia-inducible factor (HIF) pathway. HIFs are transcription factors that induce the activation of some several hundred genes in response to hypoxia [24]. Initially identified as regulators of erythropoietin (EPO), the hormone responsible for increased red blood cells in response to low oxygen levels, HIFs have since been found to regulate expression of genes that are important for angiogenesis, cellular metabolism, cardiovascular development and cardiovascular control [24–26].

In low oxygen conditions, HIFs bind DNA as heterodimeric complexes of alpha (HIF-α) and beta (HIF-β) subunits, with HIF-α being the subunit regulated by oxygen tension [27]. Higher animals have a series of isoforms for each of the HIF subunits as a result of gene evolutionary duplications [24]. In humans, there are three paralogs of HIF-α—HIF-1α, HIF-2α and HIF-3α—with the first two members being the best characterised [24, 25]. The expression of HIF-1α and HIF-2α is differentially regulated, while their balance is believed to be important for tissue-specific differences in oxygen sensing [25]. They both bind to the same DNA consensus (RCGTG) in hypoxia-response elements of the genome, but they only induce partially overlapping sets of genes [27, 28].

In normoxic conditions, the HIF-α subunit is hydroxylated by Fe(II) prolyl hydroxylase domain (PHD) enzymes (PHD1, PHD2 and PHD3 or otherwise known as Egln2, Egln1 and Egln3) that use 2-oxoglutarate and Fe^{2+} as substrates [29]. After hydroxylation by PHDs, HIF-α is recognised and bound by the von Hippel-Lindau (VHL) protein, a ubiquitin E3 ligase, which marks HIF-α for proteasomal degradation. In hypoxia, PHD enzymes are inactive allowing HIF-α subunits to translocate to the nucleus and activate HIF target genes. HIFs are further regulated by factor-inhibiting HIF (FIH)-mediated asparaginyl hydroxylation, which impairs their recruitment to transcriptional complexes [30].

Mouse models of HIF-1α and HIF-2α have illustrated that the HIF pathway is critically important for the pulmonary hypoxic response and the development of PH. Heterozygous deficiency of either HIF-1α or HIF-2α allele in mice does not affect their life span, and these animals are largely normal in unstressed, normal oxygen conditions. In response to chronic hypoxia (10% for 3 weeks), HIF-1$\alpha^{+/-}$ mice exhibit an attenuated PH with a low rise in right ventricular pressure and right ventricular hypertrophy [31]. Interestingly, heterozygous HIF-2$\alpha^{+/-}$ mice, exposed to 10% oxygen for 10 weeks, showed a complete lack of any PH manifestation [32]. Of note, animals with hetero- or homozygous mutations in stabilising HIF-2α spontaneously developed progressive PH [33]. These studies all indicate a pathological role of both HIF-α subunits in PH development.

Cell-type-specific inactivation of HIF-α with the use of a variety of promoters has also been studied but with some variable results, which may be due to the method of HIF-α manipulations and/or the use of different mouse strains [34–36]. Nevertheless, there seems to be a clear link between HIFs and PH, since studies from human genetics, including several populations that have adapted to different altitudes, have demonstrated the importance of HIF-2α in pulmonary response to hypoxia and PH pathophysiology [37].

http://dx.doi.org/10.5772/67151

The Tibetans, who have lived for at least 25,000 years in 4000 m elevation and continuously inspired partially pressured oxygen (~80 mmHg), have been identified to have a number of single-nucleotide polymorphisms in close-to-one-another loci near the gene *EPAS1*, which encodes HIF-2α [38]. HIF-2α is the subunit responsible for EPO regulation and in turn erythropoiesis. Tibetans manifest blunted PH and reduced erythropoiesis at high altitude. At sea level, they manifest a lower pulmonary arterial pressure in response to hypoxia when compared with other populations [39, 40]. Recently, a missense mutation in PHD2 (*EGLN1*) was identified which allows for increased PHD2 activity under hypoxic conditions, thereby decreasing HIF-α stabilisation and reducing erythropoiesis at altitude [41].

Further evidence for a role for HIF-2α in PH comes from another human genetic study, which showed that an activating HIF-2α mutation (G$\rightarrow$A substitution in position 2097) caused erythrocytosis with elevated total red cell volume and PH in an affected family [42].

5. VHL and pulmonary hypertension

The VHL protein is a tumour suppressor and an essential component for the clearance of HIF-α through the ubiquitin-proteasomal degradation pathway [24, 43]. A number of VHL mutations have been described that result in aberrant induction of HIF target genes, due to the loss of function of VHL and in turn to the loss of HIF-α regulation. VHL mutations are associated with VHL syndrome, which is a hereditary condition, characterised by highly vascularised tumours within specific tissues, including the renal, retinal and central nervous system [44]. However, a small number of VHL mutations (R200W, D126N, S183L, D126N) are associated with development of Chuvash polycythemia (CP) [45–47]. CP is a rare autosomal recessive condition that is endemic to the population in Chuvashia, Russia and in the island of Ischia, Italy [46, 48]. Chuvash patients manifest increased haemoglobin and haematocrit with elevated levels of EPO, as well as increased expression of vascular endothelial growth factor (VEGF) and ET-1, which are HIF-α target genes [45–49]. In addition, these patients are highly susceptible to both arterial and venous thrombosis and can develop mild to severe PH [45–49].

The importance of HIF-2α isoform in the regulation of pulmonary vascular control has also been demonstrated by the use of a mouse model of CP [50]. This model carries a hypomorphic VHL allele (with an R200W substitution) and recapitulates all symptoms of the human CP phenotype. Interestingly, when these mice are crossed with HIF-2$\alpha^{+/-}$ or HIF-1$\alpha^{+/-}$ strains for heterozygous deficiency in either of the two HIF-α, they manifest an ameliorated PH phenotype for suppressed HIF-2α, but not for HIF-1α.

Comparison of CP and HIF-2α gain-of-function mutation human phenotypes has additionally shown that the latter condition somehow manifests more moderate symptoms than the first. The explanation for this may be that, in CP, both HIF-α subunits are upregulated, and therefore, there may be an additive effect [51]. Furthermore, VHL has a number of HIF-α-independent functions that may also play a role in the CP phenotype.

6. New advances: hypoxic induction of zinc transporters

Zinc, an essential dietary element, plays an important cytoprotective role for the lung by sheltering the pulmonary epithelium from extrinsic activation of apoptotic pathways following acute lung injury [52]. Zinc transporters are responsible for zinc cellular uptake and homeostasis [53]. A recent linkage analysis study that compared a PH-resistant rat strain, Fisher 344 (F344), with the Wistar Kyoto (WKY) strain identified the gene *Slc39a12*, which encodes the ZIP12 zinc transporter, as a major regulator of hypoxia-induced pulmonary vascular remodelling [53]. In the F344 strain, this gene lacks a crucial thymidine, which leads to a frameshift mutation in exon 11 and renders translation of the protein redundant. ZIP12 is normally expressed in endothelial, interstitial and VSMCs, but its expression increases in remodelled pulmonary vessels following hypoxia-induced PH [53]. ZIP12 is likely a HIF target gene since both HIF-1α and HIF-2α were detected bound to ZIP12 hypoxia-response element. The investigators of this study further generated a ZIP12$^{-/-}$ rat model for comparison with the original F344 and WKY strains and found that genetic disruption of ZIP12 recapitulates the phenotype of the PH-resistant F344 strain under conditions of hypoxia.

Zinc-binding motifs have been considered as potential PH drug-therapeutic targets with phosphodiesterase type 5 (PDE5) and histone deacetylases as examples [54, 55]. Zinc is a structural component of a number of intracellular enzymes, transcription factors, other proteins and cofactors and is a putative drug target for PH.

7. Role of hypoxia-inducible microRNAs in pulmonary hypertension

MicroRNAs (miRNAs) are small non-coding RNA molecules (about 21 nucleotides long) that regulate gene expression post-transcriptionally. Hypoxic stimulation of a variety of human cell types has shown induction of more than 90 miRNAs [56], with altered expression of some of these miRNAs involved in VSMC remodelling and endothelial cell dysfunction in PH [57].

MiRNAs that have been causally implicated in PH include miR-204, miR-138, miR-21 and miR-130/miR-301, among others (**Table 1**). MiR-204 has been shown to be downregulated in VSMCs of patients suffering from PH, as well as in mouse models of the disease [58, 59]. The degree of miR-204 suppression has been found to be inversely proportional to the degree of pulmonary artery resistance and pressure, while compensating for the loss of miR-204 through nebulisation in PH patients has been shown to reverse the VSMC proliferative and anti-apoptotic phenotype [59]. MiR-204 is involved in the activation of the nuclear factor of activated T cell (NFAT) pathway, the Rho pathway, VSMC proliferation and resistance to apoptosis, as well as downregulation of transcripts such as bone morphogenetic protein receptor type II (BMPR2) and interleukin-6 (IL-6) [60–62]. Also, miR-204 regulates the expression of the Runt-related transcription factor 2 (RUNX2), which has been shown to stabilise HIF-1α in chondrocytes by competing with VHL [20, 63]. In the context of hypoxia, RUNX2 is upregulated, since miR-204 is downregulated, and therefore sustains HIF-1α activation,

http://dx.doi.org/10.5772/67151

MicroRNA	Change in PH	Target transcripts	Cellular function, process or pathway affected	Ref.
miR-204	↓	BMPR2, IL-6, RUNX2 among others	Activation of NFAT pathway, VSMC proliferation, resistance to apoptosis, Rho pathway, HIF-1α pathway	[20, 58–63]
miR-138	↑	HIF-1α, S100A1	HIF-1α pathway, endothelial regulation of vasomotor tone	[64]
miR-21	↑	PDCD4, SPRY2, PPARα	VSMC proliferation, resistance to apoptosis	[61, 65–67]
miR-130/301	↑	PPARγ which leads to subordinate gene targets and other miRNAs	Master regulator of cell proliferation and apoptosis in PH ↓ miR-204	[68]

Table 1. MicroRNAs that are causally implicated in PH.

which in turn contributes to aberrant VSMC proliferation, resistance to apoptosis and their transdifferentiation to osteoblast-like cells [20].

MiR-138 is upregulated by hypoxia and suppresses HIF-1α [64]. However, its upregulation also contributes to endothelial cell dysfunction in PH by downregulating the small EF-hand Ca^{2+}-binding protein S100A1 that relays Ca^{2+} oscillations, controlling vascular tone responses [64].

MiR-21 expression has been found to be upregulated in both pulmonary VSMC and endothelial cells during hypoxic conditions [61, 65]. This upregulation, in turn, leads to downregulation of programmed cell death protein 4 (PDCD4), sprouty homolog 2 (SPRY2) and peroxisome proliferator-activated receptor-α (PPARα), which when dysregulated play a role in the increased proliferation and resistance to apoptosis [65–67]. Treatment of mice with anti-miR-21 during hypoxia showed an improvement in distal pulmonary artery muscularisation [69]. However, miR-21 has also been shown to have a protective effect during PH [61]. Using VHL-null mice, IL-6 transgenic mice, pulmonary vessels from patients with PH as well as deficient (miR-21$^{-/-}$) or miR-21 overexpression (miR-21$^{+/+}$) mouse models, it has been demonstrated that miR-21 loss of function causes onset of PH [61]. Specifically, miR-21 deletion showed exaggerated pulmonary vascular remodelling, whereas in mice overexpressing miR-21, these disease-associated phenotypes were abolished [61].

The family of miR-130/301 is also upregulated in pulmonary VSMCs and the endothelium in hypoxia, as well as in the lungs of mice with PH due to chronic hypoxic exposure [68]. This upregulation is mediated by HIF-2α and Oct-4. MiR-130/301 is a master regulator miRNA subordinating other miRNA pathways, and, for instance, it suppresses miR-204 [68].

miR-223, miR-17, miR-130, miR-145, miR-424 and miR503 are also involved in the pathophysiology of PH (reviewed in Ref. [70]). So far, PH animal models have helped greatly in these studies, but the exact role and balance for each of these miRNAs in human PH have not been fully elucidated.

8. mTOR signalling in hypoxia-induced pulmonary hypertension

Mechanistic target of rapamycin (mTOR) is a cellular hub that controls growth factor signalling and nutrient sensing to regulate cell growth, proliferation, metabolism and survival [71]. mTOR is a protein kinase that is the catalytic component of two functionally distinct complexes, mTOR complex 1 (mTORC1) and mTOR complex 2 (mTORC2) [72, 73]. mTORC1 is composed of mTOR, Raptor, LST8/GβL, PRAS40 and DEP domain containing mTOR-interacting protein (DEPTOR), and its activity is stimulated by growth factor signals to regulate protein synthesis through 4E-BP1/BP2 and the S6 kinases, S6K1 and S6K2 [74, 75]. By contrast, mTORC2, which comprises mTOR, Rictor, LST8/GβL, DEPTOR, SIN1 and PRR5, regulates cytoskeletal organisation [76, 77] and has a role in phosphorylation of protein kinase C (PKC), protein kinase B (PKB) and serum- and glucocorticoid-induced protein kinase (SGK) to promote cell survival and cell cycle progression [78–80].

Aberrant mTOR activity has a well-characterised role in promoting proliferative diseases including cancer and smooth muscle cell pathologies [71]. mTORC1 signalling is activated following vascular injury promoting Vinhibitor, rapamycin, promotes smooth muscle cell (SMC) remodelling. Accordingly, mTOR inhibitors are widely used in drug-eluting stents to prevent restenosis. In addition, mTOR also regulates the differentiation state of VSMCs since the mTOR inhibitor, rapamycin, promotes SMC differentiation and expression of contractile proteins [81]. mTORC1 activity is low in differentiated contractile VSMCs but becomes activated by growth factors and is thought to contribute to the change towards a synthetic phenotype that is characterised by increased SMC proliferation and migration. As such, rapamycin analogues may have therapeutic potential for treating PH.

The relationship between hypoxic conditions and mTOR is complex and depends, in part, on cellular context. Many cell types respond to prolonged periods of hypoxia by inactivating energy-intensive processes such as protein synthesis and proliferation, and accordingly mTOR is downregulated [82]. By contrast, the vasculature responds to long-term hypoxia by promoting new blood vessel growth—angiogenesis, which in turn, restores O_2 to deprived tissues. Hypoxic stress is a key driving force in the vascular remodelling observed in pulmonary hypertension, and HIFs activate pulmonary artery endothelial and smooth muscle cell proliferation, which is mediated by both mTORC1 and mTORC2 [83–85]. Currently, the mechanisms by which hypoxia/HIFs signal to activate mTOR in ECs and VSMCs are poorly understood [86–90].

9. Conclusion

Severe PH associated with hypoxic lung disease is a life-threatening condition with poor survival rates. Despite significant advances in targeted therapeutics for PH, randomised clinical trial data for this particular group of patients are scarce, and it is not clear whether endothelin receptor antagonists will benefit patients with hypoxia-associated PH. Importantly, recent genetic studies identifying mutations in the oxygen-sensing machinery have provided new mechanistic insights into the aetiology of PH. Further studies are required to determine whether specific targeting of HIF-2α will provide additional therapeutic benefit for this complex disease.

http://dx.doi.org/10.5772/67151

Author details

Nicoletta Charolidi and Veronica A. Carroll*

*Address all correspondence to: vcarroll@sgul.ac.uk

Vascular Biology Research Centre, Molecular and Clinical Sciences Research Institute, St George's, University of London, London, UK

References

[1] Euler U, Liljestrand G. Observations on the pulmonary arterial blood pressure in the cat. Acta Physiol Scand. 1946;12:301–20.

[2] Groves BM, Reeves JT, Sutton JR, Wagner PD, Cymerman A, Malconian MK, et al. Operation Everest II: elevated high-altitude pulmonary resistance unresponsive to oxygen. J Appl Physiol (1985). 1987 Aug;63(2):521–30.

[3] Aldenderfer M. Peopling the Tibetan plateau: insights from archaeology. High Alt Med Biol. 2011;12(2):141–7.

[4] West JB, American College of Physicians, American Physiological Society. The physiologic basis of high-altitude diseases. Ann Intern Med. 2004 Nov 16;141(10):789–800.

[5] Seeger W, Adir Y, Barberà JA, Champion H, Coghlan JG, Cottin V, et al. Pulmonary hypertension in chronic lung diseases. J Am Coll Cardiol. 2013 Dec 24;62 (25 Suppl):D109–16.

[6] Wells JM, Washko GR, Han MK, Abbas N, Nath H, Mamary AJ, et al. Pulmonary arterial enlargement and acute exacerbations of COPD. N Engl J Med. 2012 Sep 6;367(10):913–21.

[7] Blanco I, Piccari L, Barberà JA. Pulmonary vasculature in COPD: the silent component. Respirology. 2016 Aug;21(6):984–94.

[8] Wells JM, Farris RF, Gosdin TA, Dransfield MT, Wood ME, Bell SC, et al. Pulmonary artery enlargement and cystic fibrosis pulmonary exacerbations: a cohort study. Lancet Respir Med. 2016 Aug;4(8):636–45.

[9] Stenmark KR, Fagan KA, Frid MG. Hypoxia-induced pulmonary vascular remodeling: cellular and molecular mechanisms. Circ Res. 2006 Sep 29;99(7):675–91.

[10] Kylhammar D, Rådegran G. The principal pathways involved in the in vivo modulation of hypoxic pulmonary vasoconstriction, pulmonary arterial remodelling and pulmonary hypertension. Acta Physiol (Oxf). 2016 Jul 6;Epub ahead of print.

[11] Stamler JS, Loh E, Roddy MA, Currie KE, Creager MA. Nitric oxide regulates basal systemic and pulmonary vascular resistance in healthy humans. Circulation. 1994 May;89(5):2035–40.

[12] Tuder RM, Cool CD, Geraci MW, Wang J, Abman SH, Wright L, et al. Prostacyclin synthase expression is decreased in lungs from patients with severe pulmonary hypertension. Am J Respir Crit Care Med. 1999 Jun;159(6):1925–32.

[13] Barberà JA, Roger N, Roca J, Rovira I, Higenbottam TW, Rodriguez-Roisin R. Worsening of pulmonary gas exchange with nitric oxide inhalation in chronic obstructive pulmonary disease. Lancet (London, England). 1996 Feb 17;347(8999):436–40.

[14] Giaid A, Yanagisawa M, Langleben D, Michel RP, Levy R, Shennib H, et al. Expression of endothelin-1 in the lungs of patients with pulmonary hypertension. N Engl J Med. 1993 Jun 17;328(24):1732–9.

[15] Bialecki RA, Fisher CS, Murdoch WW, Barthlow HG, Bertelsen DL. Functional comparison of endothelin receptors in human and rat pulmonary artery smooth muscle. Am J Physiol. 1997 Feb;272(2 Pt 1):L211–8.

[16] Fukuroda T, Fujikawa T, Ozaki S, Ishikawa K, Yano M, Nishikibe M. Clearance of circulating endothelin-1 by ETB receptors in rats. Biochem Biophys Res Commun. 1994 Mar 30;199(3):1461–5.

[17] Yang Q, Shigemura N, Underwood MJ, Hsin M, Xue H-M, Huang Y, et al. NO and EDHF pathways in pulmonary arteries and veins are impaired in COPD patients. Vascul Pharmacol. 2012;57(2–4):113–8.

[18] Owens GK, Kumar MS, Wamhoff BR. Molecular regulation of vascular smooth muscle cell differentiation in development and disease. Physiol Rev. 2004 Jul;84(3):767–801.

[19] Carlsen J, Hasseriis Andersen K, Boesgaard S, Iversen M, Steinbrüchel D, Bøgelund Andersen C. Pulmonary arterial lesions in explanted lungs after transplantation correlate with severity of pulmonary hypertension in chronic obstructive pulmonary disease. J Heart Lung Transplant. 2013 Mar;32(3):347–54.

[20] Ruffenach G, Chabot S, Tanguay VF, Courboulin A, Boucherat O, Potus F, et al. Role for Runt-related transcription factor 2 in proliferative and calcified vascular lesions in pulmonary arterial hypertension. Am J Respir Crit Care Med. 2016 Nov 15;194(10)1273–85.

[21] Santos S, Peinado VI, Ramírez J, Melgosa T, Roca J, Rodriguez-Roisin R, et al. Characterization of pulmonary vascular remodelling in and patients with mild COPD. Eur Respir J. 2002 Apr;19(4):632–8.

[22] Powell RJ, Cronenwett JL, Fillinger MF, Wagner RJ, Sampson LN. Endothelial cell modulation of smooth muscle cell morphology and organizational growth pattern. Ann Vasc Surg. 1996 Jan;10(1):4–10.

[23] Brown DJ, Rzucidlo EM, Merenick BL, Wagner RJ, Martin KA, Powell RJ. Endothelial cell activation of the smooth muscle cell phosphoinositide 3-kinase/Akt pathway promotes differentiation. J Vasc Surg. 2005 Mar;41(3):509–16.

[24] Bishop T, Ratcliffe PJ. HIF hydroxylase pathways in cardiovascular physiology and medicine. Circ Res. 2015 Jun 19;117(1):65–79.

[25] Semenza GL. Oxygen sensing, homeostasis, and disease. N Engl J Med. 2011 Aug 11;365(6):537–47.

http://dx.doi.org/10.5772/67151

[26] Maxwell PH, Pugh CW, Ratcliffe PJ. Inducible operation of the erythropoietin 3′ enhancer in multiple cell lines: evidence for a widespread oxygen-sensing mechanism. Proc Natl Acad Sci U S A. 1993 Mar 15;90(6):2423–7.

[27] Hu CJ, Wang LY, Chodosh LA, Keith B, Simon MC. Differential roles of hypoxia-inducible factor 1alpha (HIF-1alpha) and HIF-2alpha in hypoxic gene regulation. Mol Cell Biol. 2003 Dec;23(24):9361–74.

[28] Schödel J, Oikonomopoulos S, Ragoussis J, Pugh CW, Ratcliffe PJ, Mole DR. High-resolution genome-wide mapping of HIF-binding sites by ChIP-seq. Blood. 2011 Jun 9;117(23):e207–17.

[29] Bruick RK, McKnight SL. A conserved family of prolyl-4-hydroxylases that modify HIF. Science. 2001 Nov 9;294(5545):1337–40.

[30] Mahon PC, Hirota K, Semenza GL. FIH-1: a novel protein that interacts with HIF-1alpha and VHL to mediate repression of HIF-1 transcriptional activity. Genes Dev. 2001 Oct 15;15(20):2675–86.

[31] Yu AY, Shimoda LA, Iyer NV, Huso DL, Sun X, McWilliams R, et al. Impaired physiological responses to chronic hypoxia in mice partially deficient for hypoxia-inducible factor 1alpha. J Clin Invest. 1999 Mar;103(5):691–6.

[32] Brusselmans K, Compernolle V, Tjwa M, Wiesener MS, Maxwell PH, Collen D, et al. Heterozygous deficiency of hypoxia-inducible factor-2alpha protects mice against pulmonary hypertension and right ventricular dysfunction during prolonged hypoxia. J Clin Invest. 2003 May;111(10):1519–27.

[33] Tan Q, Kerestes H, Percy MJ, Pietrofesa R, Chen L, Khurana TS, et al. Erythrocytosis and pulmonary hypertension in a mouse model of human HIF2A gain of function mutation. J Biol Chem. 2013 Jun 14;288(24):17134–44.

[34] Ball MK, Waypa GB, Mungai PT, Nielsen JM, Czech L, Dudley VJ, et al. Regulation of hypoxia-induced pulmonary hypertension by vascular smooth muscle hypoxia-inducible factor-1α. Am J Respir Crit Care Med. 2014 Feb 1;189(3):314–24.

[35] Kim Y-M, Barnes EA, Alvira CM, Ying L, Reddy S, Cornfield DN. Hypoxia-inducible factor-1α in pulmonary artery smooth muscle cells lowers vascular tone by decreasing myosin light chain phosphorylation. Circ Res. 2013 Apr 26;112(9):1230–3.

[36] Skuli N, Liu L, Runge A, Wang T, Yuan L, Patel S, et al. Endothelial deletion of hypoxia-inducible factor-2alpha (HIF-2alpha) alters vascular function and tumor angiogenesis. Blood. 2009 Jul 9;114(2):469–77.

[37] Semenza GL. Hypoxia-inducible factors in physiology and medicine. Cell. 2012 Feb 3;148(3):399–408.

[38] Beall CM, Cavalleri GL, Deng L, Elston RC, Gao Y, Knight J, et al. Natural selection on EPAS1 (HIF2alpha) associated with low hemoglobin concentration in Tibetan highlanders. Proc Natl Acad Sci U S A. 2010 Jun 22;107(25):11459–64.

[39] Petousi N, Croft QP, Cavalleri GL, Cheng HY, Formenti F, Ishida K, et al. Tibetans living at sea level have a hyporesponsive hypoxia-inducible factor system and blunted physiological responses to hypoxia. J Appl Physiol. 2014 Apr 1;116(7):893–904.

[40] Simonson TS, Yang Y, Huff CD, Yun H, Qin G, Witherspoon DJ, et al. Genetic evidence for high-altitude adaptation in Tibet. Science. 2010 Jul 2;329(5987):72–5.

[41] Lorenzo FR, Huff C, Myllymäki M, Olenchock B, Swierczek S, Tashi T, et al. A genetic mechanism for Tibetan high-altitude adaptation. Nat Genet. 2014;46(9):951–6.

[42] Gale DP, Harten SK, Reid CDL, Tuddenham EG, Maxwell PH. Autosomal dominant erythrocytosis and pulmonary arterial hypertension associated with an activating HIF2 alpha mutation. Blood. 2008 Aug 1;112(3):919–21.

[43] Maxwell PH, Wiesener MS, Chang GW, Clifford SC, Vaux EC, Cockman ME, et al. The tumour suppressor protein VHL targets hypoxia-inducible factors for oxygen-dependent proteolysis. Nature. 1999 May 20;399(6733):271–5.

[44] Chittiboina P, Lonser RR. Von Hippel-Lindau disease. Handb Clin Neurol. 2015;132:139–56.

[45] Sarangi S, Lanikova L, Kapralova K, Acharya S, Swierczek S, Lipton JM, et al. The homozygous VHL(D126N) missense mutation is associated with dramatically elevated erythropoietin levels, consequent polycythemia, and early onset severe pulmonary hypertension. Pediatr Blood Cancer. 2014 Nov;61(11):2104–6.

[46] Ang SO, Chen H, Hirota K, Gordeuk VR, Jelinek J, Guan Y, et al. Disruption of oxygen homeostasis underlies congenital Chuvash polycythemia. Nat Genet. 2002 Dec;32(4):614–21.

[47] Bond J, Gale DP, Connor T, Adams S, de Boer J, Gascoyne DM, et al. Dysregulation of the HIF pathway due to VHL mutation causing severe erythrocytosis and pulmonary arterial hypertension. Blood. 2011 Mar 31;117(13):3699–701.

[48] Perrotta S, Nobili B, Ferraro M, Migliaccio C, Borriello A, Cucciolla V, et al. Von Hippel-Lindau-dependent polycythemia is endemic on the island of Ischia: identification of a novel cluster. Blood. 2006 Jan 15;107(2):514–9.

[49] Smith TG, Brooks JT, Balanos GM, Lappin TR, Layton DM, Leedham DL, et al. Mutation of von Hippel-Lindau tumour suppressor and human cardiopulmonary physiology. PLoS Med. 2006 Jul;3(7):e290.

[50] Hickey MM, Richardson T, Wang T, Mosqueira M, Arguiri E, Yu H, et al. The von Hippel-Lindau Chuvash mutation promotes pulmonary hypertension and fibrosis in mice. J Clin Invest. 2010 Mar;120(3):827–39.

[51] Formenti F, Beer PA, Croft QP, Dorrington KL, Gale DP, Lappin TRJ, et al. Cardiopulmonary function in two human disorders of the hypoxia-inducible factor (HIF) pathway: von Hippel-Lindau disease and HIF-2alpha gain-of-function mutation. FASEB J. 2011 Jun;25(6):2001–11.

[52] Zalewski PD, Forbes IJ, Betts WH. Correlation of apoptosis with change in intracellular labile Zn(II) using zinquin [(2-methyl-8-p-toluenesulphonamido-6-quinolyloxy)acetic acid], a new specific fluorescent probe for Zn(II). Biochem J. 1993 Dec 1;296(Pt 2):403-8.

[53] Zhao L, Oliver E, Maratou K, Atanur SS, Dubois OD, Cotroneo E, et al. The zinc transporter ZIP12 regulates the pulmonary vascular response to chronic hypoxia. Nature. 2015 Aug 20;524(7565):356–60.

[54] Zhao L, Mason NA, Morrell NW, Kojonazarov B, Sadykov A, Maripov A, et al. Sildenafil inhibits hypoxia-induced pulmonary hypertension. Circulation. 2001 Jul 24;104(4):424–8.

[55] Zhao L, Chen CN, Hajji N, Oliver E, Cotroneo E, Wharton J, et al. Histone deacetylation inhibition in pulmonary hypertension: therapeutic potential of valproic acid and suberoylanilide hydroxamic acid. Circulation. 2012 Jul 24;126(4):455–67.

[56] Kozomara A, Griffiths-Jones S. miRBase: annotating high confidence microRNAs using deep sequencing data. Nucleic Acids Res. 2014 Jan;42(Database issue):D68–73.

[57] White K, Loscalzo J, Chan SY. Holding our breath: the emerging and anticipated roles of microRNA in pulmonary hypertension. Pulm Circ. 2012 Jul;2(3):278–90.

[58] Caruso P, MacLean MR, Khanin R, McClure J, Soon E, Southgate M, et al. Dynamic changes in lung microRNA profiles during the development of pulmonary hypertension due to chronic hypoxia and monocrotaline. Arterioscler Thromb Vasc Biol. 2010 Apr;30(4):716–23.

[59] Courboulin A, Paulin R, Giguère NJ, Saksouk N, Perreault T, Meloche J, et al. Role for miR-204 in human pulmonary arterial hypertension. J Exp Med. 2011 Mar 14;208(3):535–48.

[60] Bonnet S, Rochefort G, Sutendra G, Archer SL, Haromy A, Webster L, et al. The nuclear factor of activated T cells in pulmonary arterial hypertension can be therapeutically targeted. Proc Natl Acad Sci U S A. 2007 Jul 3;104(27):11418–23.

[61] Parikh VN, Jin RC, Rabello S, Gulbahce N, White K, Hale A, et al. MicroRNA-21 integrates pathogenic signaling to control pulmonary hypertension: results of a network bioinformatics approach. Circulation. 2012 Mar 27;125(12):1520–32.

[62] Tuder RM, Marecki JC, Richter A, Fijalkowska I, Flores S. Pathology of pulmonary hypertension. Clin Chest Med. 2007 Mar;28(1):23–42, vii.

[63] Lee SH, Che X, Jeong JH, Choi JY, Lee YJ, Lee YH, et al. Runx2 protein stabilizes hypoxia-inducible factor-1α through competition with von Hippel-Lindau protein (pVHL) and stimulates angiogenesis in growth plate hypertrophic chondrocytes. J Biol Chem. 2012 Apr 27;287(18):14760–71.

[64] Sen A, Ren S, Lerchenmüller C, Sun J, Weiss N, Most P, et al. MicroRNA-138 regulates hypoxia-induced endothelial cell dysfunction by targeting S100A1. PLoS One. 2013 Nov 11;8(11):e78684.

[65] Sarkar J, Gou D, Turaka P, Viktorova E, Ramchandran R, Raj JU. MicroRNA-21 plays a role in hypoxia-mediated pulmonary artery smooth muscle cell proliferation and migration. Am J Physiol Lung Cell Mol Physiol. 2010 Dec;299(6):L861–71.

[66] Cheng Y, Zhu P, Yang J, Liu X, Dong S, Wang X, et al. Ischaemic preconditioning-regulated miR-21 protects heart against ischaemia/reperfusion injury via anti-apoptosis through its target PDCD4. Cardiovasc Res. 2010 Aug 1;87(3):431–9.

[67] Davis BN, Hilyard AC, Lagna G, Hata A. SMAD proteins control DROSHA-mediated microRNA maturation. Nature. 2008 Jul 3;454(7200):56–61.

[68] Bertero T, Lu Y, Annis S, Hale A, Bhat B, Saggar R, et al. Systems-level regulation of microRNA networks by miR-130/301 promotes pulmonary hypertension. J Clin Invest. 2014 Aug;124(8):3514–28.

[69] Yang S, Banerjee S, Freitas Ad, Cui H, Xie N, Abraham E, et al. miR-21 regulates chronic hypoxia-induced pulmonary vascular remodeling. Am J Physiol Lung Cell Mol Physiol. 2012 Mar 15;302(6):L521–9.

[70] Mohsenin V. The emerging role of microRNAs in hypoxia-induced pulmonary hypertension. Sleep Breath. 2016 Sep;20(3):1059–67.

[71] Laplante M, Sabatini DM. mTOR signaling in growth control and disease. Cell. 2012 Apr 13;149(2):274–93.

[72] Sciarretta S, Volpe M, Sadoshima J. Mammalian target of rapamycin signaling in cardiac physiology and disease. Circ Res. 2014 Jan 31;114(3):549–64.

[73] Ratcliffe PJ. Oxygen sensing and hypoxia signalling pathways in animals: the implications of physiology for cancer. J Physiol. 2013 Apr 15;591(8):2027–42.

[74] Corradetti MN, Guan KL. Upstream of the mammalian target of rapamycin: do all roads pass through mTOR?. Oncogene. 2006 Oct 16;25(48):6347–60.

[75] Sengupta S, Peterson TR, Sabatini DM. Regulation of the mTOR complex 1 pathway by nutrients, growth factors, and stress. Mol Cell. 2010 Oct 22;40(2):310–22.

[76] Sarbassov DD, Ali SM, Kim DH, Guertin DA, Latek RR, Erdjument-Bromage H, et al. Rictor, a novel binding partner of mTOR, defines a rapamycin-insensitive and raptor-independent pathway that regulates the cytoskeleton. Curr Biol. 2004 Jul 27;14(14):1296–302.

[77] Liu L, Das S, Losert W, Parent CA. mTORC2 regulates neutrophil chemotaxis in a cAMP- and RhoA-dependent fashion. Dev Cell. 2010 Dec 14;19(6):845–57.

[78] Sarbassov DD, Guertin DA, Ali SM, Sabatini DM. Phosphorylation and regulation of Akt/PKB by the rictor-mTOR complex. Science. 2005 Feb 18;307(5712):1098–101.

[79] García-Martínez JM, Alessi DR. mTOR complex 2 (mTORC2) controls hydrophobic motif phosphorylation and activation of serum- and glucocorticoid-induced protein kinase 1 (SGK1). Biochem J. 2008 Dec 15;416(3):375–85.

[80] Alessi DR, Andjelkovic M, Caudwell B, Cron P, Morrice N, Cohen P, et al. Mechanism of activation of protein kinase B by insulin and IGF-1. EMBO J. 1996 Dec 2;15(23):6541–51.

http://dx.doi.org/10.5772/67151

[81] Martin KA, Rzucidlo EM, Merenick BL, Fingar DC, Brown DJ, Wagner RJ, et al. The mTOR/p70 S6K1 pathway regulates vascular smooth muscle cell differentiation. Am J Physiol Cell Physiol. 2004 Mar;286(3):C507–17.

[82] Brugarolas J, Lei K, Hurley RL, Manning BD, Reiling JH, Hafen E, et al. Regulation of mTOR function in response to hypoxia by REDD1 and the TSC1/TSC2 tumor suppressor complex. Genes Dev. 2004 Dec 1;18(23):2893–904.

[83] Humar R, Kiefer FN, Berns H, Resink TJ, Battegay EJ. Hypoxia enhances vascular cell proliferation and angiogenesis in vitro via rapamycin (mTOR)-dependent signaling. FASEB J. 2002 Jun;16(8):771–80.

[84] Goncharov DA, Kudryashova TV, Ziai H, Ihida-Stansbury K, DeLisser H, Krymskaya VP, et al. Mammalian target of rapamycin complex 2 (mTORC2) coordinates pulmonary artery smooth muscle cell metabolism, proliferation, and survival in pulmonary arterial hypertension. Circulation. 2014 Feb 25;129(8):864–74.

[85] Krymskaya VP, Snow J, Cesarone G, Khavin I, Goncharov DA, Lim PN, et al. mTOR is required for pulmonary arterial vascular smooth muscle cell proliferation under chronic hypoxia. FASEB J. 2011 Jun;25(6):1922–33.

[86] Goncharova EA. mTOR and vascular remodeling in lung diseases: current challenges and therapeutic prospects. FASEB J. 2013 May;27(5):1796–807.

[87] Dai Z, Li M, Wharton J, Zhu MM, Zhao Y-Y. Prolyl-4 hydroxylase 2 (PHD2) deficiency in endothelial cells and hematopoietic cells induces obliterative vascular remodeling and severe pulmonary arterial hypertension in mice and humans through hypoxia-inducible factor-2α. Circulation. 2016 Jun 14;133(24):2447–58.

[88] Houssaini A, Abid S, Derumeaux G, Wan F, Parpaleix A, Rideau D, et al. Selective tuberous sclerosis complex 1 gene deletion in smooth muscle activates mammalian target of rapamycin signaling and induces pulmonary hypertension. Am J Respir Cell Mol Biol. 2016 Sep;55(3):352–67.

[89] Wessler JD, Steingart RM, Schwartz GK, Harvey BG, Schaffer W. Dramatic improvement in pulmonary hypertension with rapamycin. Chest. 2010 Oct;138(4):991–3.

[90] Seyfarth H-J, Hammerschmidt S, Halank M, Neuhaus P, Wirtz HR. Everolimus in patients with severe pulmonary hypertension: a safety and efficacy pilot trial. Pulm Circ. 2013 Sep;3(3):632–8.

Chapter 12

Stage-Specific Effects of Hypoxia on Interstitial Lung Disease

Sandeep Artham and Payaningal R. Somanath

Additional information is available at the end of the chapter

http://dx.doi.org/10.5772/66817

Abstract

Interstitial lung disease (ILD) comprises a group of lung diseases principally affecting the pulmonary interstitium, for example, pulmonary fibrosis. Following acute lung injury (ALI), the fate of an injured lung progressing towards either injury resolution or pulmonary fibrosis is dictated by hypoxia at various stages during the disease progression. Hypoxia that is tissue destructive at one stage of lung injury becomes beneficial at a different stage, with each hypoxic stage involving a different scheme of molecular pathways, cellular interplay and tissue remodeling. In this chapter, we provide a detailed account of hypoxia during the different stages of lung injury in ILDs, delineate the cellular and molecular mechanisms mediating tissue remodeling in the hypoxic lungs as well as the basic and clinical findings in this field with an emphasis on future therapeutics to modulate hypoxia to treat ILD.

Keywords: acute lung injury, wound resolution, hypoxia, interstitial lung disease, PAH

1. Introduction

Interstitial lung disease (ILD) comprises a group of lung diseases principally affecting the pulmonary interstitium, for example, pulmonary fibrosis [1]. An injured lung as a result of infection, inhalation of chemical, and other harmful substances either resolves over time or progresses into irreversible damage and fibrosis. Therefore, lung injury as in acute respiratory distress syndrome (ARDS), due to conditions like hypoxia can progress to interstitial lung damage or fibrosis similar to ILD-associated pulmonary fibrosis. Yet, another important pulmonary pathological condition associated with hypoxia is the pulmonary arterial hypertension (PAH) [2]. The ARDS is a devastating clinical syndrome of acute lung injury (ALI) that affects both medical and surgical patients [3]. The official definition of ARDS was first published in 1994 by

American-European Consensus conference (AECC), according to which ARDS is characterized by arterial partial pressure of oxygen to fraction of inspired oxygen [PaO2/FIO2] ≤200 mm Hg with bilateral infiltrates on frontal chest radiograph, with no evidence of left atrial hypertension. A new entity—ALI was also introduced as a condition of less severe hypoxemia [PaO2/FIO2] ≤300 mm Hg. Arterial hypoxemia that is refractory to treatment with supplemental oxygen is a characteristic feature of acute lung injury. ALI is characterized by alveolar-capillary injury, inflammation with neutrophil accumulation and release of pro-inflammatory cytokines leading to alveolar edema [3]. Patients with ALI develop hypoxia. The term ALI was eventually removed in 2011 in the updated Berlin definition of ARDS. According to Berlin definition, ARDS was classified into three mutually exclusive categories based on the degree of hypoxemia; mild (200 mm Hg < PaO2/FIO2 ≤ 300 mm Hg), moderate (100 mm Hg < PaO2/FIO2 ≤ 200 mm Hg) and severe (PaO2/FIO2 ≤ 100 mm Hg) [4]. Hypoxia may be a consequence of ALI leading to deviation in lung function and preventing repair. Hypoxia induces destructive exudative changes within the lung parenchyma, which include the following: (1) increased alveolar paracellular permeability due to hypoxia disrupted alveolar epithelial cell (AEC) cytoskeleton and tight junction (TJ) protein organization; (2) Prolonged hypoxia induces loss of stress fibers such as actin (including breakdown of spectrin), internalization of TJ protein occludin and a decrease in zona occludens-1 (ZO-1) protein levels that are associated with trans-epithelial permeability; (3) reduced efficacy of AEC to clear alveolar edema fluid as a result of decreased expression of two major proteins, the apical epithelial sodium channel (ENaC) and the basolateral Na/K-ATPase channel which are involved in transcellular sodium (Na) transport. Thus, hypoxia-mediated effects not only enhance alveolar edema but also impair alveolar edema clearance contributing to reduced alveolar gaseous exchange capacity in ALI [5].

2. Hypoxia in alveolar edema and fluid clearance in the lungs

The mechanism by which hypoxia promotes pulmonary edema is not completely understood and is still under scrutiny. Alveolar edema accumulation is a result of enhanced pulmonary vascular permeability. Vascular endothelial growth factor (VEGF) is a potent inducer of endothelial dysfunction and thus can play a crucial role in vascular permeability [6]. Since VEGF is induced in hypoxic conditions and recovery from hypoxia, its role in pulmonary vascular remodeling and enhanced alveolar edema is prominent [7]. The source of VEGF in the inflammatory milieu of lung injury includes monocytes, eosinophils and aggregated platelets. Research on hypoxia-induced VEGF expression as a cause for pathological conditions has been carried out for more than two decades now. Studies have shown that both acute and chronic hypoxia induce an upregulation in the gene expression of VEGF, and its receptors (KDR/Flk and Flt) in the animal models of prolonged hypoxia-induced pulmonary hypertension [8]. In fact, the increase in the VEGF gene expression was seen as early as 2 h upon hypoxic challenge in isolated and perfused rat lungs while chronic hypoxia resulted in greater upregulation of the VEGF receptor genes. These studies also scrutinized the mechanism by which hypoxia induces VEGF expression by examining the role of nitric oxide synthase (NOS) and hypoxia inducible factors (HIFs) as the downstream regulators [8, 9]. Studies on transcriptional regulation of VEGF by hypoxia have revealed a functional HIF-1 binding site on the rat VEGF 5′-flanking region as a possible transcriptional activator of VEGF gene by hypoxia [9]. Further studies have shown the involvement of specific regions in 3′-untranslated region (UTR) of VEGF gene in the stability of VEGF mRNA induced by hypoxia [10]. This has led to investigation of proteins that bind to this specific region to control the posttranscriptional regulation of VEGF expression. One such protein is HuR, a member of Elav-like protein family (Elav is a *Drosophila* RNA-binding protein required for neuronal differentiation). HuR was found to post-transcriptionally regulate VEGF expression by binding within four nucleotides of a canonical nonameric instability element in the VEGF AU-rich element [10]. Thus, hypoxia regulates VEGF at both transcriptional and posttranscriptional levels. Transcriptional regulation is by the hypoxia-induced transcription factor HIF-1 which activates VEGF transcription by binding to specific promoter sequences. A study exploring possible mechanisms involved in securing efficient translation of VEGF during hypoxic stress showed that internal ribosome entry site (IRES) present in the 5′-UTR of VEGF gene functions as an alternative to cap-dependent translation during such stressful conditions [11].

Becker et al. studied hypoxia-induced VEGF's role in enhancing pulmonary vascular permeability. They showed that ischemia/hypoxia-induced upregulation of VEGF mRNA and protein was associated with increased pulmonary vascular permeability [12]. Their study was also supported by several other studies which have reported an increase in vascular permeability due to exogenously administered VEGF in skin, muscle, GI tract and airways. In their study, hypoxic ischemia-enhanced VEGF expression, which was associated with increased HIF-1α protein expression and redistribution of VEGF protein to alveolar septae as demonstrated by immunohistochemical staining. This distribution of VEGF protein in the alveolar septae was further associated with increased pulmonary vascular permeability, suggesting its role in acute lung injury and alveolar edema [12]. The enhanced pulmonary vascular permeability effect of VEGF was also confirmed by another study in a sepsis-induced lung injury model, which showed that enhanced plasma VEGF level was accompanied by increased expression of vascular permeability-mediating VEGF receptor, Flt-1 and not the angiogenic-mediating receptor, Flk-1. As a result, enhanced lung edema was observed confirming the role of VEGF in causing alveolar edema [13].

Na,K-ATPase channels present in the alveolar epithelial cells play a major role in edema clearance from the alveoli [14]. Hypoxia-induced pulmonary edema also disrupts their function and inhibits edema clearance. Studies have shown that hypoxia generated reactive oxygen species (ROS) activates PKCζ (Protein Kinase C Zeta is a key regulator of critical intracellular signaling pathways induced by various extracellular stimuli), which in turn, phosphorylates the α1-subunit of Na,K-ATPase at Ser-18 site leading to its endocytosis through a clathrin-dependent mechanism and eventually to lysosomal degradation. With the loss of Na,K-ATPase, edema reabsorption is impaired and thus hypoxia not only promotes pulmonary edema but also inhibits its clearance as observed in conditions like ALI [14].

3. Hypoxia in pulmonary aquaporin's expression and edema

Aquaporins (AQPs) comprise a group of cell membrane water-transporting proteins that are involved in physiological as well as pathological fluid transport. They have been identified in the lung and are believed to play a major role in pulmonary edema [15]. AQPs can bidirectionally transport fluid across the alveolar epithelium and hence are involved in both edema formation and clearance of edema from alveoli (thus injury resolution). About 6 (AQP-1, -3, -4, -5, -8 and -9) of the 13 different AQPs are distributed in lung tissue, and it is very interesting to study how hypoxia regulates the expression of these AQPs and thus pulmonary edema formation or clearance of edema. AQPs expression could play a major role in the pathological condition of hypoxia-induced enhanced pulmonary edema and ALI [15]. Several studies have scrutinized the role of aquaporins in pulmonary edema, and the results are controversial, yet intriguing. For example, Wu et al. studied the role of AQP-1 [expressed on pulmonary endothelial cells (ECs) and alveolar type II cells] and AQP-4 (expressed throughout the airways epithelial cells) in relation to high-altitude hypoxia lung injury. They found that hypoxia-induced pulmonary edema was associated with a decreased expression of AQP-1 and no change in the expression of AQP-4 [16]. They went on to reason that hypoxia resulted in pulmonary edema as a consequence of decreased function of AQP-1, which plays a regulatory role in water clearance around the bronchi and vessels. However, the relation of AQP-1 expression and pulmonary edema, as a result of hypoxia was only correlative and the study did not use knockout models to confirm the relationship between these effects of hypoxia. On the contrary, Su et al. showed that depletion of AQP-1 does not affect isosmolar fluid clearance and had no effect on lung edema. Nevertheless, depletion of AQP-1 resulted in a 10-fold decrease in the alveolar-capillary osmotic water permeability. They concluded that depletion of AQP-1 did not have any effect on lung edema formation and resolution [17]. Several other reports have also ruled out the role of AQP-1, -4 and -5 in physiological clearance of water in the lung or the accumulation of edema in the injured lung. Another report using gene knockout mouse model of AQP5 in hypoxic conditions showed a significant increase in pulmonary edema with the loss of AQP-5 [18]. As aforementioned, a few other reports also demonstrated that upregulation and downregulation of AQPs expression is related to pulmonary edema in different kinds of lung injuries. AQP-1 has also been shown to facilitate stabilization of HIF and has been speculated that besides its role as water transporter, it could also be involved in oxygen transport [19]. Therefore, the effect of hypoxia on AQPs expression especially in the lung and its effect on pulmonary edema warrants further studies before arriving at a conclusion [16–20].

4. Hypoxia in pulmonary arterial hypertension (PAH)

Prolonged lung injury can lead to lung fibrosis as well as PAH. Hypoxia is a well-studied trigger for pulmonary vascular remodeling and PAH development [2]. In fact, hypoxia-induced PAH is an established animal model for studying the pathophysiology and therapeutic management of PAH. PAH is a refractory disease characterized by uncontrolled vascular remodeling involving enhanced proliferation and differentiation of pulmonary vascular ECs and pulmonary vascular smooth muscle cells [2]. This vascular remodeling ensues enhanced pulmonary arterial pressure (≥25 mm Hg on right heart catheterization) due to increased pulmonary vasoconstriction and increased pulmonary vascular resistance and eventually right ventricular failure [2]. Chronic hypoxia is a well-known trigger for the abovementioned events. The mechanism by which hypoxia induces PAH has been extensively studied and involves several molecular signaling pathways. Leptin, a non-glycosylated protein, synthesized and secreted by adipocytes is encoded by obese (ob) gene, which is hypoxia sensitive. HIF-1 induces the expression of ob gene in adipocytes, and clinical studies have suggested an association between plasma leptin levels and severity of PAH [21]. Results of studies scrutinizing the role of leptin signaling in hypoxia-induced PAH show that hypoxia-induced leptin expression results in pulmonary arterial smooth muscle cells (PASMCs) proliferation through ERK, STAT and AKT pathways [21]. These results were further confirmed in ob/ob mice. Obese gene knockout mice subjected to hypoxia showed an attenuated hypoxia-induced PAH that was gauged in terms of reduced right ventricular systolic pressure (RVSP) and right ventricular hypertrophy index (RVHI) when compared to wild-type (WT) mice. Thus, leptin signaling could be a potential therapeutic target to treat hypoxia-induced PAH [21]. In hypoxia-induced pulmonary hypertension, iron supplementation has been found to be beneficial [22]. A study involving human subjects in an acute model of mountain sickness has shown that iron supplementation was associated with a decrease in pulmonary arterial systolic pressure (PASP) while progressive development of iron deficiency correlated with worsening of pulmonary arterial pressure determined by echocardiography, thus suggesting a causal relationship between iron deficiency and acute hypoxic PAH [23]. Recent studies speculate that iron deficiency may worsen hypoxic pulmonary hypertension through HIFs signaling [24].

HIFs are transcription factors comprising of an O_2-sensitive α-subunit, mainly HIF-1α and HIF-2α and a constitutively expressed β-subunit which are responsible for mediating adaptive responses to hypoxia and ischemia [25]. HIF-α and HIF-β form heterodimer and induce the transcription of over 100 genes that affect cellular functions ranging from metabolism, survival, proliferation, migration and angiogenesis among several others [25]. While HIF-1α is more ubiquitously expressed, HIF-2α expression is predominant in the lung tissue [25]. Several studies have shown the mechanistic role of HIF-2α in hypoxia-induced PAH. In hypoxia-induced PAH studies, even partial deficiency of either HIF1α (HIF1$\alpha^{+/-}$) or HIF2α (HIF2$\alpha^{+/-}$), achieved using murine models, significantly decreased pulmonary arterial pressure and right ventricular hypertrophy induced by chronic hypoxia in comparison with wild-type mice that did not have any alteration in HIF1α or HIF2α expression [26]. The role of HIFs in hypoxia-induced PAH was further scrutinized and deficiency in HIFs-related beneficial effects in PAH was at least partly due to the reduced pulmonary vascular remodeling observed in these animals. Further *in vitro* analysis on PASMCs showed that HIF-1-dependent smooth muscle hypertrophy contributed to pulmonary vascular remodeling during hypoxia [26]. HIF1α is involved in hypoxia-induced PASMC depolarization, reduction in K^+ channel expression and activity and elevated intracellular calcium concentration and pH. This eventually results in altered PASMC ion homeostasis contributing to a more contractile, apoptosis resistant, proliferative and migratory phenotype [26]. Furthermore, in human PAH patients and mouse models of PAH, dysregulation of HIF pathway was reported and it has been associated with HIF-2α mutations, which was confirmed by studies where loss of one copy of HIF-2α gene was sufficient to attenuate hypoxia-induced PAH in these animal models [27]. On the other hand, HIF-2α gain of functions is associated with PAH. Studies scrutinizing the mechanism by which HIF-2α regulates hypoxic PAH have found several ways by which it mediates the hypoxic effects. In human PASMC, hypoxia increases expression of transcription factor forkhead box M1 (FoxM1), through HIF-2α, to promote PASMC proliferation [27]. Secreted matricellular protein thrombospondin-1 (TSP-1) is believed to play an important role in vascular health and disease via inhibition of vasodilation in part by limiting NO production and signaling [28]. Vascular remodeling in PAH involves the proliferation of both pulmonary artery smooth muscle cells (PASMCs) and fibroblasts apart from endothelial dysfunction. In a recent study published from our laboratory, we showed that hypoxia-induced pulmonary rarefaction and fibrosis in mice lung, and mechanistically, we found that hypoxia-induced Akt1 expression in fibroblasts was associated with enhanced TSP-1 expression resulting in fibroproliferation and fibrosis [29]. Another study has shown that hypoxia, in a HIF-2α-dependent manner, increases the expression of TSP-1 in pulmonary tissue and pulmonary artery cells which in turn contributes to enhanced endothelial permeability (mediated in part by changes in cell-cell adhesion) and accompanied by increased fibroblast and PASMC proliferation which is at least partially due to restricted adhesion of these cells in their mouse model of hypoxia-induced PAH. Also it was speculated that TSP-1 could promote hypoxic pulmonary artery contraction through enhanced TSP-1–induced endothelin-1 expression [28].

Prolyl hydroxylase domain-containing enzymes (PHDs) use molecular O_2 as a substrate to hydroxylate-specific proline residues of HIF-α which subsequently promotes HIF-α binding to von Hippel-Lindau (VHL protein) and ubiquitin E3 ligase, resulting in ubiquitination and proteasomal degradation [27]. In patients with idiopathic pulmonary fibrosis (IPF), PHD2 expression is diminished in ECs of obliterative pulmonary vessels [27]. A study using mouse model of endothelial and hematopoietic cells-specific knockdown of gene encoding PHD2 has shown that these mice spontaneously develop PAH with obliterative vascular remodeling as seen in human PAH [27]. They found that PHD2 deficiency in ECs promoted HIF-2α-mediated (and not HIF-1α) expression of CXCL12 (also known as stromal cell-derived factor 1α) that had a paracrine effect on PASMC proliferation contributing to the pathogenesis of severe PAH in this mouse model. PHD2 deficiency in ECs also promoted endothelin-1 expression that resulted in pulmonary artery-vasoconstriction. Thus, HIF-2α-mediated vascular remodeling and plexiform-like lesions formation (due to PASMC proliferation) resulted in PAH in this mouse model [27, 28]. As discussed above, prevention of PASMC apoptosis along with enhanced proliferation is an important pathological event in hypoxic PAH. Another study showed the mechanism by which hypoxia mediates this effect. In PASMCs, hypoxia induces opening of mitochondrial ATP-sensitive potassium channels (mitoK_{ATP}), which results in calcium-dependent increase in mitochondrial permeability or mitochondrial membrane transition (MPT). MPT eventually leads to loss of mitochondrial membrane potential (denoted by $\Delta\Psi$m), thus preventing the cytochrome C release from mitochondria and inhibition of cytochrome C–caspase 9 pathway induced PASMC apoptosis [30]. The involvement of mitoK_{ATP} channels in hypoxia-induced PASMC apoptosis resistance was further confirmed by administering 5-hydroxydecanoate (5-HD), a compound that prevents opening of mitoK_{ATP} channels abolishes these effects of hypoxia to a certain extent and prevents mitoK_{ATP} channels opening and PASMC apoptosis. Hypoxia-induced opening of mitoK_{ATP} was not only associated with prevention of PASMC apoptosis but also increased the production of H_2O_2 in

http://dx.doi.org/10.5772/66817

mitochondria. The effect of this ROS production was an increased transcriptional activity of AP-1, which is responsible for the proliferation of PASMCs. Thus, hypoxia through mitoK$_{ATP}$ opening prevented apoptosis and enhanced proliferation of PASMCs. As discussed, apart from proliferation of PASMCs, hypoxia-induced prevention of PASMC apoptosis also plays a major role in PAH. Another mechanism involves inhibition of the mitochondrial pro-apoptotic Bax protein expression and induction of the anti-apoptotic Bcl-2 expression, thus preventing the release of mitochondrial cytochrome C into cytoplasm and eventually inhibiting cleavage of caspase 9 resulting in PASMC apoptosis [31]. Therefore, hypoxia-HIF signaling is a potential therapeutic target to treat PAH, and several in vivo studies have demonstrated this [30–32].

5. Hypoxia and alveolar epithelial-to-mesenchymal transition (EMT)

Several groups have studied the role of hypoxia in disease progression and pathogenesis of ILDs such as pulmonary fibrosis [33, 34]. Activated myofibroblasts play an important role in the production of collagen and ECM proteins during pulmonary fibrosis. The source of these myofibroblasts are numerous, which include resident stromal fibroblasts, bone marrow-derived fibroblasts, and mesenchymal transition of epithelial and ECs [33]. Epithelial-to-mesenchymal transition (EMT) is a cellular process during which epithelial cells lose many of their epithelial characteristics such as cell-cell interaction and apicobasal polarity and acquire properties typical to mesenchymal cells. EMT is driven by a cytokine, transforming growth factor-β1 (TGF-β1) and is characterized by changes in cell morphology and acquisition of mesenchymal markers including α-smooth muscle actin (α-SMA) and vimentin as well as loss of epithelial markers such as E-cadherin [33, 34]. Active TGF-β1 binds to its receptors (transmembrane serine-threonine kinase receptor I and II), which leads to a downstream activation of the transcription factor Smad, whose target genes include α-SMA and vimentin [33]. Increasing evidence over the years has highlighted the critical role of EMT in pathological conditions such as fibrosis apart from its well-known involvement in tissue development during embryogenesis. Exposure to hypoxia during ALI could promote phenotypic changes in AEC consistent with EMT. In vitro studies on rat AEC cultured on semipermeable filters showed that prolonged hypoxic exposure (1.5% O2 for up to 12 days) induced profound changes in AEC phenotype consistent with EMT including change in cell morphology, decrease in transepithelial resistance and in the expression of epithelial markers such as zona occludens (ZO-1), E-cadherin, AQP-5, TTF-1, together with an increase in mesenchymal markers such as vimentin and α-SMA. Supporting this phenotypical switch, expression of transcription factors driving EMT such as SNAIL1, ZEB1 and TWIST1 increased after 2, 24 and 48 h of hypoxia, respectively. Hypoxia also induced expression and secretion of two EMT inducers TGF-β1 and connective tissue growth factor (CTGF) [35].

Similarly, Zhou et al. investigated the effect of hypoxia on the induction of EMT in AEC. Results from this study suggest that hypoxia induces EMT in transformed human, rat and mouse AEC lines, and freshly isolated rat type II AECs [36]. They also scrutinized the mechanism by which hypoxia induces EMT in AEC and showed the involvement of hypoxia-induced mitochondrial ROS production and HIF-1α stabilization in TGF-β1 production, resulting in EMT [37]. Treatment of cells with ROS scavenger Euk-134 or using mitochondria-deficient cells prevented hypoxia-induced EMT illustrating their importance in this cellular process. Moreover, although ROS is known to stabilize HIF-1α, their results showed that normoxic stabilization of HIF-1α failed to induce α-SMA expression, suggesting that HIF alone is not sufficient to induce EMT in AEC. Their data suggest that ROS and HIF-1α stabilization are upstream of TGF-β1 production in hypoxia-induced EMT in AEC. However, TGF-β1 can also increase ROS production and HIF-1α stabilization. TGF-β1 can either directly activate NADPH (Nicotinamide adenine dinucleotide phosphate) oxidase or upregulate gene expression of Nox4 NADPH oxidase to generate ROS [38, 39]. TGF-β1 decreases mitochondrial complex IV activity resulting in disruption of mitochondrial membrane potential and ROS production [40]. TGF-β1 was reported to stabilize HIF-1α through selective inhibition of PHD2 (a HIF-1α prolyl hydroxylase) expression thus reducing HIF-1α prolyl hydroxylation leading to its stabilization [41]. Therefore, TGF-β1 and ROS/HIF may form a feedback loop to maintain a prolonged signaling cascade initiated by either ROS/HIF or TGF-β1 leading to hypoxia-induced EMT in AECs [36].

In one interesting study, investigators evaluated the possible role of tissue hypoxia in the development of fibrotic lesions in lung fibrosis [42]. In this study, they used animal models of ALI/ARDS, in which severe inflammation progresses into the early (exudative) phase of ALI and sequentially fibrosis develops as the late (fibrotic) phase of ALI. They found intriguing effects of acute versus persistent hypoxia as seen in exudative and fibrotic phases of ALI, respectively. Acute hypoxia induced de novo Surfactant Protein-D (SP-D) expression in AECs followed by stabilization of HIF-1α expression [42]. Contrastingly, persistent hypoxia-induced HIF-1α stabilization repressed SP-D expression and enhanced the mRNA levels of an EMT-driving transcription factor TWIST, but not SNAIL. This was accompanied by phenotypic switch in the AECs exposed to persistent hypoxia (72-h hypoxia for in vitro studies) as seen by decreased E-cadherin expression and enhanced vimentin expression. SP-D is mainly derived from alveolar epithelial cells and therefore loss of its expression during persistent hypoxia along with enhanced EMT transcription factor expression clearly indicates phenotypic switch of these alveolar epithelial cells to more proliferative phenotype contributing to lung fibrosis [42].

Endothelial-to-mesenchymal transition (EndMT) is similar to EMT, which is characterized by a loss of endothelial cell-cell junctions, the acquisition of migratory properties, and phenotypic switch involving loss of endothelial-specific markers such as CD31 and vascular endothelial (VE)-cadherin expression, and the acquisition of mesenchymal markers α-SMA, and vimentin [43]. EndMT also contributes to fibrosis. The role of EndMT in pulmonary fibrosis involves phenotypic switch in the pulmonary EC lining the pulmonary capillaries. Radiation-induced pulmonary fibrosis (RIPF) may involve hypoxia-mediated EndMT as an initial pathological insult leading to fibrosis [13]. Fleckenstein and colleagues have shown that radiation during thoracic radiotherapy for lung cancer induces tissue hypoxia, in part, due to enhanced oxygen consumption by Macrophages. These macrophages are activated because of radiation-induced reduction in blood perfusion in the lungs contributing to lung injury [44]. This suggests that hypoxia plays a major role in the radiation-induced lung injury. Fleckenstein et al. also reported that hypoxia is important in triggering continuous production of fibrogenic cytokines and perpetuation of late lung tissue injury [44]. However, the precise mechanism by which hypoxia affects radiation-induced fibrosis remains elusive. EndMT of the pulmonary ECs was shown as a possible consequence of radiation-induced hypoxia resulting in lung fibrosis and injury by Choi et al. [43]. They investigated the reason behind fibrotic effects of radiation in a mouse model of RIPF and in *in vitro* studies on human pulmonary ECs. Since fibrosis is a long-term event, their investigation aimed at elucidating the mechanisms behind the early damage to ECs by radiation and its link to the later observed fibrosis. Their results indicate ECs specifically expressing hypoxic marker, CA9, just prior to the substantial fibrogenesis. They went on to show that radiation-induced vascular hypoxia-triggered EndMT in vascular ECs, and in fact, this was observed prior to the onset of alveolar EMT and thus could be a trigger to EMT as well. Thus, EndMT contributed to chronic tissue fibrosis and targeting EndMT was speculated to be a potential therapeutic target to treat RIPF [43, 44].

In conclusion, current evidences suggest that the pathogenesis of human pulmonary fibrosis might involve the recruitment of fibroblasts derived from AECs through hypoxia-induced EMT as well as fibroblasts derived from pulmonary ECs through hypoxia-induced EndMT, apart from the bone marrow-derived precursors forming the fibrotic lesions. Thus, hypoxia could contribute to the formation of fibrotic lesions in the lung and hence the pathogenesis of pulmonary fibrosis (see **Figure 1**).

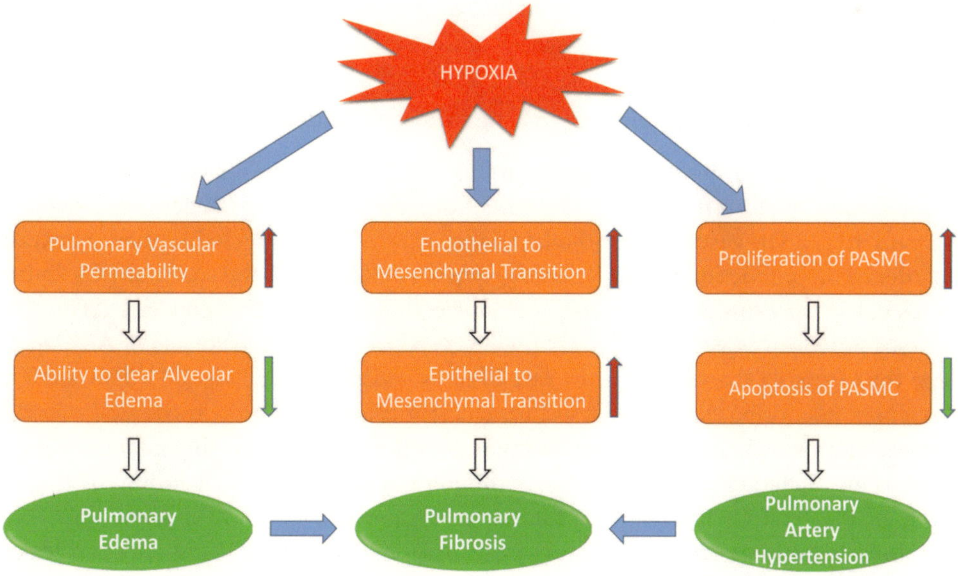

Figure 1. Summary of the effect of hypoxia on pulmonary tissue and vasculature. Hypoxia induces pulmonary edema by enhancing vascular permeability and decreasing the ability of alveolar fluid clearance. Hypoxia induces pulmonary vascular EndMT and alveolar EMT that result in myofibroblast proliferation ensuing pulmonary fibrosis. Hypoxia-induced PAH is a result of enhanced proliferation and survival of PASMCs. ALI and PAH can eventually progress to pulmonary fibrosis.

6. Hypoxia in lung injury resolution (fate of hypoxia as a consequence of pathological conditions)

While in the early stages of ALI, hypoxia plays a major role in the progression of lung injury, intriguingly in chronic pulmonary pathological conditions that ensue hypoxic milieu, and hypoxia has also been found to be involved in enhancing injury resolution. Studies indicate a protective and anti-inflammatory role of HIFs such as HIF-1α in lung protection during the early exudative phase of ALI [45–47]. As mentioned above, hypoxia inactivates PHDs and stabilizes HIF-1α [45–47]. During the acute stage of ALI, inflammation, including enhanced neutrophil activity within the alveoli, leads to an increased alveolar edema and decreased alveolar gaseous exchange capacity. HIF stabilization has been shown to have anti-inflammatory role in conditions like intestinal inflammation. The protective role of HIF activators in the treatment of inflammatory bowel disease or ischemia and reperfusion injury of several organs has been shown in several studies [48–50]. Interestingly, Eckle et al. showed the beneficial role of normoxic HIF1A stabilization in lung protection during ALI, where HIF-dependent control of alveolar-epithelial glucose metabolism function as an endogenous feedback loop to dampen lung inflammation [51]. In vivo HIF-1α increased glycolysis, lactate production and glucose flux rates in alveolar epithelium. Overall, this normoxic stabilization of HIF-1α in alveolar epithelium increased glycolytic capacity and TCA flux thus optimizing mitochondrial respiration to enhance ATP production. This HIF-dependent protection of mitochondrial function in ALI not only enhanced ATP production but also concomitantly prevented ROS accumulation and lung inflammation [51]. Hence, the role of hypoxia and subsequent HIF stabilization in reducing inflammation is prominent in resolution of ALI.

6.1. Hypoxia and adenosine signaling in lung injury resolution

Emigration of polymorphonucleated neutrophils (PMNs) through the endothelial barrier in an injured lung creates a potential for vascular fluid leakage leading to edema and decreased oxygenation [52]. The vascular endothelial adaptations to hypoxia include enhanced extracellular adenosine production during limited oxygen availability. In the vascular ECs, hypoxia induces enhanced expression of surface ectonucleotidases, CD39 that converts ATP/ADP to AMP (ectoapyrase), as well as CD73 that is involved in phosphohydrolysis of AMP to adenosine thus forming the source for extracellular adenosine production [52]. This enhanced extracellular adenosine can then signal through four different G-protein-coupled adenosine receptors, all of which are present on vascular endothelia thus enhancing adenosine signaling that is implicated in tissue protection in different models of injury including ALI. Several studies, notably couple of them from Eltzschig, H.K., et al. [52, 53], have shown the role of extracellular adenosine and its signaling in attenuating hypoxia-induced vascular leakage. They also showed that the source of ATP in hypoxic milieu is the PMNs. Hypoxia induces the production of ATP by PMNs, however, the exact mechanism by which ATP is produced still needs to be explored. This ATP is then phosphohydrolyzed as mentioned above to produce extracellular adenosine [53]. Enhanced adenosine concentrations activate adenosine receptor, (AdoRA$_{2A}$/A$_{2B}$ on ECs, which when activated increases intracellular cyclic AMP (cAMP)

http://dx.doi.org/10.5772/66817

and activates protein kinase A (PKA) to induce resealing of the endothelial-barrier [54]. The resealing of endothelial-barrier during PMN transmigration was obviated by inhibition of cAMP formation. This resealing effect is mediated by PKA-induced phosphorylation of vasodilator-stimulated phosphoprotein, a protein responsible for changes in the geometry of actin filaments and distribution of junctional proteins as a result affecting the characteristics of junctional proteins and increasing barrier function [54]. Intriguingly, adenosine not only activates the endothelial A_{2B} receptor, but also neutrophil A_2 adenosine receptor which has been shown to play an important role in limitation and termination of PMN mediated systemic inflammatory responses. Few others have also demonstrated that PMN A_2 adenosine receptor stimulation decreased leukocyte adherence and transmigration which might contribute to attenuated vascular leak associated with leukocyte accumulation [53–55]. Thus, hypoxia-induced adenosine signaling in vascular ECs and PMNs contributes to decreased vascular leak and inflammation, both of which are beneficial in inflammatory conditions such as ALI (see **Figure 2**).

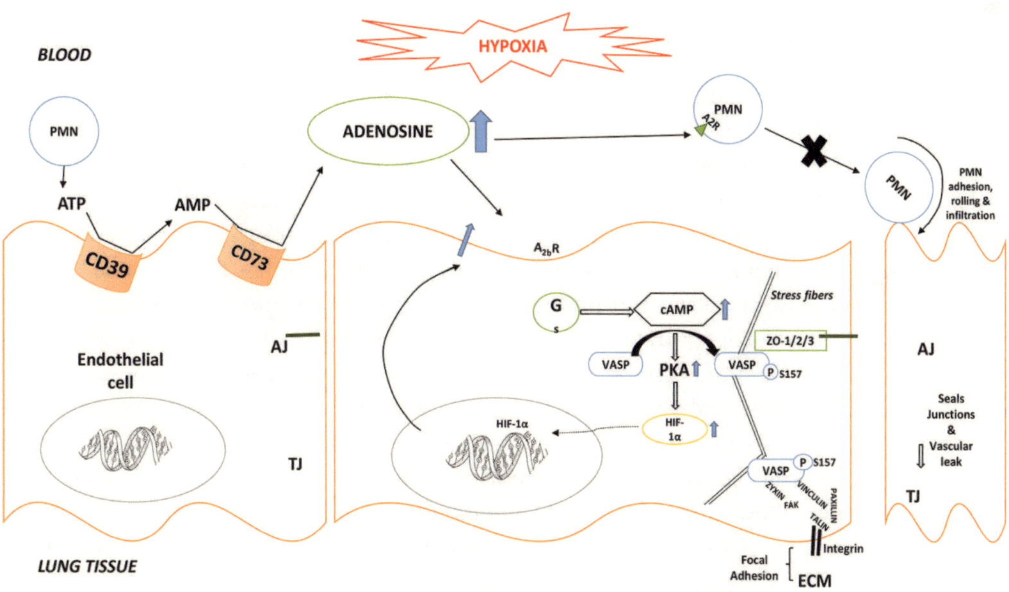

Figure 2. Hypoxia and adenosine signaling in the lungs. Hypoxia-induced extracellular adenosine production acts through adenosine receptors on ECs to enhance intracellular cAMP and PKA production. PKA catalyzes the phosphorylation of VASP, which integrates into stress fibers and helps seal the endothelial barrier by enhancing expression of AJs, TJs and also focal adhesion. PKA also enhances HIF-1A expression, which translocates into nucleus and enhances adenosine receptor transcription. Extracellular adenosine also acts on A2-receptors on PMNs and prevents their adhesion, rolling and infiltration into lung tissue. Thus, hypoxia-induced extracellular adenosine seals endothelial junctions, prevents PMN infiltration and protects lung tissue by preventing alveolar edema accumulation. PKA, protein kinase-A; PMN-polymorphonuclear neutrophils; ATP, adenosine triphosphate; AMP, adenosine monophosphate; $A_{2b}R$, adenosine 2b receptor; cAMP, cyclic AMP; VASP, vasodilator-stimulated phosphoprotein; AJ, adherent junction; TJ, tight junction and ECM, extracellular matrix.

When adenosine signaling was inhibited in transgenic mice with targeted disruption of CD73 that were subjected to hypoxia, fulminant vascular leakage, associated with severe edema and inflammation was seen [56]. Recently, studies have shown three other mechanisms by which hypoxia enhances extracellular adenosine levels, including hypoxia-mediated repression of the equilibrative nucleoside transporters (ENT-1 and ENT-2) that are responsible for adenosine transport across the membrane into the cytoplasm; HIF-1α mediated inhibition of intracellular adenosine kinase that converts intracellular adenosine to AMP and transcriptional induction of AdoRA$_{2B}$ receptor [57]. These studies indicate the protective role of adenosine signaling during hypoxia, especially in the pulmonary tissue [37]. On the other hand, chronically increased adenosine levels are detrimental as seen in pathological conditions, such as asthma and chronic obstructive pulmonary disease (COPD), and they also correlate with degree of inflammation in COPD. In order to regulate excessive adenosine signaling, chronic exposure to hypoxia eventually induces endothelial CD26 and extracellular adenosine deaminase (ADA). CD26 on EC surface acts as the ADA-complexing protein and localizes ADA accumulation on EC surface limiting extracellular adenosine accumulation during prolonged hypoxia [55].

6.2. Hypoxia and lung inflammation

Uncontrolled inflammation is one of the major players in ALI and suppression of inflammation is beneficial for injury resolution [58, 59]. Interestingly, as mentioned above, hypoxia-induced, HIF-1–mediated enhanced expression of Adenosine A$_2$ receptor on different types of immune cells, along with enhanced extracellular adenosine levels, which activate these receptors, are responsible for anti-inflammatory and tissue-protecting effects of hypoxia [58, 59]. This anti-inflammatory effect is attributed to elevated intracellular cAMP levels through activation of adenylyl cyclase. Even pharmacological immunosuppressive molecules, such as catecholamines, neuropeptides, histamine and prostaglandins are known to have their effects through elevation of cAMP levels [59]. Therefore, this extracellular adenosine serves to report excessive collateral immune damage and prevents further damage by suppressing-activated immune cells. Adenosine triggers high-affinity A$_{2A}$ adenosine receptors on activated immune cells resulting in enhanced intracellular cAMP levels to suppress these immune cells. Few studies also show that hypoxia inhibits adenosine kinase, an enzyme responsible for re-phosphorylation of adenosine to AMP, to maximize the anti-inflammatory effect [60].

6.3. Adenosine receptors in inflammation

Adenosine receptors are a family of heptahelical transmembrane G-protein-coupled purinergic receptors that are classified into four types based on the potency of agonists with respect to the intracellular production of cAMP [37]. They are A1, A$_{2A,}$ A$_{2B}$ and A3 receptors. Extracellular agonists signal through these G protein receptors and can either stimulate (Gs) or inhibit (Gi) adenylyl cyclase, an enzyme that catalyzes the formation of cAMP. Cloning experiments show that high-affinity A$_{2A}$ and low-affinity A$_{2B}$ receptors activate adenylyl cyclase (Gs) enhancing the levels of intracellular cAMP, whereas high-affinity A1 and low-affinity A3 receptors inhibit (Gi) adenylyl cyclase [37].

6.4. Hypoxia induced adenosine signaling in individual immune cells

a. *Polymorphonuclear Leukocytes (PML):* Pathological stimulation of inflammation can result in deleterious nonspecific PML bactericidal effector functions directed towards hosts' healthy tissue resulting in extensive collateral damage [54]. PMN toxic effects on microvascular endothelium are more prominent as they attach to ECs, easily because they use the same recepvtors (CR3, CD11b/CD18) that ensure PML attachment to pathogenic microorganisms [54]. Hypoxia-induced extracellular adenosine acts through adenosine receptor (high affinity A1 and A2 receptors) to mediate its anti-inflammatory effect. However, since both A1 and A2 are high affinity receptors, the overall effects of adenosine on PML might depend on the interplay between them and their expression on PML [61]. Studies show that the anti-inflammatory effects of A_{2A} receptor are to a certain extent prevented by A1 receptor, on the other hand, deleterious effects such as chemotaxis, adhesion and oxygen radical production stimulated by A1 were inhibited by A_{2A} [61, 62]. Overall, hypoxia-induced extracellular adenosine may protect the microvascular endothelium from PML by inhibiting the expression of β2-integrins and adhesion, ROS production, TNF-α production and degranulation, all of which without compromising the bactericidal function of PML such as production of bactericidal toxins and complement receptor type-3–mediated phagocytosis of bacteria [54, 63].

b. *Mononuclear phagocytes and dendritic cells:* In macrophages, activation of A1 receptor is stimulatory, while A2 receptor activation is inhibitory [54]. A_{2A} receptor activation in lipopolysaccharide (LPS)-stimulated macrophages was associated with the inhibition of IL-12 production but enhanced IL-10 secretion. In LPS-stimulated dendritic cells, adenosine enhanced A_{2A} receptor expression and intracellular cyclic AMP production along with inhibition of IL-12 production. In dendritic cells, except adenosine, other cAMP-elevating agents increase IL-10 and lower expression of MHC type II [64]. However, adenosine-mediated A_{2A} activation decreases the capacity of maturing dendritic cells to induce T-helper (Th1) polarization of native $CD4^+$ T-lymphocytes (possible anti-inflammatory effect). Upon LPS-induced differentiation of dendritic cells, A_{2A} activation favors production of CCL17 over CXCL10 chemokines [65]. Overall, these studies suggest that extracellular adenosine stimulation of adenosine receptors on antigen-presenting cells (macrophages and dendritic cells) might play an important role in the downregulation and polarization of immune response, modulation of MHC class I and II expression, and/or decrease in IL-12 and increase in IL-10 or IL-4 production to favor the initiation of a Th2 response over a Th1 response. This effect of adenosine on innate and adoptive immune system plays a crucial role in the modulation of inflammatory response [54, 64–66].

c. *Thymocytes:* The microenvironment of thymocytes is hypoxic even under normal physiological condition when compared to other lymphoid and non-lymphoid tissues [54]. Thus, the thymic environment favors increased adenosine levels and its signaling. Patients with severe combined immunodeficiency were found to be ADA deficient (enzyme responsible for decreased adenosine levels), where ADA deficient patients had developmental defects in T- and B-cells [67, 68]. This enhanced extracellular adenosine signals through A_{2A} receptor and induces apoptosis in a subset of immature thymocytes through its cAMP elevating effects. In peripheral T-cells, activation of extracellular adenosine-mediated A_{2A} receptor inhibits TCR-triggered IL-2 receptor upregulation, thereby inhibiting T-cell proliferation [69]. Other effects of adenosine signaling in $CD8^+$ cytotoxic T-lymphocytes include inhibition of inflammatory cytokine production, lethal hit delivery by granule exocytosis, as well as FasL mRNA upregulation. It is interesting to note that in human blood peripheral leukocytes, more $CD4^+$ than $CD8^+$ T-cells express A_{2A} receptor, but on activation of T-cells increased A_{2A} receptor expression is predominantly observed in $CD8^+$ T-cells. These studies suggest the variable expression of A_{2A} receptors on T-cell subset and how they favor the production of anti-inflammatory cytokines over inflammatory cytokines. Compared to T-lymphocytes, not much is known about the effects of A_{2A} receptor signaling in B-cell development, activation, antibody-production and class switching, and cytokine secretion [70].

However, it is very important to note that all the above mentioned effects of extracellular adenosine on immune cells were mostly observed in pharmacological experiments and is yet to be explored whether there are sufficient levels of extracellular adenosine in vivo to signal through A_{2A} receptor on immune cells. So far, there is no evidence of physiological downregulation of immune cells by extracellular adenosine in vivo. However, hypoxia-induced extracellular adenosine may have anti-inflammatory effects even in in vivo similar to in vitro studies [67, 71, 72].

7. Conclusions and future directions

Hypoxia, either as a consequence of the pathological condition during ILDs or as an etiology for ILDs has several roles in modulating the severity of the disease condition. Most of the effects of hypoxia are regulated through HIFs. Interestingly, stabilization of HIFs at various stages of lung injury can have different consequences either favoring injury resolution or worsening the condition. This complicates to provide a potential therapeutic target against HIFs to treat ILDs. Targeting hypoxia signaling was speculated to have therapeutic importance in inflammatory and ischemic conditions, such as inflammatory bowel disease, myocardial ischemic-reperfusion injury, ALI and so on. However, most of the clinical trials for drug discovery examined HIF inhibitors in the context of cancer treatment. Some of the examples include pharmacological HIF inhibitors such as dutasteride152 (ClinicalTrials.gov identifier: NCT00880672), topotecan153 (ClinicalTrials.gov identifier: NCT00117013), PX-478 (ClinicalTrials.gov identifier: NCT00522652) or digoxin13 (ClinicalTrials.gov identifier: NCT01763931) or the antisense oligonucleotide HIF inhibitor EZN-2968 (ClinicalTrials.gov identifier: NCT01120288). Apart from HIF inhibitors, HIF-stabilizing agents such as PHD inhibitors are also being studied as potential therapeutic targets in conditions where HIF stabilization is beneficial, such as, conditions which require enhanced angiogenesis (HIF activates VEGF and enhances angiogenesis) like bronchopulmonary dysplasia, a chronic disease effecting preterm neonates in which enhanced angiogenesis improves lung growth and function. Favoring the plethora of evidence from preclinical studies, in future, we can expect more clinical trials targeting PHD-HIF pathway as a potential therapy for ILDs and several other ischemic conditions.

http://dx.doi.org/10.5772/66817

Author details

Sandeep Artham[1] and Payaningal R. Somanath[1, 2*]

*Address all correspondence to: sshenoy@augusta.edu

1 Program in Clinical and Experimental Therapeutics, College of Pharmacy, University of Georgia and the Charlie Norwood VA Medical Center, Augusta, GA, USA

2 Department of Medicine, Vascular Biology Center and Cancer Center, Augusta University, Augusta, GA, USA

References

[1] Wallis, A. and K. Spinks, The diagnosis and management of interstitial lung diseases. BMJ, 2015. **350**: p. h2072.

[2] Archer, S.L., E.K. Weir, and M.R. Wilkins, Basic science of pulmonary arterial hypertension for clinicians: new concepts and experimental therapies. Circulation, 2010. **121**(18): p. 2045–66.

[3] Ware, L.B. and M.A. Matthay, The acute respiratory distress syndrome. N Engl J Med, 2000. **342**(18): p. 1334–49.

[4] Ranieri, V.M., et al., Acute respiratory distress syndrome: the Berlin Definition. JAMA, 2012. **307**(23): p. 2526–33.

[5] Bouvry, D., et al., Hypoxia-induced cytoskeleton disruption in alveolar epithelial cells. Am J Respir Cell Mol Biol, 2006. **35**(5): p. 519–27.

[6] Proescholdt, M.A., et al., Vascular endothelial growth factor (VEGF) modulates vascular permeability and inflammation in rat brain. J Neuropathol Exp Neurol, 1999. **58**(6): p. 613–27.

[7] Shweiki, D., et al., Vascular endothelial growth factor induced by hypoxia may mediate hypoxia-initiated angiogenesis. Nature, 1992. **359**(6398): p. 843–5.

[8] Tuder, R.M., B.E. Flook, and N.F. Voelkel, *I*ncreased gene expression for VEGF and the VEGF receptors KDR/Flk and Flt in lungs exposed to acute or to chronic hypoxia. Modulation of gene expression by nitric oxide. J Clin Invest, 1995. **95**(4): p. 1798–807.

[9] Levy, A.P., et al., Transcriptional regulation of the rat vascular endothelial growth factor gene by hypoxia. J Biol Chem, 1995. **270**(22): p. 13333–40.

[10] Levy, N.S., et al., Hypoxic stabilization of vascular endothelial growth factor mRNA by the RNA-binding protein HuR. J Biol Chem, 1998. **273**(11): p. 6417–23.

[11] Stein, I., et al., Translation of vascular endothelial growth factor mRNA by internal ribosome entry: implications for translation under hypoxia. Mol Cell Biol, 1998. **18**(6): p. 3112–9.

[12] Becker, P.M., et al., Oxygen-independent upregulation of vascular endothelial growth factor and vascular barrier dysfunction during ventilated pulmonary ischemia in isolated ferret lungs. Am J Respir Cell Mol Biol, 2000. **22**(3): p. 272–9.

[13] Jesmin, S., et al., Time-dependent alterations of VEGF and its signaling molecules in acute lung injury in a rat model of sepsis. Inflammation, 2012. **35**(2): p. 484–500.

[14] Lecuona, E., H.E. Trejo, and J.I. Sznajder, Regulation of Na,K-ATPase during acute lung injury. J Bioenerg Biomembr, 2007. **39**(5–6): p. 391–5.

[15] Borok, Z. and A.S. Verkman, Lung edema clearance: 20 years of progress: invited review: role of aquaporin water channels in fluid transport in lung and airways. J Appl Physiol (1985), 2002. **93**(6): p. 2199–206.

[16] Wu, Y., et al., Expression of aquaporin 1 and 4 in rats with acute hypoxic lung injury and its significance. Genet Mol Res, 2015. **14**(4): p. 12756–64.

[17] Su, X., et al., The role of aquaporin-1 (AQP1) expression in a murine model of lipopolysaccharide-induced acute lung injury. Respir Physiol Neurobiol, 2004. **142**(1): p. 1–11.

[18] She, J., et al., New insights of aquaporin 5 in the pathogenesis of high altitude pulmonary edema. Diagn Pathol, 2013. **8**: p. 193.

[19] Singha, O., et al., Pulmonary edema due to oral gavage in a toxicological study related to aquaporin-1, -4 and -5 expression. J Toxicol Pathol, 2013. **26**(3): p. 283–91.

[20] Echevarria, M., et al., Development of cytosolic hypoxia and hypoxia-inducible factor stabilization are facilitated by aquaporin-1 expression. J Biol Chem, 2007. **282**(41): p. 30207–15.

[21] Chai, S., et al., Leptin knockout attenuates hypoxia-induced pulmonary arterial hypertension by inhibiting proliferation of pulmonary arterial smooth muscle cells. Transl Res, 2015. **166**(6): p. 772–82.

[22] Shimoda, L.A. and G.L. Semenza, HIF and the lung: role of hypoxia-inducible factors in pulmonary development and disease. Am J Respir Crit Care Med, 2011. **183**(2): p. 152–6.

[23] Smith, T.G., et al., Effects of iron supplementation and depletion on hypoxic pulmonary hypertension: two randomized controlled trials. JAMA, 2009. **302**(13): p. 1444–50.

[24] Robinson, J.C., et al., The crossroads of iron with hypoxia and cellular metabolism. Implications in the pathobiology of pulmonary hypertension. Am J Respir Cell Mol Biol, 2014. **51**(6): p. 721–9.

[25] Brusselmans, K., et al., Heterozygous deficiency of hypoxia-inducible factor-2alpha protects mice against pulmonary hypertension and right ventricular dysfunction during prolonged hypoxia. J Clin Invest, 2003. **111**(10): p. 1519–27.

[26] Yu, A.Y., et al., Impaired physiological responses to chronic hypoxia in mice partially deficient for hypoxia-inducible factor 1alpha. J Clin Invest, 1999. **103**(5): p. 691–6.

[27] Dai, Z., et al., Prolyl-4 Hydroxylase 2 (PHD2) deficiency in endothelial cells and hematopoietic cells induces obliterative vascular remodeling and severe pulmonary arterial hypertension in mice and humans through hypoxia-inducible factor-2alpha. Circulation, 2016. **133**(24): p. 2447–58.

[28] Labrousse-Arias, D., et al., HIF-2alpha-mediated induction of pulmonary thrombospondin-1 contributes to hypoxia-driven vascular remodelling and vasoconstriction. Cardiovasc Res, 2016. **109**(1): p. 115–30.

[29] Abdalla, M., et al., The Akt inhibitor, triciribine, ameliorates chronic hypoxia-induced vascular pruning and TGFbeta-induced pulmonary fibrosis. Br J Pharmacol, 2015. **172**(16): p. 4173–88.

[30] Hu, H.L., et al., Effects of mitochondrial potassium channel and membrane potential on hypoxic human pulmonary artery smooth muscle cells. Am J Respir Cell Mol Biol, 2010. **42**(6): p. 661–6.

[31] Huang, X., et al., Salidroside attenuates chronic hypoxia-induced pulmonary hypertension via adenosine A2a receptor related mitochondria-dependent apoptosis pathway. J Mol Cell Cardiol, 2015. **82**: p. 153–66.

[32] Peng, X., et al., Involvement of calcium-sensing receptors in hypoxia-induced vascular remodeling and pulmonary hypertension by promoting phenotypic modulation of small pulmonary arteries. Mol Cell Biochem, 2014. **396**(1–2): p. 87–98.

[33] Thiery, J.P. and J.P. Sleeman, Complex networks orchestrate epithelial-mesenchymal transitions. Nat Rev Mol Cell Biol, 2006. **7**(2): p. 131–42.

[34] Zavadil, J. and E.P. Bottinger, TGF-beta and epithelial-to-mesenchymal transitions. Oncogene, 2005. **24**(37): p. 5764–74.

[35] Uzunhan, Y., et al., Mesenchymal stem cells protect from hypoxia-induced alveolar epithelial-mesenchymal transition. Am J Physiol Lung Cell Mol Physiol, 2016. **310**(5): p. L439-51.

[36] Zhou, G., et al., Hypoxia-induced alveolar epithelial-mesenchymal transition requires mitochondrial ROS and hypoxia-inducible factor *1*. Am J Physiol Lung Cell Mol Physiol, 2009. **297**(6): p. L1120–30.

[37] Ohta, A. and M. Sitkovsky, Role of G-protein-coupled adenosine receptors in downregulation of inflammation and protection from tissue damage. Nature, 2001. **414**(6866): p. 916–20.

[38] Murillo, M.M., et al., Activation of NADPH oxidase by transforming growth factor-beta in hepatocytes mediates up-regulation of epidermal growth factor receptor ligands through a nuclear factor-kappaB-dependent mechanism. Biochem J, 2007. **405**(2): p. 251–9.

[39] Sturrock, A., et al., Transforming growth factor-beta1 induces Nox4 NAD(P)H oxidase and reactive oxygen species-dependent proliferation in human pulmonary artery smooth muscle cells. Am J Physiol Lung Cell Mol Physiol, 2006. **290**(4): p. L661–l673.

[40] Yoon, Y.S., et al., TGF beta1 induces prolonged mitochondrial ROS generation through decreased complex IV activity with senescent arrest in Mv1Lu cells. Oncogene, 2005. **24**(11): p. 1895–903.

[41] McMahon, S., et al., Transforming growth factor beta1 induces hypoxia-inducible factor-1 stabilization through selective inhibition of PHD2 expression. J Biol Chem, 2006. **281**(34): p. 24171–81.

[42] Sakamoto, K., et al., Differential modulation of surfactant protein D under acute and persistent hypoxia in acute lung injury. Am J Physiol Lung Cell Mol Physiol, 2012. **303**(1): p. L43–53.

[43] Choi, S.H., et al., A Hypoxia-Induced Vascular Endothelial-to-Mesenchymal Transition in Development of Radiation-Induced Pulmonary Fibrosis. Clin Cancer Res, 2015. **21**(16): p. 3716–26.

[44] Fleckenstein, K., et al., Temporal onset of hypoxia and oxidative stress after pulmonary irradiation. Int J Radiat Oncol Biol Phys, 2007. **68**(1): p. 196–204.

[45] Kaelin, W.G., Jr. and P.J. Ratcliffe, Oxygen sensing by metazoans: the central role of the HIF hydroxylase pathway. Mol Cell, 2008. **30**(4): p. 393–402.

[46] Eltzschig, H.K., D.L. Bratton, and S.P. Colgan, Targeting hypoxia signalling for the treatment of ischaemic and inflammatory diseases. Nat Rev Drug Discov, 2014. **13**(11): p. 852–69.

[47] Vohwinkel, C.U., S. Hoegl, and H.K. Eltzschig, Hypoxia signaling during acute lung injury. J Appl Physiol (1985), 2015. **119**(10): p. 1157–63.

[48] Colgan, S.P. and H.K. Eltzschig, Adenosine and hypoxia-inducible factor signaling in intestinal injury and recovery. Annu Rev Physiol, 2012. **74**: p. 153–75.

[49] Cummins, E.P., et al., The hydroxylase inhibitor dimethyloxalylglycine is protective in a murine model of colitis. Gastroenterology, 2008. **134**(1): p. 156–65.

[50] Eltzschig, H.K. and T. Eckle, Ischemia and reperfusion--from mechanism to translation. Nat Med, 2011. **17**(11): p. 1391–401.

[51] Eckle, T., et al., HIF1A reduces acute lung injury by optimizing carbohydrate metabolism in the alveolar epithelium. PLoS Biol, 2013. **11**(9): p. e1001665.

[52] Eltzschig, H.K., et al., Coordinated adenine nucleotide phosphohydrolysis and nucleoside signaling in posthypoxic endothelium: role of ectonucleotidases and adenosine A2B receptors. J Exp Med, 2003. **198**(5): p. 783–96.

[53] Eltzschig, H.K., et al., Endogenous adenosine produced during hypoxia attenuates neutrophil accumulation: coordination by extracellular nucleotide metabolism. Blood, 2004. **104**(13): p. 3986–92.

[54] Sitkovsky, M.V., et al., Physiological control of immune response and inflammatory tissue damage by hypoxia-inducible factors and adenosine A2A receptors. Annu Rev Immunol, 2004. **22**: p. 657–82.

[55] Eltzschig, H.K., et al., Endothelial catabolism of extracellular adenosine during hypoxia: the role of surface adenosine deaminase and CD26. Blood, 2006. **108**(5): p. 1602–10.

[56] Thompson, L.F., et al., Crucial role for ecto-5'-nucleotidase (CD73) in vascular leakage during hypoxia. J Exp Med, 2004. **200**(11): p. 1395–405.

[57] Morote-Garcia, J.C., et al., HIF-1-dependent repression of adenosine kinase attenuates hypoxia-induced vascular leak. Blood, 2008. **111**(12): p. 5571–80.

[58] Clambey, E.T., et al., Hypoxia-inducible factor-1 alpha-dependent induction of FoxP3 drives regulatory T-cell abundance and function during inflammatory hypoxia of the mucosa. Proc Natl Acad Sci U S A, 2012. **109**(41): p. E2784–93.

[59] Bruzzese, L., et al., NF-kappaB enhances hypoxia-driven T-cell immunosuppression via upregulation of adenosine A(2A) receptors. Cell Signal, 2014. **26**(5): p. 1060–7.

[60] Kohler, D., et al., Inhibition of Adenosine Kinase Attenuates Acute Lung Injury. Crit Care Med, 2016. **44**(4): p. e181–9.

[61] Cronstein, B.N., et al., The adenosine/neutrophil paradox resolved: human neutrophils possess both A1 and A2 receptors that promote chemotaxis and inhibit O2 generation, respectively. J Clin Invest, 1990. **85**(4): p. 1150–7.

[62] Cronstein, B.N., et al., Adenosine: an endogenous inhibitor of neutrophil-mediated injury to endothelial cells. J Clin Invest, 1986. **78**(3): p. 760–70.

[63] Thiel, M., et al., Effects of adenosine on the functions of circulating polymorphonuclear leukocytes during hyperdynamic endotoxemia. Infect Immun, 1997. **65**(6): p. 2136–44.

[64] Panther, E., et al., Expression and function of adenosine receptors in human dendritic cells. FASEB J, 2001. **15**(11): p. 1963–70.

[65] Panther, E., et al., Adenosine affects expression of membrane molecules, cytokine and chemokine release, and the T-cell stimulatory capacity of human dendritic cells. Blood, 2003. **101**(10): p. 3985–90.

[66] Xaus, J., et al., IFN-gamma up-regulates the A2B adenosine receptor expression in macrophages: a mechanism of macrophage deactivation. J Immunol, 1999. **162**(6): p. 3607–14.

[67] Apasov, S.G. and M.V. Sitkovsky, The extracellular versus intracellular mechanisms of inhibition of TCR-triggered activation in thymocytes by adenosine under conditions of inhibited adenosine deaminase. Int Immunol, 1999. **11**(2): p. 179–89.

[68] Aldrich, M.B., et al., Adenosine deaminase-deficient mice: models for the study of lymphocyte development and adenosine signaling. Adv Exp Med Biol, 2000. **486**: p. 57–63.

[69] Huang, S., et al., Role of A2a extracellular adenosine receptor-mediated signaling in adenosine-mediated inhibition of T-cell activation and expansion. Blood, 1997. **90**(4): p. 1600–10.

[70] Kojima, H., et al., Abnormal B lymphocyte development and autoimmunity in hypoxia-inducible factor 1alpha-deficient chimeric mice. Proc Natl Acad Sci U S A, 2002. **99**(4): p. 2170–4.

[71] Hale, L.P., et al., Hypoxia in the thymus: role of oxygen tension in thymocyte survival. Am J Physiol Heart Circ Physiol, 2002. **282**(4): p. H1467–77.

[72] Caldwell, C.C., et al., Differential effects of physiologically relevant hypoxic conditions on T lymphocyte development and effector functions. J Immunol, 2001. **167**(11): p. 6140–9.

Chapter 13

Hypoxia Modulates the Adenosinergic Neural Network

Susana P. Gaytán and Rosario Pasaro

Additional information is available at the end of the chapter

http://dx.doi.org/10.5772/65242

Abstract

The aim of this study was to review the latest findings about the neural plasticity on the adenosinergic neural network after the exposition to hypoxia. Identification of the neuromorphology that supports the physiological adaptations underlying the response of organisms to environmental factors including injurious exposures (specifically hypoxia) has been one of the major research challenges in biomedicine. To know these responses would connect the metabolic needs and the vegetative neuronal networks in an integrated way. Hypoxia refers to a state in which oxygen supply is insufficient and several neural cardiorespiratory structures are responsible for correcting and preventing its effects. Although hypoxia is often a pathological condition, variations in arterial oxygen concentrations can be part of the normal physiological responses, for example, during hypoventilation training or strenuous physical exercise. Also, hypoxia is a serious consequence of preterm birth in the neonate. Neural plasticity is a persistent change in the morphology and/or function based on prior experiences, and it is crucial for understanding its effects. Plasticity is well evident when the triggering experience occurs early in life; but in the case of respiratory control plasticity, could also be present in adult life. The regulation of adenosinergic neural network maturation, especially in central cardiorespiratory areas, could provide new perspectives in respiratory new-born distress symptoms.

Keywords: hypoxia, purinergic network, adenosine, central respiratory control, neuronal plasticity

1. Introduction

One of the main functions of the cardiorespiratory system is to guarantee that all tissues are adequately oxygenated at all time, maintaining the normal mitochondrial oxidative process and ATP production. The most common electron acceptor is molecular oxygen (O_2), and when O_2 is present, the mitochondria will undergo aerobic respiration. To maintain O_2 levels, in healthy animals, ventilation is tightly controlled by a system that must maintain the precise constancy of alveolar and arterial blood gases and acid-base status, as well as minimizing the work and metabolic cost of breathing. Deviations from these normal values lead to hypoxic tissue environments [1–6].

In mammals, a lack of O_2 (hypoxia) induces acute reflexes including increasing ventilation and sympathetic tone in order to almost immediately improve the uptake and distribution of O_2 to all tissues of the organism. When the conditions of hypoxia were prolonged, during hours or days, as a defence mechanism it would induce the expression of different genes that, consequently, would modify the ATP metabolism. Indeed, all the homeostatic control of the animal would be affected and other changes would be induced such as increased ventilation, erythropoiesis and angiogenesis, all of that would results in improved O_2 tissue levels. In order to produce the complete response to hypoxia, a group of specialized cells are key to mediate these fast reflex responses. These cells are crucial because they are capable of sensing small variations of O_2, and this information is crucial to maintain O_2 homeostasis. Among the organs that respond acutely to hypoxia, the carotid body (CB) is currently attracting renewed medical interest, as its over-activation seems to be involved in the autonomous dysfunction that accompanies numerous highly prevalent disorders such as sleep apnoea, diabetes, hypertension and chronic heart failure [1–6].

The aim of this study was to review the latest findings about the neural plasticity of the adenosinergic neural network implicated in the central regulation of breathing after the exposition to hypoxia. Four types of hypoxia are currently known: first, the hypoxemic type, in which the blood O_2 levels fall down and they could not saturate the molecules of haemoglobin. Secondly, in the anaemic type, low concentrations of functional haemoglobin avoid the erythrocytes that could make an effective transportation of O_2.Thirdly, the stagnant type, in which hemodynamic is altered and the velocity and volume of the blood flow is diminished, as that occurs in shock or syncope. Finally, the histotoxic hypoxia was referred to a reduction due to a deficiency in the utilization of O_2 by the cells. To compensate for hypoxia, cardiovascular and respiratory functions are implemented increasing the cardiac rhythm, causing hypertension, modifying the ventilatory rhythm and increasing the activity of the accessory breathing muscles of neck and upper chest. As the hypoxia continues to worsen, these compensatory mechanisms would begin to fail [1–6].

All of these systemic responses are controlled by specific brain areas that integrate the information about the hypoxic conditions and conduct the changes during the hypoxic insult to initiate an adaptive process. As in other systems, the neural plasticity is a central cue for the cardiovascular and respiratory responses to the hypoxia functional adaptation. Neural plasticity implies a persistent change in the morphology and/or function based on prior experiences and it is crucial for understanding the changes in the central control of cardiorespiratory functions. Plasticity is well evident when the triggering experience occurs early in life; but in the case of respiratory central control, plasticity could also be present in adult life [3, 5, 7–11]. Since ATP production is compromised during exposure to hypoxia, it is interesting to try to discuss the possible role of the purinergic signalling, in general, and the neuronal

http://dx.doi.org/10.5772/65242

adenosinergic network, among other neural structures, responsible of the defence response against hypoxia. This interplay could confer emergent properties to the central respiratory control system. Understanding these mechanisms and their interactions may enable us to optimize hypoxia-induced plasticity as a way to improve treatments for patients that suffer from different ventilatory impairments or other related pathologies [1–6]. On the other hand, the hypoxic hypometabolism differs in adults or young animals. Indeed, it would have a more evident effect in mammals when the levels of O_2 consumption are higher (i.e. in small or young animals when they are exposed to cold). It is clear that a good strategical adaptation to low O_2 levels (hypoxia) requires coordinated down-regulation of metabolic demand, as well as tissue supply, in order to prevent a mismatch in ATP utilization and production that might end in a bioenergetic collapse. In this way, substantial experimental evidence suggests that common integrative structures are probably involved in the metabolic and ventilatory responses to hypoxia [12–15]. The synthesis of adenosine is related to the cellular ratio AMP/ATP (**Figure 1**) and, obviously, to the energy metabolism of cells. In addition, in the central nervous system (CNS), an increase in neuronal activity needs a higher expense of energy and, for this reason, the extracellular levels of adenosine would be modified. The adenosinergic system acts, in CNS, to bind adenosine to one of the different adenosine receptors (A-Rs). Usually, the increased high levels of extracellular adenosine would induce a decrease in neuronal activity. Because the cells reduce its activity, its need for energy falls down too. This nucleoside usually acts via receptor-dependent mechanisms, and could also use receptor-independent mechanisms. Anyway, its complex and wide range of actions imply that adenosine could have a significant role in the defence against cell damage in areas of increased energy requirements, in tissues as well as in recovering the normal/physiological state from a pathologic one [6, 12–22].

Furthermore, the above-mentioned hypometabolism is mediated by an activation of the chemoreceptors by depletion in the arterial O_2 partial pressure (Pa_{O_2}) among other factors. The sensing of the Pa_{O_2} is the principal afferent pathway to modify the alveolar ventilation, which assure the O_2 supply. Thus, arterial chemoreceptors (aortic bodies and CBs) serve an important role in the control of alveolar ventilation, but they also exert a powerful influence on cardiovascular function. Aortic bodies sense likewise the levels of arterial carbon dioxide partial pressure (Pa_{CO_2}) to regulate the depth and rhythm of breathing, but not changes in the blood H^+ concentration ([H^+]). To detect this last factor it is necessary to understand the role of the CB that detects all the previously described arterial variables, and, as its major quality, they do not desensitize. Finally, central chemoreceptors located on the ventrolateral surface of medulla oblongata detect changes in cerebrospinal fluid [H^+] (**Figure 1**) [5–7, 9–11].

It is obvious then that the hypoxic response is a complex effect that must be studied at different levels, including the central areas where the respiratory rhythm and pattern is generated, as well as newly described functions of the CB, the integrative nature of central chemoreceptors and the interaction between peripheral and central chemoreception. Furthermore, it must be also taken into account the metabolic signalling influence of purinergic control, in general, and, in particular, the adenosinergic influence [1, 13, 17, 18, 23, 24].

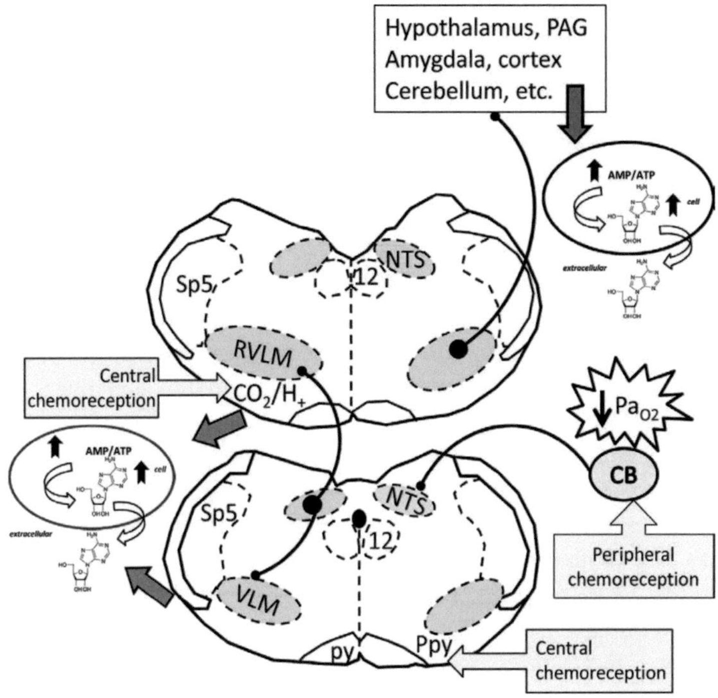

Figure 1. Schematic diagram of the hypoxic response generated at the ventrolateral medulla after the integration of peripheral and central chemoreceptors, including the role of metabolic signalling within the central neuronal network. Abbreviations: 12, hypoglossal nucleus; py, pyramidal tract; Sp5, spinal trigeminal nucleus.

2. Brain, hypoxia and pathophysiology

Normal breathing must be continuously adjusted to maintain homeostasis of arterial blood gases by means of feedback, feedforward and adaptive control strategies that depend of the brainstem respiratory network. How this process is centrally controlled is still under discussion, despite the advances (especially thanks to the development of *in vitro* preparations) that have been recently made [2, 3, 6, 7]. The precise mechanisms (cellular, synaptic and molecular) that underlie the generation and modulation of respiratory rhythm/pattern still remain largely unknown. This lack of fundamental knowledge in the field of neural control of respiration, and its relationship with other neurovegetative controls, is likely due to the complexity of the mammalian brain where synaptic connectivity between central cardiorespiratory neurons, motoneurons and their peripheral counterparts, to the present day, cannot be reliably mapped [2, 3, 7, 8].

Adaptive responses have evolved in different animal species to guarantee a sufficient supply of O_2 to tissues and to facilitate the survival of cells under transient or sustained conditions of limited O_2 availability. Although hypoxia is often related to a pathological condition, it is of great importance to recognize that variations in Pa_{O_2} can be part of normal situations that require strenuous physiological responses, for example, during hypoventilation training or intense physical exercise [4, 5, 16, 21, 25–28]. It has to be also taken into account the condition of hypercapnia that results from an excess of Pa_{CO_2}, which results in acidification of blood and tissues. The respiratory central medullary rhythm/pattern generator must respond to these chemosensory cues to maintain O_2 and carbon dioxide (CO_2) homeostasis in the blood and tissues. To do so, sensorial cells located in the periphery and CNS monitors the Pa_{O_2} and Pa_{CO_2} and initiates respiratory and autonomic reflex adjustments during hypoxic and hypercapnic. Activation of either the hypoxic or hypercapnic chemoreflex elicits both hyperventilation and sympathetic activation [4, 5, 16, 25–28]. However, the hypoxic insult is a fundamental drive to increase respiratory rate.

Traditionally, physiological research has been focused on the effect of a chronic sustained hypoxia (CH), but relatively few works were directed to the effect of periods of intermittent hypoxia that is maintained chronically. However, the different protocols resemble several pathological states that occur when patients suffer discontinuous expositions to hypoxia by malfunction of the ventilatory system. Nevertheless, these chronic intermittent hypoxia (CIH) laboratory protocols vary greatly between researches in lifespan of hypoxic exposure periods, numbers of hypoxic episodes *per day* and the total number of days of exposure. In any case, and in spite of the lack of a uniform definition, most of the recent data suggest that animals exposed to CIH would present multiple long-term pathophysiological consequences that are similar to those observed in clinic and, for that, it would be a good animal model to study different respiratory pathologies [4, 5, 16, 21, 25–28].

2.1. The role of carotid body as chemoreceptor

O_2 sensing is necessary for the activation of cardiorespiratory reflexes that permit the survival of individuals under hypoxic environments, like high altitude or pathological conditions (with reduced capacity for gas exchange between the lung alveoli and the blood). Changes are detected by the arterial chemoreceptors, in particular CB, to facilitate rapid adaptations to hypoxia including hyperventilation and sympathetic activation. The CB is located at the carotid bifurcation although its precise location varies between mammalian species. The CB is composed of functional units named glomeruli, which are clusters of cells separated by a profuse network of small capillaries and connective tissue. Each glomerulus (in close contact with blood vessels and nerve fibres) contains neuron-like glomus (or type I) cells, which can be easily identified because they are strongly dopaminergic. Glomus cells are surrounded by processes of sustentacular (type II) cells that are positive for antibodies against glial fibrillary acidic protein and other glial markers. It has been shown that type II cells, or a subpopulation of them, are quiescent stem cells that are activated under hypoxia to proliferate and differentiate into glomus and other cell types [5, 9–11]. Glomus neuron-like cells contain O_2-sensitive K^+ channels, which are inhibited by hypoxia acting through several mechanisms, including release of gaseous transmitters (NO, CO, H_2S), AMP-activated protein kinases and/or reactive oxygen species. Finally, it has been demonstrated that CBs are polymodal receptors that would respond not only to modifications in Pa_{O_2}, Pa_{CO_2} and H^+, but also to stimuli as K^+, several neurotransmitters (i.e. norepinephrine), changes in temperature and osmolarity, as well as variations in the levels of glucose or insulin. Furthermore, reductions in CB blood flow (in addition to a decrease in Pa_{O_2}) also provide powerful CB stimulation and remodelling over time [5, 9–11].

The feedback from the CB is sent to the cardiorespiratory centres in the medulla oblongata via the afferent branches of the glossopharyngeal nerve. The afferent neurons to CB have their somas in the petrosal ganglion. This ganglion is anatomically distinct in several species of mammals like cat and rabbit, but in others (i.e. rat) it is part of a structure that includes the jugular and nodose ganglia. Their afferent fibres project to the commissural or medial subnuclei of the nucleus tractus solitarius (NTS) (**Figure 1**) that convey sensory information regarding cardiorespiratory homeostasis in the form of graded action potential frequencies in fibres of the carotid sinus branch of the ninth cranial (glossopharyngeal) nerve. The efferent innervation arises primarily from the sympathetic fibres originating from the superior cervical ganglion constituting the ganglio-glomerular nerve. Efferent innervation may best be considered as a modulating influence affecting the CB chemosensitivity largely, but not solely, via a modulation of CB blood flow [5, 7–11, 29, 30].

2.2. Central integrative chemoreception process

The brainstem is the central structure that operates the integrative process of the different chemoreceptors and baroreceptors inputs and which also generates the respiratory rhythm/pattern. From these structures it should be outlined that the NTS is composed of a series of clusters of neuronal cell bodies forming a vertical column of grey matter embedded in the dorsal medulla oblongata. The NTS projects to, among other regions, the reticular formation, parasympathetic preganglionic neurons, hypothalamus and thalamus, conforming circuits that contribute to autonomic regulation (**Figure 1**). Anatomical and physiological experiments have shown that the dorsomedial part of the NTS is the primary termination site of glossopharyngeal and vagal baroreceptors, integrating the baroreceptor afferents, while the midline area, caudal to the *calamus scriptorius*, has been identified as a primary central termination site for CB afferents. The NTS neurons are stimulated by hypoxia or hypercapnia, and most profoundly by a combination of both. Under normal or pathological conditions, CB information reaches the respiratory pattern generator neuronal network via NTS glutamatergic neurons, which also target the rostral ventrolateral medulla oblongata (RVLM) presympathetic neurons, thereby raising sympathetic nerve activity (**Figure 1**). For that, NTS second-order neurons could induce chemoreceptor reflex responses that include hyperpnoea, bradycardia and a sympathetically mediated vasoconstriction for a long-term acclimatization to hypoxia [5, 7, 9–11, 29, 30].

Other group of neurons to be highlighted is the RVLM, containing several functionally distinct types of neurons, which control and orchestrate cardiovascular and respiratory responses to hypoxia and hypercapnia (**Figure 1**) [3, 7, 8, 29, 30]. At this level, chemoreceptors regulate presympathetic neurons and cardiovagal preganglionic neurons indirectly via inputs from the neurons related to the respiratory pattern generator. Secondary effects of chemoreceptors on the autonomic outflows result from changes in lung stretch afferent and baroreceptor activity [3, 7, 8, 29, 30].

On the other hand, central respiratory chemosensitivity is caused by direct effects of cerebrospinal [H^+] on neurons and indirect effects of CO_2 via astrocytes. Central respiratory chemoreceptors are not definitively identified but several brainstem areas have been demonstrated to have a role as chemoreceptor. First, the retrotrapezoid nucleus (RTN), located at the rostral end of RVLM, is a particularly strong candidate (**Figure 1**). Indeed, the absence of RTN likely causes severe central apnoeas in congenital central hypoventilation syndrome. The RTN chemoreceptor neurons provide a CO_2/H^+-dependent drive to breathe and serve as an integrator centre of convergence of chemosensory information from other central and peripheral sites, including the CBs. Finally, the RTN chemosensitive neurons also appear to serve as important sites of integration of several stimuli, as these neurons are significantly modulated by inputs from vagal-mediated pulmonary stretch receptors and from the hypothalamus [29, 30].

Another cluster of RVLM cells (constituted by a population of C1 catecholaminergic neurons) controls sympathetic vasomotor tone in resting and in hypoxic and hypercapnic conditions, including the peripheral chemoreflex [29, 30]. The increased sympathetic outflow elicited by peripheral chemoreceptors is mediated primarily by activation of the presympathetic neurons of the RVLM, the majority of which are C1 neurons. In fact, the cardiorespiratory effects of peripheral chemoreceptors are mediated in part by the direct glutamatergic inputs from the NTS to C1 neurons (**Figure 1**) [2, 3, 7, 8, 29, 30].

Recently, the description of the structures related to the respiratory rhythmogenesis has improved with the advent of the *in vitro* neonatal rodent brainstem preparation [31]. This recording technique has allowed for precise identification of specific medullary sites for separate but coupled rhythm generation or "oscillators". These neurons reside in the pre-Bötzinger complex and in the parafacial respiratory group (pFRG) located in the RVLM [29, 30]. The most exciting result so far was the finding that some inspiratory neurons in RVLM act as inspiratory pacemakers; they continue to produce rhythmic bursts of potentials even when the synaptic connections are blocked [2]. Although the inspiratory pacemaker neurons do not constitute a well-defined group within the medulla, this group of neurons named pre-Bötzinger complex certainly play an important role in the generation and/or modulation of the breathing rhythm [2]. Of the several models proposed for generating respiratory rhythm, the most promising appears to be a hybrid model, which combines emergent properties of networks of synaptic connections and intrinsic membrane properties of individual neurons together with independent pacemaker-type neurons [1– 3, 7, 8, 23, 29, 30].

Furthermore, several facts support that the pFRG/RTN complex is likely to be the major site of central CO_2 chemo-responsiveness. First, pFRG/RTN is characterized by glutamatergic interneurons that strongly express Phox2b (that codes for the homeodomain transcription factor expressed exclusively in the nervous system, in most neurons that control the viscera, like cardiovascular, digestive and respiratory systems). Besides, the Phox2b neurons are part of an uninterrupted chain of neurons in a circuit that includes the CBs and their afferents as well as the NTS projections to the RTN. The functional consequences of this linkage are that stimulation of the peripheral chemoreceptors enhances the slope of the central CO_2 ventilatory response,and conversely, inhibition of the CBs reduces the slope of the central CO_2 response [1–3, 7, 8, 23, 29, 30].

Another interesting central chemosensitive area is the caudal parapyramidal (Ppy), located near the ventral surface of the medulla, at the level of the pyramidal decussation and may function as well as the pFRG/RTN complex (**Figure 1**). Furthermore, medullary neurons activated in response to hypercapnia were only found in the Ppy area. Nevertheless, neurons in both regions, RTN and PPy, could belong to the same cell population based on their histochemical and physiological properties and their location, near the medullary surface that facilitates the sensing of the arterial composition [1, 23].

In any case, the brainstem cardiorespiratory control areas are connected with other areas such as periaqueductal gray (PAG), hypothalamus, amygdala, cortex and cerebellum (**Figure 1**). These areas also exert influences over the respiratory rhythm/pattern generator. In this way, it has been found, from data obtained by clinical evidences in patients submitted to deep brain stimulation (by means of stimulating electrodes that recorded field potentials during neurosurgical procedures), that the PAG and the subthalamic nucleus have a key role in activating the central command of cardiorespiratory responses to stress. The PAG is an integrative structure that maintains a wide network of connectivity with different neural systems, such as prefrontal cortex, hypothalamus and nociceptive pathways. Moreover, the PAG efferent projections also addressed to the medullary cardiorespiratory control areas. Finally, anatomical evidences support the connectivity to amygdala and cortex from RVLM and neurons of the respiratory pattern generator that supports, among others effects, the vegetative correlate of emotions or learning (**Figure 1**) [3, 7, 8, 30, 31].

All of the above described structures are part of an extended neuronal network that participates in the regulation and integration of cardiovascular and respiratory functions. From all of the neurotransmitters shared by this complex neuronal network, the purinergic network is one of the choices to regulate the physiologic responses to hypoxia. Recent evidence suggests that ATP-mediated purinergic signalling at the level of the RVLM coordinates cardiorespiratory responses triggered by hypoxia and hypercapnia by activating RTN and C1 neurons, respectively. For all of that, the role of ATP-mediated signalling in the RVLM must be critical for cardiovascular and respiratory activities (**Figure 1**) [3, 7, 8, 29, 30].

2.3. Pathophysiological responses to hypoxia

Since the condition in which the whole body (or a region) was exposed to variations in arterial O_2 concentrations can be part of the normal physiology, a mild and non-damaging intermittent hypoxia (IH) is used intentionally, for example, during altitude training to develop an athletic performance adaptation at both the systemic and cellular level [4, 5, 16, 21, 26–28]. However, hypoxia is a deprivation of adequate O_2 supply at the tissue level and, often, a pathological condition with very serious consequences of preterm birth in the neonate, for example. The main cause for this pathology is that the lungs of the human foetus are among the last organs to develop during pregnancy. The perinatal hypoxic-ischemic cerebral injuries found in the clinic are a main problem of paediatrics because of its severe consequences for the posterior development of the infants, such as the appearances of cerebral paralysis. Accumulating evidence points to an evolving process of brain injury after intrapartum hypoxia-ischemia, initiated *in utero* and extending into a recovery period. This process in the neonate originates numerous functional deficits, such as impaired resting ventilation and ventilatory response to hypoxia [17, 28, 31, 32].

On the other hand, abnormalities or mutations of the medullary neuronal breathing rhythm/pattern networks may also have a great impact on the progress of human diseases in children or adults. Failures in the breathing pattern with severe consequences are well-documented. These problems, often cause CO_2 retention in awake, and in particular, in sleeping subjects, that could be associated to neurodegenerative diseases such as Parkinson's disease, amyotrophic lateral sclerosis or post-polio syndrome. It is also been proved that these breathing alterations are often associated to medullary and multiple system atrophy of patients. These syndromes have been linked to deficits in neurons related with the respiratory control in the pre-Bötzinger complex, pontine raphe and adjacent areas. Obviously, an understanding of how the response to hypoxia is organized and when or why the system become maladapted and could induce cell damage is extremely important for knowing how to fight against the diseases in the future [4, 5, 16, 21, 26–28].

It is well known that disruption of the drive to breathe is thought to contribute to the mortality of certain pathologies, including stroke or epilepsy, and it is the cause of sudden infant death syndrome (SIDS) [1–6]. In the case of SIDS, it has generally been accepted that, in the absence of trauma, children death occurs to either respiratory or circulatory failure. The events appear to be a sequential process, first hypoxia occurs, and then there must be a failure to recover from hypoxia. The failure to recover could occur when the infant does not arouse from sleep and/or self-resuscitation mechanisms fail. For that, it has been proposed that there should be three necessary components for development of SIDS: congenital or acquired vulnerability, a critical "time-window" during maturational development and an acute stressor. The arousal response is essential for avoiding the hypoxic conditions due to certain microenvironments that could cause the loss of consciousness or the risk of dying. A failure of the neural system that would induce the arousal response from sleep, in the hypoxic condition, could be related to the progress or, in certain cases, the fatal result in diagnosed SIDS. However, these kinds of malfunctions do not explain all the process that should appear in SIDS. In fact, it seems clear that an initial respiratory failure and hypoxemia ignites the sequence of responses that, dramatically, may cause the death. Respiratory chemoreceptor studies on infants at risk for SIDS have suggested that a decreased sensitivity to CO_2 could play a causal role in these deaths [1–6, 33].

Concerning CB function, there is a significant increase in sensitivity of the peripheral chemoreceptors during the first few weeks of life and it has been frequently shown that CB denervation in animal models is followed by hypoventilation and sudden death later on. Therefore, these denervated animals for the most part are markedly symptomatic prior to death. The principal problem in translating these results to humans is that SIDS infants do not appear to have any symptoms before death. This fact implies that it could be a problem related to the central integration of CB information in SIDS, but its role is still under discussion. However,

CB must be taken into account in the pathogeny of SIDS, because a partial decrease in the sensitivity to hypercapnia or hypoxemia would be a causal role in this syndrome [2, 33].

Several studies indicate that changes in the strength and/or pattern of respiratory-sympathetic coupling may have pathological implications in the control of arterial pressure levels. Such dysfunctions can be observed in the experimental condition of CIH, and also is commonly observed in patients suffering from obstructive sleep apnoea (OSA). OSA consists of a repetitive obstruction of the upper airways during sleep. Each obstruction causes an episode of hypoxia leading to a picture of CIH causing a fall in the Pa_{O_2} and arterial haemoglobin saturation. OSA is characterized by repetitive collapse or near collapse of the upper airway during sleep, and these repetitive events impose substantial adverse effects on multiple organ systems. As a result of these mechanical changes in the airway, hypoxemia and hypercapnia develop, which further stimulate respiratory effort. Without airway opening the increased drive is ineffective at increasing ventilation. Hypoxic episodes stimulate the CB, triggering an increased motor muscles towards the inspiratory output and an arousal reaction, which together solve the obstruction [1–6]. Following even very brief periods of IH interspersed with normoxia, hyperventilation and increased sympathetic activity are sustained over an hour or more (i.e. the so-called long-term facilitation). Central adaptive responses occur following CIH in the persistent elevation of tonic hyperactivity of neurons at the level of the hypothalamus and other structures [4, 16, 21, 26–28]. As OSA progresses, it frequently generates a syndrome with associated pathologies at different systems: cardiovascular (hypertension and augmented acute vascular accidents), hepato-metabolic (insulin resistance, glucose intolerance, fatty liver disease) and neuropsychiatric (anxiety, depression and cognitive-executive deficits). Clinical and experimental studies indicate that CIH is an important event in the occurrence of OSA-associated pathologies because it causes CB sensitization [1–6]. The process probably includes increasing CB chemoreceptor input to the brainstem leading to an exaggerated sympathetic tone, which generates hypertension and subsequent cardiovascular and metabolic pathologies. In OSA patients, the repetitive respiratory events lead to IH and CO_2 retention, both of which can augment sympathetic nerve activity via stimulation of central and peripheral chemoreceptors. Conditions of hypoxia, both chronic and intermittent lack of O_2, seem to induce CNS plasticity of respiratory and sympathetic functions neuronal networks and metabolic changes that could also lead to pathological states [4, 5, 27, 28].

3. Purinergic neuronal networks and hypoxia

ATP is released in an activity-dependent manner from different cell types in the brain, fulfilling different roles as a neurotransmitter, neuromodulator, in astrocyte-to-neuron communication, propagating astrocytic responses and modulating microglia responses. So, purinergic signalling has been found to contribute at all levels of the nervous system, including enteric, autonomic and central [34–38]. The term purinergic receptor was classically introduced to name specific classes of membrane receptors that mediate the release of ATP (P2 receptors) or adenosine (P1 receptors). The group of adenosine P1 receptors (A1-R, A2a-R, A2b-R, A3-R) are expressed on presynaptic and postsynaptic neurons, on astrocytes, microglia and mature and precursor oligodendrocytes. The mechanisms of ATP signalling are equally diverse, acting by means of P2 receptors, including ionotropic (P2X-R) and metabotropic (P2Y-R) subtypes, as well as varying methods of transmission, including vesicular, volume-regulated anion channel and gap junction hemichannel release of ATP from neuronal and non-neuronal cells [34–38].

ATP is involved in central respiratory control and may mediate changes in the activity of medullary respiratory neurons during hypercapnia. The P2 receptor family comprises seven ionotropic P2X-R subunits (P2X1-7), forming both homomeric or heteromeric receptors and eight metabotropic P2Y-R subtypes (P2Y1, 2, 4, 6, 11, 12, 13, 14). The brain displays a robust mRNA expression, an intense binding, and immunoreactivity for both P2X-R and P2Y-R in neuronal and non-neuronal elements, although the role of central P2-R remains ill defined. The ATP-mediated signalling in respiratory control and central chemoreception is associated to the profile of the P2X2-R subunit. This subunit is expressed, by physiologically identified respiratory neurons, in areas of the ventral medulla, the pontine locus coeruleus, the NTS, and the raphe nuclei. There are several evidences that sustain the hypothesis that purinergic signalling could play a central role in the mechanisms underlying the chemosensitivity of RVLM (**Figure 1**). It has been demonstrated the responses evoked by ATP in neurons expressing P2X-Rs to changes in extracellular [H^+]. In that way, this evidence supports the putative mechanism of chemosensitivity of RVLM cells, and it would be necessary the tonic release of ATP. This may be the case, when P2-R blockade reduces the baseline firing of RVLM respiratory neurones. The modulation of P2X2-R function, evoked by acidification of the extracellular environment during hypercapnia, contributes to the changes in activity of the RVLM respiratory neurones that express these receptors [34–38].

Furthermore, it has been shown that several medullary areas may have chemosensitive responses mediated by ATP. In this way, experiments made in brain slices using cell-attached recordings of membrane potentials have shown that CO_2/H^+-receptive NTS neurons are activated by focal ATP applications. However, it has been evidenced that purinergic P2-R blockade did not affect their CO_2/H^+ responsiveness [38]. On the other hand, CO_2/H^+-sensitive raphe neurons were unaffected by ATP or P2-R blockade [34, 38]. When the experiments where realized *in vivo*, ATP injection into the NTS increased cardiorespiratory activity; however, injections of a P2-R antagonist into this area did not change the baseline breathing or the CO_2/H^+ responsiveness [34, 38]. Indeed, a significant proportion of respiratory neurones located in the vicinity of the Bötzinger and pre-Bötzinger areas express the P2X2-R subunit and respond with an increase in discharge during ATP application. This fact could mean that purinergic signalling plays an additional role in the generation and shaping of central respiratory output, as well as premotoneurons that are responsible for transmitting this rhythm to the spinal motoneurons controlling the diaphragm and intercostal muscles [34–38].

Finally, as above stated, RVLM contributes to peripheral chemoreceptor modulation of breathing and blood pressure, by chemosensitive RTN neurons and presympathetic C1 neurons, respectively, and these neurons are activated by purinergic agonists. In contrast, the blockade of P2-Rs in the RVLM blunted cardiorespiratory responses to peripheral chemoreceptor activation in anesthetized rats [34–38]. RTN neuronal activity was found to be independent of temperature and stimulus strength and was wholly retained when synaptic activity was blocked using high-Mg^{++}, low-Ca^{++} solution. In the RTN, mechanisms of chemoreception involved direct H^+-mediated activation of chemosensitive neurons and indirect modulation by purinergic signalling. This modulation implies a CO_2/H^+-evoked ATP release by RTN astrocytes, contributing to respiratory drive. ATP injection into the RTN increased breathing and blood pressure by a P2-R dependent mechanism, at the cellular and systems level [38]. However, because the results using antagonists of P2-R and focal injections did not elucidate the cells that were responsible, it is necessary more experimental evidence to determine the putative chemoreceptors and, if it is the case, the above observed effects could be indirect ones. Nevertheless, purinergic signalling also modulates the activity of CO_2/H^+-sensitive neurons at least in two other brainstem regions thought to contribute to central chemoreception (i.e. the caudal NTS and medullary raphe). In any case, these evidences suggest that purinergic signalling is a unique feature of RTN chemoreception and point out to a unique CO_2/H^+ sensing mechanism in the RTN [34–38].

4. Adenosine receptors, brain development and pathophysiological hypoxic response

The role of adenosine, as an extracellular signalling molecule, was defined after the observations of the ability of purines to control the functioning of the heart. Adenosine modulates the activity of the nervous system at cellular level both presynaptically by inhibiting or facilitating transmitter release, and postsynaptically by hyperpolarising or depolarising neurons, as well as exerting non-synaptic effects (i.e. on glial cells). It is usually assumed that adenosinergic signalling provides a neuroprotective role. However, several researches have shown that, under determined circumstances, changes in the levels of adenosine could have the opposite effects, contributing to neuronal damage and cell death [6, 12–15, 19–22]. These two ways of actions could be determined by the union of adenosine to different subtypes of A-Rs. Furthermore, changes in the levels of expression of the different subtypes, interactions between these receptors, differential actions on neuronal and glial cells and several "time-windows" (that are critical during development) could also provide different actions at different events, as well as adenosinergic agonist and antagonist compounds administration. Moreover, adenosine do not work isolated, and, in spite of this, it is still unclear if the role of A-R subtypes (A1-R and A2-R) in the control of neuroprotection is mostly due to the control of glutamatergic transmission. Another possible role of adenosine is that its protection is mediated by one of the homeostatic roles of its receptors, such as control of metabolism, neuroglial communication, inflammatory response, neurogenesis or mechanism of action of growth factors [6, 12–15, 19–22].

Adenosine acts in parallel as a neuromodulator and as a homeostatic modulator in the CNS [6, 12–22]. The adenosine role as a neuromodulator is especially important around the time of birth and is involved in the suppression of foetal and neonatal breathing, particularly during hypoxia when extracellular levels of this nucleoside rapidly increase. Apnoea of prematurity, defined as cessation of breathing lasting longer than 15 s and accompanied by bradycardia or hypoxia, is common occurring in 85% of infants born less than 34-week gestation. Preterm birth constitutes approximately 6–12% of all births in industrialized countries and accounts for 70% of neonatal mortality and 75% of neonatal morbidity [6, 12–21]. Depending on gestational age and birth weight, preterm infants present a wide range of abnormal physiological responses due to their immature organ systems [17, 28, 31, 32]. During development A1-Rs are especially important, being the earliest receptors expressed in the embryonic brain and heart. A1-R activation potently inhibits the development of axons and can lead to leukomalacia [18, 32].

The most common method of treatment of the apnoeas of prematurity is continuous positive airway pressure and administration of a methylxanthine. The family of methylxanthines includes caffeine (1, 3, 7-trimethylxanthine), one of the most popular human stimulants, and all of them derivate from xanthine, that is a purine present in human and other organism's tissues and fluids. This group of alkaloids has therapeutically been used for their effects stimulating respiratory function by means of its excitatory effects on the CNS, because of its capacity to suppress respiratory depression, reduce periodic breathing and enhance diaphragmatic activity. Caffeine also increases ventilatory drive and improves sensitivity and/or responsiveness to changes in the level of Pa_{O_2} [6, 12–22]. The discovery that methylxanthines acted as antagonists of adenosine receptors represented a crucial step to establish the idea that adenosine indeed acted as an extracellular signalling molecule operating on selective receptors. Caffeine, at high doses, can also inhibit phosphodiesterases, block GABAa receptors or cause a release of intracellular Ca^{++}. Furthermore, caffeine acts on the respiratory cycle by antagonizing the actions of endogenous A1-R, A2a-R or A2b-R [6, 12–22]. Studies on A1-R have demonstrated that these receptors are found at high density in the brainstem and hypothalamus while A2a-Rs are widely distributed in the medulla [14, 17, 18]. Animal studies have shown that caffeine treatment alters A-R expression and distribution, cause transient motor impairments and could also be neurotoxic to the newborn. In rats, limited exposure to therapeutic doses of caffeine during early life (postnatal days 3–6, P3–P6) changes the distribution, density and sensitivity of A1-Rs in several regions of the CNS; these changes could persist until adulthood. Caffeine treatment at P2–P6 mimics the clinical use of caffeine in human neonates. Since the relative level of maturation of the CNS in newborn rats in the first week of life is similar to that of a premature newborn human between 20 and 40 weeks postconception, newborn rats could serve as a suitable animal model to test the potential impact of perinatal caffeine treatment on the adenosinergic system. The oral administration of caffeine in critical periods of newborn rat and immunohistological experiments showed an increase of A1-R labelling in restricted cardiorespiratory related areas. These labelled structures were the anterior hypothalamic area, ventromedial hypothalamic nucleus, parabrachial complex and ventrolateral medulla of the caffeine-treated group at P6. For the subtype A2a-R, it was found a moderate increase of immunolabelling in pontomedullary and other hypothalamic areas also related to vegetative functions. Indeed, increased A1-R and A2a-R gene expression was observed in both the brainstem and hypothalamus at P5. These results showed an up-regulation of adenosinergic maturation in central cardiorespiratory areas when the animals were caffeine treated in the neonatal period and could explain the pharmacological effects observed in caffeine treated premature infants, and it would also imply that caffeine mediated a modification of the postnatal development of the adenosinergic system during a critical period or "time-window" [6, 12–22]. To date, human data show that such caffeine treatment has no major side effects on neurodevelopmental outcome in children in the 38–42 weeks following birth and up to 2 years after the treatment. However, further research is required to determine the long-term pathologic and functional effects of caffeine and the combination of caffeine and other substances on the developing immature brain [6, 12–22].

Anyway, adenosine, is not only crucial in development, it also mediates multifactorial forms of ventilatory responses. The reduced hypoxic ventilatory response could be attributed to depressed adenosinergic peripheral excitatory mechanisms and to enhanced adenosinergic central depression mechanisms, both of which contribute to the blunted ventilatory response in different metabolic states (**Figure 1**). Several important groups of clinical studies, in which the adenosinergic network role has been demonstrated, are related to OSA, asthma and interstitial lung disease such as idiopathic pulmonary fibrosis (IPF) [1–6]. Levels of adenosine receptors are altered in the lungs of asthmatics and OSA patients and a recent study has shown that the A2b-R is increased in remodelled airway epithelial cells of rapidly progressing IPF patients [6, 12–22]. Furthermore, CIH (as an experimental OSA model) elicits phrenic long-term facilitation by an adenosine-dependent mechanism [2, 6, 12–22]. All of the above are interesting evidences about the mechanisms that support and induce inflammatory and tissue remodelling processes in these pathological states; however, it is necessary to do more research on the pathways that provoke their progressive and chronic evolution. For example, there are already implemented several models of deregulated or overactive wound healing pathways to explain how these processes contribute to an excessive remodelling response such as seen in chronic lung disease [2, 6, 12–22]. Consistent with this, adenosine levels are elevated in the lungs of patients with chronic lung disease, where it is hypothesized that adenosine regulates the balance between tissue repair and excessive airway remodelling. Furthermore, it has been demonstrated that exogenous adenosine treatment can elicit acute bronchoconstriction in patients with asthma or OSA [1–6]. In contrast, the administration of adenosine to healthy subject did not affect them, suggesting a fundamental difference with respect to adenosinergic signalling in the treated patients. The differential response could be mediated by the activation of A-Rs that would modify the activity of different cell types that play a central role in chronic lung disease. These groups of possible targets include mast cells, eosinophils, macrophages, airway epithelial cells, pulmonary fibroblasts and airway smooth muscle cells. Indeed, recent studies directly demonstrate that adenosine is involved in the regulation of pulmonary fibrosis. Lastly, there are correlations between the degree of inflammation and damage and adenosine accumulations in adenosine deaminase-deficient individuals. Furthermore, purinergic metabolism and signalling components are altered in a manner that promotes adenosine production in tissue samples from patients with OSA and IPF. These modifications were related to the very important changes found in the expression of the promoter molecules of inflammatory process that could be induced by A2b-R signalling. Finally, it was interesting to point out that it has been demonstrated that activation of A2b-Rs can

http://dx.doi.org/10.5772/65242

influence the production of inflammatory and fibrotic mediators from macrophages isolated from these patients [6, 12–22].

All of the above findings suggest that adenosine-based therapeutics may be beneficial in the treatment of chronic lung diseases such as OSA and IPF. On the other hand, it is known that inflammation-induced release of prostaglandin E_2 changes breathing patterns and the response to CO_2 levels. This bioactive eicosanoid regulates many biologically important processes as a potent activator of several signalling pathways, through four distinct G-protein-coupled receptors. All of this alters neural network activity in the pre-Bötzinger rhythm-generating complex and in the chemosensitive brainstem respiratory regions, thereby increasing sigh frequency and the depth of inspiration with implications for inspiration and sighs throughout life, and the ability to autoresuscitate when breathing fails [2, 6, 7, 12–15, 19–22, 29, 30].

5. Conclusion

Identification of the neurophysiological mechanisms underlying the response of organisms to environmental factors, in particular, to injurious exposures like hypoxia, represents one of the most important research problems in biomedicine. Neural plasticity, as a persistent change in the morphology and/or function based on prior experiences, is crucial for understanding the effects of O_2 supply changes over neuronal networks. Plasticity is well evident when the triggering experience occurs early in life; but in the case of respiratory control plasticity, could also be present in adult life. The regulation of adenosinergic neural network maturation, especially in central cardiorespiratory areas, could provide new perspectives in respiratory newborn distress symptoms. Adenosine acts as an extracellular signalling molecule operating on selective receptors. Regulation of adenosinergic maturation in central cardiorespiratory areas in caffeine-treated neonatal mammals could explain the pharmacological effects of caffeine observed in premature infants. Anyhow, the neuroplasticity observed in the cardiorespiratory network is fundamental to maintain life in many adverse conditions.

The central and peripheral chemical drive to breathe is associated with several widespread autonomic disorders. Deficits in central chemical drive are associated with central sleep apnoea, a debilitating disease with few therapies besides constant positive airway pressure. In addition, disruption of the drive to breathe is thought to contribute to mortality of certain pathologies, including SIDS, stroke and epilepsy. Finally, in OSA, certain forms of hypertension and heart failure, it has been observed sensitization of peripheral chemoreceptor drive, particularly the sympathetic component and this over-activity is thought to contribute to the pathology.

Purinergic signalling has been proposed to be an excellent system to target for therapies of numerous pathologies, mainly due to novel pharmacological agents being developed. As more detailed understanding of the purinergic mechanisms involved in the chemical drive to breathe are uncovered, these would allow to possible pharmacological treatments of the aforementioned pathologies with the newly developed purinergic agents.

Author details

Susana P. Gaytán* and Rosario Pasaro

*Address all correspondence to: sgaytan@us.es

Department of Physiology, University of Seville, Sevilla, Spain

References

[1] Barnett WH, Abdala AP, Paton JF, Rybak IA, Zoccal DB, Molkov YI. Chemoreception and neuroplasticity in respiratory circuits. Exp Neurol. 2016;4886(16): 30156-X. DOI: 10.1016/j.expneurol.2016.05.036

[2] Guyenet PG. Regulation of breathing and autonomic outflows by chemoreceptors. Compr Physiol. 2014;4(4):1511–1562. DOI: 10.1002/cphy.c140004

[3] Molkov YI, Zoccal DB, Baekey DM, Abdala AP, Machado BH, Dick TE, Paton JF, Rybak IA. Physiological and pathophysiological interactions between the respiratory central pattern generator and the sympathetic nervous system. Prog Brain Res. 2014;212:1–23. DOI: 10.1016/B978-0-444-63488-7.00001-X

[4] Pouyssegur J, López-Barneo J. Hypoxia in health and disease. Mol Aspects Med. 2016;47–48:1–2. DOI: 10.1016/j.mam.2016.02.001

[5] Quintero M, Olea E, Conde SV, Obeso A, Gallego-Martin T, Gonzalez C, Monserrat JM, Gómez-Niño A, Yubero S, Agapito T. Age protects from harmful effects produced by chronic intermittent hypoxia. J Physiol. 2016;594(6):1773–1790. DOI: 10.1113/JP270878

[6] Ribeiro JA, Sebastião AM, de Mendonça A. Adenosine receptors in the nervous system: pathophysiological implications. Prog Neurobiol. 2002;68(6):377–392. DOI:10.1016/S0301-0082(02)00155-7

[7] Dempsey JA, Smith CA. Pathophysiology of human ventilatory control. Eur Respir J. 2014;44(2):495–512. DOI: 10.1183/09031936.00048514

[8] Gaytán SP, Pasaro R. Connections of the rostral ventral respiratory neuronal cell group: an anterograde and retrograde tracing study in the rat. Brain Res Bull. 1998;47(6):625–642. DOI: 10.1016/S0361-9230(98)00125-7

[9] Julien CA, Joseph V, Bairam A. Alteration of carotid body chemoreflexes after neonatal intermittent hypoxia and caffeine treatment in rat pups. Respir Physiol Neurobiol. 2011;177(3):301–312. DOI: 10.1016/j.resp.2011.05.006

[10] López-Barneo J, González-Rodríguez P, Gao L, Fernández-Agüera MC, Pardal R, Ortega-Sáenz P. Oxygen sensing by the carotid body: mechanisms and role in

adaptation to hypoxia. Am J Physiol Cell Physiol. 2016;310(8):629–642. DOI: 10.1152/ajpcell.00265.2015

[11] López-Barneo J, Ortega-Sáenz P, González-Rodríguez P, Fernández-Agüera MC, Macías D, Pardal R, Gao L. Oxygen-sensing by arterial chemoreceptors: mechanisms and medical translation. Mol Aspects Med. 2016;47–48:90–108. DOI: 10.1016/j.mam.2015.12.002

[12] Black AM, Pandya S, Clark D, Armstrong EA, Yager JY. Effect of caffeine and morphine on the developing pre-mature brain. Brain Res. 2008;1219:136–142. DOI: 10.1016/j.brainres.2008.04.066

[13] Borea PA, Gessi S, Merighi S, Varani K. Adenosine as a multi-signalling guardian angel in human diseases: when, where and how does it exert its protective effects? Trends Pharmacol Sci. 2016;37(6):419–434. DOI: 10.1016/j.tips.2016.02.006

[14] Gomes CV, Kaster MP, Tomé AR, Agostinho PM, Cunha RA. Adenosine receptors and brain diseases: neuroprotection and neurodegeneration. Biochim Biophys Acta. 2011;1808(5):1380–1399. DOI: 10.1016/j.bbamem.2010.12.001

[15] Wardas J. Neuroprotective role of adenosine in the CNS. Pol J Pharmacol. 2002;54:313–326 ISSN 1230-6002.PMID: 12523485

[16] Bruzzese L, Rostain JC, Née L, Condo J, Mottola G, Adjriou N, Mercier L, Berge-Lefranc JL, Fromonot J, Kipson N, Lucciano M, Durand-Gorde JM, Jammes Y, Guieu R, Ruf J, Fenouillet E. Effect of hyperoxic and hyperbaric conditions on the adenosinergic pathway and CD26 expression in rat. J Appl Physiol (1985). 2015;119(2):140–147. DOI: 10.1152/japplphysiol.00223.2015

[17] Gaytan SP, Pasaro R. Neonatal caffeine treatment up-regulates adenosine receptors in brainstem and hypothalamic cardio-respiratory related nuclei of rat pups. Exp Neurol. 2012;237(2):247–259. DOI: 10.1016/j.expneurol.2012.06.028

[18] Gaytan SP, Saadani-Makki F, Bodineau L, Frugière A, Larnicol N, Pasaro R. Effect of postnatal exposure to caffeine on the pattern of adenosine A1 receptor distribution in respiration-related nuclei of the rat brainstem. Auton Neurosci. 2006;126–127:339–346. DOI: 10.1016/j.autneu.2006.03.009

[19] Lee SD, Nakano H, Farkas GA. Adenosinergic modulation of ventilation in obese zucker rats. Obes Res. 2005;13(3):545–555. DOI: 10.1038/oby.2005.58

[20] de Mendonça A, Sebastião AM, Ribeiro JA. Adenosine: does it have a neuroprotective role after all? Brain Res Brain Res Rev. 2000;33(2–3):258–274. DOI:10.1016/S0165-0173(00)00033-3

[21] Schmidt C, Bellingham MC, Richter DW. Adenosinergic modulation of respiratory neurones and hypoxic responses in the anaesthetized cat. J Physiol. 1995;483(Pt 3):769–781. PMCID: PMC1157817

[22] Zhou Y, Murthy JN, Zeng D, Belardinelli L, Blackburn MR. Alterations in adenosine metabolism and signaling in patients with chronic obstructive pulmonary disease and idiopathic pulmonary fibrosis. PLoS One. 2010;5(2):e9224. DOI: 10.1371/journal.pone.0009224

[23] Ribas-Salgueiro JL, Gaytán SP, Crego R, Pásaro R, Ribas J. Highly H^+-sensitive neurons in the caudal ventrolateral medulla of the rat. J Physiol. 2003;549(Pt 1):181–194. DOI: 10.1113/jphysiol.2002.036624

[24] Ribas-Salgueiro JL, Gaytán SP, Ribas J, Pásaro R. Characterization of efferent projections of chemosensitive neurons in the caudal parapyramidal area of the rat brain. Brain Res Bull. 2005;66(3):235–248. DOI: 10.1016/j.brainresbull.2005.05.014

[25] Kara T, Narkiewicz K, Somers VK. Chemoreflexes-physiology and clinical implications. Acta Physiol Scand. 2003;177(3):377–384. DOI: 10.1046/j.1365-201X.2003.01083.x

[26] Nichols NL, Dale EA, Mitchell GS. Severe acute intermittent hypoxia elicits phrenic long-term facilitation by a novel adenosine-dependent mechanism. J Appl Physiol. (1985). 2012;112(10):1678–1688. DOI: 10.1152/japplphysiol.00060.2012

[27] Olea E, Gaytan SP, Obeso A, Gonzalez C, Pasaro R. Interactions between postnatal sustained hypoxia and intermittent hypoxia in the adulthood to alter brainstem structures and respiratory function. Adv Exp Med Biol. 2012;758:225–231. DOI: 10.1007/978-94-007-4584-1_31

[28] Perlman JM. Intervention strategies for neonatal hypoxic-ischemic cerebral injury. Clin Ther. 2006;28(9):1353–1365. DOI: 10.1016/j.clinthera.2006.09.005

[29] Barna BF, Takakura AC, Mulkey DK, Moreira TS. Purinergic receptor blockade in the retrotrapezoid nucleus attenuates the respiratory chemoreflexes in awake rats. Acta Physiol (Oxf). 2016;217(1):80–93. DOI: 10.1111/apha.12637

[30] Forsberg D, Horn Z, Tserga E, Smedler E, Silberberg G, Shvarev Y, Kaila K, Uhlén P, Herlenius E. CO_2-evoked release of PGE2 modulates sighs and inspiration as demonstrated in brainstem organotypic culture. Elife. 2016;5(pii):e14170. DOI: 10.7554/eLife.14170

[31] Mathew OP. Apnea of prematurity: pathogenesis and management strategies. J Perinatol. 2011;31(5):302–310. DOI: 10.1038/jp.2010.126

[32] Rivkees SA, Zhao Z, Porter G, Turner C. Influences of adenosine on the fetus and newborn. Mol Genet Metab. 2001;74(1–2):160–171. DOI:10.1006/mgme.2001.3217

[33] Thach BT. The role of respiratory control disorders in SIDS. Respir Physiol Neurobiol. 2005;149(1–3):343–353. DOI: 10.1016/j.resp.2005.06.011

[34] Gourine AV, Atkinson L, Deuchars J, Spyer KM. Purinergic signalling in the medullary mechanisms of respiratory control in the rat: respiratory neurones express the P2X2 receptor subunit. J Physiol. 2003;552(Pt 1):197–211. DOI: 10.1113/jphysiol.2003.045294

[35] Moreira TS, Wenker IC, Sobrinho CR, Barna BF, Takakura AC, Mulkey DK. Independent purinergic mechanisms of central and peripheral chemoreception in the rostral ventrolateral medulla. J Physiol. 2015;593(5):1067–1074. DOI: 10.1113/jphysiol.2014.284430

[36] Pedata F, Dettori I, Coppi E, Melani A, Fusco I, Corradetti R, Pugliese AM. Purinergic signalling in brain ischemia. Neuropharmacology. 2016;104:105–130. DOI: 10.1016/j.neuropharm.2015.11.007

[37] Rodrigues RJ, Tomé AR, Cunha RA. ATP as a multi-target danger signal in the brain. Front Neurosci. 2015;9:148. DOI: 10.3389/fnins.2015.00148

[38] Sobrinho CR, Wenker IC, Poss EM, Takakura AC, Moreira TS, Mulkey DK. Purinergic signalling contributes to chemoreception in the retrotrapezoid nucleus but not the nucleus of the solitary tract or medullary raphe. J Physiol. 2014;592(6):1309–1323.DOI: 10.1113/jphysiol.2013.268490

Chapter 14

The HIF System Response to ESA Therapy in CKD-Anemia

Sandra Ribeiro, Luís Belo, Flávio Reis and
Alice Santos-Silva

Additional information is available at the end of the chapter

http://dx.doi.org/10.5772/64611

Abstract

Anemia is a common complication of chronic kidney disease (CKD) associated with disease progression and increased mortality. This anemia is mainly due to inadequate production of erythropoietin (EPO) by the failing kidneys, resulting from the reduction in renal EPO-producing cells (REPC) or from dysregulation of the hypoxia-inducible factor (HIF) system that regulates several genes related to hypoxia, angiogenesis, fibrosis and glucose metabolism, among others. In this chapter, we present a review on the HIF system in CKD-anemia, the HIF response to erythropoiesis-stimulating agents (ESA) therapy and its potential involvement in the development of ESA resistance by enhancing kidney fibrosis and inflammation. Due to concerns related to ESA use, new drugs to correct anemia are under study, being the prolyl hydroxylase inhibitors the most promising candidates.

Keywords: chronic kidney disease, erythropoietin resistance, fibrosis, HIF system, Hypoxia, inflammation

1. Introduction

Anemia is a common complication of chronic kidney disease (CKD) that often develops early in the course of the disease, and its frequency and severity increase with the decline of renal function [1]. This condition is associated with a decreased quality of life [2, 3], increased hospitalizations and comorbidities [4, 5], progression of renal dysfunction [6–8], enhanced cardiovascular complications [9, 10] and mortality [11–13]. The main cause for anemia in CKD patients is erythropoietin (EPO) deficit, due to decreased hormone production by the failing kidneys; other factors can also contribute to the development or worsening of CKD-anemia, such as iron deficiency, inflammation and uremic toxins, among others [14].

EPO is a glycoprotein that presents several functions acting as a hormone, cytokine or growth factor on target cells that express the EPO receptors (EPOR), through different pathways. In the bone marrow, EPO controls cell proliferation, differentiation and death of erythroid cells.

During fetal life, the majority of EPO is produced by the liver; after birth there is a switch to renal production, and in the adulthood, 90% of this hormone is produced by the kidneys, whereas the liver is a secondary site of production [15]. EPO is also expressed in the brain, spleen, lung and testis, but its contribution to serum EPO levels is not clarified [16]. The kidney cells responsible for EPO production are still under debate, but several studies showed that renal EPO-producing cells (REPC) include the peritubular fibroblast-like interstitial cells in the inner cortex and in the outer medulla [17, 18], the proximal and distal convoluted tubules and cortical collecting ducts [19]. REPC are sensitive to changes in oxygen (O_2) tension, and in conditions of hypoxia, the kidney responds increasing the number of REPC capable of producing EPO [20].

In CKD, the severity of the disease defines the kidney capacity to produce EPO [21, 22]. Indeed, patients with GFR >30 mL/min/1.73 m^2 are still able to induce a physiologic response to anemia, showed by the normal or even elevated serum EPO levels [23, 24]. Nevertheless, serum EPO levels may not be sufficient for the degree of anemia; actually, anemic patients with normal renal function may present a 10-fold to 100-fold increase in serum EPO levels [25, 26], to achieve correction of anemia.

The kidney is the major site of EPO production in the adults; however, it is possible that extrarenal sites contribute for the marked rise in plasma EPO in end-stage renal disease (ESRD) patients [27], as already showed in animal models of kidney injury [28, 29]. It was also reported that patients with anemia can switch EPO production from the kidney to the liver [30, 31], as can be shown by glycoform analysis of EPO. Indeed, the posttranslational EPO glycosylation is specific of the synthesizing cells, giving rise to different EPO glycoforms that can be used to localize EPO synthesis [30, 32].

Hypoxia regulates the EPO gene through the hypoxia-inducible factor (HIF) system [20]. This HIF system includes O_2-dependent HIF-1α, HIF-2α (also known as endothelial PAS domain-containing protein 1) and HIF-3α subunits, and the constitutively expressed HIF-1β and HIF-2β subunits (also known as aryl hydrocarbon receptor nuclear translocator). The HIF-α subunits are hydroxylated in specific proline residues, by the prolyl-4-hydroxylase (PHD) proteins that require O_2 as a co-substrate (**Figure 1**). The hydroxylated HIF-α subunit targets the von Hippel-Lindau tumor suppressor protein (VHL) to be recognized by an ubiquitin ligase complement that will induce a rapid ubiquitination and proteasomal degradation of HIF-α subunits. Under normoxia, HIF-α subunits are almost undetectable, but in hypoxic conditions, the hydroxylation by PHD proteins is inhibited; thus, the HIF-α accumulates in the cytoplasm, is translocated to the nucleus and binds to the HIF-β subunit, forming a complex that recruits the coactivators P300/CBP and activates the transcription of several genes [20].

Several genes are regulated by the HIF-1α and HIF-2α subunits (**Figure 1**), but recent studies showed that HIF-2α is the main regulator of EPO synthesis in the kidney and liver [33–35] and is also important for the regulation of several factors involved in iron homeostasis, as iron is an important element for hemoglobin (Hb) synthesis [36]. The HIF-1α subunit activates the transcription of glucose metabolism, angiogenesis and fibrosis related genes to promote wound healing [37]. The role of HIF-3α is still ambiguous and under current investigation. It is known that HIF-3α presents several isoforms with different roles [38]; the up-regulation of some HIF-3α isoforms appears to act as a negative feedback mechanism to regulate HIF-1α and/or HIF-2α subunits; however, recent studies showed that HIF-3α might share with HIF-1α the regulation of some genes [39].

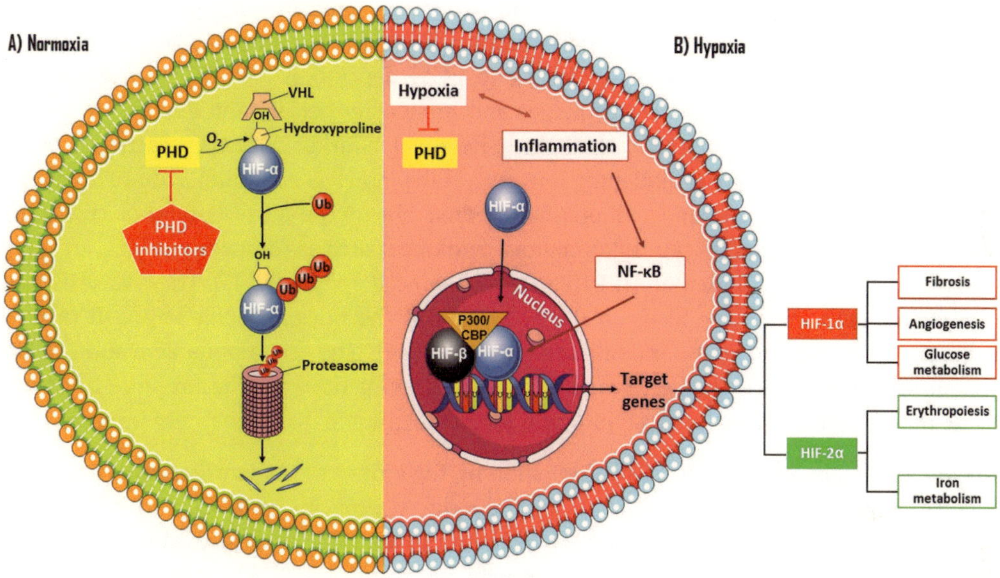

Figure 1. Regulation of hypoxia-inducible system. (A) In conditions of normoxia, the HIF-α subunits are hydroxylated, in specific proline residues by prolyl-4-hydroxylase (PHD) proteins, which recruit the von Hippel-Lindau tumor suppressor protein (VHL) a signal for rapid ubiquitination and proteasomal degradation of HIF-α subunits. PHD inhibitors are under development, as they might impair the degradation of the HIF-α subunits, improving anemia. (B) Under hypoxic conditions, the PHD proteins are inhibited, and consequently, the HIF-α subunits are not targeted by VHL protein for degradation, translocating to the nucleus and binding to the HIF-β subunit, forming a complex that recruit the coactivators P300/CBP, leading to the transcription of several genes that will depend on the type of HIF-α subunit (HIF-1α or HIF-2a) that binds to the target gene sequences. There is a crosstalk between hypoxia and inflammation, leading to the activation of the nuclear factor kappa beta (NF-κB) pathway that can also induce HIF-1α accumulation.

This chapter reviews the HIF response to erythropoiesis-stimulating agents (ESA) therapy focusing on its potential involvement in the development of ESA resistance, by enhancing kidney fibrosis and inflammation.

2. Hypoxia and progression of renal disease

Renal hypoxia is well known as an important contributor for the progression of renal disease. A study conducted in a rat model of diabetic nephropathy reported that intrarenal hypoxia develops early in the course of the disease and precedes the alterations in circulating biomarkers of kidney damage [40]. Irrespective of the initial cause of CKD, the histopathological analysis of renal biopsies showed that fibrosis is the common final pathway [41]. The underlying mechanisms are still debatable.

Glomerular injury leads to a reduction in glomerular blood flow and consequently limits blood flow into peritubular capillaries, causing hypoxia and tubulointerstitial injury [42]. After an initial injury, the tubular cells will attempt to correct and repair the injury by recruiting and activating several cells, such as macrophages, fibroblasts and epithelial tubular cells that will release pro-inflammatory cytokines and fibrosis factors, and contribute to excessive interstitial extracellular matrix (ECM) accumulation and expansion. Transforming growth factor beta (TGF-β), a recognized pro-fibrotic factor, appears to be central for fibroblast activation, proliferation and transdifferentiation, contributing to ECM deposition [43]. TGF-β also presents immunomodulatory effects on macrophages and monocyte recruitment, leading to the production of inflammatory cytokines [44]. In early renal injuries, M2-type macrophages are recruited to promote tissue remodeling; however, if the injury is continuous, more inflammatory monocytes will be recruited differentiating their phenotype into M1-type macrophages, responsible for the release of pro-inflammatory cytokines (such as tumor necrosis factor [TNF-α], interferon [IFN]-γ, interleukin (IL)-1β and IL-6) and cell apoptosis [45]. The release of these pro-inflammatory cytokines leads to the activation of the nuclear factor kappa B (NF-κB) pathway, thus amplifying the inflammatory process [44]. The continuous activation of this system will culminate with the formation of scar tissue or fibrosis. The presence of fibrotic tissue reduces the diffusion of O_2, which will further aggravate the hypoxic environment.

Anemia caused by inadequate EPO production by the kidneys also contributes to renal hypoxia. However, the mechanisms underlying the reduced capacity for EPO production by the REPC are not well understood. It has been proposed that after renal injury, REPC can suffer a transdifferentiation, called epithelial to mesenchymal transition (EMT), into myofibroblasts, losing their capacity to synthesize EPO and increasing the synthesis of collagen, contributing to the expansion of ECM [46]. Nevertheless, this EMT phenomenon was never proved in humans. The residual capacity to increase serum EPO levels when subjected to hypoxic environment or high altitudes by renal patients, even those on dialysis [47], indicates that a dysregulation of the HIF system, more than a complete loss of REPC cells, could be responsible for the reduced EPO production. Moreover, the pharmacological inhibition of the PHD in CKD patients stimulates endogenous EPO production further supporting a deranged oxygen sensing [27]. A recent study in mice by Souma et al. [48] also strengthened this hypothesis, by showing that inflammatory cytokines and/or fibrosis factors suppress HIF activation through the over-activation of PHD even under pathologic hypoxic conditions, and that the inhibition of PHD restores EPO production.

3. Erythropoiesis-stimulating agents in CKD-anemia

The standard treatment for CKD-anemia is based on pharmacological intervention, using ESA and/or iron supplementation, in order to correct and maintain Hb concentration in the range of 10–11.5g/dL [49]. ESA are medicines produced by recombinant DNA technology with similar structure and biological activity of EPO. They differ from EPO by the different patterns of glycosylation that increases their half-life.

The use of ESA has beneficial effects by correcting anemia and their associated symptoms and improving patients' quality of life [50, 51]. However, the effects of ESA on the progression of renal function are controversial. Some studies showed that after starting ESA therapy and correction of anemia, renal function declines at a slower rate, delaying the need for dialysis in pre-dialysis patients [52–54]; in opposition, other studies reported that ESA do not significantly affect renal function [55, 56].

ESA were designed to correct anemia, but some evidences showed that these drugs (and EPO) may act beyond hematopoiesis. Pleiotropic effects have been attributed to EPO and ESA, such as cytoprotection, anti-apoptosis, anti-inflammatory and angiogenesis [57]. These non-hematopoietic actions appear to result from the activation of another EPOR, a heterodimeric receptor constituted by the EPOR homodimer complexed with CD131, the common beta receptor (βCR) that is involved in granulocyte macrophage colony-stimulating factor, IL-3 and IL-5 signaling [58]. The two EPOR present different affinities for EPO; in erythroid cells picomolar concentrations of EPO are sufficient to trigger activation of the EPOR homodimer, whereas on other cells and tissues high local EPO concentrations are needed to activate EPOR heterodimer [59]. This receptor was detected in several cells and tissues, such as brain (neurons, astrocytes and microglia), kidney, female reproductive system organs, vascular endothelial cells, cardiomyocytes, lymphocytes and monocytes, among others [57].

The slower progression of renal dysfunction observed in some CKD patients may result from renoprotection of ESA therapy. Several studies on acute kidney injury (AKI) reported that a single dose of recombinant human EPO (rHuEPO) reduces kidney dysfunction through anti-apoptotic mechanisms and increases NO production, only in intact vessels [60]. ESA therapy also exerts renoprotective effects by reducing the production of pro-inflammatory cytokines (e. g., IL-1β and TNF-α), acute phase proteins [e.g., C-reactive protein (CRP)], pro-fibrotic factors (e.g., TGF-β) and oxidative stress [61]. However, these effects appear to be only achieved with low doses of ESA, as high doses increase hematocrit and may activate platelets, increasing their adhesion to the injured endothelium, contributing to hemorheologic changes [60]. Indeed, other side effects are associated with ESA therapy, namely hypertension [62] and thrombotic events [63].

Despite the benefits of ESA therapy, some concerns have emerged from studies reporting a high incidence of cardiovascular events and mortality in CKD patients treated with ESA [63, 64], independently of the type of ESA used [65, 66]. Since the introduction of ESA therapy, several clinical trials aimed to define the better Hb target/ESA dose associated with lower cardiovascular risk. Indeed, recent studies reported increased cardiovascular risk and death in patients treated with high ESA doses to achieve higher Hb levels [9, 67–69].

The need for new drugs with lower associated cardiovascular risk opened a growing area of research. The most promising are the PHD inhibitors (**Table 1**) with several compounds already under evaluation in clinical trials. Some of these compounds showed to be well tolerated, corrected anemia in non-dialysis CKD and incident dialysis patients without increasing blood pressure, and also reduced serum hepcidin levels [70–73]. However, regarding their effects in reducing cardiovascular events and slowing the progression of the renal disease, no data are still available from human studies. Yu et al. [22] showed that the administration of PHD inhibitors in a more advanced stage of CKD in the rat reduced renal fibrosis and protected renal function, whereas the administration in an early stage of CKD promoted renal fibrosis and exacerbated renal dysfunction. In another strategy to induce EPO production, the hydrodynamic gene transfer of a plasmid encoding for EPO in a rat model overexpressing TGF-β showed that this therapy increased Hb levels but had no effect on kidney fibrosis or function [74].

PHD inhibitor	Route administration	ClinicalTrials.gov Identifier
Molidustat(BAY85-3934)	Oral	• NCT02064426
Roxadustat(FG-4592)	Oral	• NCT01630889
		• NCT01887600
Vadadustat(AKB-6548)	Oral	• NCT01906489
		• NCT02648347
		• NCT02680574
GSK1278863	Oral	• NCT02689206

Table 1. Prolyl-4-hydroxylase (PHD) inhibitors in clinical trials.

4. Hyporesponsiveness to erythropoiesis-stimulating agents in CKD

The majority of CKD patients respond adequately to the currently available ESA therapy, but 5–10% of them do not respond properly, developing hyporesponsiveness to these drugs [75]. According to the KDIGO guidelines [49], CKD patients can present initial or acquired ESA hyporesponsiveness; in primary hyporesponsiveness patients, after one month of treatment with adequate weight-based ESA dose, the target Hb concentration is not achieved; in acquired ESA hyporesponsiveness, after effective treatment with stable ESA dose, achieving the target Hb concentration, the patient requires two consecutive increases (up to 50% beyond the stable dose) in ESA dose. Hyporesponsiveness (also widely referred as resistance) to ESA therapy is associated with a poor outcome, progression of renal disease, sudden death, infectious complications, sudden death and all-cause mortality, mainly due to cardiovascular events in dialysis patients [76–79]. Several causes are associated with poor response to ESA therapy, including iron deficiency, inflammation, malnutrition and hyperparathyroidism, among others [80–82].

4.1. Inflammation

A pro-inflammatory state is a hallmark of CKD, which is due to increased uremic toxins that induce the production of inflammatory cytokines. Additionally, active infections, the vascular

http://dx.doi.org/10.5772/64611

access for hemodialysis (HD) procedure and surgery-related inflammation (vascular surgery included) can also contribute to inflammation.

The activation of inflammatory cells is also associated with increased oxidative stress, favoring alterations in red blood cells (RBC) membrane, namely increased phosphatidylserine exposure, increased membrane bound Hb and increased membrane protein band 3 aggregation, all markers for RBC phagocytosis by macrophages and, thus, for a premature RBC removal [83, 84]. Uremic toxins and pro-inflammatory cytokines also inhibit erythropoiesis, through the inhibitory effect of IL-1β, TNF-α and IFN-γ on early erythroid cell stages in the bone marrow [85]. The macrophages of the bone marrow can also be stimulated to increase local pro-inflammatory cytokines, amplifying the effects of systemic inflammation [86]. In CKD patients, hepcidin synthesis is enhanced, due to the increase in Il-6, contributing for the limited iron availability for erythropoiesis [87]. Indeed, CKD patients often present with replete or even higher iron stores, alongside with inflammation and anemia. A disturbance in the crosstalk between inflammation, iron metabolism and erythropoiesis may, therefore, favor ESA hyporesponsiveness. The best predictors for ESA response appear to be IL-6 and CRP [88, 89]. Studies conducted by our group showed that HD patients with poorer response to ESA present higher levels of pro-inflammatory cytokines [90, 91]; moreover, in studies using a rat model of chronic renal failure, we found that the severity of the inflammatory state was related to the reduction in the rHuEPO response [92].

4.2. HIF system in the hyporesponsiveness to erythropoiesis-stimulating agents

Hyporesponsive patients to ESA therapy will develop anemia, and as already referred, it will promote the progression of renal disease. Tissue hypoxia is amplified according to the severity of anemia that will reduce O_2 availability to body tissues and organs. Within the kidney, the hypoxic environment leads to the activation of the HIF system, promoting the transcription of several target genes. In the hypoxic kidney, HIF-1α is essentially expressed in tubular and glomerular epithelial cells, whereas HIF-2α expression is limited to endothelial and interstitial cells [93]. The localization of these HIF-α subunits is related to their target genes.

Renal biopsies from CKD patients showed that increased expression of HIF-1α in tubular epithelial cells is correlated with the stage of renal disease [94]. It was reported that HIF-α activation in CKD rats presents dynamic changes, as it is activated in early CKD stages and suppressed in the moderate and end-stage of CKD [95]. Thus, the administration of PHD inhibitors may improve renal function in more advanced stages of CKD, while in earlier stages, the PHD inhibitors may increase renal fibrosis due to upregulation of the HIF-1α subunit [22].

HIF-1α subunit is involved in the activation of pro-fibrotic genes (**Figure 1**), including the connective tissue growth factor (CTGF) gene [96]; indeed, the plasma levels of CTGF appear as a good marker for staging diabetic nephropathy progression [97]. CTGF is a potent pro-fibrotic factor and a marker of renal fibrosis, increasing ECM production, promoting EMT, stimulating fibroblasts and potentiating TGF-β signaling [94, 98]. CTGF and TGF-β present similar effects, but TGF-β also presents immunomodulatory actions [44], recruiting macrophages to reduce the injury; however, a continuous macrophage activation leads to excessive ECM accumulation and increased release of pro-inflammatory cytokines promoting fibrosis. A study by Basu et al. [99] suggested that TGF-β can in turn induce HIF-1α activation, which would amplify cell collagen expression contributing to the progression of fibrosis.

There is also a crosstalk between HIF-1α and inflammation (**Figure 1**). Inflammation favor tissue hypoxia by several mechanisms including: impaired EPO response, iron mobilization and bone marrow erythropoiesis, reduced RBC lifespan and also increased demand for O_2 by the inflammatory cells in order to increase pro-inflammatory cytokines. However, it was also reported that NF-κB can induce HIF-1α activation due to the presence of responsive elements in the promoter of *HIF-1α* gene [100]. Another mechanism is the interaction of PHD with some effectors of the NF-κB pathway, though the exact proteins involved remain unknown [101].

The majority of the studies report a beneficial effect of ESA on renal fibrosis through several mechanisms [29, 102]. However, recently Gobe et al. [103] reported that in rat model of AKI the use of higher rHuEPO doses was associated with increased TGF-β expression, oxidative stress and stimulation of fibroblasts and EMT, contributing to the progression of the disease and gradual development of CKD in the long term. In this study, the expression of HIF-α subunits was not reported, as well as the linking between HIF activation and the alterations observed. Further studies regarding this issue are warranted.

Despite the underlying mechanism, a continuous inflammatory response favoring fibrosis and a disturbance in the HIF system creates a vicious cycle, contributing to the progression of renal disease and aggravation of renal anemia [92], and reducing the response to ESA therapy creating a scenario of hyporesponsiveness to EPO.

5. Conclusions

Anemia is a common complication in CKD patients that can be corrected by the treatment with ESA. However, the development of a hyporesponse to this therapy was associated with (i) the progression of the renal disease, due to the amplification of fibrosis and inflammation through a mechanism involving activation of HIF-1α pathway; (ii) increased risks in the development of cardiovascular disorder events and all-cause mortality in patients treated with higher doses, opened a new research field, focused on the design of more effective agents to control anemia in CKD patients, with less side effects. The use of PHD inhibitors is promising, but further is needed to confirm their effects in the reduction of cardiovascular events and progression of renal disease.

Acknowledgements

This work received financial support from FCT/MEC through national funds and co-financed by FEDER, under the Partnership Agreement PT2020 (UID/MULTI/04378/2013—POCI/01/0145/FERDER/007728, UID/NEU/04539/2013) and Norte Portugal Regional Coordination and Development Commission (CCDR-N)/NORTE2020/Portugal 2020 (Norte-01-0145-FEDER-000024).

Author details

Sandra Ribeiro[1], Luís Belo[1], Flávio Reis[2,3] and Alice Santos-Silva[1]*

*Address all correspondence to: assilva@ff.up.pt

1 Research Unit on Applied Molecular Biosciences (UCIBIO), REQUIMTE, Department of Biological Sciences, Laboratory of Biochemistry, Faculty of Pharmacy, University of Porto, Porto, Portugal

2 Laboratory of Pharmacology and Experimental Therapeutics, Institute for Biomedical Imaging and Life Sciences (IBILI), Faculty of Medicine, University of Coimbra, Coimbra, Portugal

3 Center for Neuroscience and Cell Biology, Institute for Biomedical Imaging and Life Sciences (CNC.IBILI) Research Unit, University of Coimbra, Coimbra, Portugal

References

[1] Astor BC, Muntner P, Levin A, Eustace JA, Coresh J. Association of kidney function with anemia: the Third National Health and Nutrition Examination Survey (1988–1994). Arch Intern Med. 2002;162(12):1401–8. doi:10.1001/archinte.162.12.1401

[2] Fukuhara S, Akizawa T, Morita S, Tsubakihara Y. Understanding measurements of vitality in patients with chronic kidney disease: connecting a quality-of-life scale to daily activities. PLoS One. 2012;7(7):e40455. doi:10.1371/journal.pone.0040455

[3] Bonner A, Caltabiano M, Berlund L. Quality of life, fatigue, and activity in Australians with chronic kidney disease: a longitudinal study. Nurs Health Sci. 2013;15(3):360–7. doi:10.1111/nhs.12038

[4] Staples AO, Wong CS, Smith JM, Gipson DS, Filler G, Warady BA, Martz K, Greenbaum LA. Anemia and risk of hospitalization in pediatric chronic kidney disease. Clin J Am Soc Nephrol. 2009;4(1):48–56. doi:10.2215/CJN.05301107

[5] Garlo K, Williams D, Lucas L, Wong R, Botler J, Abramson S, Parker MG. Severity of anemia predicts hospital length of stay but not readmission in patients with chronic kidney disease: a retrospective cohort study. Medicine. 2015;94(25):e964. doi:10.1097/MD.0000000000000964

[6] Warady BA, Abraham AG, Schwartz GJ, Wong CS, Munoz A, Betoko A, Mitsnefes M, Kaskel F, Greenbaum LA, Mak RH, Flynn J, Moxey-Mims MM, Furth S. Predictors of rapid progression of glomerular and nonglomerular kidney disease in children and adolescents: the chronic kidney disease in children (CKiD) cohort. Am J Kidney Dis. 2015;65(6):878–88. doi:10.1053/j.ajkd.2015.01.008

[7] Chase HS, Hirsch JS, Mohan S, Rao MK, Radhakrishnan J. Presence of early CKD-related metabolic complications predict progression of stage 3 CKD: a case-controlled study. BMC Nephrol. 2014;15:187. doi:10.1186/1471-2369-15-187

[8] Phillips JK, Boyd R, Krockenberger MB, Burgio G. Progression of anemia and its relationship with renal function, blood pressure, and erythropoietin in rats with chronic kidney disease. Vet Clin Pathol. 2015;44(3):342–54. doi:10.1111/vcp.12276

[9] McMurray JJ, Uno H, Jarolim P, Desai AS, de Zeeuw D, Eckardt KU, Ivanovich P, Levey AS, Lewis EF, McGill JB, Parfrey P, Parving HH, Toto RM, Solomon SD, Pfeffer MA. Predictors of fatal and nonfatal cardiovascular events in patients with type 2 diabetes mellitus, chronic kidney disease, and anemia: an analysis of the Trial to Reduce cardiovascular Events with Aranesp (darbepoetin-alfa) Therapy (TREAT). Am Heart J. 2011;162(4):748–55. doi:10.1016/j.ahj.2011.07.016

[10] Chang JM, Chen SC, Huang JC, Su HM, Chen HC. Anemia and left ventricular hypertrophy with renal function decline and cardiovascular events in chronic kidney disease. Am J Med Sci. 2014;347(3):183–9. doi:10.1097/MAJ.0b013e31827981be

[11] Anderson J, Glynn LG, Newell J, Iglesias AA, Reddan D, Murphy AW. The impact of renal insufficiency and anaemia on survival in patients with cardiovascular disease: a cohort study. BMC Cardiovasc Disord. 2009;9:51–8. doi:10.1186/1471-2261-9-51

[12] Nseir W, Artul S, Nasrallah N, Mograbi J, Mahamid M. Hospitalization and 1-year all-cause mortality in type 2 diabetic patients with chronic kidney disease at stages 1 and 2: effect of mild anemia. J Diabetes. 2015;8(4):502–7. doi:10.1111/1753-0407.12318

[13] Iimori S, Naito S, Noda Y, Nishida H, Kihira H, Yui N, Okado T, Sasaki S, Uchida S, Rai T. Anaemia management and mortality risk in newly visiting patients with chronic kidney disease in Japan: the CKD-ROUTE study. Nephrology (Carlton). 2015;20(9):601–8. doi:10.1111/nep.12493

[14] Lankhorst CE, Wish JB. Anemia in renal disease: diagnosis and management. Blood Rev. 2010;24(1):39–47. doi:10.1016/j.blre.2009.09.001

[15] Lacombe C, Mayeux P. Biology of erythropoietin. Haematologica. 1998;83(8):724–32.

[16] Weidemann A, Johnson RS. Nonrenal regulation of EPO synthesis. Kidney Int. 2009;75 (7):682–8. doi:10.1038/ki.2008.687

[17] Asada N, Takase M, Nakamura J, Oguchi A, Asada M, Suzuki N, Yamamura K, Nagoshi N, Shibata S, Rao TN, Fehling HJ, Fukatsu A, Minegishi N, Kita T, Kimura T, Okano H, Yamamoto M, Yanagita M. Dysfunction of fibroblasts of extrarenal origin underlies renal fibrosis and renal anemia in mice. J Clin Invest. 2011;121(10):3981–90. doi:10.1172/JCI5730157301

[18] Pan X, Suzuki N, Hirano I, Yamazaki S, Minegishi N, Yamamoto M. Isolation and characterization of renal erythropoietin-producing cells from genetically produced anemia mice. PLoS One. 2011;6(10):e25839. doi:10.1371/journal.pone.0025839

[19] Nagai T, Yasuoka Y, Izumi Y, Horikawa K, Kimura M, Nakayama Y, Uematsu T, Fukuyama T, Yamazaki T, Kohda Y, Hasuike Y, Nanami M, Kuragano T, Kobayashi N, Obinata M, Tomita K, Tanoue A, Nakanishi T, Kawahara K, Nonoguchi H. Reevaluation of erythropoietin production by the nephron. Biochem Biophys Res Commun. 2014;449 (2):222–8. doi:10.1016/j.bbrc.2014.05.014

[20] Haase VH. Regulation of erythropoiesis by hypoxia-inducible factors. Blood Rev. 2013;27(1):41–53. doi:10.1016/j.blre.2012.12.003

[21] Sanada S, Toyama H, Ejima Y, Matsubara M. Potential for erythropoietin synthesis in kidney of uraemic rat alters depending on severity of renal failure. Nephrology (Carlton). 2009;14(8):735–42. doi:10.1111/j.1440-1797.2009.01110.x

[22] Yu X, Fang Y, Liu H, Zhu J, Zou J, Xu X, Jiang S, Ding X. The balance of beneficial and deleterious effects of hypoxia-inducible factor activation by prolyl hydroxylase inhibitor in rat remnant kidney depends on the timing of administration. Nephrol Dial Transplant. 2012;27(8):3110–9. doi:10.1093/ndt/gfr754

[23] Fehr T, Ammann P, Garzoni D, Korte W, Fierz W, Rickli H, Wuthrich RP. Interpretation of erythropoietin levels in patients with various degrees of renal insufficiency and anemia. Kidney Int. 2004;66(3):1206–11. doi:10.1111/j.1523-1755.2004.00880.x

[24] Mercadal L, Metzger M, Casadevall N, Haymann JP, Karras A, Boffa JJ, Flamant M, Vrtovsnik F, Stengel B, Froissart M. Timing and determinants of erythropoietin deficiency in chronic kidney disease. Clin J Am Soc Nephrol. 2012;7(1):35–42. doi:10.2215/CJN.04690511

[25] Artunc F, Risler T. Serum erythropoietin concentrations and responses to anaemia in patients with or without chronic kidney disease. Nephrol Dial Transplant. 2007;22 (10):2900–8. doi:10.1093/ndt/gfm316

[26] Sato Y, Yanagita M. Renal anemia: from incurable to curable. Am J Physiol Renal Physiol. 2013;305(9):F1239–48. doi:10.1152/ajprenal.00233.2013

[27] Bernhardt WM, Wiesener MS, Scigalla P, Chou J, Schmieder RE, Gunzler V, Eckardt KU. Inhibition of prolyl hydroxylases increases erythropoietin production in ESRD. J Am Soc Nephrol. 2010;21(12):2151–6. doi:10.1681/ASN.2010010116

[28] Garrido P, Ribeiro S, Fernandes J, Vala H, Bronze-da-Rocha E, Rocha-Pereira P, Belo L, Costa E, Santos-Silva A, Reis F. Iron-hepcidin dysmetabolism, anemia and renal hypoxia, inflammation and fibrosis in the remnant kidney rat model. PLoS One. 2015;10(4): e0124048. doi:10.1371/journal.pone.0124048

[29] Ribeiro S, Garrido P, Fernandes J, Vala H, Rocha-Pereira P, Costa E, Belo L, Reis F, Santos-Silva A. Renal risk-benefit determinants of recombinant human erythropoietin therapy in the remnant kidney rat model—hypertension, anaemia, inflammation and drug dose. Clin Exp Pharmacol Physiol. 2016;43(3):343–54. doi:10.1111/1440-1681.12541

[30] Lonnberg M, Garle M, Lonnberg L, Birgegard G. Patients with anaemia can shift from kidney to liver production of erythropoietin as shown by glycoform analysis. J Pharm Biomed Anal. 2013;81–2:187–92. doi:10.1016/j.jpba.2013.04.009

[31] de Seigneux S, Lundby AK, Berchtold L, Berg AH, Saudan P, Lundby C. Increased synthesis of liver erythropoietin with CKD. J Am Soc Nephrol. 2016;27(8):2265–9. doi:10.1681/ASN.2015050508

[32] Lundby AK, Keiser S, Siebenmann C, Schaffer L, Lundby C. Kidney-synthesized erythropoietin is the main source for the hypoxia-induced increase in plasma erythropoietin in adult humans. Eur J Appl Physiol. 2014;114(6):1107–11. doi:10.1007/s00421-014-2844-7

[33] Percy MJ, Furlow PW, Lucas GS, Li X, Lappin TR, McMullin MF, Lee FS. A gain-of-function mutation in the HIF2A gene in familial erythrocytosis. N Engl J Med. 2008;358(2):162–8. doi:10.1056/NEJMoa073123

[34] Paliege A, Rosenberger C, Bondke A, Sciesielski L, Shina A, Heyman SN, Flippin LA, Arend M, Klaus SJ, Bachmann S. Hypoxia-inducible factor-2alpha-expressing interstitial fibroblasts are the only renal cells that express erythropoietin under hypoxia-inducible factor stabilization. Kidney Int. 2010;77(4):312–8. doi:10.1038/ki.2009.460

[35] Kapitsinou PP, Liu Q, Unger TL, Rha J, Davidoff O, Keith B, Epstein JA, Moores SL, Erickson-Miller CL, Haase VH. Hepatic HIF-2 regulates erythropoietic responses to hypoxia in renal anemia. Blood. 2010;116(16):3039–48. doi:10.1182/blood-2010-02-270322

[36] Peyssonnaux C, Zinkernagel AS, Schuepbach RA, Rankin E, Vaulont S, Haase VH, Nizet V, Johnson RS. Regulation of iron homeostasis by the hypoxia-inducible transcription factors (HIFs). J Clin Invest. 2007;117(7):1926–32. doi:10.1172/JCI31370

[37] Kumar H, Choi DK. Hypoxia inducible factor pathway and physiological adaptation: a cell survival pathway? Mediators Inflamm. 2015;2015:584758. doi:10.1155/2015/584758

[38] Heikkila M, Pasanen A, Kivirikko KI, Myllyharju J. Roles of the human hypoxia-inducible factor (HIF)-3alpha variants in the hypoxia response. Cell Mol Life Sci. 2011;68(23):3885–901. doi:10.1007/s00018-011-0679-5

[39] Ravenna L, Salvatori L, Russo MA. HIF3alpha: the little we know. FEBS J. 2016;283(6):993–1003. doi:10.1111/febs.13572

[40] Franzen S, Pihl L, Khan N, Gustafsson H, Palm F. Pronounced kidney hypoxia precedes albuminuria in type 1 diabetic mice. Am J Physiol Renal Physiol. 2016;310(9):F807–9. doi:10.1152/ajprenal.00049.2016

[41] Kriz W, LeHir M. Pathways to nephron loss starting from glomerular diseases-insights from animal models. Kidney Int. 2005;67(2):404–19. doi:10.1111/j.1523-1755.2005.67097.x

[42] Schlondorff DO. Overview of factors contributing to the pathophysiology of progressive renal disease. Kidney Int. 2008;74(7):860–6. doi:10.1038/ki.2008.351

[43] Thakur S, Viswanadhapalli S, Kopp JB, Shi Q, Barnes JL, Block K, Gorin Y, Abboud HE. Activation of AMP-activated protein kinase prevents TGF-beta1-induced epithelial-mesenchymal transition and myofibroblast activation. Am J Pathol. 2015;185(8):2168–80. doi:10.1016/j.ajpath.2015.04.014

[44] Lopez-Hernandez FJ, Lopez-Novoa JM. Role of TGF-beta in chronic kidney disease: an integration of tubular, glomerular and vascular effects. Cell Tissue Res. 2012;347(1): 141–54. doi:10.1007/s00441-011-1275-6

[45] Fujiu K, Manabe I, Nagai R. Renal collecting duct epithelial cells regulate inflammation in tubulointerstitial damage in mice. J Clin Invest. 2011;121(9):3425–41. doi:10.1172/JCI57582

[46] LeBleu VS, Taduri G, O'Connell J, Teng Y, Cooke VG, Woda C, Sugimoto H, Kalluri R. Origin and function of myofibroblasts in kidney fibrosis. Nat Med. 2013;19(8):1047–53. doi:10.1038/nm.3218

[47] Brookhart MA, Bradbury BD, Avorn J, Schneeweiss S, Winkelmayer WC. The effect of altitude change on anemia treatment response in hemodialysis patients. Am J Epidemiol. 2011;173(7):768–77. doi:10.1093/aje/kwq423

[48] Souma T, Nezu M, Nakano D, Yamazaki S, Hirano I, Sekine H, Dan T, Takeda K, Fong GH, Nishiyama A, Ito S, Miyata T, Yamamoto M, Suzuki N. Erythropoietin synthesis in renal myofibroblasts is restored by activation of hypoxia signaling. J Am Soc Nephrol. 2016;27(2):428–38. doi:10.1681/ASN.2014121184

[49] Kidney Disease: Improving Global Outcomes (KDIGO) Anemia Work Group. KDIGO Clinical practice guideline for anemia in chronic kidney disease. Kidney Int Suppl. 2012;2:279–335. doi:10.1038/kisup.2012.37

[50] Foley RN, Curtis BM, Parfrey PS. Erythropoietin therapy, hemoglobin targets, and quality of life in healthy hemodialysis patients: a randomized trial. Clin J Am Soc Nephrol. 2009;4(4):726–33. doi:10.2215/CJN.04950908

[51] Johansen KL, Finkelstein FO, Revicki DA, Evans C, Wan S, Gitlin M, Agodoa IL. Systematic review of the impact of erythropoiesis-stimulating agents on fatigue in dialysis patients. Nephrol Dial Transplant. 2012;27(6):2418–25. doi:10.1093/ndt/gfr697

[52] Gouva C, Nikolopoulos P, Ioannidis JP, Siamopoulos KC. Treating anemia early in renal failure patients slows the decline of renal function: a randomized controlled trial. Kidney Int. 2004;66(2):753–60. doi:10.1111/j.1523-1755.2004.00797.x

[53] Dean BB, Dylan M, Gano A Jr, Knight K, Ofman JJ, Levine BS. Erythropoiesis-stimulating protein therapy and the decline of renal function: a retrospective analysis of patients with chronic kidney disease. Curr Med Res Opin. 2005;21(7):981–7. doi:10.1185/030079905X49644

[54] Palazzuoli A, Silverberg D, Iovine F, Capobianco S, Giannotti G, Calabro A, Campagna SM, Nuti R. Erythropoietin improves anemia exercise tolerance and renal function and reduces B-type natriuretic peptide and hospitalization in patients with heart failure and anemia. Am Heart J. 2006;152(6):1096e9–15. doi:10.1016/j.ahj.2006.08.005

[55] Villar E, Lievre M, Kessler M, Lemaitre V, Alamartine E, Rodier M, Francois M, Zaoui P, Moranne O, Choukroun G, Guerraoui A, Jolivot A, Janin G, Branger B, Heng AE,

Boudray C, Bissery A, Rabilloud M, Pouteil-Noble C. Anemia normalization in patients with type 2 diabetes and chronic kidney disease: results of the NEPHRODIAB2 randomized trial. J Diabetes Complications. 2011;25(4):237–43. doi:10.1016/j.jdiacomp.2011.03.003

[56] Covic A, Nistor I, Donciu MD, Dumea R, Bolignano D, Goldsmith D. Erythropoiesis-stimulating agents (ESA) for preventing the progression of chronic kidney disease: a meta-analysis of 19 studies. Am J Nephrol. 2014;40(3):263–79. doi:10.1159/000366025

[57] Ogunshola OO, Bogdanova AY. Epo and non-hematopoietic cells: what do we know? Methods Mol Biol. 2013;982:13–41. doi:10.1007/978-1-62703-308-4_2

[58] Brines M, Grasso G, Fiordaliso F, Sfacteria A, Ghezzi P, Fratelli M, Latini R, Xie QW, Smart J, Su-Rick CJ, Pobre E, Diaz D, Gomez D, Hand C, Coleman T, Cerami A. Erythropoietin mediates tissue protection through an erythropoietin and common beta-subunit heteroreceptor. Proc Natl Acad Sci USA. 2004;101(41):14907–12. doi:10.1073/pnas.0406491101

[59] Brines M. The therapeutic potential of erythropoiesis-stimulating agents for tissue protection: a tale of two receptors. Blood Purif. 2010;29(2):86–92. doi:10.1159/000245630

[60] Bahlmann FH, Fliser D. Erythropoietin and renoprotection. Curr Opin Nephrol Hypertens. 2009;18(1):15–20. doi:10.1097/MNH.0b013e32831a9dde.00041552-200901000-00005 [pii]

[61] Bartnicki P, Kowalczyk M, Rysz J. The influence of the pleiotropic action of erythropoietin and its derivatives on nephroprotection. Med Sci Monit. 2013;19:599–605. doi:10.12659/MSM.889023

[62] Suttorp MM, Hoekstra T, Mittelman M, Ott I, Franssen CF, Dekker FW. Effect of erythropoiesis-stimulating agents on blood pressure in pre-dialysis patients. PLoS One. 2013;8(12):e84848. doi:10.1371/journal.pone.0084848

[63] Vinhas J, Barreto C, Assuncao J, Parreira L, Vaz A. Treatment of anaemia with erythropoiesis-stimulating agents in patients with chronic kidney disease does not lower mortality and may increase cardiovascular risk: a meta-analysis. Nephron Clin Pract. 2012;121(3–4):c95–101. doi:10.1159/000345158

[64] Jackevicius CA, Fan CS, Warner A. Clinical outcomes of erythropoietin use in heart failure patients with anemia of chronic kidney disease. J Card Fail. 2014;20(5):327–33. doi:10.1016/j.cardfail.2014.02.001

[65] Alsalimy N, Awaisu A. Methoxy polyethylene glycol-epoetin beta versus darbepoetin alfa for anemia in non-dialysis-dependent CKD: a systematic review. Int J Clin Pharm. 2014;36(6):1115–25. doi:10.1007/s11096-014-0023-x

[66] Winkelmayer WC, Chang TI, Mitani AA, Wilhelm-Leen ER, Ding V, Chertow GM, Brookhart MA, Goldstein BA. Longer-term outcomes of darbepoetin alfa versus epoetin alfa in patients with ESRD initiating hemodialysis: a quasi-experimental cohort study. Am J Kidney Dis. 2015;66(1):106–13. doi:10.1053/j.ajkd.2015.02.339

[67] Besarab A, Bolton WK, Browne JK, Egrie JC, Nissenson AR, Okamoto DM, Schwab SJ, Goodkin DA. The effects of normal as compared with low hematocrit values in patients with cardiac disease who are receiving hemodialysis and epoetin. N Engl J Med. 1998;339(9):584–90. doi:10.1056/NEJM199808273390903

[68] Drueke TB, Locatelli F, Clyne N, Eckardt KU, Macdougall IC, Tsakiris D, Burger HU, Scherhag A. Normalization of hemoglobin level in patients with chronic kidney disease and anemia. N Engl J Med. 2006;355(20):2071–84. doi:10.1056/NEJMoa062276

[69] Singh AK, Szczech L, Tang KL, Barnhart H, Sapp S, Wolfson M, Reddan D. Correction of anemia with epoetin alfa in chronic kidney disease. N Engl J Med. 2006;355(20):2085–98. doi:10.1056/NEJMoa065485

[70] Flamme I, Oehme F, Ellinghaus P, Jeske M, Keldenich J, Thuss U. Mimicking hypoxia to treat anemia: HIF-stabilizer BAY 85-3934 (Molidustat) stimulates erythropoietin production without hypertensive effects. PLoS One. 2014;9(11):e111838. doi:10.1371/journal.pone.0111838

[71] Provenzano R, Besarab A, Sun CH, Diamond SA, Durham JH, Cangiano JL, Aiello JR, Novak JE, Lee T, Leong R, Roberts BK, Saikali KG, Hemmerich S, Szczech LA, Yu KH, Neff TB. Oral hypoxia-inducible factor prolyl hydroxylase inhibitor roxadustat (FG-4592) for the treatment of anemia in patients with CKD. Clin J Am Soc Nephrol. 2016;11(6):982–91. doi:10.2215/CJN.06890615

[72] Besarab A, Chernyavskaya E, Motylev I, Shutov E, Kumbar LM, Gurevich K, Chan DT, Leong R, Poole L, Zhong M, Saikali KG, Franco M, Hemmerich S, Yu KH, Neff TB. Roxadustat (FG-4592): correction of anemia in incident dialysis patients. J Am Soc Nephrol. 2016;27(4):1225–33. doi:10.1681/ASN.2015030241

[73] Brigandi RA, Johnson B, Oei C, Westerman M, Olbina G, de Zoysa J, Roger SD, Sahay M, Cross N, McMahon L, Guptha V, Smolyarchuk EA, Singh N, Russ SF, Kumar S. A novel hypoxia-inducible factor-prolyl hydroxylase inhibitor (GSK1278863) for anemia in CKD: a 28-day, phase 2A randomized trial. Am J Kidney Dis. 2016;67(6):861–71. doi:10.1053/j.ajkd.2015.11.021

[74] Pedersen L, Wogensen L, Marcussen N, Cecchi CR, Dalsgaard T, Dagnaes-Hansen F. Restoration of haemoglobin level using hydrodynamic gene therapy with erythropoietin does not alleviate the disease progression in an anaemic mouse model for TGFbeta1-induced chronic kidney disease. PLoS One. 2015;10(6):e0128367. doi:10.1371/journal.pone.0128367

[75] KDOQI and National Kidney Foundation. KDOQI clinical practice guidelines and clinical practice recommendations for anemia in chronic kidney disease. Am J Kidney Dis. 2006;47:S11–145. doi:10.1053/j.ajkd.2006.03.010

[76] Panichi V, Rosati A, Bigazzi R, Paoletti S, Mantuano E, Beati S, Marchetti V, Bernabini G, Grazi G, Rizza GM, Migliori M, Giusti R, Lippi A, Casani A, Barsotti G, Tetta C. Anaemia and resistance to erythropoiesis-stimulating agents as prognostic factors in haemodialysis

patients: results from the RISCAVID study. Nephrol Dial Transplant. 2011;26(8):2641–8. doi:10.1093/ndt/gfq802

[77] Okazaki M, Komatsu M, Kawaguchi H, Tsuchiya K, Nitta K. Erythropoietin resistance index and the all-cause mortality of chronic hemodialysis patients. Blood Purif. 2014;37 (2):106–12. doi:10.1159/000358215

[78] Schneider A, Gutjahr-Lengsfeld L, Ritz E, Scharnagl H, Gelbrich G, Pilz S, Macdougall IC, Wanner C, Drechsler C. Longitudinal assessments of erythropoietin-stimulating agent responsiveness and the association with specific clinical outcomes in dialysis patients. Nephron Clin Pract. 2014;128:147–52. doi:10.1159/000367975

[79] Minutolo R, Conte G, Cianciaruso B, Bellizzi V, Camocardi A, De Paola L, De Nicola L. Hyporesponsiveness to erythropoiesis-stimulating agents and renal survival in non-dialysis CKD patients. Nephrol Dial Transplant. 2012;27(7):2880–6. doi:10.1093/ndt/gfs007

[80] Rossert J, Gassmann-Mayer C, Frei D, McClellan W. Prevalence and predictors of epoetin hyporesponsiveness in chronic kidney disease patients. Nephrol Dial Transplant. 2007;22(3):794–800. doi:10.1093/ndt/gfl716

[81] Gaweda AE, Goldsmith LJ, Brier ME, Aronoff GR. Iron, inflammation, dialysis adequacy, nutritional status, and hyperparathyroidism modify erythropoietic response. Clin J Am Soc Nephrol. 2010;5(4):576–81. doi:10.2215/CJN.04710709

[82] Sibbel SP, Koro CE, Brunelli SM, Cobitz AR. Characterization of chronic and acute ESA hyporesponse: a retrospective cohort study of hemodialysis patients. BMC Nephrol. 2015;16:144–53. doi:10.1186/s12882-015-0138-x

[83] Nangaku M, Mimura I, Yamaguchi J, Higashijima Y, Wada T, Tanaka T. Role of uremic toxins in erythropoiesis-stimulating agent resistance in chronic kidney disease and dialysis patients. J Ren Nutr. 2015;25(2):160–3. doi:10.1053/j.jrn.2014.10.011

[84] Straat M, van Bruggen R, de Korte D, Juffermans NP. Red blood cell clearance in inflammation. Transfus Med Hemother. 2012;39(5):353–61. doi:10.1159/000342229

[85] Chawla LS, Krishnan M. Causes and consequences of inflammation on anemia management in hemodialysis patients. Hemodial Int. 2009;13(2):222–34. doi:10.1111/j.1542-4758.2009.00352.x

[86] Hom J, Dulmovits BM, Mohandas N, Blanc L. The erythroblastic island as an emerging paradigm in the anemia of inflammation. Immunol Res. 2015;63:75–89. doi:10.1007/s12026-015-8697-2

[87] Costa E, Swinkels DW, Laarakkers CM, Rocha-Pereira P, Rocha S, Reis F, Teixeira F, Miranda V, do Sameiro Faria M, Loureiro A, Quintanilha A, Belo L, Santos-Silva A. Hepcidin serum levels and resistance to recombinant human erythropoietin therapy in haemodialysis patients. Acta Haematol. 2009;122(4):226–9. doi:10.1159/000253590

[88] Won HS, Kim HG, Yun YS, Jeon EK, Ko YH, Kim YS, Kim YO, Yoon SA. IL-6 is an independent risk factor for resistance to erythropoiesis-stimulating agents in

hemodialysis patients without iron deficiency. Hemodial Int. 2012;16(1):31–7. doi:10.1111/j.1542-4758.2011.00635.x

[89] Kimachi M, Fukuma S, Yamazaki S, Yamamoto Y, Akizawa T, Akiba T, Saito A, Fukuhara S. Minor elevation in C-reactive protein levels predicts incidence of erythropoiesis-stimulating agent hyporesponsiveness among hemodialysis patients. Nephron. 2015;131(2):123–30. doi:10.1159/000438870

[90] Costa E, Rocha S, Rocha-Pereira P, Nascimento H, Castro E, Miranda V, Faria Mdo S, Loureiro A, Quintanilha A, Belo L, Santos-Silva A. Neutrophil activation and resistance to recombinant human erythropoietin therapy in hemodialysis patients. Am J Nephrol. 2008;28(6):935–40. doi:10.1159/000142147

[91] do Sameiro-Faria M, Ribeiro S, Costa E, Mendonca D, Teixeira L, Rocha-Pereira P, Fernandes J, Nascimento H, Kohlova M, Reis F, Amado L, Bronze-da-Rocha E, Miranda V, Quintanilha A, Belo L, Santos-Silva A. Risk factors for mortality in hemodialysis patients: two-year follow-up study. Dis Markers. 2013;35(6):791–8. doi:10.1155/2013/518945

[92] Ribeiro S, Garrido P, Fernandes J, Vala H, Rocha-Pereira P, Costa E, Belo L, Reis F, Santos-Silva A. Pathological and molecular mechanisms underlying resistance to recombinant human erythropoietin therapy in the remnant kidney rat model of chronic kidney disease associated anemia. Biochimie. 2016;125:150–62. doi:10.1016/j.biochi.2016.03.012

[93] Rosenberger C, Mandriota S, Jurgensen JS, Wiesener MS, Horstrup JH, Frei U, Ratcliffe PJ, Maxwell PH, Bachmann S, Eckardt KU. Expression of hypoxia-inducible factor-1alpha and -2alpha in hypoxic and ischemic rat kidneys. J Am Soc Nephrol. 2002;13(7):1721–32. doi:10.1097/01.ASN.0000017223.49823.2A

[94] Higgins DF, Kimura K, Bernhardt WM, Shrimanker N, Akai Y, Hohenstein B, Saito Y, Johnson RS, Kretzler M, Cohen CD, Eckardt KU, Iwano M, Haase VH. Hypoxia promotes fibrogenesis in vivo via HIF-1 stimulation of epithelial-to-mesenchymal transition. J Clin Invest. 2007;117(12):3810–20. doi:10.1172/JCI30487

[95] Yu X, Fang Y, Ding X, Liu H, Zhu J, Zou J, Xu X, Zhong Y. Transient hypoxia-inducible factor activation in rat renal ablation and reduced fibrosis with L-mimosine. Nephrology (Carlton). 2012;17(1):58–67. doi:10.1111/j.1440-1797.2011.01498.x

[96] Higgins DF, Biju MP, Akai Y, Wutz A, Johnson RS, Haase VH. Hypoxic induction of Ctgf is directly mediated by Hif-1. Am J Physiol Renal Physiol. 2004;287(6):F1223–32. doi:10.1152/ajprenal.00245.2004

[97] Slagman MC, Nguyen TQ, Waanders F, Vogt L, Hemmelder MH, Laverman GD, Goldschmeding R, Navis G. Effects of antiproteinuric intervention on elevated connective tissue growth factor (CTGF/CCN-2) plasma and urine levels in nondiabetic nephropathy. Clin J Am Soc Nephrol. 2011;6(8):1845–50. doi:10.2215/CJN.08190910

[98] Okada H, Kikuta T, Kobayashi T, Inoue T, Kanno Y, Takigawa M, Sugaya T, Kopp JB, Suzuki H. Connective tissue growth factor expressed in tubular epithelium plays a

pivotal role in renal fibrogenesis. J Am Soc Nephrol. 2005;16(1):133–43. doi:10.1681/ASN.2004040339

[99] Basu RK, Hubchak S, Hayashida T, Runyan CE, Schumacker PT, Schnaper HW. Interdependence of HIF-1alpha and TGF-beta/Smad3 signaling in normoxic and hypoxic renal epithelial cell collagen expression. Am J Physiol Renal Physiol. 2011;300(4): F898–905. doi:10.1152/ajprenal.00335.2010

[100] Haase VH. Inflammation and hypoxia in the kidney: friends or foes? Kidney Int. 2015;88 (2):213–5. doi:10.1038/ki.2015.89

[101] Scholz CC, Cavadas MA, Tambuwala MM, Hams E, Rodriguez J, von Kriegsheim A, Cotter P, Bruning U, Fallon PG, Cheong A, Cummins EP, Taylor CT. Regulation of IL-1beta-induced NF-kappaB by hydroxylases links key hypoxic and inflammatory signaling pathways. Proc Natl Acad Sci USA. 2013;110(46):18490–5. doi:10.1073/pnas.13097 18110

[102] Nasri H. Renal cell protection of erythropoietin beyond correcting the anemia in chronic kidney disease patients. Cell J. 2014;15(4):378–80.

[103] Gobe GC, Bennett NC, West M, Colditz P, Brown L, Vesey DA, Johnson DW. Increased progression to kidney fibrosis after erythropoietin is used as a treatment for acute kidney injury. Am J Physiol Renal Physiol. 2014;306(6):F681–92. doi:10.1152/ajprenal.00 241.2013

Chapter 15

Role of the Hypoxia-Inducible Factor in Periodontal Inflammation

Xiao Xiao Wang, Yu Chen and Wai Keung Leung

Additional information is available at the end of the chapter

http://dx.doi.org/10.5772/66037

Abstract

Human periodontitis is a chronic inflammatory disease induced by opportunistic Gram-negative anaerobic bacteria at the tooth-supporting apparatus. Within the gingivitis-affected sulcus or periodontal pocket, the resident anaerobic bacteria interact with the host inflammatory reactions leading to a lower oxygen or hypoxic environment. A cellular/tissue oxygen-sensing mechanism and its appropriate regulation are needed to assist tissue adaptation to natural/pathology-induced variations in oxygen availability. In this chapter, we reviewed the biological relevance of hypoxia in periodontal/oral cellular development, epithelial barrier function, periodontal inflammation, and immunity. The role of hypoxia-inducible factor-1α in pathogen-host cross talk and alveolar bone homeostasis was also discussed. The naturally occurring pathophysiological process of hypoxia appeared to entail fundamental relevance for periodontal defense and regeneration.

Keywords: cell hypoxia, chronic periodontitis, hypoxia-inducible factor-1, alpha subunit

1. Introduction

Regardless of the oxygen sources, when an animal acquires oxygen through its breathing apparatus, the oxygen will have to pass under a reducing partial oxygen pressure (pO_2) gradient from the source via circulation to different organs and then tissues and cells. In mammals, such as rats, inspired pO_2 is around 21.3 kPa at sea level. When blood flows through the alveolar capillaries, it drops to approximately 14 kPa and is then progressively reduced to 2.1, 1.3, and 0.27–3.3 kPa in the spleen, thymus, and retina, respectively [1, 2], while in the brain, it may be as low as 0.05–1.07 kPa, depending on the cranial location [3].

Due to the colonization by subgingival biofilm, oxygen is persistently consumed to various extents by the facultative anaerobic microbes within the periodontal sulcus (2.33–8.40 kPa). In the gingivitis-affected sulcus or periodontal pocket, the inflammation induced by the residential anaerobic bacteria with or without microulcerations or wounding leads to an even lower oxygen tension [4]. At the tissue level, the availability of oxygen is dependent on the distance from the oxygen-supplying blood vessels. Although the diffusion distance of oxygen *in vivo* is estimated to be 100–200 μm, a pO_2 of almost zero has been recorded in tissues 100 μm away from the nourishing blood vessels [5]. Therefore, a cellular/tissue oxygen-sensing mechanism is needed to assist tissue adaptation to nature/pathology-induced variations in oxygen availability.

In humans, a drop in oxygen concentration in the atmosphere is sensed by the carotid body at the bifurcation of the carotid arteries, which then increases the rate and depth of breathing. At the levels of tissues and cells, including the human periodontium, such adaptive responses to low oxygen tension or hypoxia are mainly mediated through a key cellular transcription factor named the hypoxia-inducible factor (HIF) [6].

2. Hypoxia in the oral/periodontal environment

Oxygen is an essential molecule for survival. Mammals—including humans—depend on oxygen for electron transport, oxidative phosphorylation, and energy generation. Variations in tissue oxygen needs are attributed to a number of physiological or pathological states, meaning that the tissues concerned have to be able to adapt to various O_2 environments including hypoxia. To survive, mammalian cells evolved in such a way that cellular O_2 availability or homeostasis could be monitored and tightly regulated [7]. This is made possible by a cellular HIF system. Cellular hypoxia, or a lower than "normal" concentration of O_2 in cells, occurs commonly and could induce significant changes, immediate or delayed, on cellular processes, including cell growth and apoptosis, cell proliferation and survival, pH regulation and energy metabolism, cell migration, matrix and barrier function, angiogenesis, and vasomotor regulation [8–13]. These biological processes involve active responses by the body to secure an additional oxygen supply via circulation. Such dynamic processes of cellular/tissue oxygen monitoring, O_2 consumption, and delivery, corresponding to the respective cellular/tissue functional state, are tightly controlled to ensure proper survival of the multicellular organism concerned [14].

As described earlier, the normal tissue/cellular pO_2 levels in mammals are dependent on their location and physiology and, hence, vary among different human body compartments and cell/tissue conditions [15]. Hypoxia in oral cells/tissues is, in fact, a common occurrence [6]. The local hypoxic microenvironment is considered a consequence of growth/development, wound healing, smoking habits, or concurrent oral inflammation/infection/diseases.

Taking oral cellular development/regeneration as an example, the blood vessel network is promoted by vascular endothelial growth factors (VEGF) secreted by stem cells from apical papilla under hypoxia, suggesting a role of hypoxia in pulp revascularization and bioengineered pulp

http://dx.doi.org/10.5772/66037

replacements [16]. On the other hand, it is reported that extreme hypoxia-like response induced by the chemical cobalt chloride ($CoCl_2$) could stimulate periodontal ligament (PDL) stem cell cytotoxicity through mitochondria-apoptotic and autophagic pathways involving HIF-1α [17]. During pathological processes, it is reported that a low oxygen level may regulate cell migration of oral cancer cells, thus influencing the invasion and metastasis in malignant oral lesions [18].

With reference to growth, increasing evidence shows that certain hormonal regulation could be interfered with hypoxia or HIF [19]. For instance, it is reported that growth hormone expression in lymphocytes and parathyroid hormone-related protein in articular chondrocytes can be induced by hypoxia [20, 21]. We postulate that if similar biology could be expressed in the head and neck region, HIF or hypoxia may bring profound effects on the growth and development of orofacial structures.

3. Hypoxia and chronic periodontal inflammation

Metabolic shifts under hypoxia are common occurrences in the periodontal inflammatory process as a result of the imbalance between the tissue oxygen supply and consumption [22]. The accumulation of intracellular HIF-1 promotes the transcription of a spectrum of genes to maintain cellular homeostasis. Hypoxia induces the expression of a number of angiogenic factors to improve the blood supply in needed areas including inflamed periodontium [6]. These include VEGF, platelet-derived growth factor (PDGF), and angioprotein-1 and -2. Related genes produce controlling perfusion, such as the PDGF-β receptor, cyclooxygenase-2, and nitric oxide synthase (NOS), of which NOS modulates vascular smooth muscle cells' functions and reacts to changes in the cellular HIF-1 level [23]. Moreover, HIF activation promotes a metabolic switch to reduce oxygen consumption by shifting energy metabolism from aerobic respiration to glycolysis. Activation of HIF also upregulates the expression of pyruvate dehydrogenase kinase, which reduces the incorporation of pyruvate into the citric acid cycle [24]. This metabolic switch is essential for the hosts' defense because such HIF-1α–regulated glycolytic metabolism is required in B cell development [25] and T cell metabolism [26].

Under a chronic inflammatory state, hypoxia induces protective cellular responses or a local defense. However, if the cause of inflammation cannot be eradicated, such hypoxic cell/tissue reactions contribute to the pathophysiology of inflammation and, hence, disease pathogenesis [27]. A similar scenario can be observed within the human periodontium in periodontitis. Periodontitis is characterized by chronic inflammation of the tooth-supporting tissues, initiated by a multitude of Gram-negative anaerobic pathogens including *Aggregatibacter actinomycetemcomitans*, *Porphyromonas gingivalis*, *Tannerella forsythia*, *Treponema denticola*, and so on [28]. At sites where a chronic inflammatory reaction could be found, oxygen consumption is elevated and blood perfusion is stimulated, but the actual local microcirculation could be compromised [29]. This local tissue pO_2 change is partly due to increased oxygen consumption, including oxygen usage by both resident cells and infiltrated defense cells, and partly because of diminished oxygen availability due to endothelial damage and vasoconstricted microcirculation.

Local hypoxia in periodontitis in turn enhances the anaerobic Gram-negative pathogens' survival and further lowers the oxygen tension at the vicinity. The tissue hypoxia in periodontal disease has been characterized by increased HIF-1α protein that is detectable in periodontitis-affected tissue biopsies using Western blot and anti–HIF-1α immunostaining [6, 30]. Myeloid cell lineage of HIF-1$\alpha^{-/-}$ (deprived) mice had impaired immune effector molecules, such as nitric oxide (NO) and tumor necrosis factor-alpha (TNF-α) production, thus reducing their bactericidal capability [31]. Therefore, the ability to adapt to a reduced oxygen supply, which maintains immune cell surveillance capability in all tissue environments, is important and necessary in the successful elimination of pathogens [32].

Proinflammatory cytokines and matrix metalloproteinases (MMPs) act as mediators for the inflammation process or play a role in extracellular matrix degradation, respectively. Researchers often investigate the levels of such biological markers in the periodontium in attempts to gauge the severity of periodontal disease and monitor periodontal treatment outcomes [33]. Recent studies reported that a hypoxic environment may upregulate proinflammatory cytokines and MMPs' expression from host cells during periodontal disease [34]. The idea was that hypoxia further encourages lipopolysaccharide (LPS)-induced TNF-α, interleukin-1β, and interleukin 6 (IL-6) expressions via LPS toll-like receptor (TLR) interaction that, in turn, activates the nuclear factor kappa B (NF-κB) pathway in human PDL cells upon exposure to the aforementioned Gram-negative bacterial surface component [35–37].

At the collagen destruction front, periodontal epithelial cells could produce MMPs in response to bacteria-induced activation of pathogen-associated molecular patterns (PAMP) including TLRs. These host enzymes contribute to the extracellular matrix degradation that accommodates local inflammatory reactions, as well as the later tissue remodeling that ensues once inflammation stops [38, 39]. Inhibition of HIF-1α activity by chetomin, a *Chaetomium* metabolite that can incapacitate tumor cells' hypoxic adaptation or knockdown HIF-1α gene expression by small, interfering RNA, could markedly attenuate the production of LPS- and nicotine-stimulated MMPs and prostaglandin E_2 from PDL cells. Such observations suggest the possibility of HIF-1α being a potential target in periodontal tissue destruction associated with smoking and dental plaque [40]. Further supporting the idea that hypoxia may be one of the key biological responses in periodontal inflammation.

Certain periodontopathogens, other than acting as effective mediators of periodontal inflammation, are capable of doing more harm to a host under a low pO_2 environment. For instance, *P. gingivalis* LPS under hypoxia increases PDL fibroblasts' oxidative stress and induces a reduction of catalase, indicating a collapse of the protective machinery favoring the increase in reactive oxygen species (ROS) and the progression of inflammatory oral diseases [41].

Considering the healing of oral wounds, several studies reported that the biological process in general could be enhanced or accelerated under hypoxia via HIF-1 [42, 43]. For example, the wound healing of rat palatal mucosa was enhanced by the hydroxylase inhibitor dimethyloxalylglycine, a HIF-1α stabilizer, under a hypoxic environment, and this enzyme was reported to induce hypoxia-mimetic angiogenesis [44]. With reference to hard tissue healing, $CoCl_2$ triggered the expression of angiogenic mediators and bone turnover-related genes, which promoted fracture healing and repair *in vivo* [45]. The research report also indicated that, during distraction osteogenesis, an angiogenic effect and bone healing could be promoted by conditioned media collected from dental pulp cells under hypoxia [46]. These findings implied the possibility that a low tissue oxygen level may act as a biological signal, promoting soft and hard tissue healing, including that of the orofacial regions, mediated through inflammation.

4. Hypoxia and periodontal immunity

Hypoxic responses or HIF is reported to be strongly related to innate human responses, with low oxygen modulating energy metabolism and various genes' expression within defense cells that, in turn, dictate the immune performance and the host protection outcomes [47]. The biological impact of low pO_2 on T cells' functions was reflected by the HIF-1– and adenosine receptor–modulated effects [48]. Indeed, both lymphocytes and myeloid cells were affected and the hypoxia-induced adaptive immune response changes would interfere or affect the innate immunity. The relevance of hypoxia in pathological processes was well established upon the appreciation that wounds, infectious loci, and tumor growth each involved extremely low oxygen tension [1].

It has been well appreciated that low oxygen tension is common at inflamed periodontitis sites [4]; thus, the corresponding local immune responses must adapt to the hypoxic challenges. As mentioned above, hypoxia plays an important role in modulating the cellular activities of innate and adaptive immunity, so the impact of low pO_2 in periodontal immune responses is quite significant.

Oral innate immunity is the first line of defense against periodontopathogens, which functions to recognize, attenuate, and eliminate the nonself invaders and to trigger downstream immune responses. Granulocytes and monocytes/macrophages are the main cell types for innate periodontal immunity [49, 50]. When extensive inflammation takes place, these cells have to travel into the tissue compartment with low pO_2 (i.e., the infected area) to provide defense and wall-off the invasion. To prevent the invasion, intense energy metabolism has to occur within the involved innate defense cells. An appropriate hypoxic cellular reaction and adaptation is, therefore, very important in the periodontal innate immune cells, which develop functional and survival responses regulated by the oxygen sensor HIF [51].

Defense cells rely heavily on glycolysis for the production of ATP to compensate for the limited oxidative metabolism in hypoxia. Immune cell energy metabolism appeared to significantly influence its corresponding response. As a critical modulator for the expression of glycolytic enzymes, the absence of HIF-1α leads to a significant reduction of ATP availability in myeloid cells [52]. It was reported that a knockdown of HIF-1α protein led to a nullified IL-6 production when exposed to LPS, suggesting that HIF-1α supported the LPS-dependent expression of IL-6 that, in turn, prevented the depletion of ATP and, therefore, protected myeloid cells against LPS/TLR4-induced apoptosis [53]. In human monocytes, LPS and hypoxia synergistically activated HIF-1 through p44/42 mitogen-activated protein kinases (MAPK) and NF-κB; however, repetitive exposure to LPS could induce tolerance to bacterial endotoxins and, hence, impair corresponding HIF-1α induction, which reduces the ability of monocytic cells to survive and function under low oxygen [54, 55].

To combat invading pathogens, HIF also promotes polymorphonuclear neutrophil (PMN) recruitment via the restoration of blood flow at inflamed tissues and enhances neovascularization. With hypoxia, the HIF restored perfusion also facilitates PMNs' diapedesis [56, 57]. Furthermore, PMN apoptosis was attenuated under hypoxia, with HIF-1α reported to be a protective factor in the regulation of its functional longevity [58]. Such longevity regulation involved NF-κB signaling that was found to be essential in constitutive HIF-1 protein translation [58, 59].

The cellular stress-related transcription factor NF-κB is closely related to hypoxia despite the fact that the relationship is not yet completely understood. It was reported that classical or canonical NF-κB activation under the stress of hypoxia often involves the activation of transforming growth factor-B-activating kinase and the inhibitor of κB kinase (IKK) complex [60]. In addition to classical NF-κB signaling, the noncanonical NF-κB pathway could be activated by hypoxia independent of HIF-1α via NF-κB-inducing kinase and IKK homodimer activation [61]. ROS, a key inflammatory regulator in chronic periodontal inflammation, is confirmed to mediate HIF-1α induction dependent on NF-κB [62].

Dendritic cells (DCs), a group of professional antigen-presenting cells, are key members that enable cross talk between the innate and adaptive immune systems. They present an antigen to activate naive lymphocytes and assist in the development of specific adaptive immune responses to pathogens. Hypoxia has been found to play an important role in the maturation and cytokines release of DCs, but the mechanism of the related divergent effects still remains controversial [63]. Studies found that the knockdown of HIF-1α in DCs inhibited their maturation and significantly impaired their capability to stimulate allogeneic T cells, probably because of the reliance on the HIF-controlled glycolysis [64, 65]. In contrast, it is reported that low oxygen tension inhibited the DCs' defense against LPS, but strongly upregulated the production of proinflammatory cytokines in the cells involved [66]. Similar results can be observed in the human antifungal response: hypoxia at the site of *Aspergillus fumigatus* infection inhibited the full activation and function of DCs [67]. These findings suggest that hypoxia may function as a regulator against DCs' mediated immune overreaction.

Lymphocytes are known to be involved in periodontal tissues' health homeostasis, and their functional upset was believed to be associated with periodontal pathogenesis. An HIF-1α deficiency was associated with abnormal B cell development, which led to autoimmunity in a mouse model [68]. A recent study also indicated that T cells' HIF-1α regulation played a critical role in avoiding cardiac damage in diabetic mice [69]. We postulated that a similar protection mechanism may be called to function in diabetic periodontium. Therefore, hypoxia or HIF-1α regulation in DCs and lymphocytes may confer a marked impact on the innate and adaptive cellular immunity in periodontal tissues, with the exact mechanism yet to be elucidated.

5. HIF and epithelial barrier function

The human periodontium is a unique environment for microorganisms. One special characteristic is the nonshedding tooth's hard tissue surface, allowing microorganisms to remain *in situ*. To counter the invasion of possible pathogens, the corresponding epithelial tissues build up an effective barrier against the colonizing microbes [70]. With appropriate daily oral hygiene, the continued host-bacteria interaction maintains the periodontium in health or low grade/subclinical inflammation. Those who have inadequate oral hygiene tip the balance toward a proinflammatory state, resulting in inflammatory responses that present clinically as gingivitis. Due to poor oral hygiene and inherited or acquired risks, approximately 20% of the human population, develop chronic periodontal inflammation with tissue destruction resulting in what is known as periodontitis [71]. Regardless of the host-parasitic interaction outcomes, humans and their complex residential microflora have coevolved over time [72].

TLRs on the periodontal/gingival epithelial cells recognize the conserved molecular patterns on pathogenic bacteria that are also known as PAMP, limiting invasion of the microbes, and help to maintain oral health [73]. Other than providing a physical barrier to the outside world, the skin and mucosal membrane produce a number of antimicrobial peptides (AMPs). The AMPs have a broad activity spectrum against both Gram-negative and Gram-positive bacteria colonization, enveloped viruses, fungi, and even transformed or cancerous cells.

It has become clear that AMPs, such as defensins and the cathelicidins family of peptides—especially LL-37, play important roles independently or together in maintaining oral health, including antimicrobial effects and mediating chemotaxis of the immune cells [74, 75]. Researchers reported that a deficit of cathelicidin allowed infection by *A. actinomycetemcomitans* and the development of severe periodontitis [76].

The epithelial cells in both oral mucosa and the gut are relatively hypoxic [4, 77]. The corresponding oxygen gradient between the epithelium and subepithelial perfusion in turn provides a matching cellular HIF-1α gradient in the tissues involved and perhaps the respective physiological function in cellular homeostasis. In human intestine, when the oxygen supply was impaired due to stasis of the local perfusion, the affected site would be left with increased susceptibility to infection [78]. As such, appropriate adaptive response to hypoxia at the epithelial barriers is vital. HIF-1α functions as an intracellular pO_2 sensor, enabling appropriate adaptive responses for cell survival. Using prolyl hydroxylase inhibitor or AKB-4924, a HIF-1α stabilizing agent, production of cathelicidin and β-defensin in uroepithelial cells was significantly enhanced, and *Escherichia coli* infection was deterred [79]. On the other hand, a deletion of HIF-1α in skin keratinocytes decreased the production of cathelicidin and led to increased susceptibility of infection by a group of *A. Streptococcus* [80]. Naturally occurring low-grade hypoxic reaction and hence HIF-1 accumulation in gut/urogenital/skin epithelia followed by corresponding HIF-1 downstream genes expression were recently postulated to be a key concept that underpin biological barrier function of intestinal epithelium [77, 81]. If in case the same biological process is also in action at the dentogingival junction, HIF-1 would contribute in the periodontal epithelial barrier function that maintains periodontal health and prevents oral pathogenic microorganism invasion.

Besides AMPs, there are also many factors regulated by HIF at the periodontal epithelial barrier. For instance, trefoil factors (TFF), secreted molecules from mucous epithelia, were involved in oral protection against tissue damage and immune response [82, 83]. Their expression was influenced by cellular pO_2 levels. It was reported that HIF-1 mediated the induction of TFF gene expression and provided an adaptive link for the maintenance of the barrier function during hypoxia of gastric/intestinal lining cells [84, 85]. Salivary mucins form a protective layer on the oral surfaces including that of oral sulcular and junctional epithelia, which serve as a physical barrier against bacterial invasion and function as essential antimicrobial macromolecules [86, 87]. Similar to TFF, mucins' production was upregulated in hypoxia [88]. This evidence indicated that the epithelial barrier cells' HIF regulation may constitute an important defense mechanism. Such oral protective machinery could contribute an additional local defense mechanism against periodontal diseases.

6. HIF in the periodontopathogen-host cross talk

Hypoxia is common in the inflammatory microenvironment, and appropriate cellular responses to hypoxia contribute to mucosal defense through the oxygen-sensitive transcription regulator HIF-1α. Hypoxia increases the expression of certain TLRs on human gingival keratinocytes [89], the interaction of low oxygen with appropriate bacteria ligands *in vivo* could potentially enhance the production of cytokines and antimicrobial peptides and thus, in theory, could help to eliminate or reduce the pathogen-related concerns.

The human periodontium is persistently exposed to risks of infection; the source is the commensal and pathogenic oral microorganisms constituting the dental plaque adhering onto teeth. Bacterial components, such as LPS and peptidoglycans, released by bacteria recognized by TLRs on the surface of host cells could instigate the inflammatory reaction cascade [38]. Under steady-state conditions, activation of TLRs by commensal bacteria is critical for the maintenance of oral health [73]. Thus, TLRs provide the first line of defense in periodontal health maintenance. When stimulated, such as via TLRs recognition, PMNs exhibit increased chemotaxis and proinflammatory cytokine production [90].

Our group previously reported that bacterial components may induce HIF-1α accumulation during periodontal disease pathogenesis independent of hypoxia [91]. An immunoprecipitation experiment showed that human gingival fibroblasts' HIF-1α accumulation was induced by LPS in the dose- and time-dependent manner. The accumulation of HIF-1α may be modulated by TLRs and pattern recognition in certain ways, since a TLR4 neutralizing antibody could attenuate such an effect from *E. coli* LPS. Moreover, the expression of TLR4, CD14, and MD-2 in both human gingival keratinocytes and fibroblasts is confirmed, and the TLR4 protein expression in periodontal epithelial compartments appeared different *in vivo*, indicating that LPS sensing in the dentogingival front in health could be heterogeneous in nature [92].

A recent study on oral squamous cell carcinoma provided a novel mechanism of HIF-1 and TLRs' interplay. It was reported that the activation of TLR3 and TLR4 stimulated the expression of HIF-1 through NF-κB, while HIF-1 accumulation increased the expression of TLR3 and TLR4 through direct promoter binding [93]. This observation provided evidence that the TLR3/4-NF-κB pathway may form a positive feedback loop with HIF-1, which theoretically could also happen in the periodontal tissue. Further investigations are needed to confirm such a postulation.

7. HIF and bone homeostasis

HIF appears to play important functional roles in bone homeostasis. The regulatory system seemed complex because HIF is known to stimulate both bone resorption and regeneration, the two essential biological processes in bone homeostasis/repair.

It is reported that a lack of oxygen in periodontal tissues may contribute to alveolar bone resorption and, in theory, accelerated periodontitis [94]. Chromatin immunoprecipitation showed that HIF-1α binds to the receptor activator of the NF-κB ligand (RANKL) promoter region, and mutations of the putative HIF-1α binding site prevented hypoxia-induced RANKL transcriptional promotion, thus suggesting that HIF-1α mediates hypoxia-induced upregulation of RANKL expression and enhanced osteoclastogenesis [95]. Furthermore, it was reported that hypoxia triggered the differentiation of peripheral mononuclear blood cells into functional osteoclasts in a HIF-dependent manner [96].

Conversely, in recent studies, HIF-1α was considered to be a critical mediator of neoangiogenesis required for bone regeneration. Exposure of PDL stem cells to hypoxia improved their osteogenic potential, mineralization and paracrine release, and the mitogen-activated protein kinase kinase/extracellular signal-regulated kinase, and p38 MAPK signaling pathways were involved [97–99]. It was suggested that HIF, HIF mimicking agents, or HIF stabilizing agents were considered triggers for the initiation and promotion of angiogenic-osteogenic coupling [100, 101]. A recent animal study reported new bone and vessels formation induced by the overexpression of HIF-1α via adenovirus, leading to enhanced alveolar bone defect regeneration [102]. A similar result was reported from a study investigating bone loss arrest in ovariectomized C57BL/6 J mice via activated HIF-1α and Wnt/β-catenin signaling pathways [103]. Cementoblastic differentiation of human dental stem cells, a key cellular mechanism concerning periodontal regeneration, was reported to be stimulated by hypoxia in an HIF-1-dependent manner [104].

Taken together, these reports suggested that HIF-1α plays a part in alveolar bone homeostasis, resorption, or periodontal regeneration, while the exact nature of HIF-1α's roles in these processes and the way in which the related pathophysiological processes were regulated warrants further investigations.

8. Conclusions

It seems that tissue/cellular hypoxia, or more specifically, expression of HIF-1α, is involved in periodontal inflammation. HIF-1 not only mediates the host's immune response, providing defense against microbial invaders and maintaining periodontal health, but also could facilitate periodontal-supporting tissue breakdown and, hence, the progression of periodontitis.

Putting all currently available information together, it appears that hypoxia could bring either beneficial or detrimental effects on periodontal health. At the present juncture, we hypothesize that similar to the intestines, a low-grade hypoxia or low level of HIF-1 is expressed in the human periodontium for baseline defense or to act as a surveillance "alarm" against significant invasion or periodontitis. A successful immune response that associates with appropriate HIF-1 mediated biological reactions would result in periodontal health maintenance. Over- or underactivation of the immune system with or without the corresponding dysregulation of HIF-1 biology in tissues as well as alveolar bone, however, could give rise to periodontal tissue damages. We also postulate that other risk indicators related to progression of periodontitis, such as smoking and diabetes mellitus, under the influence of periodontal plaque biofilm, may exert their harmful effects via inappropriate activation of the HIF pathway. Effects of these risks indicators are particular relevant as they often undermine proper periodontal healing/regeneration after therapy [105].

The mechanisms underlying the role of HIF-1 and periodontal defense/pathogenesis, however, remain elusive. Further investigations are, therefore, required in these directions to decipher what leads to the unfavorable immune reactions in periodontal inflammation and the reasons why that came about. Such new knowledge not only fosters the further understanding of human periodontal disease pathogenesis, but may provide novel therapeutic strategies that take advantage of the new understandings of periodontal HIF biology, an important element relevant for periodontal defense and regeneration.

Acknowledgments

The work described in this paper was substantially supported by grants from the Research Grants Council of the Hong Kong Special Administrative Region, China (HKU 17113114), the University of Hong Kong Small Project Funding (201007176307, 201109176129), and Seed Funding (200911159126).

Author details

Xiao Xiao Wang[1], Yu Chen[2,†] and Wai Keung Leung[2,*]

*Address all correspondence to: ewkleung@hku.hk

1 Guanghua School of Stomatology, Provincial Key Laboratory of Stomatology, Sun Yat-sen University, Guangzhou, Guangdong, PR China

2 Faculty of Dentistry, The University of Hong Kong, Hong Kong SAR, PR China

† Current address: Department of Periodontology, Nanjing Stomatology Hospital, Nanjing, Jiangsu Province, PR China

References

[1] Braun RD, Lanzen JL, Snyder SA, Dewhirst MW. Comparison of tumor and normal tissue oxygen tension measurements using OxyLite or microelectrodes in rodents. Am J Physiol Heart Circ Physiol. 2001;280(6):H2533–44.

[2] Yu DY, Cringle SJ. Retinal degeneration and local oxygen metabolism. Exp Eye Res. 2005;80(6):745–51.

[3] Erecinska M, Silver IA. Tissue oxygen tension and brain sensitivity to hypoxia. Respir Physiol. 2001;128(3):263–76.

[4] Mettraux GR, Gusberti FA, Graf H. Oxygen tension (pO_2) in untreated human periodontal pockets. J Periodontol. 1984;55(9):516–21.

[5] Zhu H, Bunn HF. Oxygen sensing and signaling: impact on the regulation of physiologically important genes. Respir Physiol. 1999;115(2):239–47.

[6] Ng KT, Li JP, Ng KM, Tipoe GL, Leung WK, Fung ML. Expression of hypoxia-inducible factor-1alpha in human periodontal tissue. J Periodontol. 2011;82(1):136–41.

[7] Piruat JI, López-Barneo J. Oxygen tension regulates mitochondrial DNA-encoded complex I gene expression. J Biol Chem. 2005;280(52):42676–84.

[8] Semba H, Takeda N, Isagawa T, Sugiura Y, Honda K, Wake M, et al. HIF-1alpha-PDK1 axis-induced active glycolysis plays an essential role in macrophage migratory capacity. Nat Commun. 2016;7:11635.

[9] Wu D, Chen B, Cui F, He X, Wang W, Wang M. Hypoxia-induced microRNA-301b regulates apoptosis by targeting Bim in lung cancer. Cell Prolif. 2016;49(4):476–83.

[10] Li X, Liu Y, Ma H, Guan Y, Cao Y, Tian Y, et al. Enhancement of glucose metabolism via PGC-1alpha participates in the cardioprotection of chronic intermittent hypobaric hypoxia. Front Physiol. 2016;7:219.

[11] Katayama K, Ishida K, Saito M, Koike T, Ogoh S. Hypoxia attenuates cardiopulmonary reflex control of sympathetic nerve activity during mild dynamic leg exercise. Exp Physiol. 2016;101(3):377–86.

[12] Hyun SW, Jung YS. Hypoxia induces FoxO3a-mediated dysfunction of blood-brain barrier. Biochem Biophys Res Commun. 2014;450(4):1638–42.

[13] McDonald PC, Chafe SC, Dedhar S. Overcoming hypoxia-mediated tumor progression: combinatorial approaches targeting pH regulation, angiogenesis and immune dysfunction. Front Cell Dev Biol. 2016;4:27.

[14] Pugh CW. Modulation of the hypoxic response. Adv Exp Med Biol. 2016;903:259–71.

[15] Ward JP. Oxygen sensors in context. Biochim Biophys Acta. 2008;1777(1):1–14.

[16] Yuan C, Wang P, Zhu L, Dissanayaka WL, Green DW, Tong EH, et al. Coculture of stem cells from apical papilla and human umbilical vein endothelial cell under hypoxia

increases the formation of three-dimensional vessel-like structures in vitro. Tissue Eng Part A. 2015;21(5–6):1163–72.

[17] Song ZC, Zhou W, Shu R, Ni J. Hypoxia induces apoptosis and autophagic cell death in human periodontal ligament cells through HIF-1alpha pathway. Cell Prolif. 2012;45(3):239–48.

[18] Teppo S, Sundquist E, Vered M, Holappa H, Parkkisenniemi J, Rinaldi T, et al. The hypoxic tumor microenvironment regulates invasion of aggressive oral carcinoma cells. Exp Cell Res. 2013;319(4):376–89.

[19] Dehne N, Fuhrmann D, Brüne B. Hypoxia-inducible factor (HIF) in hormone signaling during health and disease. Cardiovasc Hematol Agents Med Chem. 2013;11(2):125–35.

[20] Weigent DA. Hypoxia and cytoplasmic alkalinization upregulate growth hormone expression in lymphocytes. Cell Immunol. 2013;282(1):9–16.

[21] Pelosi M, Lazzarano S, Thoms BL, Murphy CL. Parathyroid hormone-related protein is induced by hypoxia and promotes expression of the differentiated phenotype of human articular chondrocytes. Clin Sci (Lond). 2013;125(10):461–70.

[22] Gordon HA, Rovin S, Bruckner G. Blood flow, collagen components of oral tissue and salivary kallikrein in young to senescent, germfree and conventional rats. A study on the etiologic factors of periodontal disease. Gerontology. 1978;24(1):1–11.

[23] Fong GH. Mechanisms of adaptive angiogenesis to tissue hypoxia. Angiogenesis. 2008;11(2):121–40.

[24] Kim JW, Tchernyshyov I, Semenza GL, Dang CV. HIF-1-mediated expression of pyruvate dehydrogenase kinase: a metabolic switch required for cellular adaptation to hypoxia. Cell Metab. 2006;3(3):177–85.

[25] Kojima H, Kobayashi A, Sakurai D, Kanno Y, Hase H, Takahashi R, et al. Differentiation stage-specific requirement in hypoxia-inducible factor-1alpha-regulated glycolytic pathway during murine B cell development in bone marrow. J Immunol. 2010;184(1):154–63.

[26] Phan AT, Goldrath AW. Hypoxia-inducible factors regulate T cell metabolism and function. Mol Immunol. 2015;68(2 Pt C):527–35.

[27] Semenza GL. Oxygen sensing, hypoxia-inducible factors, and disease pathophysiology. Annu Rev Pathol. 2014;9:47–71.

[28] Oliveira RR, Fermiano D, Feres M, Figueiredo LC, Teles FR, Soares GM, et al. Levels of candidate periodontal pathogens in subgingival biofilm. J Dent Res. 2016;95(6):711–8.

[29] Karhausen J, Haase VH, Colgan SP. Inflammatory hypoxia: role of hypoxia-inducible factor. Cell Cycle. 2005;4(2):256–8.

[30] Vasconcelos RC, Costa Ade L, Freitas Rde A, Bezerra BA, Santos BR, Pinto LP, et al. Immunoexpression of HIF-1alpha and VEGF in periodontal disease and healthy gingival tissues. Braz Dent J. 2016;27(2):117–22.

[31] Peyssonnaux C, Datta V, Cramer T, Doedens A, Theodorakis EA, Gallo RL, et al. HIF-1alpha expression regulates the bactericidal capacity of phagocytes. J Clin Invest. Jul 2005;115(7):1806–15.

[32] Dehne N, Brune B. HIF-1 in the inflammatory microenvironment. Exp Cell Res. 2009;315(11):1791–7.

[33] Boronat-Catala M, Catala-Pizarro M, Bagan Sebastian JV. Salivary and crevicular fluid interleukins in gingivitis. J Clin Exp Dent. 2014;6(2):e175–9.

[34] Ozcan E, Saygun NI, Serdar MA, Bengi VU, Kantarci A. Non-surgical periodontal therapy reduces saliva adipokines and matrix metalloproteinases levels in periodontitis. J Periodontol. 2016;87(8):934-43.

[35] Pumklin J, Bhalang K, Pavasant P. Hypoxia enhances the effect of lipopolysaccharide stimulated IL-1beta expression in human periodontal ligament cells. Odontology. 2016;104(3):338-46.

[36] Golz L, Memmert S, Rath-Deschner B, Jager A, Appel T, Baumgarten G, et al. Hypoxia and *P. gingivalis* synergistically induce HIF-1 and NF-kappa B activation in PDL cells and periodontal diseases. Mediators Inflamm. 2015;2015:438085.

[37] Jian C, Li C, Ren Y, He Y, Li Y, Feng X, et al. Hypoxia augments lipopolysaccharide-induced cytokine expression in periodontal ligament cells. Inflammation. 2014;37(5):1413–23.

[38] Mahanonda R, Pichyangkul S. Toll-like receptors and their role in periodontal health and disease. Periodontol 2000. 2007;43:41–55.

[39] Li W, Zhu Y, Singh P, Ajmera DH, Song J, Ji P. Association of common variants in MMPs with periodontitis risk. Dis Markers. 2016;2016:1545974.

[40] Kim YS, Shin SI, Kang KL, Chung JH, Herr Y, Bae WJ, et al. Nicotine and lipopolysaccharide stimulate the production of MMPs and prostaglandin E2 by hypoxia-inducible factor-1alpha up-regulation in human periodontal ligament cells. J Periodontal Res. 2012;47(6):719–28.

[41] Golz L, Memmert S, Rath-Deschner B, Jager A, Appel T, Baumgarten G, et al. LPS from *P. gingivalis* and hypoxia increases oxidative stress in periodontal ligament fibroblasts and contributes to periodontitis. Mediators Inflamm. 2014;2014:986264.

[42] Duscher D, Maan ZN, Whittam AJ, Sorkin M, Hu MS, Walmsley GG, et al. Fibroblast-specific deletion of hypoxia inducible factor-1 critically impairs murine cutaneous neovascularization and wound healing. Plast Reconstr Surg. 2015;136(5):1004–13.

[43] Tong C, Hao H, Xia L, Liu J, Ti D, Dong L, et al. Hypoxia pretreatment of bone marrow-derived mesenchymal stem cells seeded in a collagen-chitosan sponge scaffold promotes skin wound healing in diabetic rats with hindlimb ischemia. Wound Repair Regen. 2016;24(1):45–56.

[44] Zhu T, Park HC, Son KM, Yang HC. Effects of dimethyloxalylglycine on wound healing of palatal mucosa in a rat model. BMC Oral Health. 2015;15:60.

[45] Huang J, Liu L, Feng M, An S, Zhou M, Li Z, et al. Effect of $CoCl_2$ on fracture repair in a rat model of bone fracture. Mol Med Rep. 2015;12(4):5951–6.

[46] Fujio M, Xing Z, Sharabi N, Xue Y, Yamamoto A, Hibi H, et al. Conditioned media from hypoxic-cultured human dental pulp cells promotes bone healing during distraction osteogenesis. J Tissue Eng Regen Med. 2015; DOI: 10.1002/term.2109

[47] Nizet V, Johnson RS. Interdependence of hypoxic and innate immune responses. Nat Rev Immunol. 2009;9(9):609–17.

[48] Sitkovsky M, Lukashev D. Regulation of immune cells by local-tissue oxygen tension: HIF1 alpha and adenosine receptors. Nat Rev Immunol. 2005;5(9):712–21.

[49] Huang X, Yu T, Ma C, Wang Y, Xie B, Xuan D, et al. Macrophages play a key role in the obesity induced periodontal innate immune dysfunction via NLRP3 pathway. J Periodontol. 2016;23:1–18; DOI: 10.1902/jop.2016.160102

[50] Hajishengallis G, Chavakis T, Hajishengallis E, Lambris JD. Neutrophil homeostasis and inflammation: novel paradigms from studying periodontitis. J Leukoc Biol. 2015;98(4):539–48.

[51] Walmsley SR, Cadwallader KA, Chilvers ER. The role of HIF-1alpha in myeloid cell inflammation. Trends Immunol. 2005;26(8):434–9.

[52] Gale DP, Maxwell PH. The role of HIF in immunity. Int J Biochem Cell Biol. 2010;42(4):486–94.

[53] Lall H, Coughlan K, Sumbayev VV. HIF-1alpha protein is an essential factor for protection of myeloid cells against LPS-induced depletion of ATP and apoptosis that supports toll-like receptor 4-mediated production of IL-6. Mol Immunol. 2008;45(11):3045–9.

[54] Frede S, Stockmann C, Winning S, Freitag P, Fandrey J. Hypoxia-inducible factor (HIF) 1alpha accumulation and HIF target gene expression are impaired after induction of endotoxin tolerance. J Immunol. 2009;182(10):6470–6.

[55] Frede S, Stockmann C, Freitag P, Fandrey J. Bacterial lipopolysaccharide induces HIF-1 activation in human monocytes via p44/42 MAPK and NF-kappa B. Biochem J. 2006;396(3):517–27.

[56] Kong T, Eltzschig HK, Karhausen J, Colgan SP, Shelley CS. Leukocyte adhesion during hypoxia is mediated by HIF-1-dependent induction of beta 2 integrin gene expression. Proc Natl Acad Sci U S A. 2004;101(28):10440–5.

[57] Massena S, Christoffersson G, Vagesjo E, Seignez C, Gustafsson K, Binet F, et al. Identification and characterization of VEGF-A-responsive neutrophils expressing CD49d, VEGFR1, and CXCR4 in mice and humans. Blood. 2015;126(17):2016–26.

[58] Walmsley SR, Print C, Farahi N, Peyssonnaux C, Johnson RS, Cramer T, et al. Hypoxia-induced neutrophil survival is mediated by HIF-1alpha-dependent NF-kappa B activity. J Exp Med. 2005;201(1):105–15.

[59] Rius J, Guma M, Schachtrup C, Akassoglou K, Zinkernagel AS, Nizet V, et al. NF-kappa B links innate immunity to the hypoxic response through transcriptional regulation of HIF-1alpha. Nature. 2008;453(7196):807–11.

[60] Belaiba RS, Bonello S, Zahringer C, Schmidt S, Hess J, Kietzmann T, et al. Hypoxia up-regulates hypoxia-inducible factor-1alpha transcription by involving phosphatidylino-sitol 3-kinase and nuclear factor kappa B in pulmonary artery smooth muscle cells. Mol Biol Cell. 2007;18(12):4691–7.

[61] Yeramian A, Santacana M, Sorolla A, Llobet D, Encinas M, Velasco A, et al. Nuclear factor-kappa B2/p100 promotes endometrial carcinoma cell survival under hypoxia in a HIF-1alpha independent manner. Lab Invest. 2011;91(6):859–71.

[62] Bonello S, Zahringer C, BelAiba RS, Djordjevic T, Hess J, Michiels C, et al. Reactive oxygen species activate the HIF-1alpha promoter via a functional NFkappa B site. Arterioscler Thromb Vasc Biol. 2007;27(4):755–61.

[63] O'Neill LA, Pearce EJ. Immunometabolism governs dendritic cell and macrophage function. J Exp Med. 2016;213(1):15–23.

[64] Fluck K, Breves G, Fandrey J, Winning S. Hypoxia-inducible factor 1 in dendritic cells is crucial for the activation of protective regulatory T cells in murine colitis. Mucosal Immunol. 2016;9(2):379–90.

[65] Jantsch J, Chakravortty D, Turza N, Prechtel AT, Buchholz B, Gerlach RG, et al. Hypoxia and hypoxia-inducible factor-1 alpha modulate lipopolysaccharide-induced dendritic cell activation and function. J Immunol. 2008;180(7):4697–705.

[66] Mancino A, Schioppa T, Larghi P, Pasqualini F, Nebuloni M, Chen IH, et al. Divergent effects of hypoxia on dendritic cell functions. Blood. 2008;112(9):3723–34.

[67] Fliesser M, Wallstein M, Kurzai O, Einsele H, Loffler J. Hypoxia attenuates anti-*Aspergillus fumigatus* immune responses initiated by human dendritic cells. Mycoses. 2016;59(8):503–8.

[68] Kojima H, Gu H, Nomura S, Caldwell CC, Kobata T, Carmeliet P, et al. Abnormal B lymphocyte development and autoimmunity in hypoxia-inducible factor 1 alpha-deficient chimeric mice. Proc Natl Acad Sci U S A. 2002;99(4):2170–4.

[69] Lin Y, Tang Y, Wang F. The protective effect of HIF-1alpha in T lymphocytes on cardiac damage in diabetic mice. Ann Clin Lab Sci. 2016;46(1):32–43.

[70] Groeger SE, Meyle J. Epithelial barrier and oral bacterial infection. Periodontol 2000. 2015;69(1):46–67.

[71] Ng SKS, Leung WK. A community study on the relationship between stress, coping, affective dispositions and periodontal attachment loss. Community Dent Oral Epidemiol. 2006;34(4):252–66.

[72] Ostaff MJ, Stange EF, Wehkamp J. Antimicrobial peptides and gut microbiota in homeostasis and pathology. EMBO Mol Med. 2013;5(10):1465–83.

[73] Hans M, Hans VM. Toll-like receptors and their dual role in periodontitis: a review. J Oral Sci. 2011;53(3):263–71.

[74] Greer A, Zenobia C, Darveau RP. Defensins and LL-37: a review of function in the gingival epithelium. Periodontol 2000. 2013;63(1):67–79.

[75] Turkoglu O, Emingil G, Kutukculer N, Atilla G. Gingival crevicular fluid levels of cathelicidin LL-37 and interleukin-18 in patients with chronic periodontitis. J Periodontol. 2009;80(6):969–76.

[76] Eick S, Puklo M, Adamowicz K, Kantyka T, Hiemstra P, Stennicke H, et al. Lack of cathelicidin processing in Papillon-Lefevre syndrome patients reveals essential role of LL-37 in periodontal homeostasis. Orphanet J Rare Dis. 2014;9:148.

[77] Colgan SP, Taylor CT. Hypoxia: an alarm signal during intestinal inflammation. Nat Rev Gastroenterol Hepatol. 2010;7(5):281–287.

[78] Szabo S. "Gastric cytoprotection" is still relevant. J Gastroenterol Hepatol. 2014;29(Suppl 4):124–32.

[79] Lin AE, Beasley FC, Olson J, Keller N, Shalwitz RA, Hannan TJ, et al. Role of hypoxia inducible factor-1 alpha (HIF-1α) in innate defense against uropathogenic *Escherichia coli* infection. PLoS Pathog. 2015;11(4):e1004818.

[80] Peyssonnaux C, Boutin AT, Zinkernagel AS, Datta V, Nizet V, Johnson RS. Critical role of HIF-1alpha in keratinocyte defense against bacterial infection. J Invest Dermatol. 2008;128(8):1964–8.

[81] Shehade H, Oldenhove G, Moser M. Hypoxia in the intestine or solid tumors: a beneficial or deleterious alarm signal? Eur J Immunol. 2014;44(9):2550–7.

[82] Choudhary A, Smitha CN, Suresh DK. Trefoils: an unexplored natural protective shield of oral cavity. J Oral Biol Craniofac Res. 2015;5(3):226–31.

[83] Chaiyarit P, Chayasadom A, Wara-Aswapati N, Hormdee D, Sittisomwong S, Nakaresisoon S, et al. Trefoil factors in saliva and gingival tissues of patients with chronic periodontitis. J Periodontol. 2012;83(9):1129–38.

[84] Hernandez C, Santamatilde E, McCreath KJ, Cervera AM, Diez I, Ortiz-Masia D, et al. Induction of trefoil factor (TFF)1, TFF2 and TFF3 by hypoxia is mediated by hypoxia inducible factor-1: implications for gastric mucosal healing. Br J Pharmacol. 2009;156(2):262–72.

[85] Furuta GT, Turner JR, Taylor CT, Hershberg RM, Comerford K, Narravula S, et al. Hypoxia-inducible factor 1-dependent induction of intestinal trefoil factor protects barrier function during hypoxia. J Exp Med. 2001;193(9):1027–34.

[86] Kejriwal S, Bhandary R, Thomas B, Kumari S. Estimation of levels of salivary mucin, amylase and total protein in gingivitis and chronic periodontitis patients. J Clin Diagn Res. 2014;8(10):ZC56–60.

[87] Sanchez GA, Miozza VA, Delgado A, Busch L. Relationship between salivary mucin or amylase and the periodontal status. Oral Dis. 2013;19(6):585–91.

[88] Zhou X, Tu J, Li Q, Kolosov VP, Perelman JM. Hypoxia induces mucin expression and secretion in human bronchial epithelial cells. Transl Res. 2012;160(6):419–27.

[89] Chen Y. Hypoxia and *E. coli* LPS-induced periodontal resident cells PAMP expressions: implication for periodontitis pathogenesis. Ph. D. Dissertation, The University of Hong Kong, 2015.

[90] Alvarez ME, Fuxman Bass JI, Geffner JR, Fernandez Calotti PX, Costas M, Coso OA, et al. Neutrophil signaling pathways activated by bacterial DNA stimulation. J Immunol. 2006;177(6):4037–46.

[91] Li JP, Li FY, Xu A, Cheng B, Tsao SW, Fung ML, et al. Lipopolysaccharide and hypoxia-induced HIF-1 activation in human gingival fibroblasts. J Periodontol. 2012;83(6):816–24.

[92] Li JP, Chen Y, Ng CH, Fung ML, Xu A, Cheng B, et al. Differential expression of toll-like receptor 4 in healthy and diseased human gingiva. J Periodontal Res. 2014;49(6):845–54.

[93] Shengwei H, Wenguang X, Zhiyong W, Xiaofeng Q, Yufeng W, Yanhong N, et al. Crosstalk between the HIF-1 and toll-like receptor/nuclear factor-κB pathways in the oral squamous cell carcinoma microenvironment. Oncotarget. 2016; DOI: 10.18632/oncotarget.9329

[94] Yu XJ, Xiao CJ, Du YM, Liu S, Du Y, Li S. Effect of hypoxia on the expression of RANKL/OPG in human periodontal ligament cells in vitro. Int J Clin Exp Pathol. 2015;8(10):12929–35.

[95] Park HJ, Baek KH, Lee HL, Kwon A, Hwang HR, Qadir AS, et al. Hypoxia inducible factor-1α directly induces the expression of receptor activator of nuclear factor-κB ligand in periodontal ligament fibroblasts. Mol Cells. 2011;31(6):573–8.

[96] Dandajena TC, Ihnat MA, Disch B, Thorpe J, Currier GF. Hypoxia triggers a HIF-mediated differentiation of peripheral blood mononuclear cells into osteoclasts. Orthod Craniofac Res. 2012;15(1):1–9.

[97] Wu Y, Yang Y, Yang P, Gu Y, Zhao Z, Tan L, et al. The osteogenic differentiation of PDLSCs is mediated through MEK/ERK and p38 MAPK signalling under hypoxia. Arch Oral Biol. 2013;58(10):1357–68.

[98] Wu Y, Cao H, Yang Y, Zhou Y, Gu Y, Zhao X, et al. Effects of vascular endothelial cells on osteogenic differentiation of noncontact co-cultured periodontal ligament stem cells under hypoxia. J Periodontal Res. 2013;48(1):52–65.

[99] Zhao L, Wu Y, Tan L, Xu Z, Wang J, Zhao Z, et al. Coculture with endothelial cells enhances osteogenic differentiation of periodontal ligament stem cells via cyclooxygenase-2/prostaglandin E2/vascular endothelial growth factor signaling under hypoxia. J Periodontol. 2013;84(12):1847–57.

[100] Mamalis AA, Cochran DL. The therapeutic potential of oxygen tension manipulation via hypoxia inducible factors and mimicking agents in guided bone regeneration. A review.. Arch Oral Biol. 2011;56(12):1466–75.

[101] Ding H, Gao YS, Wang Y, Hu C, Sun Y, Zhang C. Dimethyloxaloylglycine increases the bone healing capacity of adipose-derived stem cells by promoting osteogenic differentiation and angiogenic potential. Stem Cells Dev. 2014;23(9):990–1000.

[102] Zhang Y, Huang J, Wang C, Hu C, Li G, Xu L. Application of HIF-1alpha by gene therapy enhances angiogenesis and osteogenesis in alveolar bone defect regeneration. J Gene Med. 2016;18(4–6):57–64.

[103] Peng J, Lai ZG, Fang ZL, Xing S, Hui K, Hao C, et al. Dimethyloxalylglycine prevents bone loss in ovariectomized C57BL/6 J mice through enhanced angiogenesis and osteogenesis. PLoS One. 2014;9(11):e112744.

[104] Choi H, Jin H, Kim JY, Lim KT, Choung HW, Park JY, et al. Hypoxia promotes CEMP1 expression and induces cementoblastic differentiation of human dental stem cells in an HIF-1-dependent manner. Tissue Eng Part A. 2014;20(1–2):410–23.

[105] Grossi SG, Skrepcinski FB, DeCaro T, Zambon JJ, Cummins D, Genco RJ. Response to periodontal therapy in diabetics and smokers. J Periodontol. 1996;67(10 Suppl):1094–102.

Chapter 16

Interplay between Hypoxia, Inflammation and Adipocyte Remodeling in the Metabolic Syndrome

Ana Marina Andrei, Anca Berbecaru-Iovan,
Felix Rareş Ioan Din-Anghel,
Camelia Elena Stănciulescu, Sorin Berbecaru-Iovan,
Ileana Monica Baniță and Cătălina Gabriela Pisoschi

Additional information is available at the end of the chapter

http://dx.doi.org/10.5772/65491

Abstract

Obesity, a major social and health problem in many countries, is due to the accumulation of white adipose tissue in subcutaneous and visceral depots. The discovery of adipocytes capacity of synthesis of numerous adipocytokines and growth factors and the cross talk between adipocytes and cells of the adipose stromo-vascular fraction had highlighted the role of adipose tissue dysfunction in obesity. In visceral obesity the unbalanced synthesis of pro- and anti-inflammatory adipocytokines contributes to the development of the metabolic syndrome which cumulates the factors that increase the risk for ischemic heart disease and cerebral stroke. Adipose tissue accumulation is associated with a state of chronic inflammation, and local hypoxia is considered its underlying cause due to the hypertrophic or/and the hyperplasic growth of the fat pad. Adipose tissue hypoxia is one of the first pathophysiological changes and was placed as a missing link between obesity and low-grade inflammation present in the metabolic syndrome. Hypoxia is a major trigger for adipose tissue remodeling including adipocyte death, inflammation, tissue fibrosis, and angiogenesis. Recently, the role of hypoxia in brown adipose tissue dysfunction, a tissue presumed as the biologic counterbalance of the metabolic disturbances in human obesity, is discussed.

Keywords: adipose tissue, hypoxia, inflammation, metabolic syndrome, fibrosis, angiogenesis

1. Introduction

Until two decades ago, the adipose tissue has been considered one of the least dynamic structures of the mammalian organism involved exclusively in fat storage. Some key events have changed this mechanistic point of view, and now the whole fat of an organism is viewed as a complex organ composed of at least two main varieties of adipose tissues: the white adipose tissue (WAT) containing unilocular adipocytes and the brown adipose tissue (BAT) formed by multilocular adipocytes. Besides this different type of adipocytes, both tissues contain a non-adipocitary stromo-vascular fraction that includes undifferentiated cells, preadipocytes, fibroblasts, inflammatory cells, and various amounts of vessels and nerves. The adult adipose organ is divided into two types of depots: subcutaneous/peripheral and visceral/central constituted of lobules of unilocular adipocytes sustained by the stromo-vascular fraction well vascularized and innervated [1–5].

A significant development in the knowledge of adipose tissue is related to its function as an endocrine organ, both types of tissues being able to elaborate adipocytokines, humoral factors with various metabolic, vascular, pro-inflammatory, and anti-inflammatory roles [2, 4].

The accumulation of WAT in physiological depots leads to obesity characterized by an increase of the body mass index (BMI) over 30 kg/m^2 [6]. Obesity became a major social and health problem in many countries (between one quarter and one third of the population), a recent report of the World Health Organization (WHO) mentioning more than 1.9 billion of adult overweight subjects worldwide, more than 600 millions being obese [7]. From a pathogenically point of view, the quality and the distribution of adipose tissue seem to be more important in triggering the metabolic syndrome than the quantity of the fat per se. A direct relationship is accepted between abdominal/visceral fat accumulation—apple-shaped obesity—and the emergence and development of the metabolic syndrome or abdominal and pelvic cancers. Unbalanced synthesis of pro- and anti-inflammatory adipocytokines in visceral obesity contributes to the development of many features of the metabolic syndrome which cumulates the factors that increase the risk for ischemic heart disease and cerebral stroke: apple-shaped fat deposition, impaired glucose metabolism, dyslipidemia, and high blood pressure [8–10]. Pear-shaped obesity—i.e., subcutaneous fat accumulation—has a minimal risk for the development of such pathologies even at the same BMI greater than 30 kg/m^2 [11–13].

Hypoxia is one of the mechanisms responsible for the development of the metabolic changes and the pro-inflammatory milieu of white adipose tissue in obesity [3].

Tissue partial O_2 pressure (pO_2) reflects the balance between O_2 delivery and consumption, and continuous, chronic low O_2 tension occurs as a tissue inability to provide adequate compensatory vascular supply [3, 14, 15]. Obviously, adipose tissue hypoxia has a polymorphic feature since it depends on the adipose tissue blood flow regulation, different between the adipose phenotype WAT or BAT, the adipose fat pad localization, subcutaneous or visceral, and the delay of time between the onset of hypoxia and its quantification.

In healthy lean young adult, the pO_2 in adipose tissue is considered 55–60 mm Hg [14, 16] similar to the general tissue oxygenation [4], but important differences were reported in obese subjects. Oxygen supply was found markedly lower (44.7 mm Hg) in obese subjects in fasting and postprandial status than in lean subjects (55.4 mmHg) [14, 17], but Goossens et al. [18] found that in WAT of obese subjects the pO_2 was even higher (67.4 mmHg) than lean (46.8 mmHg). Of note, the pO_2 is not in a direct relation with the surface of the vascular network in the adipose pad. Capillary density for both subcutaneous and visceral depots is lower in obese human than in lean, but in lean subjects, the density is greater in visceral location [14, 19]. Even if BAT adipose tissue is more vascularized than WAT, it was indicated that obesity also causes BAT hypoxia, the same response being noted in multilocular adipocytes that became larger in obese animals [20]. Interestingly, BAT hypoxia seems to be temperature-dependent. Xue et al. proved that there is no hypoxia in mice housed at 30°C, but it appears in animals living at 4°C [21].

Adipose tissue is one of the most plastic organs in adults gifted with the ability of a continuous remodeling—extends or regresses depending on nutrient intake. The plasticity of any tissue is due to its capacity of extending vasculature which requires the cross talk between adipocytes and stromal and endothelial cells in the case of adipose tissue.

There are several arguments in favor of this "hypoxia concept." Normally, each adipocyte is surrounded by capillaries, and it is widely accepted that WAT is poorly oxygenated in obese individuals because adipocytes may be up to 200 μm, so larger than the normal diffusion distance of oxygen within tissues. As adipose tissue mass rapidly increases, clusters of unilocular adipocyte distance from the vessels and pockets of hypoxia are generated [22]. Another cause presumed for adipose tissue hypoxia is the loss of endothelial cells usually associated with the damage of parenchymal cells in other tissues. Recently, the interest in brown adipose tissue (BAT) increased, and studies have indicated that obesity determines also BAT hypoxia and the loss of its thermogenic capacity [20].

Chronic adipose tissue hypoxia has been suggested to be part of the pathogenesis of adipocyte dysfunction [14, 23, 24]. Local hypoxia triggers the generation of reactive oxygen species (ROS) and endoplasmic reticulum (ER) stress [25] and initiates the inflammatory response able to regulate the balance between angiogenic factors and inhibitors in order to stimulate angiogenesis and increase blood flow. The paucity of endothelial barrier is associated with the release of profibrogenic and pro-inflammatory cytokines and an augmented influx of inflammatory cells [26]. There is considerable evidence that obese adipose tissue is markedly infiltrated with macrophages which participate in the inflammatory pathways and are very important in adipose tissue remodeling, macrophage infiltration being signalized by lipid-overloaded adipocytes necrosis. Numerous reports emphasized that visceral adipose tissue in obese individuals is more fibrotic than that of lean subjects [27–29].

Normally, BAT and WAT produce various pro-angiogenic factors and cytokines able to induce remodeling of the vasculature, and as a response to hypoxia, an unbalanced production of these multiple bioactive pro-angiogenic and antiapoptotic growth factors synthesized by the adipose stromal cells may occur. Local hypoxia in obese is the underlying cause of an increase of macrophage cell number accompanied by the state of chronic inflammation and impaired adipokine secretion. Hypoxia promotes the delivery of many adipocytokines related to inflammation and tissue remodeling needed for angiogenesis to the ischemic tissue, such as macrophage migration inhibitory factor (MIF), granulocyte-macrophage colony-stimulating factor (GM-CSF), matrix metalloproteinases MMP-2 and MMP-9, transforming growth factor (TGF)-β, vascular endothelial growth factor (VEGF), interleukins (IL-1, IL-6, IL-10), tumor necrosis factor (TNF)-α, angiopoietin-like (Angptl)-4, and leptin [4, 15, 22, 30–32].

This chapter summarizes the potential links between hypoxia, inflammation, adipocyte hypertrophy, and macrophage infiltration of adipose tissue and the effects of inflammatory mediators on its remodeling.

2. Essentials of adipose organ structure and functions

The adult adipose organ is composed by two types of adipose depots divided into adipose lobules of (i) unilocular adipose tissue (WAT—white adipose tissue) composed of unilocular cells and (ii) brown adipose tissue (BAT), formed by multilocular adipocytes (**Figure 1a** and **b**).

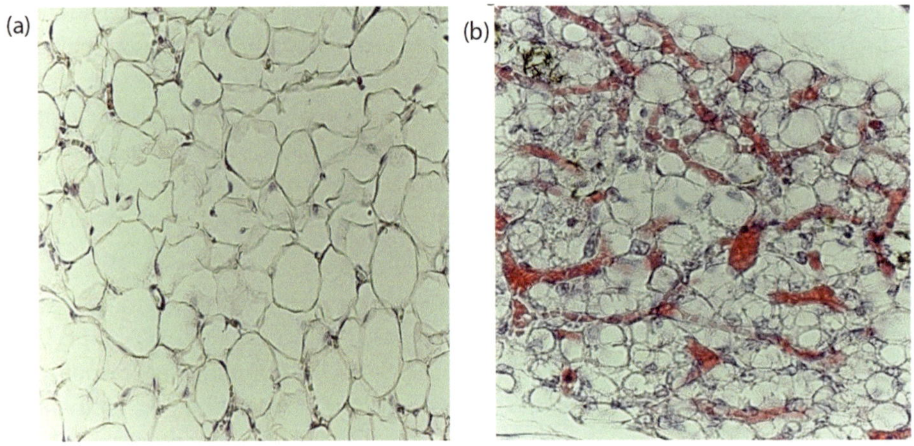

Figure 1. (a) Human adult subcutaneous WAT (hematoxylin and eosin staining, ob. ×40) and (b) human newborn visceral adipose depot with unilocular WAT and multilocular BAT adipocytes (hematoxylin and eosin staining, ob. ×20).

Both types of cells organized into adipose lobules are sustained by the stromo-vascular fraction well vascularized and innervated [11, 33]. Anatomically, WAT depots are located primarily in two major areas—subcutaneous/peripheral and visceral/central, which differ in the composition of the stromo-vascular fraction [34, 35]. Although at a first view the adipose tissue looks quite simple, a deeper molecular analysis revealed a high heterogeneity of cells. With respect to adipose cells, recent research identified both in rodent and men, the third type of adipocytes with common features of WAT and BAT adipocytes named "brite" or "beige" cells.

BAT, so named because of its yellow-brown color in vivo due to a very rich vascularization, is distinguishable morphologically from WAT by its cytoplasmic multiple droplets of stored triglycerides, while WAT contains a single large droplet. The multilocular cells are rich in mitochondria containing the uncoupling protein (UCP)1 which is uniquely present in BAT and therefore considered a marker for it (**Figure 2**).

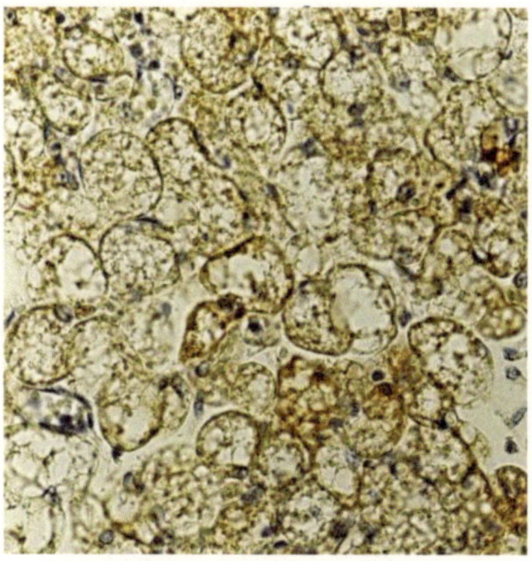

Figure 2. Newborn human brown adipocytes labeled with UCP1 (IHC, ob. ×40).

In humans, two types of BAT are present: (i) the classical (or constitutive BAT—cBAT) that is fully developed at birth and then reduced to remain in human adult only in a symmetrical cervical position and around the clavicles as very recently localized by PET/CT scanning, and the second type of brown adipocytes named "beige" or "brite" (brown in white), inducible or recruitable BAT (rBAT). This is composed of isolated brown multilocular cells resident between white cells mainly in subcutaneous depots [36, 37]. WAT is recognized as the site of fat storage, while BAT acts, as in rodents, as a heat-generating tissue through uncoupled oxidative phosphorylation which involves the action of UCP1 [38].

The functional complexity of adipose tissue is also due to the heterogeneity of cell phenotypes located in the non-adipocitary stromo-vascular fraction that includes undifferentiated or mesenchymal cells, preadipocytes, fibroblasts, and inflammatory cells (macrophages, lymphocytes, and mast cells). These cells are surrounded by a very complex network of vessels and nerves. The vascular network is more developed and branched in BAT than in WAT [39]. Normal metabolic functions and their imbalance involve a cross talk between adipocytes and the cells from the stromo-vascular fraction mediated by the components of adipose tissue extracellular matrix (ECM).

WAT secretoma. The discovery of leptin by Friedman in 1994 initiated the recognition of white adipocytes as major endocrine cells that secrete numerous bioactive molecules: lipids (such as free fatty acids mobilized in lipolysis, prostaglandins, and endocannabinoids) and proteins (termed "adipokines" or "adipocytokines" with metabolic and pro-/anti-inflammatory functions) [40]. Several adipocytokines are listed in **Table 1**. Impaired production of adipokines is associated with the pathogenesis of obesity-related disorders—type 2 diabetes mellitus, metabolic syndrome, cardiovascular diseases, and certain types of cancer [2, 41–44]. Generally, blood adipocytokine levels rise with the increase of fat mass except for adiponectin and omentin levels which are reported to be lower in obese and overweight subjects [31, 45, 46].

Adipocytokine	Function
Leptin	Feeding behavior, fat mass, pro-angiogenic
Adiponectin	Insulin sensitivity, anti-inflammatory, pro-angiogenic
Resistin	Insulin resistance, pro-inflammatory, antiangiogenic
Visfatin (pre-B-cell colony-enhancing factor, PBEF)	Insulin resistance, pro-inflammatory
Vaspin (visceral adipose tissue-derived serpin)	Insulin resistance
Omentin	Insulin resistance
Retinol-binding protein (RBP)-4	Insulin resistance
Serum amyloid A	Insulin resistance, pro-inflammatory
Cholesteryl ester transfer protein (CETP)	Lipid metabolism
Lipoprotein lipase (LPL)	Lipid metabolism
Adipocyte fatty acid-binding protein (A-FABP)-4	Lipid metabolism
Perilipin	Lipid metabolism
Apelin	Vasodilatation, pro-angiogenic
Angiotensinogen	Regulation of blood pressure
Angiotensin II	Regulation of blood pressure
Adipsin (adipocyte trypsin/complement factor D)	Lipid and glucose metabolism, inflammation
Tumor necrosis factor (TNF)-α	Pro-inflammatory
Interleukin 6 (IL-6)	Pro-inflammatory
C-reactive protein (CRP)	Pro-inflammatory
Plasminogen activator inhibitor (PAI)-1	Fibrinolysis, pro-angiogenic
Monocyte chemoattractant protein (MCP)-1	Macrophage activation
Intercellular adhesion molecule (ICAM)-1	Macrophage activation
Fibroblast growth factor (FGF)-2	Pro-angiogenic
Hepatocyte growth factor (HGF)	Pro-angiogenic
Platelet-derived growth factor (PDGF)	Pro-angiogenic
Vascular endothelial growth factor (VEGF)	Pro-angiogenic
Transforming growth factor (TGF)-β	Inflammation, fibrosis
Matrix metalloproteinases (MMPs)	Pro- and antiangiogenic, ECM remodeling
Tissue inhibitor of metalloproteinases (TIMPs)	Antiangiogenic, ECM remosdeling

Table 1. Adipocytokines and their main biological effects (adapted with permission from [31]).

Leptin and adiponectin are the most important hormones secreted by white adipocytes with multiple metabolic roles (regulating appetite and energy balance, insulin sensitivity) but also encompass angiogenic and anti-inflammatory actions [2, 4]. Leptin increases the vascular permeability in adipose tissue and influences microvessels density [47].

Adiponectin is regarded as a link between obesity and related metabolic disorders because it improves glucose and lipid metabolism and prevents inflammation [15]. There are many other members of the "adipokinome" involved in the inflammatory response: tumor necrosis factor (TNF)-α, interleukins (IL-6, IL-8, IL-10), monocyte chemoattractant protein (MCP)-1, and macrophage migration inhibitory factor (MIF) [4, 15, 22]. Besides the adipocytes, many other cells from the stromo-vascular fraction secrete inflammatory cytokines and chemokines in response to adipocyte hypertrophy or hypoxic conditions. Other adipokines related to inflammation include several crucial angiogenic factors, such as vascular endothelial growth factor (VEGF), hepatocyte growth factor (HGF)-1, angiopoetin-2, nerve growth factor (NGF), plasminogen activator inhibitor (PAI)-1, apelin, and adipsin [4, 30–32]. The release of numerous inflammatory adipocytokines is markedly increased in obesity-related diseases. Subcutaneous and visceral adipose tissue display differences in their adipokinome. Even if the results of in vitro and in vivo studies are controversial, it can be assumed, for example, that leptin and adiponectin are mainly produced in vivo by the subcutaneous adipocytes, while others (angiotensinogen, A-fatty acid-binding protein (FABP)-4, IL-6) are secreted at higher levels in visceral adipose tissue [48–51].

3. Adipose tissue dysfunction and hypoxia

Adipocyte capacity of synthesis corroborated with the clinical observation that a proportion of obese individuals seem to be protected against metabolic syndrome [52] had highlighted the role of adipose tissue dysfunction in obesity. Obesity is so long considered a genetic predisposition that promotes the excess of energy intake or the scarce energy expenditure.

In humans, the adipose tissue from the two main locations (subcutaneous and visceral) shows anatomical and functional differences (in contrast to subcutaneous adipose tissue, abdominal depots drain directly onto the portal circulation [31]) and different gene expressions.

Oxygen is a main nutritional factor without which oxidation of nutrients in aerobic tissues cannot take place. The decrease of oxygen level in various tissues can occur even if the total amount provided to the organism is not reduced [20]. Evinced hypoxia that follows low oxygen tension has numerous implications for cellular metabolism and transcriptional program [27]. Recent research suggests that adipose tissue hypoxia occurs in obese mice and even in human subjects. In obese rodents the existence of hypoxia was demonstrated by qualitative reaction (using hypoxic cell markers, such as pimonidazole—PIMO) or quantitative technique using needle-type oxygen sensors [3, 15, 22, 23]. In human obese subjects, the results are more controversial since normoxia and even hyperoxia have been reported in various experiments [18, 20, 53].

Chronic hypoxia has been suggested to be part of the pathogenic pathways leading to adipose tissue dysfunction [14, 23, 24].

Local hypoxia triggers the main alterations defining the adipose tissue dysfunction: generation of ROS and oxidative stress [54], ER stress [25], adipocyte death [55], inhibition of adiponectin expression [55, 56], and leptin hyperproduction [57] and initiates the inflammatory response able to regulate the balance between angiogenic and inhibitor factors in order to stimulate angiogenesis and increase blood flow.

More causes of adipose tissue hypoxia are discussed, this concept being related to the histological changes of the adipose obese tissue—hyperplasia and adipocyte hypertrophy. Reduction of blood supply in adipose pads is a common mechanism of tissue hypoxia. Reduced adipose tissue blood flow in obese rats and humans was reported many years ago (Larsen et al, 1966, West et al., 1987 cited by [26]), being associated with insulin resistance in obese individuals [17, 18]. Adipose tissue angiogenesis is insufficient to maintain normoxia in the growing number of fat-storing cells in adipose depots as they are in obesity. Histological analysis has demonstrated a scarce capillary network in abdominal subcutaneous depots in obese subjects compared to the leans [14, 18].

A second cause is related to the increased size of adipocytes—hypertrophy—reaching in obese subjects a diameter larger than 150–200 μm [45]. This exceeds the normal capacity of oxygen diffusion through the tissue (100–200 μm), and oxygenation of adipose tissue will be compromised [58].

Hypoxia-inducible factor (HIF)-1 is the key transcriptional factor involved in response to hypoxia, which moves into the nucleus and binds to hypoxia-response elements from a myriad of target genes to initiate their transcription [3]. Both murine and human adipocytes exhibit extensive functional changes in culture in response to HIF-1, which alters the expression of up to 1300 genes [59]. These include genes encoding key adipokines, such as leptin, apelin, visfatin, TNF-α, IL-1, IL-6, VEGF, angiopoietin-like protein (Angptl)-4, MIF, PAI-1, and matrix metalloproteinases 2 and 9 (MMP-2, MMP-9), which are upregulated, and adiponectin, peroxisome proliferator-activated receptor (PPAR)-γ which is downregulated [3, 20, 55, 60, 61].

Hypoxia alters genes encoding key proteins for metabolic processes: glucose uptake, glycolysis, oxidative metabolism, lipolysis, and lipogenesis. Glucose uptake into adipocytes is stimulated by hypoxia because the expression of GLUT transporters is upregulated [20, 55, 62]. A switch from aerobic to anaerobic metabolism in hypoxic adipocytes is sustained by the increased activity of some glycolytic enzymes (e.g., phosphofructokinase [63]) and a net lactate release. Many studies focused on hypoxia-induced derangements of lipid metabolism reporting an increased lipolysis rather than unchanged but reduced lipogenesis in hypoxic adipocytes [64–66].

It seems that various degrees of adipose tissue hypoxia have different metabolic effects, and it is supposed also that subcutaneous and visceral adipocytes respond differently to factors that mediate tissue hypoxia. A recent study demonstrated that hypercaloric diet induces more severe hypoxia in mesenteric adipose tissue of mice than in the subcutaneous one [67].

Another direct effect of hypoxia is induction of insulin resistance via the upregulation of certain adipokines, the impairment of insulin-signaling pathway being a key change for white adipocyte dysfunction in obese subjects [3, 4].

Adipose tissue is one of the most plastic entities of an organism in terms of growth in the childhood and even in the adulthood in normal and pathological conditions, responding rapidly and dynamically to nutrient excess or starvation. Nor normal or pathological tissue, therefore nor the adipose tissue, is able to grow, develop, and function in the absence of an appropriate vascular network. Therefore, the hypoxia-induced expression of VEGF, the main angiogenic factor, and of certain adipokines, such as angiopoietin-2, Angptl-4, and leptin, sustains the stimulation of angiogenesis in obese adipose tissue [68–70]. Experimental data emphasize the induction of a pro-fibrotic switch of the transcriptional program in hypoxic adipocytes, fibrosis being another feature of adipose tissue dysfunction in obesity [29, 71]. Preadipocytes, pro-inflammatory cells, and fibroblasts from WAT as well as adipocytes respond to hypoxic conditions, favoring cellular events that lead to inflammation and fibrosis. Biostatistical analysis of WAT transcriptome had demonstrated a positive correlation between fat mass, degree of inflammation, and synthesis of ECM in obesity complications [72].

4. WAT hypoxia: a link between obesity and inflammation

The necessary link between abdominal (visceral or central) obesity and the development of type 2 diabetes and metabolic syndrome (which includes atherosclerosis, hypertension, and hyperlipidemia) due to the expanding fat mass and adipose tissue dysfunction was first demonstrated by Spiegelman's group [73, 74]. The mild inflammation status of the adipose tissue in obese subjects is induced by the peculiar role occupied by TNF-α, a 26 kDa transmembrane protein secreted as a cytokine and acting as an endotoxin-induced factor causing necrosis of tumors in vitro and cachexia in vivo, so naturally linked to the energy homeostasis [1]. They discovered that TNF-α is an active biofactor secreted by adipocytes and stromovascular cells positively correlated with obesity and insulin resistance.

Many signaling pathways have been proposed to be involved in the pathogenesis of obesity-associated inflammation called also "metaflammation" [75] such as (i) activation of toll-like receptor 4 (TLR4) by free fatty acids released after lipolysis [76], (ii) activation of protein kinase C (PKC) by diacylglicerol and ceramide [77]), (iii) induction of ER stress [25, 78] and oxidative stress [79], and (iv) adipocyte death [39]. Recent research data suggest that adipose tissue hypoxia is one of the first pathophysiological changes and was placed as a missing link between obesity and low-grade inflammation [61, 80].

Clinical and physiological data argue that in the whole organism the oxygen level is not the same in all the tissues nor constant for the same tissue and an isolate organ or tissue may lack oxygen even if the total supply is not compromised. This seems to be the case of the hypoxia inside the WAT human depots, the expanding adipose lobules or hypertrophic adipocytes resting isolated in pockets of tissue that lack the vascular supply, while other areas could be in normoxia or even hyperoxia [20]. The lack of oxygen perfusion for the hypertrophic adipocytes made them necrotic and finally they died. Dead adipocytes and free lipid droplets liberatedly act as recruitment factors for macrophages [39]. Besides adipocytes, preadipocytes and macrophages (the main players in WAT inflammatory response stimulating the inflammatory state in adipose tissue by the release of pro-inflammatory cytokines, such as TNF-α and interleukins) also respond to hypoxia. For such controversial results regarding the hypoxia in human adipose tissue, one must consider the technique accuracy and the methodological issues, minding that the same depot could be polarized toward hypoxic areas or inflamed and hypervascularized nests. Such a clustered differentiation is not unique in the adipose tissue since data demonstrated that in obese adipose tissue the switch from M2a macrophages discriminative for lean mice to M1 inflammatory phenotype takes place in well-defined spatiotemporal areas inside the same adipose depot [81].

In order to assess the involvement of TLR signaling in inflammation in obesity-related diseases, we analyzed the expression of TLR-2, TLR-4, TNF-α, and CD-68 in subcutaneous and visceral adipose depots from lean, obese, and obese diabetic subjects. We observed that both types of depots showed an increased number of small- and medium-dilated vessels with many CD68-positive cells [82]. In the peritoneal depots, we observed leukocyte margination with CD68-positive cells, but we didn't notice the presence of macrophages crowns in none of the samples analyzed, as Cinti and coworkers found in adipose tissue with hypertrophic cells [39]. Data obtained proved that same cells from the visceral adipose depots of obese and obese-diabetic patients, mainly macrophages, intravascular leukocytes, and endothelial cells, showed a positive reaction for both TLR-4 and TNF-α [82], proving that TLR4 activation contributes to the inflammatory process in obesity and the onset of the metabolic syndrome (**Figure 3**).

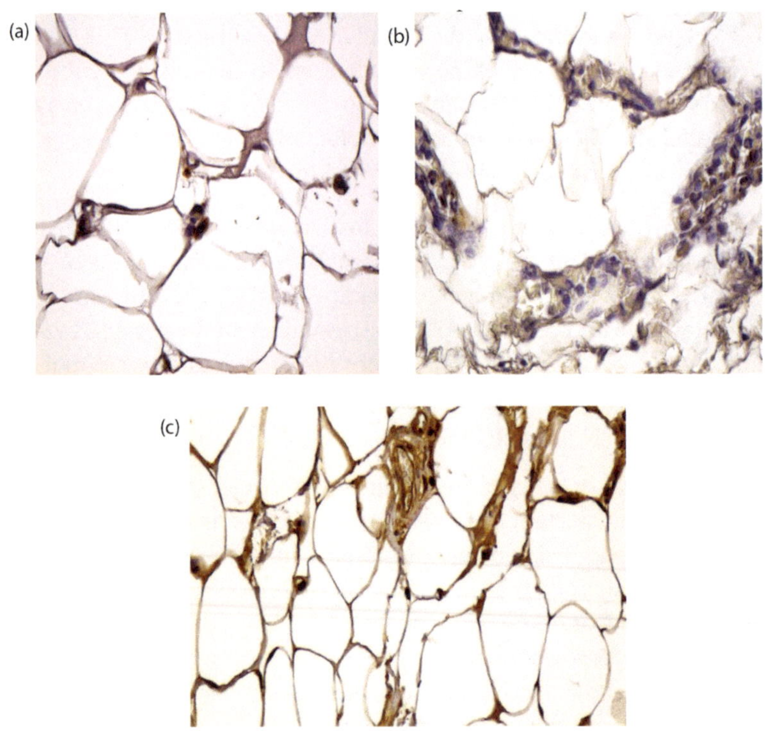

Figure 3. Immunostaining for CD68, TLR-4, and TNF-α of visceral obese adipose depots. (a) CD68-positive leukocytes between adipocytes (ob. ×40) in adipose peritoneal depots, (b) TLR-4-positive leukocytes and endothelial cells (ob. ×40), (c) intense-positive TNF-α reaction in visceral depots (ob. ×40).

http://dx.doi.org/10.5772/65491

Summarizing the data linking the cellular and molecular alterations of the adipose tissue in obesity to the adipose tissue dysfunction, among the three events highlighted—oxidative stress, ER stress, and local hypoxia—hypoxia might be the first in a logical chronologically order, since it promotes oxidative and ER stress. In obesity, quick changes from normoxia/ hyperoxia to hypoxia would be needed in order to induce oxidative stress [16]. Adipose tissue hypoxia induces inflammation through activation of two main transcription factors, HIF-1α and nuclear factor (NF)-KB, each of them activating transcription of a variety of genes encoding angiogenic and/or pro-inflammatory adipocytokines [26, 83]. Available data demonstrate that in rodent, HIF-1α upregulation starts in the first 1–3 days after the administration of a high-fat diet, before inflammation and insulin resistance develop [15, 19, 84].

5. Hypoxia: a major trigger for adipose tissue remodeling

Adipose tissue hypoxia is a concept that can practically explain the main alterations defining the adipose tissue dysfunction due to obesity: chronic inflammation, leptin expression, adiponectin reduction, adipocyte death followed by the invasion of monocytes and activation of macrophages, elevated lipolysis and adipocyte insulin resistance, and increased activity of ROS [3, 15, 55]. This entire cellular and molecular imbalance is followed by a compulsory adipose depot remodeling. The concept of remodeling of adipose tissue refers, as in all other entities, to the turnover of the cells and of the ECM in response to the requirement for growth and expansion of the adipose depots [85]. The molecules (cytokines, adipokines, growth factors, and proteases) involved in adipose tissue remodeling are synthesized and act as a permanent result of the cross talk between adipocytes and stromal cells.

5.1. Adipocyte death and inflammation

Adipocyte death is accepted as the main trigger for the adipose tissue remodeling [84], but the cause of this event is not consensual: the adipocyte size or the hypoxic milieu. In mice a positive robust correlation exists between adipocyte size and adipocyte death [39]. Consecutively macrophages are accumulating in crown-like structures being a source of numerous pro-inflammatory cytokines. A difference in the incidence of dead adipocytes was noted, the intra-abdominal cells being more susceptible than those of the inguinal depots. The clearance of the cellular detritus by the macrophages is the trigger for a homeostatic remodeling program that will allow the further expansion of the adipose depots that include matrix remodeling and vasculogenesis. Foci of adipocyte death are therefore areas where macrophages promote obesity-associated inflammation [39]. Interestingly, adipocyte loss is associated with phenotypic changes in stromal monocytic-macrophage cells. In a chronologically sequence, after the scavenging, the place occupied by the huge dead adipocytes was taken by small-size adipocytes, and the former hypertrophic adipose tissue became hyperplasic (Faust et al., 1984 cited by [84]). As a new study demonstrated that the macrophages are crowded in foci of hypoxic tissue, a second theory emphasizes that adipocyte death is caused by the hypoxia and the macrophages are trapped into the hypoxic areas by MIF [65, 86].

5.2. Hypoxia underpins adipose tissue fibrosis

There are several recent studies involving fibrosis of adipose depots in installing hypoxia and insulin resistance [27, 28, 87].

Scherer's research group proposed that in adipose obese tissues hypoxia is the most important driving force downstreaming the events associated with inflammation and fibrosis [27]. They found that in adipose tissue from the transgenic mice HIF-1α-ΔODD, in which a dominant-active deletion mutation of HIF-1α is overexpressed, fed with a hypercaloric diet, the transcription factor HIF-1α failed to promote the pro-angiogenic program by targeting genes, such as VEGF-A. Moreover, in these mice HIF-1α induces the fibrotic program by an increased synthesis of fibrotic proteins, such as lysyl oxidase (LOX), type I and type III collagens, tissue inhibitor of matrix metalloproteinases (TIMP)-1, and connective tissue growth factor (CTGF). Histology performed with trichromic staining revealed thick fibrotic streaks composed of type I collagen fibers, similar results being reported also for the adipose pads from obese human subjects [88].

LOX is a known target gene of HIF-1α, and in adipose tissue of ob/ob transgenic mouse, LOX is found in increased level compared to wild type [27]. LOX cross-links elastin and collagens in ECM and creates ECM-resistant bands of fibrosis. In adipose tissue of ob/ob mouse, these collagen bundle "streaks" are found outside the "crown-like" structures previously described [27, 39, 84]. The conclusion derived was that collagen synthesis and deposition could be anterior to the accumulation of macrophages surrounding the adipose cells because hypoxia-induced fibrotic program develops shortly after the high-fat diet is established [27]. So adipose tissue fibrosis is not necessarily induced by inflammation but could be rather an upstream phenomenon through the synthesis of HIF-1α and LOX.

From a different point of view, like in other tissues, adipose tissue fibrosis develops as a result of a persistent inflammation and a failure of the normal tissue repair with *restitutio ad integrum*.

Interestingly, fibrosis of adipose depots in obesity seems to display an otherwise intensity as the inflammation and hypoxia, those visceral seeming to be not only less fibrotic than those peripheral but also with a different distribution of collagen fibers, especially pericellular or intraparenchymatous [28]. As the visceral depots are more inflamed than the subcutaneous depots as we showed [88], this observation contradicts the accepted biological sequence that fibrosis develops as a result of an excessive and altered ECM synthesis and storage by resident cells activated in an inflammatory environment. This abnormal amount of fibrotic matrix in the subcutaneous adipose tissue could be explained if we keep in mind the histology of the host tissue where the adipose depots expand (the subcutaneous adipose tissue develops toward a much more dense tissue than the visceral one). In obese subjects fibrosis accumulates in pericellular areas—lining each adipose cell or a group of cells (interstitial fibrosis) and around the vessels (**Figure 4**).

Collagen phenotypes are also different, types I, III, and VI being present in pericellular position but only I and III form thick bundles appearing as interlobular septa surrounding more cells [28]. In visceral (omental) depots, the accumulation of fibers in pericellular position is associated with small adipocyte size and a lowest quantity of circulating triglycerides, proving that the subjects with smaller adipocytes have a less adverse metabolic profile [27, 89], so fibrosis may act as a protective reaction. In the adipose depots, the significance of type VI collagen seems to be peculiar, since its appearance changes dramatically through adipogenesis [90]. Transgenic mouse col 6KO ob/ob shows reduced necrotic cell death and consumes only a half of the amount of food that ob/ob strain [91] and type VI collagen levels correlate with hyperglycemia and insulin resistance [87, 92]. Obese humans expressed higher levels of type VI collagen and macrophage markers [92].

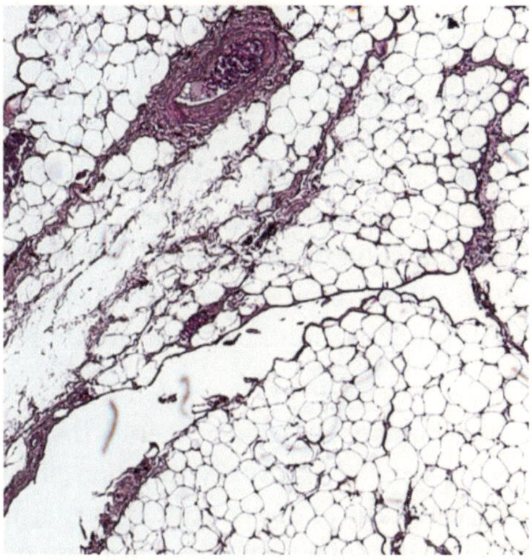

Figure 4. Pericellular and interstitial fibrosis in a visceral adipose depot from an adult obese subject (ob. ×20).

5.3. Hypoxia-induced angiogenesis in white adipose tissue

Being a compulsory condition for the expansion of any tissue, angiogenesis is a very limited process in normal adulthood (in endometrial cyclic physiology or wound healing), and the endothelial cells of the adult capillary network are in a relatively quiescent state.

In adipose tissue, angiogenesis is a very complex phenomenon regulated by a lot of molecules (hormones, cytokines, and growth factors) secreted by the stromo-vascular cells, including endothelial cells, and also by the adipocytes and preadipocytes [93, 94].

During adipose depot development, adipogenesis and vasculogenesis are temporally and spatially dependent, and in an adipose depot, the vascular network seems to act as a self-stop for the adipose expansion, since the inhibition of angiogenesis reduces the adipose tissue mass [95, 96].

In hypoxia induced by a high caloric intake, the vascular network does not progress uniformly between depots, due to the differences between the initial degree of vascularization and the rate/capacity of neovascularization during adipose tissue expansion. Hypoxia is more severe in mesenteric visceral depots than in subcutaneous [67], and at the same time, human visceral depots reveal a greater capillary density and angiogenic capacity than the subcutaneous adipose tissue [97, 98]. In their study using CD31+/CD34+ immunolabeling, Villaret and coworkers revealed that in obesity the capillary network is more developed and endothelial cell number is greater in visceral than in subcutaneous adipose depots, so increased hypoxia of visceral adipose tissue is not necessarily a consequence of capillary rarefaction [98]. The pro-angiogenic and pro-inflammatory phenotype of visceral adipose tissue could be related to endothelial cell senescence proved by an altered expression of some senescence markers such as IGFBP3, γH2AX, and SIRT1. They postulated at least two main causes for endothelial cell senescence in visceral adipose tissue: increased cell replication and oxidative stress [98]. Hyperplasia of obese visceral adipose tissue is responsible for an increased secretion of VEGF-A2 that stimulates endothelial cell proliferation.

The compensatory angiogenesis could prevent the metabolic disturbances induced by the hypoxia. It seems that not in all conditions the expansion of adipose tissue is associated with inflammation if an appropriate capillary bed is developed. If this condition is satisfied, the obese subjects are termed "metabolically healthy obese" because they may expand their adipocyte depots without inflammation consequences. This kind of expansion is associated with an enlargement of a given fat pad through recruitment of new adipocytes along with an adequate development of the vasculature, minimal associated fibrosis, and the lack of hypoxia and inflammation [83, 99].

The effects of hypoxia for obese humans have been recently disputed, the reactions triggered by the oxygen deprivation being a matter of severity, duration, and environment, since results between in vitro experiments, cell cultures under acute hypoxia, animal models, and human obese subjects are different. In recent studies, opposite data are reported by Goossens's research group. Their experiments revealed an increased pO_2 in obese insulin-resistant subjects and a positive correlation between pO_2 and gene expression for pro-inflammatory markers and an inverse association between pO_2 and peripheral insulin sensitivity [18]. In another experiment, after exposing mice at normoxia and hypoxia for the same duration of time, the authors reported a decrease in adipocyte size, macrophages infiltration, and inflammatory cell genes in adipose tissue from hypoxic animals [100]. The same results were reported for obese men exposed for 10 nights to hypoxia consecutively followed by increased insulin sensitivity [101]. Moreover, it was presumed that the obstructive sleep apnea could be a protective mechanism to maintain energy homeostasis in obese subjects [102, 103]. Angiogenesis in hypoxic tissues is controlled by HIF-1α, so-called the master regulatory of cellular and tissue response to hypoxic stress. In adipose hypoxic tissue, HIF-1 induces angiogenesis by upregulating VEGF gene. VEGF-A is the only endothelial growth factor that stimulates ECM degradation, proliferation, migration, and tube formation of endothelial cells [104]. VEGF secretion is regulated also by insulin stimulation, growth factor, and cytokines, such as PDGF, EGF, TNF-α, TGF-α, and IL-1β [99, 104].

As we showed in a previous study, VEGF immunohistochemical expression was higher in the adipose tissue of obese and obese-diabetic patients, especially in peritoneal depots. In normal weight subjects, both peripheral and central depots were VEGF negative [88].

It was demonstrated that an overexpression of VEGF in transgenic animals increased the vascularization and reversed the metabolic dysfunctions induced by a hypercaloric diet [80].

http://dx.doi.org/10.5772/65491

Recently, it had been claimed that the mechanism of VEGF promoting angiogenesis in adipose tissue is controlled by HIF-1β, while HIF-1α seems to regulate vascularization in BAT but not in WAT and additionally to promote WAT inflammation [105].

Adipokines, such as leptin and adiponectin, have also angiogenic properties that are stimulated in metabolically challenging conditions: leptin stimulates the angiogenic program upregulating VEGF expression, increases the vascular permeability by the formation of fenestrations in endothelial cells, and influences microvessel density [106]. For adiponectin, the results are conflicting: one supposed to be antiangiogenic because it inhibits endothelial cell migration and proliferation in vitro and neoangiogenesis in vivo [107] and others pro-angiogenic [99, 108].

6. Hypoxia: a trigger for BAT whitening and WAT browning

BAT presence has been reported once for small rodents and newborns, but recently, evidence for metabolically active BAT in adult humans has been reported [109]. BAT activation under β-adrenergic signaling is important for heat generation through uncoupled oxidative phosphorylation as a result of activation of non-shivering thermogenesis [110]. For this function, an important blood supply is required to provide the amount of oxygen and nutrients, and therefore BAT is much more vascularized than WAT. In relation to energy balance, an inverse relationship is accepted between BMI and age, BAT being less active in older subjects and in obese [111, 112]. Recent experiments highlighted the importance of hypoxia in BAT dysfunction too, the lack of an adequate BAT vascularization being involved in the overall dysfunction of the adipose organ in obesity [20]. BAT activity reduces the development of metabolic syndrome, and its activation increases insulin sensitivity and contributes to glucose homeostasis [113]. Having a high oxidative capacity, it is presumed that BAT is a contributor to systemic metabolic homeostasis, and this function was impaired in obesity, as demonstrated in the experiment performed by Shimizu and coworkers [114]. They proved in mice that obesity affects the density of the capillary network in BAT much more than in WAT and induced hypoxia in this organ. This elegant experiment shows in a very credible manner that the transition of phenotype from brown to white adipocytes is induced by the diminution of vascularization, a reverse mechanism of BAT differentiation observed in fetal development when the appearance of multilocularity is anticipated by the branching of the capillary loops (personal unpublished data). This vascular dysfunction is followed by the "whitening of the brown fat" (diminished β-adrenergic signaling, the appearance of enlarged lipid droplets in the cells and loss of mitochondria) and can impact obesity and obesity-related diseases [115]. HIF-1α increased level and suppression of UCP1 gene were observed in hypoxic BAT [114]. The same influences that hypoxia exerts on gene expression in WAT have been reported also for BAT, such as increased expression of leptin, VEGF, IL-6, and GLUT1. Due to loss of mitochondria, high glucose uptake will be accompanied by the same switch to anaerobic glycolysis as in WAT. Besides triggering inflammation in macrophages, lactate is supposed to be involved also in "browning of the white fat," recent experimental data proving that in vitro lactate induces the expression of genes encoding UCP1 and proteins involved in mitochondrial oxidation in mice and human white adipocytes [116]. Same authors demonstrated that lactate also controls the browning process in vivo because it regulates Ucp1 expression in a PPAR-δ-dependent manner, the combination of lactate and PPAR-δ ligand rosiglitazone constituting a strong inducer of an increased expression of some mitochondrial oxidation markers in mice white adipose depots [116]. Based on this observation, one can assume that lactate could be responsible for the recruitment of "brite" cells. In light of these results, the recruitment and activation of BAT are regarded as a potential new target for strategies to counteract obesity-induced changes.

In conclusion, hypoxia could be regarded as the leading cause of adipose tissue remodeling rather than as a consequence of the functional changes in the adipose organ. Due to the interplay between hypoxia, inflammation, and angiogenesis, targeting hypoxia pathways could be a valuable therapeutic approach to reduce the clinical consequences of the metabolic syndrome.

Author details

Ana Marina Andrei, Anca Berbecaru-Iovan, Felix Rareş Ioan Din-Anghel, Camelia Elena Stănciulescu, Sorin Berbecaru-Iovan, Ileana Monica Baniţă* and Cătălina Gabriela Pisoschi

*Address all correspondence to: monica.banita@yahoo.com

University of Medicine and Pharmacy of Craiova, Craiova, Dolj County, Romania

References

[1] Kershaw EE, Flier JS: Adipose Tissue as an Endocrine Organ. J Clin Endocrinol Metab. 2004;89(6):2548–2556. DOI:10.1210/jc.2004-0395

[2] Trayhurn P: Endocrine and signalling role of adipose tissue: new perspectives on fat. Acta Physiol Scand. 2005;184:285-293. DOI: 10.1111/j.1365-201X.2005.01468.x

[3] Trayhurn P, Wang B, Wood IS: Hypoxia and the endocrine and signalling role o white adipose tissue. Arch Physiol Biochem. 2008;114(4):267-276. DOI: 10.1080/13813450802 306602

[4] Trayhurn P: Hypoxia and adipose tissue function and dysfunction in obesity. Physiol Rev. 2013;93(1):1-21. DOI: 10.1152/physrev.00017.2012

[5] Berg AH, Scherer PE: Adipose tissue, inflammation, and cardiovascular disease. Circ Res 2005;96:939-949. DOI: 10.1161/01.RES.0000163635.62927.34

[6] McGee DL. Diverse Populations Collaboration: body mass index and mortality: a meta-analysis based on person-level data from twenty-six observational studies. Ann Epidemiol. 2005;15(2):87-97. DOI:10.1016/j.annepidem.2004.05.012

[7] http://www.who.int/mediacentre/factsheets/fs311/en/

[8] Kissebah AH, Vydelingum N, Murray R, Evans DJ, Hartz AJ, Kalkhoff RK, Adams PW: Relation of body fat distribution to metabolic complications of obesity. J Clin Endocrinol Metab. 1982;54(2):254-260. DOI:10.1210/jcem-54-2-254

[9] Carey VJ, Walters EE, Colditz GA, Solomon CG, Willet WC, Rosner BA, Speizer FE, Manson AE: Body fat distribution and risk of non-insulin-dependent diabetes mellitus in women, The Nurses' Health Study. Am J Epidemiol. 1997;145(7):614-619.

[10] Eckel RH: Obesity. Circulation. 2005;111(15):e257-259. DOI: 10.1161/01.CIR.0000163653.38992.E5

[11] Gesta S, Tseng YH, Kahn CR: Developmental origin of fat: tracking obesity to its source. Cell. 2007;131(2):242-256. DOI:10.1016/j.cell.2007.10.004

[12] Janssen I, Katzmarzyk PT, Ross R: Body mass index, waist circumference, and health risk: evidence in support of current National Institutes of Health guidelines. Arch Intern Med. 2002;162(18):2074-2079.

[13] Khandekar MJ, Cohen P, Spiegelman BM: Molecular mechanisms of cancer development in obesity. Nat Rev Cancer. 2011;11(12):886-895. DOI: 10.1038/nrc3174

[14] Pasarica M, Sereda OR, Redman LM, Albarado DC, Hymel DT, Roan LE, Rood JC, Burk DH, Smith SR: Reduced adipose tissue oxygenation in human obesity: evidence for rarefaction, macrophage chemotaxis, and inflammation without an angiogenic response. Diabetes. 2009;58:718–725. DOI:10.2337/db08-1098

[15] Hossogai N, Fukuhara A, Oshima K, Miyata Y, Tanaka S, Segawa K, Furukawa S, Tochino Y, Komuro R, Matsuda M, Shimomura I: Adipose tissue hypoxia in obesity and its impact on adipocytokine dysregulation. Diabetes. 2007;56:901-911. DOI:10.2337/db06-0911

[16] Netzer N, Gatterer H, Faulhaber M, Burtscher M, Pramsohler S, Pesta D: Hypoxia, oxidative stress and fat, Biomolecules. 2015;5(2):1143-1150. DOI:10.3390/biom5021143

[17] Karpe F, Fielding BA, Ilic V, Macdonald IA, Summers LK, Frayn KN: Impaired postprandial adipose tissue blood flow response is related to aspects of insulin sensitivity. Diabetes. 2002; 51:2467–2473. DOI:10.2337/diabetes.51.8.2467

[18] Goossens GH, Bizzarri A, Venteclef N, Essers Y, Cleutjens JP, Konings E, Jocken JWE, Čajlaković M, Ribitsch V, Clément K, Blaak EE: Increased adipose tissue oxygen tension in obese compared with lean men is accompanied by insulin resistance, impaired adipose tissue capillarization, and inflammation. Circulation. 2011;124:67–76. DOI: 10.1161/CIRCULATIONAHA.111.027813

[19] O'Rourke RW, Metcalf MD, White AE, Madala A, Winters BR, Maizlin II, Jobe BA, Roberts CT Jr, Slifka MK, Marks DL: Depot-specific differences in inflammatory mediators and a role for NK cells and IFN-gamma in inflammation in human adipose tissue. Int J Obes (Lond). 2009;33(9):978-990. DOI: 10.1038/ijo.2009.133

[20] Trayhurn P, Alomar SY: Oxygen deprivation and the cellular response to hypoxia in adipocytes—perspectives on white and brown adipose tissues in obesity. Front Endocrinol (Lausanne). 2015;6:19. DOI: 10.3389/fendo.2015.00019.eCollection.2015

[21] Xue Y, Petrovic N, Cao R, Larsson O, Lim S, Chen S, Feldmann HM, Liang Z, Zhu Z, Nedergaard J, Cannon B, Cao Y: Hypoxia-independent angiogenesis in adipose tissues during cold acclimation. Cell Metab. 2009;9(1):99-109. DOI: 10.1016/j.cmet.2008.11.009

[22] Trayhurn P, Wood IS: Adipokines: inflammation and the pleiotropic role of white adipose tissue. Br J Nutr. 2004; 92(3):347-355

[23] Ye J, Gao Z, Yin J, He Q: Hypoxia is a potential risk factor for chronic inflammation and adiponectin reduction in adipose tissue of ob/ob and dietary obese mice. Am J Physiol Endocrinol Metab. 2007; 293(4):E1118-1128. DOI: 10.1152/ajpendo.00435.2007

[24] Wood IS, de Heredia FP, Wang B, Trayhurn P. Cellular hypoxia and adipose tissue dysfunction in obesity. Proc. Nutr. Soc. 2009; 68(4):370-377. DOI: 10.1017/S0029665109990206

[25] Koumenis C, Naczki C, Koritzinsky M, Rastani S, Diehl A, Sonenberg N, Koromilas A, Wouters BG: Regulation of protein synthesis by hypoxia via activation of the endoplasmic reticulum kinase PERK and phosphorylation of the translation initiation factor eIF2alpha. Mol Cell Biol. 2002; 22:7405–7416

[26] Ye J, Gimble JM: Regulation of stem cell differentiation in adipose tissue by chronic inflammation. Clin Exp Pharmacol Physiol. 2011;38(12):872–878. DOI:10.1111/j.1440-1681.2011.05596.x

[27] Halberg N, Khan T, Trujillo ME, Wernstedt-Asterholm I, Attie AD, Sherwani S, Wang ZV, Landskroner-Eiger S, Dineen S, Magalang UJ, Brekken RA, Scherer PE: Hypoxia-inducible factor 1 alpha induces fibrosis and insulin resistance in white adipose tissue. Mol Cell Biol. 2009;29(16):4467-4483.

[28] Divoux A, Tordjman J, Lacasa D, Veyrie N, Hugol D, Aissat A, Basdevant A, Guerre-Millo M, Poitou C, Zucker JD, Bedossa P, Clement K: Fibrosis in human adipose tissue: composition, distribution, and link with lipid metabolism and fat mass loss. Diabetes. 2010; 59:2817-2825. DOI: 10.2337/db10-0585

[29] Reggio S, Pellegrinelli V, Clement K, Tordjman J: Fibrosis as a cause or a consequence of white adipose tissue inflammation in obesity. Curr Obes Rep. 2013;2:1-9. DOI: 10.1007/s13679-012-0037-4

[30] Kunduzova O, Alet N, Delesque-Touchard N, Millet L, Castan-Laurell I, Muller C, Dray C, Schaeffer P, Herault JP, Savi P, Bono F, Valet P. Apelin/APJ signaling system: a

potential link between adipose tissue and endothelial angiogenic processes. FASEB J. 2008; 22(12):4146-53. DOI: 10.1096/fj.07-104018

[31] Hajer GR, van Haeften TW, Visseren FLJ. Adipose tissue dysfunction in obesity, diabetes and vascular diseases. Eur Heart J. 2008;29(24):2959-2971. DOI: 10.1093/eurheartj/ehn387

[32] Cao Y. Adipose tissue angiogenesis as a therapeutic target for obesity and metabolic diseases. Nat Rev Drug Discov. 2010;9(2):107-15. DOI: 10.1038/nrd3055

[33] Cinti S: The adipose organ: morphological perspectives of adipose tissues. Proc Nutr Soc. 2001;60(3):319-328

[34] Cinti S: Adipocyte differentiation and transdifferentiation: plasticity of the adipose organ. J Endocrinol Invest. 2002;25(10):823-835. DOI:10.1007/BF03344046

[35] Frontini A, Cinti S: Distribution and development of brown adipocytes in the murine and human adipose organ. Cell Metab. 2010; 11(4):253-256. DOI:10.1016/j.cmet.2010.03.004

[36] Petrovic N, Walden TB, Shabalina IG, Timmons JA, Cannon B, Nedergaard J: Chronic peroxisome proliferator-activated receptor gamma (PPARgamma) activation of epididymally derived white adipocyte cultures reveals a population of thermogenically competent, UCP1-containing adipocytes molecularly distinct from classic brown adipocytes. J Biol Chem. 2010;285(10):7153-7164. DOI: 10.1074/jbc.M109.053942

[37] Seale P: Transcriptional control of brown adipocyte development and thermogenesis. Int J Obes (Lond). 2010;34 Suppl 1:S17-22. DOI: 10.1038/ijo.2010.178

[38] Chechi K, Carpentier AC, Richard D: Understanding the brown adipocyte as a contributor to energy homeostasis. Trends Endocrinol Metab. 2013;24(8):408-420. DOI: 10.1016/j.tem.2013.04.002

[39] Cinti S, Mitchell G, Barbatelli G, Murano I, Ceresi E, Faloia E, Wang S, Fortier M, Greenberg AS, Obin MS: Adipocyte death defines macrophage localization and function in adipose tissue of obese mice and humans. J Lipid Res. 2005;46(11):2347-2355. DOI:10.1194/jlr.M500294-JLR200

[40] Zhang YY, Proenca R, Maffei M, Barone M, Leopold L, Friedman JM: Positional cloning of the mouse obese gene and its human homolog. Nature. 1994; 372:425-432. DOI: 10.1038/372425a0

[41] Kahn BB, Flier JS: Obesity and insulin resistance. J Clin Invest. 2000;106(4):473-481. DOI: 10.1172/JCI10842

[42] Hotamisligil GS: Inflammation and metabolic disorders. Nature. 2006; 444:860-867. DOI:10.1038/nature05485

[43] Rosen ED, Spiegelman BM: Adipocytes as regulators of energy balance and glucose homeostasis. Nature 2006, 444:847-853. DOI:10.1038/nature05483

[44] Antuna-Puente B, Feve B, Fellahi S, Bastard JP: Adipokines: the missing link between insulin resistance and obesity. Diabetes Metab. 2008;34(1):2-11. DOI: 10.1016/j.diabet.2007.09.004

[45] Skurk T, Alberti-Huber C, Herder C, Hauner H: Relationship between adipocyte size and adipokine expression and secretion. J Clin Endocrinol Metab. 2007; 92:1023–1033. DOI: 10.1210/jc.2006-1055

[46] de Souza Batista CM, Yang RZ, Lee MJ, Glynn NM, Yu DZ, Pray J, Ndubuizu K, Patil S, Schwartz A, Kligman M, Fried SK, Gong DW, Shuldiner AR, Pollin TI, McLenithan JC: Omentin plasma level and gene expression are decreased in obesity. Diabetes. 2007;56:1655-1661. DOI: 10.2337/db06-1506

[47] Cao R, Brakenhielm E, Wahlestedt C, Thyberg J, Cao Y: Leptin induces vascular permeability and synergistically stimulates angiogenesis with FGF-2 and VEGF. Proc Natl Acad Sci USA. 2001;98(11):6390-6395. DOI:10.1073/pnas.101564798

[48] Gabrielsson BG, Johansson JM, Lonn M, Jernas M, Olbers T, Peltonen M, Larsson I, Lonn L, Sjostrom L, Carlsson LM: High expression of complement components in omental adipose tissue in obese men. Obes Res. 2003;11:699-708. DOI: 10.1038/oby.2003.100

[49] Dusserre E, Moulin P, Vidal H: Differences in mRNA expression of the proteins secreted by the adipocytes in human subcutaneous and visceral adipose tissues. Biochim Biophys Acta. 2000;1500:88-96.

[50] Tanko LB, Bruun JM, Alexandersen P, Bagger YZ, Richelsen B, Christiansen C, Larsen PJ: Novel associations between bioavailable estradiol and adipokines in elderly women with different phenotypes of obesity: implications for atherogenesis. Circulation. 2004;110:2246-2252. DOI: 10.1161/01.CIR.0000144470.55149.E5

[51] Fontana L, Eagon JC, Trujillo ME, Scherer PE, Klein S: Visceral fat adipokine secretion is associated with systemic inflammation in obese humans. Diabetes. 2007;56:1010-1013. DOI: 10.2337/db06-1656

[52] Blüher M: Adipose tissue dysfunction contributes to obesity related metabolic diseases. Best Pract Res Clin Endocrinol Metab. 2013;27:163-177. DOI:10.1016/j.beem.2013.02.005

[53] Hodson L, Humphreys SM, Karpe F, Frayn KN: Metabolic signatures of human adipose tissue hypoxia in obesity. Diabetes. 2013;62(5):1417-1425. DOI:10.2337/db12-1032

[54] Zhang L, Ebenezer PJ, Dasuri K, Fernandez-Kim SO, Francis J, Mariappan N, Gao Z, Ye J, Bruce-Keller AJ, Keller JN: Aging is associated with hypoxia and oxidative stress in adipose tissue: Implications for adipose function. Am J Physiol Endocrinol Metab. 2011;301(4):E599-607. DOI: 10.1152/ajpendo.00059.2011

[55] Ye J: Emerging role of adipose tissue hypoxia in obesity and insulin resistance. Int J Obes (Lond). 2009;33(1): 54–66. DOI:10.1038/ijo.2008.229

[56] Chen B, Lam KS, Wang Y, Wu D, Lam MC, Shen J, Wong L, Hoo RL, Zhang J, Xu A: Hypoxia dysregulates the production of adiponectin and plasminogen activator inhibitor-1 independent of reactive oxygen species in adipocytes. Biochem Biophys Res Commun. 2006;341(2):549-556. DOI: 10.1016/j.bbrc.2006.01.004

[57] Ambrosini G, Nath AK, Sierra-Honigmann MR, Flores-Riveros J: Transcriptional activation of the human leptin gene in response to hypoxia. Involvement of hypoxia-inducible factor 1. J Biol Chem. 2002;277:34601–34609. DOI: 10.1074/jbc.M205172200

[58] Blüher M, Wilson-Fritch L, Leszyk J, Laustsen PG, Corvera S, Kahn CR: Role of insulin action and cell size on protein expression patterns in adipocytes. J Biol Chem. 2004; 279:31902–1909. DOI: 10.1074/jbc.M404570200

[59] Mazzatti D, Lim FL, O'Hara A, Wood IS, Trayhurn P: A microarray analysis of the hypoxia-induced modulation of gene expression in human adipocytes. Arch Physiol Biochem. 2012;118:112-120. DOI:10.3109/13813455.2012.654611

[60] Rayalam S, Della-Fera MA, Krieg PA, Cox CM, Robins A, Baile CA: A putative role for apelin in the etiology of obesity. Biochem Biophys Res Commun. 2008;368(3):815-819. DOI:10.1016/j.bbrc.2008.02.2008

[61] Trayhurn P: Hypoxia and adipocyte physiology: Implications for adipose tissue dysfunction in obesity. Ann Rev Nutr. 2014;34:207-236. DOI: 10.1146/annurev-nutr-071812-161156

[62] Wood IS, Wang B, Lorente-Cebrian S, Trayhurn P: Hypoxia increases expression of selective facilitative glucose transporters (GLUT) and 2-deoxy-d-glucose uptake in human adipocytes. Biochem Biophys Res Commun. 2007;361:468-473. DOI: 10.016/j.bbrc.2007.07.032

[63] Rocha S: Gene regulation under low oxygen: holding your breath for transcription. Trends Biochem Sci. 2007;32:389-397. DOI:10.1016/j.tibs.2007.06.005

[64] De Glisezinski I, Crampes F, Harant I, Havlik P, Gardette B, Jammes Y, Souberbielle JC, Richalet JP, Riviere D: Decrease of subcutaneous adipose tissue lipolysis after exposure to hypoxia during a simulated ascent of Mt. Everest. Pflugers Arch. 1999;439:134-140.

[65] Yin J, Gao Z, He Q, Zhou D, Guo Z, Ye J: Role of hypoxia in obesity-induced disorders of glucose and lipid metabolism in adipose tissue. Am J Physiol Endocrinol Metab. 2009; 296:E333-E342. DOI: 10.1152/ajpendo.90760.2008

[66] O'Rourke RW, Meyer KA, Gaston G, White AE, Lumeng CN, Marks DL: Hexosamine biosynthesis is a possible mechanism underlying hypoxia's effects on lipid metabolism in human adipocytes. PLoS One.2013;8:e71165. DOI: 10.1371/journal.pone.0071165

[67] Michailidou Z, Turban S, Miller E, Zou X, Schrader J, Ratcliffe PJ, Hadoke PW, Walker BR, Iredale JP, Morton NM, Seckl JR: Increased angiogenesis protects against adipose hypoxia and fibrosis in metabolic disease-resistant 11β-hydroxysteroid dehydrogenase

type 1 (HSD1)-deficient mice. J Biol Chem. 2012;287(6):4188-4197. DOI: 10.1074/jbc.M111.259325.

[68] Bouloumié A, Drexler HCA, Lafontan M, Busse R: Leptin, the product of Ob gene, promotes angiogenesis. Circ Res. 1998; 83:1059-1066.

[69] Zhu H, Li J, Qin W, Yang Y, He X, Wan D, Gu J: Cloning of a novel gene, ANGPTL4 and the functional study in angiogenesis. Zhonghua Yi Xue Za Zhi. 2002;82:94-99.

[70] Ledoux S, Queguiner, Msika S, Calderari S, Rufat P, Gasc JM, Corvol P, Larger E: Angiogenesis associated with visceral and subcutaneous adipose tissue in severe human obesity. Diabetes. 2008;57:3247-3257. DOI:10.2237/db07-1812

[71] Sun K, Tordjman J, Clement K, Scherer PE: Fibrosis and adipose tissue dysfunction. Cell Metab. 2013;18:470-477. DOI:10.1016/j.cmet.2013.06.016

[72] Mutch DM, Tordjman J, Pelloux V, Hanczar B, Henegar C, Poitou C, Veyrie N, Zucker JD, Clément K: Needle and surgical biopsy techniques differentially affect adipose tissue gene expression profiles. Am J Clin Nutr. 2009;89:51-57. DOI: 10.3945/ajcn.2008.26802

[73] Hotamisligil GS, Shargill NS, Spiegelman BM: Adipose expression of tumor necrosis factor-alpha: direct role in obesity-linked insulin resistance. Science. 1993;259(5091):87-91.

[74] Hotamisligil GS, Arner P, Caro JF, Atkinson RL, Spiegelman BM: Increased adipose tissue expression of tumor necrosis factor-alpha in human obesity and insulin resistance. J Clin Invest. 1995;95(5):2409-2415. DOI:10.1172/JCI117936

[75] Gregor MF, Hotamisligil GS: Adipocyte stress: the endoplasmic reticulum and metabolic disease. J Lipid Res. 2007;48:1905-1914. DOI:10.1194/jlr.R700007-JLR200

[76] Shi H, Cave B, Inouye K, Bjørbaek C, Flier JS: Overexpression of suppressor of cytokine signaling 3 in adipose tissue causes local but not systemic insulin resistance. Diabetes. 2006;55(3):699-707.

[77] Yu C, Chen Y, Cline GW, Zhang D, Zong H, Wang Y, Bergeron R, Kim JK, Cushman SW, Cooney GJ, Atcheson B, White MF, Kraegen EW, Shulman GI: Mechanism by which fatty acids inhibit insulin activation of insulin receptor substrate-1 (IRS-1)-associated phosphatidylinositol 3-kinase activity in muscle. J Biol Chem. 2002;277(52):50230-50236. DOI:10.1074/jbc.M200958200

[78] Özcan U, Cao Q, Yilmaz E, Lee AW, Iwakoshi NN, Özdelen E, Tuncman G, Görgün C, Glimcher LH, Hotamisligil GS: Endoplasmic reticulum stress links obesity, insulin action, and type 2 diabetes. Science. 2004;306(5695):457-461. DOI:10.1126/science.1103160

[79] Houstis N, Rosen ED, Lander ES: Reactive oxygen species have a causal role in multiple forms of insulin resistance. Nature. 2006;440(7086):944-948. DOI:10.1038/nature04634

[80] Lefere S, Van Steenkiste C, Verhelst X, Van Vlierberghe H, Devisscher L, Geerts A: Hypoxia-regulated mechanisms in the pathogenesis of obesity and non-alcoholic fatty liver disease. Cell Mol Life Sci. 2016; April 18. DOI: 10.1007/s00018-016-2222-1

[81] Lumeng CN, DelProposto JB, Westcott DJ, Saltiel AR: Phenotypic switching of adipose tissue macrophages with obesity is generated by spatiotemporal differences in macrophage subtypes. Diabetes. 2008;57(12):3239-3246. DOI: 10.2337/db08-0872

[82] Fusaru AM, Stănciulescu CE, Surlin V, Taisescu C, Bold A, Pop OT, Baniţă IM, Crăiţoiu S, Pisoschi CG: Role of innate immune receptors TLR2 and TLR4 as mediators of the inflammatory reaction in human visceral adipose tissue. Rom J Morphol Embryol. 2012;53(3 Suppl):693-701.

[83] Sun K, Kusminski CM, Scherer PE: Adipose tissue remodeling and obesity. J Clin Invest. 2011;121(6):2094-2101. DOI: 10.1172/JCI45887

[84] Strissel KJ, Stancheva Z, Miyoshi H, Perfield JW, DeFuria J, Jick Z, Greenberg AS, Obin MS: Adipocyte death, adipose tissue remodeling, and obesity complications. Diabetes. 2007;56(12):2910-2918. DOI:10.2337/db07-0767

[85] Lee MJ, Wu Y, Fried SK: Adipose tissue remodeling in pathophysiology of obesity. Curr Opin Clin Nutr Metab Care. 2010;13(4):371–376. DOI: 10.1097/MCO.0b013e32833aabef

[86] Rausch ME, Weisberg S, Vardhana P, Tortoriello DV: Obesity in C57BL/6 J mice is characterized by adipose tissue hypoxia and cytotoxic T-cell infiltration. Int J Obes (Lond). 2008;32(3):451-463. DOI: 10.1038/sj.ijo.0803744

[87] Chun TH: Peri-adipocyte ECM remodeling in obesity and adipose tissue fibrosis. Adipocyte. 2012; 1(2): 89–95. DOI:10.4161/adip.19752

[88] Fusaru AM, Pisoschi CG, Bold A, Taisescu C, Stănescu R, Hîncu M, Crăiţoiu S, Baniţă IM: Hypoxia induced VEGF synthesis in visceral adipose depots of obese diabetic patients. Rom J Morphol Embryol. 2012;53(4):903-909.

[89] Hoffstedt J, Arner E, Wahrenberg H, Andersson DP, Qvisth V, Löfgren P, Rydén M, Thörne A, Wirén M, Palmér M, Thorell A, Toft E, Arner P. Regional impact of adipose tissue morphology on the metabolic profile in morbid obesity. Diabetologia. 2010;53(12):2496-2503. DOI: 10.1007/s00125-010-1889-3.

[90] Nakajima I, Muroya S, Tanabe R, Chikuni K: Extracellular matrix development during differentiation into adipocytes with a unique increase in type V and VI collagen. Biol Cell. 2002;94(3):197-203.

[91] Khan T, Muise ES, Iyengar P, Wang ZV, Chandalia M, Abate N, Zhang BB, Bonaldo P, Chua S, Scherer PE: Metabolic dysregulation and adipose tissue fibrosis: role of collagen VI. Mol Cell Biol. 2009;(6):1575-1591. DOI: 10.1128/MCB.01300-08

[92] Spencer M, Yao-Borengasser A, Unal R, Rasouli N, Gurley CM, Zhu B, Peterson CA, Kern PA: Adipose tissue macrophages in insulin-resistant subjects are associated with

collagen VI and fibrosis and demonstrate alternative activation. Am J Physiol Endocrinol Metab. 2010;299(6):E1016-1027. DOI:10.1152/ajpendo.00329.2010

[93] Rehman J, Traktuev D, Li J, Merfeld-Clauss S, Temm-Grove CJ, Bovenkerk JE, Pell CL, Johnstone BH, Considine RV, March KL: Secretion of angiogenic and antiapoptotic factors by human adipose stromal cells. Circulation. 2004;109(10):1292-1298. DOI: 10.1161/01.CIR. 0000121425.42966.F1

[94] Halberg N, Wernstedt-Asterholm I, Scherer PE: The adipocyte as an endocrine cell. Endocrinol Metab Clin North Am. 2008;37(3):753-768, x-xi. DOI: 10.1016/j.ecl. 2008.07.002

[95] Rupnick MA, Panigrahy D, Zhang CY, Dallabrida SM, Lowell BB, Langer R, Folkman MJ: Adipose tissue mass can be regulated through the vasculature. Proc Natl Acad Sci USA. 2002;99(16):10730-10735. DOI:10.1073/pnas.162349799

[96] Bråkenhielm E, Cao R, Gao B, Angelin B, Cannon B, Parini P, Cao Y: Angiogenesis inhibitor, TNP-470, prevents diet-induced and genetic obesity in mice. Circ Res. 2004;94(12):1579-1588. DOI: 10.1161/01.RES.0000132745.76882.70

[97] Gealekman O, Burkart A, Chouinard M, Nicoloro SM, Straubhaar J, Corvera S: Enhanced angiogenesis in obesity and in response to PPAR gamma activators through adipocyte VEGF and ANGPTL4 production. Am J Physiol Endocrinol Metab. 2008;295(5):E1056-1064. DOI: 10.1152/ajpendo.90345.2008

[98] Villaret A, Galitzky J, Decaunes P, Estève D, Marques MA, Sengenès C, Chiotasso P, Tchkonia T, Lafontan M, Kirkland JL, Bouloumié A: Adipose tissue endothelial cells from obese human subjects: differences among depots in angiogenic, metabolic, and inflammatory gene expression and cellular senescence. Diabetes. 2010;59(11): 2755-2763. DOI:10.2337/db10-0398

[99] Sun K, Wernstedt Asterholm I, Kusminski CM, Bueno AC, Wang ZV, Pollard JW, Brekken RA, Scherer PE: Dichotomous effects of VEGF-A on adipose tissue dysfunction. Proc Natl Acad Sci USA. 2012;109(15):5874-5879. DOI:10.1073/pnas.1200447109

[100] van den Borst B, Schols AM, de Theije C, Boots AW, Kohler SE, Goossens GH, Gosker HR: Characterization of the inflammatory and metabolic profile of adipose tissue in a mouse model of chronic hypoxia. J Appl Physiol. 2013;114:1619–1628. DOI: 10.1152/japplphysiol.00460.2012

[101] Lecoultre V, Peterson CM, Covington JD, Ebenezer PJ, Frost EA, Schwarz JM, Ravussin E: Ten nights of moderate hypoxia improves insulin sensitivity in obese humans. Diabetes Care. 2013;36:e197–198. DOI:10.2337/dc13-1350

[102] Ye J. Hypoxia in obesity - from bench to bedside. J Transl Med. 2012; 10(Suppl 2): A20. DOI: 10.1186/1479-5876-10-S2-A20

[103] Goossens GH, Blaak EE: Adipose tissue dysfunction and impaired metabolic health in human obesity: a matter of oxygen? Front Endocrinol. 2015;6:55. DOI:10.3389/fendo.2015.00055

[104] Liekens S, De Clercq E, Neyts J: Angiogenesis: regulators and clinical applications. Biochem Pharmacol. 2001;61(3):253-270

[105] Zhang X, Lam KS, Ye H, Chung SK, Zhou M, Wang Y, Xu A: Adipose tissue-specific inhibition of hypoxia-inducible factor 1{alpha} induces obesity and glucose intolerance by impeding energy expenditure in mice. J Biol Chem. 2010;285(43):32869-32877. DOI: 10.1074/jbc.M110.135509

[106] Christiaens V, Lijnen HR: Angiogenesis and development of adipose tissue. Mol Cell Endocrinol. 2010;318(1-2):2-9. DOI: 10.1016/j.mce.2009.08.006

[107] Brakenhielm E, Veitonmaki N, Cao R, Kihara S, Matsuzawa Y, Zhivotovsky B, Funahashi T, Cao Y: Adiponectin-induced antiangiogenesis and antitumor activity involve caspase-mediated endothelial cell apoptosis. Proc Natl Acad Sci USA. 2004;101(8): 2476-2481

[108] Kobayashi H, Ouchi N, Kihara S, Walsh K, Kumada M, Abe Y, Funahashi T, Matsuzawa Y: Selective suppression of endothelial cell apoptosis by the high molecular weight form of adiponectin. Circ Res. 2004;94(4):e27-31

[109] Zingaretti MC, Crosta F, Vitali A, Guerrieri M, Frontini A, Cannon B, Nedergaard J, Cinti S: The presence of UCP1 demonstrates that metabolically active adipose tissue in the neck of adult humans truly represents brown adipose tissue. FASEB J. 2009;23(9): 3113-3120. DOI: 10.1096/fj.09-133546

[110] Cannon B, Nedergaard J: Brown adipose tissue: function and physiological significance. Physiol Rev. 2004;84:277–359. DOI:10.1152/physrev.00015.2003

[111] Lee P, Greenfield JR, Ho KKY, Fulham MJ: A critical appraisal of the prevalence and metabolic significance of brown adipose tissue in adult humans. Am J Physiol Endocrinol Metab. 2010;299:E601–606. DOI:10.1152/ajpendo.00298.2010

[112] Pfannenberg C, Werner MK, Ripkens S, Stef I, Deckert A, Schmadl M, Reimold M, Häring HU, Claussen CD, Stefan N: Impact of age on the relationships of brown adipose tissue with sex and adiposity in humans. Diabetes. 2010;59:1789–1793. DOI:10.2337/db10-0004

[113] Stanford KI, Middelbeek RJ, Townsend KL, An D, Nygaard EB, Hitchcox KM, Markan KR, Nakano K, Hirshman MF, Tseng YH, Goodyear LJ: Brown adipose tissue regulates glucose homeostasis and insulin sensitivity. J Clin Invest. 2013;123:215–223. DOI: 10.1172/JCI62308

[114] Shimizu I, Aprahamian T, Kikuchi R, Shimizu A, Papanicolaou KN, MacLauchlan S, Maruyama S, Walsh K: Vascular rarefaction mediates whitening of brown fat in obesity. J Clin Invest. 2014;124:2099–2112. DOI:10.1172/JCI71643

[115] Shimizu I, Walsh K: The whitening of brown fat and its implications for weight management in obesity. Curr Obes Rep.2015 ;4:224-228. DOI:10.1007/s13679-015-0157-8

[116] Carrière A, Jeanson Y, Berger-Müller S, André M, Chenouard V, Arnaud E, Barreau C, Walther R, Galinier A, Wdziekonski B, Villageois P, Louche K, Collas P, Moro C, Dani C, Villarroya F, Casteilla L: Browning of white adipose cells by intermediate metabolites: an adaptive mechanism to alleviate redox pressure. Diabetes. 2014 ;63:3253–3265. DOI:10.2337/db13-1885

Chapter 17

Epigenetic Programming of Cardiovascular Disease by Perinatal Hypoxia and Fetal Growth Restriction

Paola Casanello, Emilio A. Herrera and
Bernardo J. Krause

Additional information is available at the end of the chapter

http://dx.doi.org/10.5772/66740

Abstract

Most of the worldwide deaths in patients with non-communicable diseases are due to cardiovascular and metabolic diseases, which are determined by a mix of environmental, genetic and epigenetic factors, and by their interactions. The aetiology of most cardiovascular diseases has been partially linked with *in utero* adverse conditions that may increase the risk of developing diseases later in life, known as Developmental Origins of Health and Disease (DOHaD). Perinatal hypoxia can program the fetal and postnatal developmental patterns, resulting in permanent modifications of cells, organs and systems function. In spite of the vast evidence obtained from human and animal studies linking development under adverse intrauterine conditions with increased cardiovascular risk, still few is known about the specific effects of intrauterine oxygen deficiency and the related pathogenic mechanisms. Currently, the most accepted processes that program cellular function are epigenetic mechanisms which determine gene expression in a cell-specific fashion. In this chapter we will review the current literature regarding the perinatal exposure to chronic hypoxia and Fetal Growth Restriction (FGR) in humans and animals and how this impinges the cardiovascular physiology through epigenetic, biochemical, morphologic and pathophysiologic modifications that translate into diseases blasting at postnatal life.

Keywords: hypoxia, programming, vascular function, oxidative stress, epigenetics, chronic diseases

1. Introduction

The worldwide prevalence of cardiovascular diseases (CVDs) and metabolic syndrome ranges between 20 and 40%. These figures are likely to rise over the next decades [1, 2]. Genetic changes associated with the traits of the metabolic syndrome and cardiovascular diseases are able to explain a small proportion of cases [3], suggesting the presence of other contributory factors in these conditions. Epidemiologic studies in the late 1980s in the UK revealed a strong correlation with perinatal and fetal growth patterns. Fetal growth restriction (FGR) is thus associated with an increased risk of developing adult cardiometabolic diseases [4]. Multiple reports from across the world have documented the association between intrauterine growth mediators in early life with lifelong health. These are now recognized to be important risks in the development of non-communicable diseases in adult life. This concept so-called "Fetal Programming" has evolved into "Developmental Origins of Health and Disease" (DOHaD), which we refer as Intrauterine Programming (IUP) [5] for the purpose of this chapter. The present efforts in this field are focused on unveiling the physiological and molecular mechanisms, which drive IUP, and exploring opportunities to prevent or revert the long-term consequences. The physiologic and biochemical changes that explain IUP relate to the timing and stage of development when the insult takes place; the earlier in development, the stronger the long-term effects [5]. Conversely, the long-term consequences of IUP and reproducibility of the related phenotypes suggest that epigenetic mechanisms may underlay the altered "cell programming" [6].

2. Fetal growth restriction

Fetal growth restriction (FGR) is clinically defined by a fetal weight below the 10th percentile of normal for gestational age, but in a generic manner, FGR is a condition in which the potential growth of the fetus is negatively influenced by environmental and maternal factors [7]. The short-term consequences of FGR are LBW and the corresponding phenotype, which is associated with increased perinatal morbidity and mortality [8]. The long-term effects include a two- to threefold increase in the risk of developing cardiovascular disease (hypertension and coronary heart disease) in adult life [9]. The higher CVD risk in adults resulting from FGR can be traced back to a reduced arterial compliance in pre-pubertal subjects [10] and a decreased peripheral endothelial-dependent vascular relaxation at birth [11]. Moreover, studies in human placentae show that FGR-related endothelial dysfunction can also be detected in chorionic and umbilical arteries [12, 13]. Notably, we have recently demonstrated the presence of functional and epigenetic markers of endothelial dysfunction in systemic and umbilical arteries from FGR guinea pigs. The presence of these comparable markers suggests that umbilical artery endothelial cells (ECs) may be useful to explore the endothelial function of the fetus. The etiology of FGR in humans is not fully understood; however, there are known maternal risk factors such as living at high altitude, malnutrition, smoking, stress, and vascular dysfunction [14] which induce placental dysfunction and consequently fetal growth restriction. Presently, oxygen, glucose, free radicals, amino acids, and hormones have been shown to play an important role in modulating fetal growth and development. These factors are dynamically regulated throughout gestation [15]. In the earlier stages, limitations in oxygen supply promote trophoblast proliferation; however, persistence in a hypoxic environment as occurs in FGR harms trophoblast invasion and the transformation of spiral arteries leading to a vascular dysfunction of the placenta and impaired fetal growth. Thus, chronic hypoxia and oxidative stress have an important role in the placental dysfunction observed in FGR [15]. Several studies on humans confirm the presence of molecular markers of oxidative stress in the FGR placentae, the fetus, and the mother [16–19]. Impaired placental vascular function has also been proposed to play a role in FGR, conditioned by augmented synthesis and response to vasoconstrictors [20] and limited action of vasodilators [13], as well as by an increased inhibition of endothelial-dependent relaxation mediated by prooxidants [21].

Appropriate maternal nutrient supply to the fetus is key for its development. Several approaches limiting maternal supply (i.e., diet restriction) and placental nutrient transfer have been used to alter the normal fetal growth rate and development. In order to address this issue, various animal models (sheep, rat, rabbit, and guinea pig) have been developed, where placental dysfunction is induced by a reduction in uterine blood flow [22, 23]. We have recently developed a novel model of FGR in guinea pigs, by a progressive bilateral occlusion of the uterine arteries during the second half of gestation that gradually alters placental vascular resistance [24]. Several aspects suggest that this model is relevant to human clinical significance. For instance, guinea pigs present a decreased fetal abdominal growth and impaired placental blood flow adaptation during gestation, with a preserved brain blood flow and development, translating into an asymmetric FGR. Additionally, higher resistance to blood flow in the umbilical arteries can be observed. These are relevant clinical markers of FGR. However, most of mammalian models that develop placental insufficiency present a mixed effect of undernutrition, hypoxia, and oxidative stress [22]. Therefore, complementary models on chick embryos have been used to isolate the unique fetal effects of hypoxia during development from maternal responses [22]. Interestingly, the follow-up of the chickens gestated under hypoxia has shown important insights into the pathophysiological mechanisms that impair the cardiovascular function. For instance, Tintu et al. showed that developmental hypoxia induces cardiomyopathy associated with left ventricular dilatation, reduced ventricular wall mass, and increased apoptosis [25]. These responses were coupled with pump dysfunction, decreased ejection fractions, and diastolic dysfunction, which persisted in adulthood. Further, Salinas et al. showed marked cardiovascular morphostructural changes in high-altitude chicks, which were reverted either by incubation at low altitude or by oxygen supplementation [26]. Notably, Herrera et al. followed up these chicks to adulthood describing cardiac impairment in the capacity to response to pressor challenges [27]. In addition to the cardiovascular system, several organs/functions are affected during developmental hypoxia such as central nervous system, lung, and systemic metabolism. As well as in mammalian physiology, it seems that oxidative stress might be key in establishing the impairments induced by developmental hypoxia [28].

2.1. Hypoxia and oxidative stress in FGR

Hypoxia is defined as a limited oxygen (O_2) supply relative to the physiological demands of a tissue, organ, or organism. This is a restrictive condition frequently seen in the hypobaric environment (hypoxia of high altitude) or by a diminished oxygen delivery. At lowlands, hypoxia is a restrictive condition often faced during fetal life, either by maternal, umbilical-placental, or fetal conditions. Placental insufficiency leads to fetal growth restriction due to a chronic decrease in fetoplacental perfusion. This situation affects simultaneously O_2 and nutrient supply to the fetus [29], overlapping conditions that become difficult to isolate in order to assess the specific effect of O_2 deficiency in determining vascular impairment. Using avian models of FGR has served to establish that chronic hypoxia, independent of nutrition, plays a crucial role in vascular programming [30, 31]. Studies of vascular function during fetal life show remarkable similarities between the effect of hypoxia in chick embryos and placental insufficiency in mammals [26, 28]; they have also served to assess the long-term consequences [27]. In both cases (chick embryos and mammalian fetuses), the presence of endothelial dysfunction and vascular remodeling is observed mainly in peripheral arteries. The mechanism by which hypoxia induces cell damage in either case is the result of an increased generation of reactive oxygen species (ROS) due to an incomplete reduction of oxygen [15, 32].

The imbalance between endogenous antioxidant defenses and reactive oxygen species, where ROS overwhelms the antioxidant capacity, has been termed "oxidative stress" [33]. ROS includes a wide variety of highly reactive molecules, such as superoxide anion ($\cdot O_2^-$), hydrogen peroxide (H_2O_2), ·NO, peroxynitrite (ONOO-), organic hydroperoxide (ROOH), hypochlorous acid (HOCl), and hydroxyl (·OH), alkoxy (RO·), and peroxy radicals (ROO·) [34]. Superoxide is the main ROS acting at the vascular level; it derives from the enzymatic activity of NOX (NADPH oxidases), XOR (xanthine oxidases), mitochondrial complexes I and III, uncoupled eNOS, and iNOS. In the case of NOS, ROS generation can occur because of reduced L-arginine (substrate) or BH_4 (cofactor) availability [33], uncoupling eNOS enzymes. Consequently, NOS-derived $\cdot O_2^-$ rapidly reacts with NO generating ONOO-, which reduces NO levels and modifies the structure of proteins, lipids, and DNA, causing endothelial dysfunction. Thus, increased oxidative stress exerts a negative effect on eNOS activity and NO bioavailability at multiple levels [33].

In FGR, compelling data show that oxidative stress in parallel to chronic hypoxia contributes to vascular dysfunction in the mother, placenta, and fetus [14]. In fact, short-term hypoxia induces eNOS expression and activation in human umbilical artery endothelial cells (HUAECs) [35], while in FGR HUAEC, there is reduced eNOS activation [13]. Conversely, FGR subjects present at birth increased levels of lipid peroxidation and decreased the activity of antioxidant enzymes and circulating mediators [36]. Additionally, markers of oxidative stress have been positively associated with increased umbilical artery pulsatility index, particularly in pregnancies affected by FGR [37]. We recently addressed the role of oxidative stress in FGR by treating pregnant guinea pigs with N-acetyl cysteine, a glutathione precursor, during the second half of gestation. Our results show that maternal treatment with NAC restores fetal growth by increasing placental efficiency and reverses endothelial dysfunction in FGR guinea pigs [38]. Similarly, *in ovo* melatonin administration to chronic hypoxic chick embryos reduces the levels of oxidative stress markers (i.e., lipid peroxidation and protein nitration), by increasing the expression of glutathione peroxidase (GPx), an antioxidant enzyme [28]. This effect is associated with improved endothelial function and reversal of fetal hypoxia-induced vascular remodeling; however, melatonin does not prevent FGR. Even more, in a chronic hypoxic sheep model, melatonin decreased maternal oxidative stress but simultaneously enhanced fetal growth restriction [39]. In summary, these data suggest that hypoxia and oxidative stress participate in the genesis of FGR-induced vascular dysfunction.

However, there is a need for further studies addressing the precise molecular mechanisms and effective treatments for hypoxic FGR and IUP.

At a molecular level, transcription factors nuclear factor kappa B (NFκB) [34] and nuclear factor E2-related factor 2 (Nrf2) implicated in oxidative stress [34, 40] participate in promoting and reducing cellular oxidative stress, respectively. Interestingly, Nrf2 presents the suggested properties of an oxidative stress sensor. Nrf2 is normally bound to Keap1, which targets the complex to proteasome degradation; however, a prooxidant milieu induces the oxidation of two cysteine residues in Keap1 and the release of Nrf2 that subsequently translocate to the nucleus [34]. The antioxidant response triggered by Nrf2 includes the expression of NAD(P)H dehydrogenase quinone 1 (NQO1), heme-oxygenase (HO), and other antioxidant enzymes [40]. Studies show that Nrf2-induced expression of NQO1 and HO-1 improves endothelial dysfunction increasing eNOS efficiency. However, there is no information addressing whether changes in the expression of genes involved in the antioxidant defense are present in early stages of endothelial dysfunction in FGR and whether they can be modulated during gestation.

3. Epigenetics and endothelial programming in FGR

Alteration in fetal development and IUP results in permanent changes in the physiological responses to different stressors across the life course. Undoubtedly, this represents a potential "handicap" for long-term health. Growing evidence in humans from individuals with altered fetal growth, and from animal models associated with the development of later cardiometabolic alterations, confirms the presence of epigenetic markers in different cell types [41]. Epigenetics can be considered as "chromosome-based mechanisms that modify the phenotypic plasticity of a cell or organism" [6]. Development itself is controlled by epigenetic mechanisms, which regulate cell differentiation and record environmental signals under physiologic [42] and/or pathologic conditions [43]. These epigenetic mechanisms include DNA methylation, a plethora of histone posttranslational modifications (PTM) (acetylation, methylation, phosphorylation, and others), ATP-dependent chromatin modifications, and noncoding RNAs [44].

3.1. DNA methylation

In higher animals, DNA is methylated via an enzymatic activity that transfers a methyl group to the 5′ position of cytosine ring on CpG dinucleotide generating 5-methyl-cytosine, a reaction catalyzed by two different families of DNA methyltransferases (DNMTs), named DNMT1 and DNMT3 (DNMT3a and DNMT3b) encoded by three different genes [45]. The role of DNMT1 is to preserve the DNA methylation pattern after DNA replication during mitotic cell division as well as after fertilization [46], a process guided by the presence of hemi-methylated CpGs, which are recognized by DNMT1 in dsDNA [47]. Additionally, DNMT3a and DNMT3b catalyze *de novo* methylation allowing the establishment of new DNA methylation patterns during gametogenesis, embryonic development, and cell differentiation [46, 48]. Interestingly, the genome of different cell types from a single subject presents a high DNA methylation density;

however, larger differences occur in the promoter regions of genes representing less than 5% of the total genomic DNA methylation [49]. Nonetheless, these subtle differences are likely controlling most cell-specific proteins expression at the whole organism level [50]. It is commonly accepted that DNA methylation represents a hallmark of reduced gene expression and long-term gene silencing [51, 52]; however, it is worth noting that growing evidence suggests a more dynamic role for this mechanism in the regulation of gene expression [51].

3.2. Histone posttranslational modifications

The protein structural unit of the chromosomes, the nucleosome, is formed by two copies of four histones proteins named H2A, H2B, H3, and H4. Additionally, these proteins present a globular domain to interact with other histones, and a flexible tail that participates actively in the interaction with DNA. Unlike DNA methylation, histone posttranslational modifications (PTMs) are more dynamic and do not give a straight idea regarding gene silencing or activation [52]. Moreover, histone PTMs are closely related with the context in which they take place and the presence of additional PTMs, suggesting the existence of a "histone code." Up to date, more than 50 enzymes that catalyze diverse histone modifications have been identified and classified according to the reaction they carry out [53]. **Histone acetylation** occurs in lysine residues (K) and involves the transference of an acetyl group from acetyl-CoA. In mammals, this reaction is carried out by three families of histone acetyl-transferases (HAT) named GNAT, MYST, and CBP/p300 [54]. This modification is considered an activator of gene expression, due to the fact that it stabilizes the positive charge of the lysine in the histone, reducing its affinity for DNA, avoiding the formation of highly compacted chromatin. The best characterized acetylations are those that take place in lysine 9 (K9), K14, K18, and K56 in histone 3 (H3) and K5, K8, K13, and K16 in H4 [55]. At least four types of **histone deacetylases** (HDAC I, II, III y IV) have been identified, which catalyze the reverse reaction of that done by the **histone acetyl-transferase**. This enzymatic reaction is related to gene silencing, progression of cell cycle, differentiation, and the response induced by DNA damage [56]. HDAC activity can be induced in response to DNA methylation, once repressor proteins that bind CpGs (MCP) are recruited. The latter have a site of interaction with several HDACs, suggesting that gene silencing could result from a combined action of DNA and histone modifications [51, 57].

3.3. Noncoding RNAs

The idea that noncoding RNAs could regulate the expression of genes was first proposed in the early 1960s [58], with a substantial progress in this field during the last decade. Less than 5% of the transcribed RNA encodes proteins; thus, most of them correspond to noncoding RNAs (ncRNAs) involved mainly in the regulation of gene expression [59, 60]. "Long" ncRNA (lncRNA), small interfering RNA (siRNA), and micro-RNA (miRNA) are the main regulatory ncRNAs. The lncRNA regulates the expression of a specific gene complementary either through chromatin remodeling, alternative mRNA processing (splicing), or siRNA generation [59]. Conversely, siRNA and miRNAs are interference RNA-based epigenetic mechanisms,

http://dx.doi.org/10.5772/66740

which silence genes via noncoding RNAs of ~21 bp. To date, more than a thousand noncoding miRNAs have been reported. These are transcribed by the RNA polymerase II and encoded by specific genes (~70%) or, in lesser amounts, within the intronic regions of gene encoding proteins. Micro-RNAs are transcribed as pre-miRNA and initially processed in the nucleus by the DROSHA-DGCR8 complex. Subsequently, they are exported to the cytoplasm for miRNA maturation by the action of the complex formed by the DICER1 protein and RNase IIIa IIIb [61]. This processing leads to a single-strand RNA, which is incorporated into the "protein-induced silencing complex miRNA" (miRISC), which binds to a complementary region in a target mRNA. It has been proposed that a full complementarity between the miRNA and mRNA leads to degradation of the mRNA, while partial complementarity suppresses translation [62]. Notably, a single miRNA can regulate the expression of multiple mRNAs often associated signaling pathways or metabolic processes, while several miRNAs may converge in the regulation of a single mRNA constituting a complex mechanism for gene expression regulation [61, 62].

3.4. Epigenetics in endothelial physiology

Vascular development and endothelial differentiation and function require a fine epigenetic tuning, suggesting that epigenetic mechanisms play a key role in the IUP-associated vascular dysfunction [6]. The first stages of vascular development are determined by genetic factors, while the next processes that take place (i.e., blood vessel structure, identity, and function) are influenced/determined by hemodynamic factors, ROS, and oxygen levels [63, 64]. Considering that the effect of endothelial-specific transcription factors such as KLF2 and HoxA9 does not explain the protein expression levels present in this cell type [65], an "endothelial epigenetic code" regulating the expression of crucial genes has been suggested [52, 66]. Growing evidence shows that DNA methylation, histone PTM, and miRNAs [67] play an important role in the embryonic origins of endothelial cells (EC), as well as their homeostasis during life. The epigenetic regulation of *NOS3* gene has been extensively studied in EC and non-EC, showing that ECs have a distinctive pattern of DNA methylation and histone PTMs [65]. Conversely, the decreased expression of eNOS in HUVEC exposed to acute hypoxia is controlled by the overexpression of a natural cis-antisense noncoding RNA called sONE [68] and changes in histone PTM which occur specifically at the promoter of eNOS [69]. Similarly, in the endothelium, hypoxia and oxidative stress regulate the expression of several miRNAs that modify the expression of eNOS and other enzymes related to its short- and long-term function [70]. In support of this notion, we have recently demonstrated that eNOS-induced NO enhances arginase-2 expression by epigenetic modifications in the histones residing at *ARG2* gene promoter [71]. In summary, these data show that EC-specific eNOS expression, as well as other genes related with the L-arginine/NO pathway, is effectively controlled by multiple epigenetic mechanisms which are strongly influenced by hypoxia.

3.5. Epigenetics and endothelial dysfunction

Diverse studies show that epigenetic mechanisms can increase the risk or directly participate in the development of vascular diseases. In humans, ECs from atherosclerotic plaques have decreased levels of estrogen receptor-β along with increased DNA methylation at the promoter region of this gene, compared with nonatherosclerotic plaques cells [72]. Further studies in mice [73] and swine [74] have demonstrated that disturbed flow induces genome-wide changes in the DNA methylation of EC in vivo and in vitro, an effect that would be dependent on DNMT1 expression and that mainly affects genes related to oxidative stress. Conversely, abrogation of *Nos3* promoter DNA methylation increases basal eNOS mRNA expression in vitro and protects against hind limb ischemia injury in vivo [75]. Similarly, growing evidence suggests a central role of miRNAs in the genesis of cardiometabolic dysfunction, also proposed as sensitive molecular markers of vascular disease [76]. In fact, we recently reported that circulating levels of miRNA Let-7 and miR-126 are associated with different traits of cardiometabolic dysfunction in children as well as have a predictive value for metabolic syndrome in these subjects [77]. Comparable results in adults with type 2 diabetes have been reported, where increased levels of miR-21 and decreased levels of miR-126 correlated with cardiovascular and inflammatory complications [78].

In the context of IUP of endothelial dysfunction in rats, it has been shown that brief exposure to hypoxia at the end of gestation induces pulmonary vascular dysfunction in the newborn, which associates with increased eNOS expression accompanied by decreased DNA methylation in *Nos3* gene promoter [79]. Similarly, we reported a few years ago for the first time the presence of an altered epigenetic programming of eNOS expression in EC derived from human umbilical arteries of FGR patients [12]. Notably, the altered expression of eNOS was reversed by silencing DNMT1 expression in FGR EC, which restored the DNA methylation pattern at *NOS3* promoter, as well as the regulation of eNOS expression induced by hypoxia [12]. Furthermore, using a guinea pig model of FGR, we compared the eNOS expression and DNA methylation pattern at *Nos3* promoter to clarify whether these epigenetic changes occurring in umbilical EC would represent changes that take place in systemic arteries (i.e., aorta and femoral) [38]. We found comparable changes in eNOS expression which were associated with specific changes in DNA methylation of *Nos3* promoter in the different FGR EC studied, suggesting the presence of a common programming of endothelial dysfunction in the umbilical-placental and systemic circulation. Of note, maternal treatment with an antioxidant (NAC) prevented this epigenetic programming, restoring the eNOS mRNA levels to values observed in control fetuses. Similar studies have shown the beneficial effects of antioxidants during development, showing clear evidences that ROS have causal roles in cardiovascular programming [32]. In addition, several authors have shown that ROS may induce important epigenetic modifications that determined cardiovascular dysfunction later in life. Hypoxia and oxidative stress have been shown to be present in several conditions during pregnancy, such as preeclampsia, placental insufficiency, and high-altitude pregnancies [80]. In addition, assisted reproductive technologies induce hypoxic conditions at very early stages of development. All of the above studies have suggested epigenetic modifications of the eNOS gene [80, 81]. Conversely, the response to hypoxia and oxidative stress is primarily mediated by the hypoxia-inducible transcription factor (HIF), which is regulated by the oxygen-sensing HIF hydroxylases, members of the 2-oxoglutarate (2OG)-dependent oxygen-

http://dx.doi.org/10.5772/66740

ase family. Similarly, there are demethylases from the same family modulating methylation levels. Both systems, a transcription factor and an epigenetic regulator, are being regulated by hypoxia [82]. Further, HIF-1α has been suggested as an epigenetic modulator determining chromatin remodeling of hypoxia-responsive elements (HREs) sites [83]. Interestingly, in this report, a marked hyperacetylation of histones H3 and H4 was observed in the placental growth factor (Plgf) intron in hypoxic conditions. Further studies are needed to determine the interaction of transcription factors and epigenetic regulation, which might be an efficient way of controlling gene expression.

Another epigenetic regulatory mechanism is the miRNAs in the IUP. Present evidence suggests that miRNAs could be transferred across the placenta [84] with important consequences on fetal and maternal physiology. In humans, circulating levels of miR-21 during gestation in the mother positively correlate with evidence of fetal hypoxia [85] and evidence from in vitro studies show the participation of miR-21 in the FGR placental vascular dysfunction [86, 87]. By contrast, placental miR-126 levels negatively correlate with the FGR severity [88]. Studies in umbilical endothelium from swine fetuses have shown that the expression of miRNA that targets eNOS and VEGF pathways can be modulated by maternal supplementation with an L-arginine precursor [89]. Similarly, undernutrition decreases and programs at long term the expression of an anti-remodeling miRNA and this effect is prevented by the *in utero* inhibition of corticosteroid synthesis in pregnant rats [90].

4. Potential role of hypoxia-induced miRNAs, miR-21 and miR-126, on the endothelial dysfunction in FGR

As previously discussed, ncRNAs constitute an important epigenetic mechanism, which mainly regulates RNA translation; notably miR-21 and miR-126 represent two potential miRNAs with a crucial role in the endothelium. In fact, both miRNAs are abundantly expressed in cultured endothelium [91] and respond to hypoxia with a substantial increase in miR-21 and miR-126 levels, representing ~40% of all the miRNAs present in this cell type [92]. In contrast to most miRNAs, miR-126 and miR-21 are encoded within the intronic region of genes coding for proteins. MiR-126 is encoded in the seventh intron of the gene for the endothelial-specific protein epidermal growth factor-like domain 7 (Egfl7) and its expression is partially (~30%) dependent on transcription factors that bind to the promoter region of this Egfl7 [93]. Additionally, miR-126 expression is regulated, independently of Egfl7, by the DNA methylation status of a miR-126-specific promoter located in intron 7 of Egfl7 [94], as well as the binding of Nrf2 to this region in response to oxidative stress [95]. Preliminary data from our group show that FGR human endothelial cells present increased levels of DNA methylation in miR-126 promoter, suggesting an epigenetic programming of this miRNA in FGR endothelium. Conversely, miR-21 is encoded in the 11th intron of the stress-induced protein TMEM49, but its expression is completely controlled by a specific promoter in the intron 10 of TMEM49 with predicted binding sites for transcription factors that respond to oxidative stress and inflammation [96, 97]. This suggests that the expression of miR-21 and miR-126 could be regulated by epigenetic modifications present in their specific intronic promoters.

It has been proposed that miR-126 is an endothelial-specific miRNA which promotes angiogenic activation in progenitor cells during early development, as well as vascular repair in adult subjects, while in mature endothelial cells, it has an anti-atherogenic effect maintaining endothelial quiescence and preventing inflammation [67]. In ob/ob mice, antioxidant treatment induces a miR-126-dependent anti-inflammatory and antioxidant vascular response [98], an effect also observed in HUVEC [99]. Both miRNAs, miR-21 and miR-126, are upregulated by unidirectional shear stress, protecting EC from apoptosis and increasing the activation of eNOS [100]. However, in oscillatory shear stress conditions, increased levels of miR-21 promote the expression of pro-inflammatory mediators [101]. Thus, it has been proposed that miR-21 has a dual effect on vascular function: over a short time, it protects against hypoxia and ischemia [70, 102–104], and over the longer term, leads to endothelial dysfunction, apoptosis [70, 102, 105, 106], and eNOS dysfunction. The latter would occur by targeting the expression of antioxidant enzymes [70], as well as enhancing the levels of the endogenous eNOS inhibitor asymmetric dimethyl arginine (ADMA) by downregulating the expression of the enzyme dimethyl arginine dimethylaminohydrolase 1 (DDAH1) [105, 107, 108]. These data suggest that the dynamic regulation of miR-21 and miR-126 could participate in the early defense of the endothelium to hypoxia and oxidative stress; nonetheless, they prime endothelial dysfunction over the long term. Thus, increased levels of miR-21 and decreased expression of miR-126 observed in FGR placentae at term could represent a consequence rather than a cause of the hypoxia-induced endothelial dysfunction.

5. Conclusions

The programming of vascular, particularly endothelial dysfunction by hypoxia in FGR is an important issue in fetal-maternal medicine up to date. Currently, there is a serious need to undercover the real impact of hypoxia as a driving force to perinatal and postnatal cardiovascular and metabolic diseases, pointing out the main proposed mechanisms. The reviewed data support the notion that epigenetic mechanisms contribute to defining and regulating vascular responses to pathological stimuli (leading to FGR). However, evidence of how fetal exposure to hypoxia and oxidative stress lead to epigenetic modifications remains elusive.

Therefore, new knowledge on the role of epigenetic mechanisms involved in the long-term vascular function is crucial to understand and put into context adequate interventions. The timing of the vascular adaptations and epigenetic responses is one of the most relevant questions that need to be answered in order to prioritize clinical approaches to early diagnose and treat such perinatal conditions, limiting postnatal cardiometabolic risk in the progeny.

http://dx.doi.org/10.5772/66740

Author details

Paola Casanello[1, 2*], Emilio A. Herrera[3] and Bernardo J. Krause[1]

*Address all correspondence to: paolacasanello@gmail.com

1 Division of Pediatrics, Department of Neonatology, The Pontifical Catholic University of Chile, Santiago, Chile

2 Division of Obstetrics & Gynecology, School of Medicine, The Pontifical Catholic University of Chile, Santiago, Chile

3 Pathophysiology Program, Biomedical Sciences Institute (ICBM), Faculty of Medicine, University of Chile, Santiago, Chile

References

[1] Alberti KG, Eckel RH, Grundy SM, Zimmet PZ, Cleeman JI, Donato KA, Fruchart JC, James WP, Loria CM, Smith SC, Jr.: Harmonizing the metabolic syndrome: a joint interim statement of the International Diabetes Federation Task Force on Epidemiology and Prevention; National Heart, Lung, and Blood Institute; American Heart Association; World Heart Federation; International Atherosclerosis Society; and International Association for the Study of Obesity. Circulation 2009, 120:1640–5.

[2] Escobedo J, Schargrodsky H, Champagne B, Silva H, Boissonnet CP, Vinueza R, Torres M, Hernandez R, Wilson E: Prevalence of the metabolic syndrome in Latin America and its association with sub-clinical carotid atherosclerosis: the CARMELA cross sectional study. Cardiovasc Diabetol 2009, 8:52.

[3] El Shamieh S, Visvikis-Siest S: Genetic biomarkers of hypertension and future challenges integrating epigenomics. Clin Chim Acta 2012, 414:259–65.

[4] Barker DJ: Birth weight and hypertension. Hypertension 2006, 48:357–8.

[5] Hanson MA, Gluckman PD: Early developmental conditioning of later health and disease: physiology or pathophysiology? Physiol Rev 2014, 94:1027–76.

[6] Krause B, Sobrevia L, Casanello P: Epigenetics: new concepts of old phenomena in vascular physiology. Curr Vasc Pharmacol 2009, 7:513–20.

[7] Zhang J, Merialdi M, Platt LD, Kramer MS: Defining normal and abnormal fetal growth: promises and challenges. Am J Obstet Gynecol 2010, 202:522–8.

[8] Romo A, Carceller R, Tobajas J: Intrauterine growth retardation (IUGR): epidemiology and etiology. Pediatr Endocrinol Rev 2009, 6(Suppl 3):332–6.

[9] Cohen E, Wong FY, Horne RS, Yiallourou SR: Intrauterine growth restriction: impact on cardiovascular development and function throughout infancy. Pediatr Res 2016; 79(6):821–30.

[10] Martin H, Hu J, Gennser G, Norman M: Impaired endothelial function and increased carotid stiffness in 9-year-old children with low birthweight. Circulation 2000, 102:2739–44.

[11] Martin H, Gazelius B, Norman M: Impaired acetylcholine-induced vascular relaxation in low birth weight infants: implications for adult hypertension? Pediatr Res 2000, 47:457–62.

[12] Krause BJ, Costello PM, Munoz-Urrutia E, Lillycrop KA, Hanson MA, Casanello P: Role of DNA methyltransferase 1 on the altered eNOS expression in human umbilical endothelium from intrauterine growth restricted fetuses. Epigenetics: Official Journal of the DNA Methylation Society 2013, 8:944–52.

[13] Krause BJ, Carrasco-Wong I, Caniuguir A, Carvajal J, Farias M, Casanello P: Endothelial eNOS/arginase imbalance contributes to vascular dysfunction in IUGR umbilical and placental vessels. Placenta 2013, 34:20–8.

[14] Roberts JM: Pathophysiology of ischemic placental disease. Semin Perinatol 2014, 38:139–45.

[15] Herrera EA, Krause B, Ebensperger G, Reyes RV, Casanello P, Parra-Cordero M, Llanos AJ: The placental pursuit for an adequate oxidant balance between the mother and the fetus. Frontiers Pharmacol 2014, 5:149.

[16] Takagi Y, Nikaido T, Toki T, Kita N, Kanai M, Ashida T, Ohira S, Konishi I: Levels of oxidative stress and redox-related molecules in the placenta in preeclampsia and fetal growth restriction. Virchows Archiv: Int J Pathol 2004, 444:49–55.

[17] Biri A, Bozkurt N, Turp A, Kavutcu M, Himmetoglu O, Durak I: Role of oxidative stress in intrauterine growth restriction. Gynecol Obstet Invest 2007, 64:187–92.

[18] Bar-Or D, Heyborne KD, Bar-Or R, Rael LT, Winkler JV, Navot D: Cysteinylation of maternal plasma albumin and its association with intrauterine growth restriction. Prenatal Diag 2005, 25:245–9.

[19] Potdar N, Singh R, Mistry V, Evans MD, Farmer PB, Konje JC, Cooke MS: First-trimester increase in oxidative stress and risk of small-for-gestational-age fetus. Bjog 2009, 116:637–42.

[20] Wareing M, Greenwood SL, Fyfe GK, Baker PN: Reactivity of human placental chorionic plate vessels from pregnancies complicated by intrauterine growth restriction (IUGR). Biol Reprod 2006, 75:518–23.

[21] Schneider D, Hernandez C, Farias M, Uauy R, Krause BJ, Casanello P: Oxidative stress as common trait of endothelial dysfunction in chorionic arteries from fetuses with IUGR and LGA. Placenta 2015, 36:552–8.

[22] Swanson AM, David AL: Animal models of fetal growth restriction: Considerations for translational medicine. Placenta 2015, 36:623–30.

[23] Carter AM: Animal models of human placentation--a review. Placenta 2007, 28(Suppl A):S41–7.

[24] Herrera EA, Alegria R, Farias M, Diaz-Lopez F, Hernandez C, Uauy R, Regnault TR, Casanello P, Krause BJ: Assessment of in vivo fetal growth and placental vascular function in a novel intrauterine growth restriction model of progressive uterine artery occlusion in guinea pigs. J Physiol 2016, 594:1553–61.

[25] Tintu AN, Noble FA, Rouwet EV: Hypoxia disturbs fetal hemodynamics and growth. Endothelium 2007, 14:353–60.

[26] Salinas CE, Blanco CE, Villena M, Camm EJ, Tuckett JD, Weerakkody RA, Kane AD, Shelley AM, Wooding FB, Quy M, Giussani DA: Cardiac and vascular disease prior to hatching in chick embryos incubated at high altitude. J Dev Orig Health Dis 2010, 1:60–6.

[27] Herrera EA, Salinas CE, Blanco CE, Villena M, Giussani DA: High altitude hypoxia and blood pressure dysregulation in adult chickens. J Dev Origins Health Dis 2013, 4:69–76.

[28] Itani N, Skeffington KL, Beck C, Niu YG, Giussani DA: Melatonin rescues cardiovascular dysfunction during hypoxic development in the chick embryo. J Pineal Res 2016, 60:16–26.

[29] Marsal K: Obstetric management of intrauterine growth restriction. Best Pract Res Clin Obstet Gynaecol 2009, 23:857–70.

[30] Giussani DA, Salinas CE, Villena M, Blanco CE: The role of oxygen in prenatal growth: studies in the chick embryo. J Physiol Lond 2007, 585:911–7.

[31] Miller SL, Green LR, Peebles DM, Hanson MA, Blanco CE: Effects of chronic hypoxia and protein malnutrition on growth in the developing chick. Am J Obstet Gynecol 2002, 186:261–7.

[32] Giussani DA, Camm EJ, Niu Y, Richter HG, Blanco CE, Gottschalk R, Blake EZ, Horder KA, Thakor AS, Hansell JA, Kane AD, Wooding FB, Cross CM, Herrera EA: Developmental programming of cardiovascular dysfunction by prenatal hypoxia and oxidative stress. PLoS One 2012, 7:e31017.

[33] Forstermann U: Nitric oxide and oxidative stress in vascular disease. Pflugers Arch 2010, 459:923–39.

[34] Brigelius-Flohe R, Flohe L: Basic principles and emerging concepts in the redox control of transcription factors. Antioxid Redox Signal 2011, 15:2335–81.

[35] Krause BJ, Prieto CP, Munoz-Urrutia E, San Martin S, Sobrevia L, Casanello P: Role of arginase-2 and eNOS in the differential vascular reactivity and hypoxia-induced endothelial response in umbilical arteries and veins. Placenta 2012, 33:360–6.

[36] Leduc L, Delvin E, Ouellet A, Garofalo C, Grenierd E, Morin L, Dube J, Bouity-Voubou M, Moutquin JM, Fouron JC, Klam S, Levy E: Oxidized low-density lipoproteins in cord blood from neonates with intra-uterine growth restriction. Eur J Obst Gynecol Rep Biol 2011, 156:46–9.

[37] Guven ESG, Karcaaltincaba D, Kandemir O, Kiykac S, Mentese A: Cord blood oxidative stress markers correlate with umbilical artery pulsatility in fetal growth restriction. J Matern-Fetal Neo M 2013, 26:576–80.

[38] Herrera EA, Cifuentes-Zuniga F, Figueroa E, Villanueva C, Hernandez C, Alegria R, Arroyo V, Penaloza E, Farias M, Uauy R, Casanello P, Krause BJ: N-acetyl cysteine, a glutathione precursor, reverts vascular dysfunction and endothelial epigenetic programming in intrauterine growth restricted guinea pigs. J Physiol 2016, doi: 10.1113/JP273396

[39] Gonzalez-Candia A, Veliz M, Araya C, Quezada S, Ebensperger G, Seron-Ferre M, Reyes RV, Llanos AJ, Herrera EA: Potential adverse effects of antenatal melatonin as a treatment for intrauterine growth restriction: findings in pregnant sheep. Am J Obstet Gynecol 2016, 215:245 e1–7.

[40] McSweeney SR, Warabi E, Siow RC: Nrf2 as an endothelial mechanosensitive transcription factor: going with the flow. Hypertension 2016, 67:20–9.

[41] Hanson M, Godfrey KM, Lillycrop KA, Burdge GC, Gluckman PD: Developmental plasticity and developmental origins of non-communicable disease: Theoretical considerations and epigenetic mechanisms. Prog Biophys Mol Biol 2011, 106:272–80.

[42] Ohtani K, Dimmeler S: Epigenetic regulation of cardiovascular differentiation. Cardiovasc Res 2011, 90:404–12.

[43] Ordovas JM, Smith CE: Epigenetics and cardiovascular disease. Nat Rev Cardiol 2010, 7:510–9.

[44] Kim JK, Samaranayake M, Pradhan S: Epigenetic mechanisms in mammals. Cell Mol Life Sci 2009, 66:596–612.

[45] Goll MG, Bestor TH: Eukaryotic cytosine methyltransferases. Annu Rev Biochem 2005, 74:481–514.

[46] Reik W: Stability and flexibility of epigenetic gene regulation in mammalian development. Nature 2007, 447:425–32.

[47] Buryanov YI, Shevchuk TV: DNA methyltransferases and structural-functional specificity of eukaryotic DNA modification. Biochemistry (Mosc) 2005, 70:730–42.

[48] Collas P, Noer A, Timoskainen S: Programming the genome in embryonic and somatic stem cells. J Cell Mol Med 2007, 11:602–20.

[49] Suzuki MM, Bird A: DNA methylation landscapes: provocative insights from epigenomics. Nat Rev Genet 2008, 9:465–76.

[50] Illingworth RS, Bird AP: CpG islands – 'a rough guide'. FEBS Lett 2009, 583:1713–20.

[51] Klose RJ, Bird AP: Genomic DNA methylation: the mark and its mediators. Trends Biochem Sci 2006, 31:89–97.

[52] Kimura A, Matsubara K, Horikoshi M: A decade of histone acetylation: marking eukaryotic chromosomes with specific codes. J Biochem 2005, 138:647–62.

[53] Jenuwein T, Allis CD: Translating the histone code. Science 2001, 293:1074–80.

[54] Wang GG, Allis CD, Chi P: Chromatin remodeling and cancer, Part I: covalent histone modifications. Trends Mol Med 2007, 13:363–72.

[55] Berger SL: The complex language of chromatin regulation during transcription. Nature 2007, 447:407–12.

[56] Thiagalingam S, Cheng KH, Lee HJ, Mineva N, Thiagalingam A, Ponte JF: Histone deacetylases: unique players in shaping the epigenetic histone code. Ann N Y Acad Sci 2003, 983:84–100.

[57] Matouk CC, Marsden PA: Epigenetic regulation of vascular endothelial gene expression. Circ Res 2008, 102:873–87.

[58] Britten RJ, Davidson EH: Gene regulation for higher cells: a theory. Science 1969, 165:349–57.

[59] Kaikkonen MU, Lam MT, Glass CK: Non-coding RNAs as regulators of gene expression and epigenetics. Cardiovasc Res 2011, 90:430–40.

[60] Deng K, Wang H, Guo X, Xia J: The cross talk between long, non-coding RNAs and microRNAs in gastric cancer. Acta Biochim Biophys Sin 2016;48(2):111–6.

[61] Lin S, Gregory RI: MicroRNA biogenesis pathways in cancer. Nat Rev Cancer 2015, 15:321–33.

[62] Afonso-Grunz F, Muller S: Principles of miRNA-mRNA interactions: beyond sequence complementarity. Cell Mol Life Sci 2015, 72:3127–41.

[63] le Noble F, Klein C, Tintu A, Pries A, Buschmann I: Neural guidance molecules, tip cells, and mechanical factors in vascular development. Cardiovasc Res 2008, 78:232–41.

[64] Ribatti D, Nico B, Crivellato E: Morphological and molecular aspects of physiological vascular morphogenesis. Angiogenesis 2009, 12:101–11.

[65] Fish JE, Marsden PA: Endothelial nitric oxide synthase: insight into cell-specific gene regulation in the vascular endothelium. Cell Mol Life Sci 2006, 63:144–62.

[66] Illi B, Colussi C, Rosati J, Spallotta F, Nanni S, Farsetti A, Capogrossi MC, Gaetano C: NO points to epigenetics in vascular development. Cardiovasc Res 2011, 90:447–56.

[67] Chistiakov DA, Orekhov AN, Bobryshev YV: The role of miR-126 in embryonic angiogenesis, adult vascular homeostasis, and vascular repair and its alterations in atherosclerotic disease. J Mol Cell Cardiol 2016, 97:47–55.

[68] Fish JE, Matouk CC, Yeboah E, Bevan SC, Khan M, Patil K, Ohh M, Marsden PA: Hypoxia-inducible expression of a natural cis-antisense transcript inhibits endothelial nitric-oxide synthase. J Biol Chem 2007, 282:15652–66.

[69] Fish JE, Yan MS, Matouk CC, St Bernard R, Ho JJ, Gavryushova A, Srivastava D, Marsden PA: Hypoxic repression of endothelial nitric-oxide synthase transcription is coupled with eviction of promoter histones. J Biol Chem 2010, 285:810–26.

[70] Marin T, Gongol B, Chen Z, Woo B, Subramaniam S, Chien S, Shyy JY: Mechanosensitive microRNAs-role in endothelial responses to shear stress and redox state. Free Radic Biol Med 2013, 64:61–8.

[71] Krause BJ, Hernandez C, Caniuguir A, Vasquez-Devaud P, Carrasco-Wong I, Uauy R, Casanello P: Arginase-2 is cooperatively up-regulated by nitric oxide and histone deacetylase inhibition in human umbilical artery endothelial cells. Biochem Pharmacol 2016, 99:53–9.

[72] Kim J, Kim JY, Song KS, Lee YH, Seo JS, Jelinek J, Goldschmidt-Clermont PJ, Issa JP: Epigenetic changes in estrogen receptor beta gene in atherosclerotic cardiovascular tissues and in-vitro vascular senescence. Biochim Biophys Acta 2007, 1772:72–80.

[73] Dunn J, Qiu H, Kim S, Jjingo D, Hoffman R, Kim CW, Jang I, Son DJ, Kim D, Pan C, Fan Y, Jordan IK, Jo H: Flow-dependent epigenetic DNA methylation regulates endothelial gene expression and atherosclerosis. J Clin Invest 2014, 124:3187–99.

[74] Jiang YZ, Manduchi E, Stoeckert CJ, Jr., Davies PF: Arterial endothelial methylome: differential DNA methylation in athero-susceptible disturbed flow regions in vivo. BMC Gen 2015, 16:506.

[75] Rao X, Zhong J, Zhang S, Zhang Y, Yu Q, Yang P, Wang MH, Fulton DJ, Shi H, Dong Z, Wang D, Wang CY: Loss of methyl-CpG-binding domain protein 2 enhances endothelial angiogenesis and protects mice against hind-limb ischemic injury. Circulation 2011, 123:2964–74.

[76] Navickas R, Gal D, Laucevicius A, Taparauskaite A, Zdanyte M, Holvoet P: Identifying circulating microRNAs as biomarkers of cardiovascular disease: a systematic review. Cardiovasc Res 2016.

[77] Krause BJ, Carrasco-Wong I, Dominguez A, Arnaiz P, Farias M, Barja S, Mardones F, Casanello P: Micro-RNAs Let7e and 126 in plasma as markers of metabolic dysfunction in 10 to 12 years old children. PLoS One 2015, 10:e0128140.

[78] Olivieri F, Spazzafumo L, Bonafe M, Recchioni R, Prattichizzo F, Marcheselli F, Micolucci L, Mensa E, Giuliani A, Santini G, Gobbi M, Lazzarini R, Boemi M, Testa R, Antonicelli R, Procopio AD, Bonfigli AR: MiR-21-5p and miR-126a-3p levels in plasma and circulating angiogenic cells: relationship with type 2 diabetes complications. Oncotarget 2015, 6:35372–82.

[79] Xu XF, Ma XL, Shen Z, Wu XL, Cheng F, Du LZ: Epigenetic regulation of the endothelial nitric oxide synthase gene in persistent pulmonary hypertension of the newborn rat. J Hypertens 2010, 28:2227–35.

[80] Sartori C, Rimoldi SF, Rexhaj E, Allemann Y, Scherrer U: Epigenetics in cardiovascular regulation. Adv Exp Med Biol 2016, 903:55–62.

[81] Rexhaj E, Paoloni-Giacobino A, Rimoldi SF, Fuster DG, Anderegg M, Somm E, Bouillet E, Allemann Y, Sartori C, Scherrer U: Mice generated by in vitro fertilization exhibit vascular dysfunction and shortened life span. J Clin Invest 2013, 123:5052–60.

[82] Hancock RL, Dunne K, Walport LJ, Flashman E, Kawamura A: Epigenetic regulation by histone demethylases in hypoxia. Epigenomics 2015, 7:791–811.

[83] Tudisco L, Della Ragione F, Tarallo V, Apicella I, D'Esposito M, Matarazzo MR, De Falco S: Epigenetic control of hypoxia inducible factor-1alpha-dependent expression of placental growth factor in hypoxic conditions. Epigen Off J DNA Meth Soc 2014, 9:600–10.

[84] Li J, Zhang Y, Li D, Liu Y, Chu D, Jiang X, Hou D, Zen K, Zhang CY: Small non-coding RNAs transfer through mammalian placenta and directly regulate fetal gene expression. Protein Cell 2015, 6:391–6.

[85] Whitehead CL, Teh WT, Walker SP, Leung C, Larmour L, Tong S: Circulating MicroRNAs in maternal blood as potential biomarkers for fetal hypoxia in-utero. PLoS One 2013, 8:e78487.

[86] Cindrova-Davies T, Herrera EA, Niu Y, Kingdom J, Giussani DA, Burton GJ: Reduced cystathionine gamma-lyase and increased miR-21 expression are associated with increased vascular resistance in growth-restricted pregnancies: hydrogen sulfide as a placental vasodilator. Am J Pathol 2013, 182:1448–58.

[87] Maccani MA, Padbury JF, Marsit CJ: miR-16 and miR-21 expression in the placenta is associated with fetal growth. PLoS One 2011, 6:e21210.

[88] Hromadnikova I, Kotlabova K, Hympanova L, Krofta L: Cardiovascular and cerebrovascular disease associated microRNAs are dysregulated in placental tissues affected with gestational hypertension, preeclampsia and intrauterine growth restriction. PLoS One 2015, 10:e0138383.

[89] Liu XD, Wu X, Yin YL, Liu YQ, Geng MM, Yang HS, Blachier F, Wu GY: Effects of dietary L-arginine or N-carbamylglutamate supplementation during late gestation of sows on the miR-15b/16, miR-221/222, VEGFA and eNOS expression in umbilical vein. Amino Acids 2012, 42:2111–9.

[90] Khorram O, Chuang TD, Pearce WJ: Long-term effects of maternal undernutrition on offspring carotid artery remodeling: role of miR-29c. J Dev Orig Health Dis 2015, 6:342–9.

[91] Guduric-Fuchs J, O'Connor A, Cullen A, Harwood L, Medina RJ, O'Neill CL, Stitt AW, Curtis TM, Simpson DA: Deep sequencing reveals predominant expression of miR-21 amongst the small non-coding RNAs in retinal microvascular endothelial cells. J Cell Biochem 2012, 113:2098–111.

[92] Voellenkle C, Rooij J, Guffanti A, Brini E, Fasanaro P, Isaia E, Croft L, David M, Capogrossi MC, Moles A, Felsani A, Martelli F: Deep-sequencing of endothelial cells exposed to hypoxia reveals the complexity of known and novel microRNAs. RNA 2012, 18:472–84.

[93] Harris TA, Yamakuchi M, Kondo M, Oettgen P, Lowenstein CJ: Ets-1 and Ets-2 regulate the expression of microRNA-126 in endothelial cells. Arterioscler Thromb Vasc Biol 2010, 30:1990–7.

[94] Watanabe K, Emoto N, Hamano E, Sunohara M, Kawakami M, Kage H, Kitano K, Nakajima J, Goto A, Fukayama M, Nagase T, Yatomi Y, Ohishi N, Takai D: Genome structure-based screening identified epigenetically silenced microRNA associated with invasiveness in non-small-cell lung cancer. Int J Cancer 2012, 130:2580–90.

[95] Kuosmanen SM, Viitala S, Laitinen T, Perakyla M, Polonen P, Kansanen E, Leinonen H, Raju S, Wienecke-Baldacchino A, Narvanen A, Poso A, Heinaniemi M, Heikkinen S, Levonen AL: The effects of sequence variation on genome-wide NRF2 binding – new target genes and regulatory SNPs. Nucl Acid Res 2016, 44:1760–75.

[96] Ribas J, Lupold SE: The transcriptional regulation of miR-21, its multiple transcripts, and their implication in prostate cancer. Cell Cycle 2010, 9:923–9.

[97] Kumarswamy R, Volkmann I, Thum T: Regulation and function of miRNA-21 in health and disease. RNA Biol 2011, 8:706–13.

[98] Togliatto G, Trombetta A, Dentelli P, Gallo S, Rosso A, Cotogni P, Granata R, Falcioni R, Delale T, Ghigo E, Brizzi MF: Unacylated ghrelin induces oxidative stress resistance in a glucose intolerance and peripheral artery disease mouse model by restoring endothelial cell miR-126 expression. Diabetes 2015, 64:1370–82.

[99] Sui XQ, Xu ZM, Xie MB, Pei DA: Resveratrol inhibits hydrogen peroxide-induced apoptosis in endothelial cells via the activation of PI3K/Akt by miR-126. J Atheroscler Thromb 2014, 21:108–18.

[100] Weber M, Baker MB, Moore JP, Searles CD: MiR-21 is induced in endothelial cells by shear stress and modulates apoptosis and eNOS activity. Biochem Biophys Res Commun 2010, 393:643–8.

http://dx.doi.org/10.5772/66740

[101] Zhou J, Wang KC, Wu W, Subramaniam S, Shyy JY, Chiu JJ, Li JY, Chien S. MicroRNA-21 targets peroxisome proliferators-activated receptor-{alpha} in an autoregulatory loop to modulate flow-induced endothelial inflammation. Proc Natl Acad Sci U S A 2011;108(25):10355-60.

[102] Xu X, Kriegel AJ, Jiao X, Liu H, Bai X, Olson J, Liang M, Ding X: miR-21 in ischemia/reperfusion injury: a double-edged sword? Physiol Gen 2014, 46:789–97.

[103] Ge X, Han Z, Chen F, Wang H, Zhang B, Jiang R, Lei P, Zhang J: MiR-21 alleviates secondary blood-brain barrier damage after traumatic brain injury in rats. Brain Res 2015, 1603:150–7.

[104] Qiao S, Olson JM, Paterson M, Yan Y, Zaja I, Liu Y, Riess ML, Kersten JR, Liang M, Warltier DC, Bosnjak ZJ, Ge ZD: MicroRNA-21 Mediates isoflurane-induced cardioprotection against ischemia-reperfusion injury via Akt/nitric oxide synthase/mitochondrial permeability transition pore pathway. Anesthesiology 2015, 123:786–98.

[105] Iannone L, Zhao L, Dubois O, Duluc L, Rhodes CJ, Wharton J, Wilkins MR, Leiper J, Wojciak-Stothard B: miR-21/DDAH1 pathway regulates pulmonary vascular responses to hypoxia. Biochem J 2014, 462:103–12.

[106] White K, Dempsie Y, Caruso P, Wallace E, McDonald RA, Stevens H, Hatley ME, Van Rooij E, Morrell NW, MacLean MR, Baker AH: Endothelial apoptosis in pulmonary hypertension is controlled by a microRNA/programmed cell death 4/caspase-3 axis. Hypertension 2014, 64:185–94.

[107] Chen L, Zhou JP, Kuang DB, Tang J, Li YJ, Chen XP: 4-HNE increases intracellular ADMA levels in cultured HUVECs: evidence for miR-21-dependent mechanisms. PLoS One 2013, 8:e64148.

[108] Zhao C, Li T, Han B, Yue W, Shi L, Wang H, Guo Y, Lu Z: DDAH1 deficiency promotes intracellular oxidative stress and cell apoptosis via a miR-21-dependent pathway in mouse embryonic fibroblasts. Free Radic Biol Med 2016, 92:50–60.

Chapter 18

The Critical Role of Hypoxia in Tumor-Mediated Immunosuppression

Nassera Aouali, Manon Bosseler, Delphine Sauvage, Kris Van Moer, Guy Berchem and Bassam Janji

Additional information is available at the end of the chapter

http://dx.doi.org/10.5772/65383

Abstract

Underestimated for a long time, the involvement of the microenvironment has been proven essential for a better understanding of the cancer development. In keeping with this, the tumor is not considered anymore as a mass of malignant cells, but rather as an organ composed of various malignant and nonmalignant cell populations interacting with each other to create the tumor microenvironment. The tumor immune contexture plays a critical role in shaping the tumor immune response, and it is now well supported that such an immune response is impacted by the hypoxic stress within the tumor microenvironment. Tumor hypoxia is closely linked to tumor progression, metastasis, treatment failure, and escape from immune surveillance. Thus, hypoxia seems to be a key factor involved in creating an immune-suppressive tumor by multiple overlapping mechanisms, including the impairment of the function of cytotoxic immune cells, increasing the immunosuppressive properties of immunosuppressive cells, and activating resistance mechanism in the tumor cells. In this chapter, we review some recent findings describing how hypoxic stress in the tumor microenvironment hijacks the antitumor immune response.

Keywords: cancer, hypoxia, immune response, tumor microenvironment, autophagy, tumor plasticity, tumor heterogeneity

1. Introduction

Malignant cells are part of cellular and microenvironmental complexes which both define the initiation, progression, and maintenance of the malignant phenotype. In turn, malignant cells participate in creating a hostile microenvironment characterized by hypoxic areas within the tumors. Indeed, the oxygen level in the hypoxic tumor is usually lower than that of corresponding normal tissue. The oxygenation level of tumor is likely depending on (i) the initial oxygenation of the tissue; (ii) the degree of the tumor heterogeneity; (iii) the tumor size and stage. **Table 1** summarizes the percentage of oxygen level reported as a median in some healthy organs and their corresponding tumors, as defined by several studies.

Healthy tissue/corresponding cancer	% of oxygen (Median)
Brain/brain tumor	4.6/1.7
Breast/breast cancer	8.5/1.5
Cervix/cervical cancer	9.5/1.2
Kidney cortex/renal cancer	7.0/1.3
Liver/liver cancer	4.0–7.3/0.8
Lung/nonsmall cell lung carcinoma	5.6/2.2
Pancreas/pancreatic tumor	7.5/0.3
Rectal mucosa/rectal carcinoma	3.9/1.8

Table 1. Comparison of the percentage (%) of oxygen level in different healthy tissues and in their corresponding cancers.

It is now widely appreciated that hypoxia is one of the most relevant factor involved in the impairment of the antitumor immune response by damping the cytotoxic function of immune cells. There are numerous studies supporting that hypoxic stress leads to the establishment of immune tolerance of tumor cells by preventing the migration and the homing of immune effector cells into established tumors. Furthermore, hypoxia can also drive tumor cell plasticity and functional heterogeneity and, thus, favors the emergence of more aggressive tumors. Many strategies are emerging for targeting intratumor hypoxia in order to change the immunosuppressive properties of the tumor to a microenvironment able to support antitumor immunity.

2. Hypoxia is the major factor of the tumor microenvironment

The long-lasting tumor immunology research has validated the concept of tumor immunosurveillance. The tumor immunosurveillance consists in the fact that cytotoxic immune cells recognize nascent transformed cells and destroy them before they become clinically apparent. Several types of immune cells are involved in the control of tumors such as immune effector and immune suppressor cells. Thus, cytotoxic T lymphocytes (CTL) belong to the adaptive immune system and they are able to recognize tumor antigens through the T-cell receptor (TCR) [1]. The antigens expressed exclusively by tumor cells are called tumor-specific antigens [2]. In addition to CTL, the tumor immune surveillance involves natural killer (NK) cells that belong to the innate immune system [1]. NK cells recognize tumor cells by mechanisms

http://dx.doi.org/10.5772/65383

called "missing-self" and "induced-self" [3]. Briefly, NK cells are regulated by a balance of inhibitory and activating signals of surface receptors. Thus, NK cells can kill their target cell depending on the recognized ligand(s). The identification of activating or inhibitory ligands allows NK cells to distinguish between "self" versus "nonself" and "self" versus "altered self" by "missing-self" and "induced-self" recognitions. Indeed, the protection of normal cells from NK cell killing is achieved by balancing the stimulatory signals delivered by stimulatory ligands with inhibitory signals delivered by self MHC class I molecules. When the expression of self MHC class I molecules is lost following cell transformation or infection, the stimulatory signals delivered by the target cell remain unbalanced, leading to the activation of NK cells and lysis of target cells (known as missing-self recognition). Under some circumstances, transformed or infected cells overexpress stimulatory ligands that overcome the inhibitory signals leading to target cell lysis (known as induced-self recognition). It has been reported that both missing-self and induced-self recognition could operate simultaneously. In this case, NK cells display a high ability to discriminate between normal and transformed target cells [4].

In addition to cytotoxic immune cells, the tumor immune contexture contains immune suppressive cells such as myeloid-derived suppressor cells (MDSC) able to inhibit the function of immune effectors. Macrophages and neutrophil granulocytes are also involved in antitumor immunity [5]. These cells display tumor antigens and can stimulate other immune cells such as CTL, NK cells, or antigen-presenting cells (APC) [6]. Although both CTL and NK cells kill their target following the establishment of immunological synapse (IS) [7], the molecular mechanism by which they recognize their target tumor cells is fundamentally different. Two major pathways are used by CTL and NK cells to recognize and destroy tumor cells: (i) through the release by immune cells of cytotoxic granules containing perforin and granzymes and these cytotoxic granules are captured by tumor cells to induce cell death by apoptosis [8], and (ii) through tumor necrosis factor (TNF) superfamily-dependent mechanism [9].

It has been proposed that despite the powerful ability of the immune system to attack cancer cells, tumors can outmaneuver the immune effectors cells and escape the immune surveillance. It is now well documented that the ability of tumor cells to escape immune cell control is most likely resulted from the activation of several resistance mechanisms to evade effective and functional host immune response. Therefore, it stands to reason that established tumors, displaying multiple resistance mechanism, are likely not fully controlled by the immune system. In keeping with this, it is strongly believed that clinically detected cancers have most likely evaded effective antitumor immune responses. Recently, it has been reported that in addition to its role in protecting host against tumor development, the immune system can under certain circumstances sculpt the immunogenic phenotype of well-developed tumors. Such a mechanism favors the emergence of resistant tumor cell clones [10]. Accumulating experimental and clinical evidence suggest that the resistance mechanisms activated in tumor cells are multifactorial and that such resistance mechanisms are primarily evolved and activated in the tumor microenvironment [11]. It appears that hypoxia is the major tumor microenvironmental factor involved in the alteration of the transcriptome and the metabolome of tumor cells as well as their proliferation, survival, and invasion [12].

In this chapter, we summarize some recent findings describing how hypoxic stress in the tumor microenvironment regulates the antitumor immune response and leads to tumor escape from immunosurveillance. We focus on how hypoxia confers resistance to immune attack and impairs tumor cell killing mediated by CTL and NK cells.

2.1. Hypoxia and hypoxia-inducible factors (HIF) regulation

Tumor cells are able to adapt to hypoxic stress through the regulation of the hypoxia inducible factor family of transcription factors (HIFs) [13]. It has been reported for a large number of human cancers that HIFs were overexpressed and such overexpression is associated with poor response to treatment [14]. Moreover, evidence showed a clear positive correlation between enhanced hypoxic expression of HIFs and mortality [13]. Therefore, inhibition of HIFs could represent a novel approach to improve cancer therapies. Currently, efforts are being actively pursued to identify inhibitors of HIFs and to test their efficacy as anticancer therapeutics.

Three isoforms of HIF have been identified: HIF-1, HIF-2, and HIF-3. The hypoxia-inducible factor-1 (HIF-1) is the major factor mediating adaptive responses to changes in tissue oxygen level [15]. Indeed, HIF-1 is a heterodimer composed of a constitutively expressed HIF-1β subunit and an O_2-dependent regulated HIF-1α subunit. HIF-1α is a DNA-binding basic helix-loop helix of the PAS family [Per (period circadian protein); Arnt (aryl hydrocarbon receptor nuclear translocator protein); Sim (single-minded protein)] [16]. HIF-1α contains two oxygen-dependent degradation domains (ODDD), one in the N-terminal (N-ODDD) moiety and one in the C-terminal moiety (C-ODDD) [17, 18]. It also contains two transactivation domains (TADs), one N-terminal, which overlaps with the C-ODDD, and one C-terminal [19].

2.2. Regulation of HIF-1 level

The expression level of HIF-1α is determined by the rates of protein synthesis and protein degradation. While the synthesis of HIF-1α is regulated in an O_2-independent manner, its degradation is primarily regulated via an O_2-dependent mechanism. Thus, normoxic cells constantly synthesize HIF-1α protein and degrade it rapidly [17]. It has been shown that under normoxic conditions HIF-1α has a short half-life of less than 5 min [20]. However, under hypoxia or low oxygen level, the degradation of HIF-1α is blocked or dramatically decreased [21]. Under normoxia, HIF-1α is hydroxylated on proline residue 402 and/or 564 in the ODDD by prolyl hydroxylase domain protein 2 (PHD2) [17, 22]. Such oxygen-dependent hydroxylation of HIF-1α results in its binding to the von Hippel-Lindau tumor suppressor protein (pVHL). pVHL is the recognition component of an E3 ubiquitin-protein ligase complex that targets HIF-1α for proteolysis by the ubiquitin-proteasome pathway [23].

Enzymes regulating HIF-1α proteasomal degradation were first identified to be related to egl-9 in caenorhabditis elegans and to termed prolyl hydroxylase domain (PHD) enzymes (PHD1, PHD-2, and PHD3) [24, 25]. PHD2 uses oxygen as a substrate, and thus, its activity is inhibited under hypoxic conditions [25]. The inhibition of PHD2 leads to the inhibition of prolyl hydroxylation of HIF-1α and subsequently to the inhibition of HIF-1α-dependent proteasomal degradation. Consequently, HIF-1α rapidly accumulates in the cytoplasm, translocates to the nucleus and dimerizes with HIF-1β. The HIF-1α/HIF-1β heteromeric dimer binds to the hypoxia responsive element (HRE) in target genes, recruits coactivators and activates transcription [14] (**Figure 1A**).

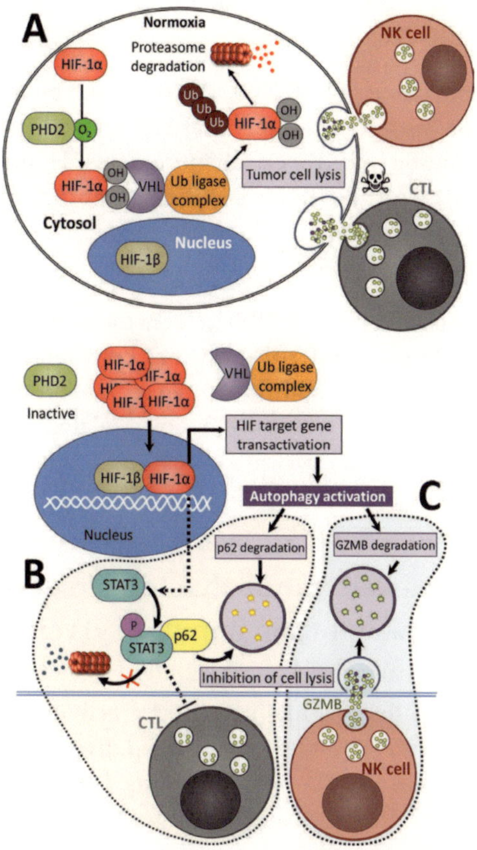

Figure 1. The role of hypoxic stress in the impairment CTL and NK-cell mediated lysis. (A) Under normoxia, the oxygen-sensitive prolyl hydroxylase domain protein 2 (PHD2) hydroxylates HIF-1α subunit. Hydroxylated HIF-1 interacted with Von Hippel-Lindau protein (VHL), subjected to ubiquitination and subsequently degraded by the ubiquitin-proteasome system. Under hypoxic stress, the function of PHD2 protein is blocked, HIF-1α is therefore stabilized and translocated to the nucleus to form heterodimeric complex with HIF-1β to transcriptionally induce the expression of HIF-target genes involved in several pathways such as autophagy. (B) Under hypoxia, STAT3 is phosphorylated at Ser-705 residue in a HIF-dependent manner by a mechanism which is not fully understood. (C) The hypoxia-dependent induction of autophagy leads to the degradation of the adaptor protein p62/SQSTM1, involved in targeting phospho-STAT3 to the ubiquitin proteasome system for degradation. Thus, targeting autophagy accumulated p62/SQSTM1 and therefore accelerated the degradation of phospho-STAT3. The degradation of phospho-STAT3 restores CTL-mediated lysis of tumor cells. In addition, the induction of autophagy in hypoxic tumor cells leads to the selective degradation of granzyme B (GZMB), a serine protease released by natural killer (NK) cells and contained in the cytotoxic granules. Such degradation inhibits NK-mediated lysis of tumor cells.

Using genomewide chromatin immunoprecipitation combined with DNA microarray (ChIP-chip) or DNA sequencing (ChIP-seq) analysis, it has been shown that more than 800 genes involved in several cell functions are direct targets of HIF [26, 27]. HIF-1 activates the expression of these genes by binding to a 50 base pair cis-acting HRE located in their enhancer and promoter regions [28]. The HREs of all these genes contain the core sequence 5′-[A/G]CGT-3′, which in most cases is ACGTG [29]. It has been reported that HIF transcription factors preferentially bind to specific bases in the 5′ and 3′ proximity of the core that has led to define the following HRE consensus sequence [T/G/C][A/G]CGTG[CGA][GTC][GTC][CTG] [29].

Similar to HIF-1α, the stabilization of HIF-2α is also regulated by oxygen-dependent hydroxylation [30]. This could be related to the fact that HIF-1α and HIF-2α displayed a similar structure of their DNA binding and dimerization domains. However, the major difference between the structure of HIF-1α and HIF-2α is in their transactivation domains [31]. In terms of genes expression, both HIF-1α and HIF-2α share overlapping target genes, and each one also regulates a set of unique targets [32].

In sharp contrast with HIF-1α and HIF-2α, HIF-3α lacks the transactivation domain and could function as an inhibitor of HIF-1α and HIF-2α. It has been reported that the expression of HIF-3α is regulated by HIF-1 [33]. In addition to the regulation of the expression of a large number of genes, HIF family members regulate hypoxia-related microRNAs (HRM) [34] and some chromatin modifying enzymes [35].

3. Intra-tumor hypoxia: a key feature that triggers several resistance mechanisms of tumor evasion from immune surveillance

It has been clearly established that the immune effector activity and the antitumor immune response are significantly regulated by hypoxia. Indeed, hypoxia, via HIF-1α, decreases the susceptibility of lung cancer cells to CTL-mediated killing. It appears that the resistance to CTL is related to the effect of HIF-1α to induce the phosphorylation of signal transducer and activator of transcription 3 (STAT3) in tumor cells by a mechanism involving the vascular endothelial growth factor (VEGF) secretion. These data suggest that following its translocation to the nucleus, HIF-1α cooperates with pSTAT3 to impair lung carcinoma cell susceptibility to CTL-mediated killing [36] (**Figure 1B**). More recently, it has been shown that the expression of the phosphorylated form of STAT3 at Ser-705 residue is tightly controlled by the induction of autophagy in hypoxic tumor cells as the accumulation of pSTAT3 was no longer observed when autophagy was targeted genetically in tumor cells [37]. Autophagy is a catabolic cell degradation process. Autophagy plays an essential role in preventing accumulation of altered cell components [38] and as an adaptive metabolic response to provide nutrients. Recently, an unexpected role of autophagy in shaping the antitumor immune response [39] and the acquisition of resistance to TNFα has been shown [40]. Autophagy is activated under stress conditions such as hypoxia, nutrient starvation, growth factor withdrawal, and endoplasmic reticulum stress. It has been reported that the molecular mechanism by which autophagy regulates the pSTAT3 level involves the protein p62/SQSTM1 the ubiquitin proteasome system [37, 41].

Another study showed that in addition to the mechanism described earlier, it has been shown that the stem cell self-renewal transcription factor NANOG is also involved in the regulation of CTL-mediated tumor cell lysis [42, 43]. Hypoxia regulates NANOG at both transcriptional and translational levels and targeting NANOG in hypoxic cells restored CTL-mediated tumor cell killing. Furthermore, NANOG depletion results in the inhibition of STAT3 phosphorylation and its nuclear translocation. The hypoxia-induced microRNA (miR)-210 is also involved in the regulation of CTL-mediated tumor cells lysis. In fact, HIF-1 induces the expression of miR-210 which subsequently targets nonreceptor protein tyrosine phosphatase type 1 (PTPN1), homeobox A1 (HOXA1), and tumor protein p53-inducible protein 11 (TP53I11), and thereby decreases tumor cell susceptibility to CTL [44]. In the context of NK-mediated tumor cell lysis, it has been described that hypoxia increases the shedding of the major histocompatibility complex (MHC) class I polypeptide-related sequence A (MICA), a ligand for the activating receptor natural killer group 2 member D (NKG2D), on the surface of prostate cancer cells leading to an impairment of NO signaling [45] and subsequent escape of tumor cells from NK- and CTL-mediated killing. MICA expression is also downregulated by HIF-1 in osteosarcoma cells resulting in tumor resistance to NK-mediated lysis [46]. Through the activation of autophagy, it has been recently reported that melanoma and breast tumor cells escape NK-mediated lysis and that targeting autophagy in hypoxic tumor cells was sufficient to restore NK-mediated lysis. In this study, it has been shown that the activation of autophagy under hypoxia was responsible for the degradation of NK-derived granzyme B making hypoxic tumor cells less sensitive to NK-mediated killing [39, 47, 48] (**Figure 1C**). In line with the studies described earlier, it is now well admitted that hypoxic stress in the tumor microenvironment is a key factor involved in the control of antitumor immune response. Beside its role in impairing the function of cytotoxic immune cells, the immunosuppressive effect of hypoxia contributes to the emergence of resistant tumor cells that compromise the effectiveness of the anti-tumor immune response [49].

4. Hypoxia and tumor cell heterogeneity and plasticity

Solid tumors frequently reveal pronounced tumor cell heterogeneity with regards to cell organization, cell morphology, cell size, and nuclei morphology [50]. The molecular mechanisms underlying the phenotypic heterogeneity involve genetic, epigenetic, and environmental factors. It is now well established that hypoxia is an important contributor to intra- and intertumor cell heterogeneity [15, 51] by altering the expression of specific genes involved in cellular phenotype. In this respect, it has been reported that neuroblastoma cells and breast cancer cells lose their differentiated gene expression patterns and develop stem cell-like phenotypes under hypoxic stress [52, 53]. As a low stage of differentiation in neuroblastoma and breast cancer is associated with poor prognosis, it is strongly believed that, in addition to its contribution to tumor heterogeneity, hypoxia-dependent induction of tumor cell dedifferentiation contributes to tumor cell plasticity and aggressiveness.

Several lines of evidence suggest that tumor microenvironment drives stem cell renewal and differentiation. Indeed, poorly vascularized tumors contain hypoxic regions with undifferentiated 'stem-like' tumor cells that survive under control of HIFs [54]. It has been reported that hypoxic stress in colon cancer inhibits the differentiation of tumor cells and maintains their stem-like phenotype [55]. In addition, myofibroblasts stromal cells secrete factors involved in maintaining cancer stem cells (CSC) population in colon cancer [56]. Furthermore, stromal cells drive a CSC phenotype on differentiated cancer cells, allowing a transient morphological heterogeneity observed in several cancers. In this regard, transient phenotypic changes from epithelial to mesenchymal (epithelial-mesenchymal transition (EMT)) or mesenchymal to epithelial (mesenchymal to epithelial transitions (MET)) phenotype, are initially considered as conversions facilitating cell plasticity but have recently gained appreciation as events involved in tumor heterogeneity [57]. In the context of tumor immunity, recent evidence revealed that tumor cell plasticity has serious implications in terms of immunological recognition and killing of the tumor, since such tumor cell plasticity may lead to the emergence of immunoresistant variants [58].

Although the role of the immune system in inhibiting early stages of tumor growth is well established, it is now strongly suggested that the immune system can also facilitate the advanced stages of tumor progression by sculpting the immunogenic phenotype of a developing tumor to favor the emergence of immune-resistant tumor cell variants. This has led to the concept of "immunoediting" which encompasses three phases: elimination, equilibrium, and escape. Thus, immunoediting allows tumors to evade immune destruction by becoming less immunogenic or more immunosuppressive [59]. Such adaptability, achieved through cell reprogramming, reflects an important property of tumors called immune-induced plasticity. While the molecular basis of immune-dependent induction of tumor cell plasticity and its effective contribution to the selection of tumor aggressive variants is still elusive, recent findings have revealed that activated CD8+ T cells can stimulate mammary epithelial tumor cells to undergo EMT and acquire the increased tumorigenic capability and therapy resistance of breast CSCs [60]. In this regard, it has been shown that reciprocal interactions between melanoma and immune cells enhances tumor cell plasticity and drives therapy resistance [61]. Based on these data, it is now well defined that targeting phenotypic plasticity should be considered for the development of novel therapeutic strategies with the ultimate goal to prevent the establishment of a more aggressive phenotype of cancer cells.

5. The clinical significance of targeting hypoxia

For many years, the major issue in the field of cancer immunity was to understand how cancer cells manage to evade immune surveillance despite the presence of a competent immune system. To address this issue, the major focus was on the mechanisms by which tumor cells escape cytotoxic immune cell recognition without considering the impact of the tumor microenvironment. This could partially explain why despite intense investigation, the gains provided by immunotherapy until recently are relatively modest. In addition, accumulating evidence suggests that tumor cell resistance mechanisms are likely evolved in the hypoxic tumor microenvironment. In keeping with this, it is therefore more accurate to consider cancer as a disease of the microenvironment rather than a disease of cells. Although remarkable progresses have been achieved over the past two decades regarding the impact of the tumor microenvironment in cancer biology and treatment, its contribution in the development of tumor resistance to immune cell killing remains fragmented.

Emerging data indicates that hypoxia stress within the tumor microenvironment is a key factor involved in the impairment of the antitumor immune response. [62] Therefore, a deep understanding of the molecular mechanism by which hypoxia induces tumor resistance may contribute to the development of more effective tumor immunotherapies.

Consistent with the fact that hypoxia-dependent overexpression of HIF-1α is associated with an increased patient mortality in several cancer types, it stands to reason that inhibition of HIF-1 activity in preclinical studies would have marked effects on tumor growth and survival. In keeping with this, efforts are underway to identify selective inhibitors of HIF-1 and to assess their efficacy as anticancer therapeutics. Currently, two main approaches are used to target hypoxia in tumors, namely bioreductive prodrugs, and inhibitors of molecular targets upon which hypoxic cell survival depends [63, 64]. However, several lines of evidence indicate that the HIF pathway is technically extremely challenging to target. Indeed, the first evidence is that transcription factors in general, including HIF, have long been considered "undruggable," and therefore, no specific inhibitor of HIF has been brought to the market so far. The second evidence is that multiple levels of regulation and signaling pathways converge on and emerge from HIF [65]. Nevertheless, based on the molecular mechanism of HIF-1 protein, it has been suggested that small molecules could be used to inhibit HIF-1 activity through a variety of mechanisms including inhibition of (i) HIF-1α protein synthesis; (ii) HIF-1α protein stabilization; (iii) HIF-1α/β dimerization, and (iv) HIF-1/DNA binding. Two comprehensive recent reviews summarize these mechanisms in detail and give fairly exhaustive lists of the small-molecule inhibitors for each level [15, 66].

Using a cell-based assay, several small-molecule inhibitors of HIF-1 activity have been identified. Briefly, topoisomerase I inhibitors block the expression of HIF-1α via an undefined mechanism [67]. The small molecule YC-1 (3-(5′-hydroxy-methyl-2′-furyl)-1-benzylindazole) was also shown to reduce the level of HIF-1α by a mechanism that has not been established but at least is known to work independently from its function as a stimulator of soluble guanylate-cyclase activity [68]. YC-1 is not in clinical use. The HSP90 inhibitor 17-allyl-aminogeldanamycin (17-AAG) has been reported to induce the degradation of HIF-1α in a VHL-independent manner [69–71]. PX-12 (thioredoxin-1 redox inhibitor) and PX-478 are both inhibitors of HIF-1α protein expression and HIF-1-mediated transactivation [72, 73]. Finally, the disruptor of microtubule polymerization 2-methoxyoestradiol (2ME2) is able to decrease the expression of HIF-1α. Currently, only topoisomerase I inhibitors, camptothecin and topotecan, are clinically approved agents, PX-478, 2ME2, and 17-AAG are under evaluation in clinical trials, whereas YC-1 and thioredoxin-1 inhibitors are not in clinical use.

Despite of the anticancer effects of these agents could be related, in part, to their inhibition of HIF-1, it seems that none of these drugs specifically targets HIF-1. Although such lack of selectivity does not disqualify these drugs as anticancer agents, it enhances the difficulty to correlate molecular and clinical responses in patients. Therefore, the identification of more selective HIF-1 inhibitors in the near future is required and more investigation needs to be done to identify novel potent and more specific inhibitors targeting clearly defined points in the HIF pathway.

Acknowledgements

This work was supported by grants from the Luxembourg Institute of Health (LECR 2013 11 05), Fondation Cancer (FC/2016/01) and Kriibskrank Kanner Foundation, Luxembourg.

Author details

Nassera Aouali[1], Manon Bosseler[1], Delphine Sauvage[1], Kris Van Moer[1], Guy Berchem[1,2] and Bassam Janji[1*]

*Address all correspondence to: bassam.janji@lih.lu

1 Laboratory of Experimental Cancer Research, Department of Oncology, Luxembourg Institute of Health, Luxembourg City, Luxembourg

2 Luxembourg Hospital Center, Department of Hemato-Oncology, Luxembourg City, Luxembourg

References

[1] Smyth, M.J., D.I. Godfrey, and J.A. Trapani. A fresh look at tumor immunosurveillance and immunotherapy. Nat Immunol, 2001. 2(4): p. 293-9.

[2] Rosenberg, S.A.. Progress in human tumour immunology and immunotherapy. Nature, 2001. 411(6835): p. 380-4.

[3] Watzl, C. and E.O. Long. Exposing tumor cells to killer cell attack. Nat Med, 2000. 6(8): p. 867-8.

[4] Raulet, D.H. and R.E. Vance. Self-tolerance of natural killer cells. Nat Rev Immunol, 2006. 6(7): p. 520-31.

[5] Di Carlo, E., G. Forni, P. Lollini, M.P. Colombo, A. Modesti, and P. Musiani. The intriguing role of polymorphonuclear neutrophils in antitumor reactions. Blood, 2001. 97(2): p. 339-45.

[6] Allavena, P., G. Germano, F. Marchesi, and A. Mantovani. Chemokines in cancer related inflammation. Exp Cell Res, 2011. 317(5): p. 664-73.

[7] Grakoui, A., S.K. Bromley, C. Sumen, M.M. Davis, A.S. Shaw, P.M. Allen, and M.L. Dustin. The immunological synapse: a molecular machine controlling T cell activation. Science, 1999. 285(5425): p. 221-7.

[8] Shresta, S., D.M. MacIvor, J.W. Heusel, J.H. Russell, and T.J. Ley. Natural killer and lymphokine-activated killer cells require granzyme B for the rapid induction of apoptosis in susceptible target cells. Proc Natl Acad Sci USA, 1995. 92(12): p. 5679-83.

[9] Cullen, S.P., M. Brunet, and S.J. Martin. Granzymes in cancer and immunity. Cell Death Differ, 2010. 17(4): p. 616-23.

[10] Hamai, A., H. Benlalam, F. Meslin, M. Hasmim, T. Carre, I. Akalay, B. Janji, G. Berchem, M.Z. Noman, and S. Chouaib. Immune surveillance of human cancer: if the cytotoxic T-lymphocytes play the music, does the tumoral system call the tune? Tissue Antigens, 2010. 75(1): p. 1-8.

[11] Whiteside, T.L. The tumor microenvironment and its role in promoting tumor growth. Oncogene, 2008. 27(45): p. 5904-12.

[12] Majmundar, A.J., W.J. Wong, and M.C. Simon. Hypoxia-inducible factors and the response to hypoxic stress. Mol Cell, 2010. 40(2): p. 294-309.

[13] Semenza, G.L. Hypoxia-inducible factors: mediators of cancer progression and targets for cancer therapy. Trends Pharmacol Sci, 2012. 33(4): p. 207-14.

[14] Semenza, G.L. Defining the role of hypoxia-inducible factor 1 in cancer biology and therapeutics. Oncogene, 2010. 29(5): p. 625-34.

[15] Semenza, G.L. Targeting HIF-1 for cancer therapy. Nat Rev Cancer, 2003. 3(10): p. 721-32.

[16] Wang, G.L., B.H. Jiang, E.A. Rue, and G.L. Semenza. Hypoxia-inducible factor 1 is a basic-helix-loop-helix-PAS heterodimer regulated by cellular O_2 tension. Proc Natl Acad Sci USA, 1995. 92(12): p. 5510-4.

[17] Huang, L.E., J. Gu, M. Schau, and H.F. Bunn. Regulation of hypoxia-inducible factor 1alpha is mediated by an O_2-dependent degradation domain via the ubiquitin-proteasome pathway. Proc Natl Acad Sci USA, 1998. 95(14): p. 7987-92.

[18] Pugh, C.W., C.C. Tan, R.W. Jones, and P.J. Ratcliffe. Functional analysis of an oxygen-regulated transcriptional enhancer lying 3' to the mouse erythropoietin gene. Proc Natl Acad Sci USA, 1991. 88(23): p. 10553-7.

[19] Jiang, B.H., J.Z. Zheng, S.W. Leung, R. Roe, and G.L. Semenza. Transactivation and inhibitory domains of hypoxia-inducible factor 1alpha. Modulation of transcriptional activity by oxygen tension. J Biol Chem, 1997. 272(31): p. 19253-60.

[20] Jewell, U.R., I. Kvietikova, A. Scheid, C. Bauer, R.H. Wenger, and M. Gassmann. Induction of HIF-1alpha in response to hypoxia is instantaneous. FASEB J, 2001. 15(7): p. 1312-4.

[21] Jiang, B.H., G.L. Semenza, C. Bauer, and H.H. Marti. Hypoxia-inducible factor 1 levels vary exponentially over a physiologically relevant range of O_2 tension. Am J Physiol, 1996. 271(4 Pt 1): p. C1172-80.

[22] Ivan, M., K. Kondo, H. Yang, W. Kim, J. Valiando, M. Ohh, A. Salic, J.M. Asara, W.S. Lane, and W.G. Kaelin, Jr. HIFalpha targeted for VHL-mediated destruction by proline hydroxylation: implications for O_2 sensing. Science, 2001. 292(5516): p. 464-8.

[23] Salceda, S. and J. Caro. Hypoxia-inducible factor 1alpha (HIF-1alpha) protein is rapidly degraded by the ubiquitin-proteasome system under normoxic conditions. Its stabilization by hypoxia depends on redox-induced changes. J Biol Chem, 1997. 272(36): p. 22642-7.

[24] Bruick, R.K. and S.L. McKnight. A conserved family of prolyl-4-hydroxylases that modify HIF. Science, 2001. 294(5545): p. 1337-40.

[25] Epstein, A.C., J.M. Gleadle, L.A. McNeill, K.S. Hewitson, J. O'Rourke, D.R. Mole, M. Mukherji, E. Metzen, M.I. Wilson, A. Dhanda, Y.M. Tian, N. Masson, D.L. Hamilton, P. Jaakkola, R. Barstead, J. Hodgkin, P.H. Maxwell, C.W. Pugh, C.J. Schofield, and P.J. Ratcliffe. C. elegans EGL-9 and mammalian homologs define a family of dioxygenases that regulate HIF by prolyl hydroxylation. Cell, 2001. 107(1): p. 43-54.

[26] Schodel, J., S. Oikonomopoulos, J. Ragoussis, C.W. Pugh, P.J. Ratcliffe, and D.R. Mole. High-resolution genome-wide mapping of HIF-binding sites by ChIP-seq. Blood, 2011. 117(23): p. e207-17.

[27] Xia, X., M.E. Lemieux, W. Li, J.S. Carroll, M. Brown, X.S. Liu, and A.L. Kung. Integrative analysis of HIF binding and transactivation reveals its role in maintaining histone methylation homeostasis. Proc Natl Acad Sci U S A, 2009. 106(11): p. 4260-5.

[28] Semenza, G.L., M.K. Nejfelt, S.M. Chi, and S.E. Antonarakis. Hypoxia-inducible nuclear factors bind to an enhancer element located 3' to the human erythropoietin gene. Proc Natl Acad Sci U S A, 1991. 88(13): p. 5680-4.

[29] Wenger, R.H. and M. Gassmann. Oxygen(es) and the hypoxia-inducible factor-1. Biol Chem, 1997. 378(7): p. 609-16.

[30] Patel, S.A. and M.C. Simon. Biology of hypoxia-inducible factor-2alpha in development and disease. Cell Death Differ, 2008. 15(4): p. 628-34.

[31] Hu, C.J., A. Sataur, L. Wang, H. Chen, and M.C. Simon. The N-terminal transactivation domain confers target gene specificity of hypoxia-inducible factors HIF-1alpha and HIF-2alpha. Mol Biol Cell, 2007. 18(11): p. 4528-42.

[32] Lau, K.W., Y.M. Tian, R.R. Raval, P.J. Ratcliffe, and C.W. Pugh. Target gene selectivity of hypoxia-inducible factor-alpha in renal cancer cells is conveyed by post-DNA-binding mechanisms. Br J Cancer, 2007. 96(8): p. 1284-92.

[33] Makino, Y., R. Cao, K. Svensson, G. Bertilsson, M. Asman, H. Tanaka, Y. Cao, A. Berkenstam, and L. Poellinger. Inhibitory PAS domain protein is a negative regulator of hypoxia-inducible gene expression. Nature, 2001. 414(6863): p. 550-4.

[34] Kulshreshtha, R., R.V. Davuluri, G.A. Calin, and M. Ivan. A microRNA component of the hypoxic response. Cell Death Differ, 2008. 15(4): p. 667-71.

[35] Wu, M.Z., Y.P. Tsai, M.H. Yang, C.H. Huang, S.Y. Chang, C.C. Chang, S.C. Teng, and K.J. Wu. Interplay between HDAC3 and WDR5 is essential for hypoxia-induced epithelial-mesenchymal transition. Mol Cell, 2011. 43(5): p. 811-22.

[36] Noman, M.Z., S. Buart, J. Van Pelt, C. Richon, M. Hasmim, N. Leleu, W.M. Suchorska, A. Jalil, Y. Lecluse, F. El Hage, M. Giuliani, C. Pichon, B. Azzarone, N. Mazure, P. Romero, F. Mami-Chouaib, and S. Chouaib. The cooperative induction of hypoxia-inducible factor-1 alpha and STAT3 during hypoxia induced an impairment of tumor susceptibility to CTL-mediated cell lysis. J Immunol, 2009. 182(6): p. 3510-21.

[37] Noman, M.Z., B. Janji, B. Kaminska, K. Van Moer, S. Pierson, P. Przanowski, S. Buart, G. Berchem, P. Romero, F. Mami-Chouaib, and S. Chouaib. Blocking hypoxia-induced autophagy in tumors restores cytotoxic T-cell activity and promotes regression. Cancer Res, 2011. 71(18): p. 5976-86.

[38] Mathew, R. and E. White. Autophagy, stress, and cancer metabolism: what doesn't kill you makes you stronger. Cold Spring Harb Symp Quant Biol, 2011. 76: p. 389-96.

[39] Viry, E., J. Baginska, G. Berchem, M.Z. Noman, S. Medves, S. Chouaib, and B. Janji. Autophagic degradation of GZMB/granzyme B: a new mechanism of hypoxic tumor cell escape from natural killer cell-mediated lysis. Autophagy, 2014. 10(1): p. 173-5.

[40] Moussay, E., T. Kaoma, J. Baginska, A. Muller, K. Van Moer, N. Nicot, P.V. Nazarov, L. Vallar, S. Chouaib, G. Berchem, and B. Janji. The acquisition of resistance to TNFalpha in breast cancer cells is associated with constitutive activation of autophagy as revealed by a transcriptome analysis using a custom microarray. Autophagy, 2011. 7(7): p. 760-70.

[41] Noman, M.Z., B. Janji, G. Berchem, F. Mami-Chouaib, and S. Chouaib. Hypoxia-induced autophagy: a new player in cancer immunotherapy? Autophagy, 2012. 8(4): p. 704-6.

[42] Hasmim, M., M.Z. Noman, J. Lauriol, H. Benlalam, A. Mallavialle, F. Rosselli, F. Mami-Chouaib, C. Alcaide-Loridan, and S. Chouaib. Hypoxia-dependent inhibition of tumor cell susceptibility to CTL-mediated lysis involves NANOG induction in target cells. J Immunol, 2011. 187(8): p. 4031-9.

[43] Hasmim, M., M.Z. Noman, Y. Messai, D. Bordereaux, G. Gros, V. Baud, and S. Chouaib. Cutting edge: hypoxia-induced Nanog favors the intratumoral infiltration of regulatory T cells and macrophages via direct regulation of TGF-beta1. J Immunol, 2013. 191(12): p. 5802-6.

[44] Noman, M.Z., S. Buart, P. Romero, S. Ketari, B. Janji, B. Mari, F. Mami-Chouaib, and S. Chouaib. Hypoxia-inducible miR-210 regulates the susceptibility of tumor cells to lysis by cytotoxic T cells. Cancer Res, 2012. 72(18): p. 4629-41.

[45] Siemens, D.R., N. Hu, A.K. Sheikhi, E. Chung, L.J. Frederiksen, H. Pross, and C.H. Graham. Hypoxia increases tumor cell shedding of MHC class I chain-related molecule: role of nitric oxide. Cancer Res, 2008. 68(12): p. 4746-53.

[46] Yamada, N., K. Yamanegi, H. Ohyama, M. Hata, K. Nakasho, H. Futani, H. Okamura, and N. Terada. Hypoxia downregulates the expression of cell surface MICA without increasing soluble MICA in osteosarcoma cells in a HIF-1alpha-dependent manner. Int J Oncol, 2012. 41(6): p. 2005-12.

[47] Baginska, J., E. Viry, J. Paggetti, S. Medves, G. Berchem, E. Moussay, and B. Janji. The critical role of the tumor microenvironment in shaping natural killer cell-mediated anti-tumor immunity. Front Immunol, 2013. 4: p. 490.

[48] Viry, E., J. Paggetti, J. Baginska, T. Mgrditchian, G. Berchem, E. Moussay, and B. Janji. Autophagy: an adaptive metabolic response to stress shaping the antitumor immunity. Biochem Pharmacol, 2014. 92(1): p. 31-42.

[49] Baginska, J., E. Viry, G. Berchem, A. Poli, M.Z. Noman, K. van Moer, S. Medves, J. Zimmer, A. Oudin, S.P. Niclou, R.C. Bleackley, I.S. Goping, S. Chouaib, and B. Janji. Granzyme B degradation by autophagy decreases tumor cell susceptibility to natural killer-mediated lysis under hypoxia. Proc Natl Acad Sci USA, 2013. 110(43): p. 17450-5.

[50] Axelson, H., E. Fredlund, M. Ovenberger, G. Landberg, and S. Pahlman. Hypoxia-induced dedifferentiation of tumor cells—a mechanism behind heterogeneity and aggressiveness of solid tumors. Semin Cell Dev Biol, 2005. 16(4-5): p. 554-63.

[51] Harris, A.L. Hypoxia—a key regulatory factor in tumour growth. Nat Rev Cancer, 2002. 2(1): p. 38-47.

[52] Jogi, A., I. Ora, H. Nilsson, A. Lindeheim, Y. Makino, L. Poellinger, H. Axelson, and S. Pahlman. Hypoxia alters gene expression in human neuroblastoma cells toward an immature and neural crest-like phenotype. Proc Natl Acad Sci USA, 2002. 99(10): p. 7021-6.

[53] Helczynska, K., A. Kronblad, A. Jogi, E. Nilsson, S. Beckman, G. Landberg, and S. Pahlman. Hypoxia promotes a dedifferentiated phenotype in ductal breast carcinoma in situ. Cancer Res, 2003. 63(7): p. 1441-4.

[54] Kim, Y., Q. Lin, P.M. Glazer, and Z. Yun. Hypoxic tumor microenvironment and cancer cell differentiation. Curr Mol Med, 2009. 9(4): p. 425-34.

[55] Yeung, T.M., S.C. Gandhi, and W.F. Bodmer. Hypoxia and lineage specification of cell line-derived colorectal cancer stem cells. Proc Natl Acad Sci USA, 2011. 108(11): p. 4382-7.

[56] Vermeulen, L., E.M.F. De Sousa, M. van der Heijden, K. Cameron, J.H. de Jong, T. Borovski, J.B. Tuynman, M. Todaro, C. Merz, H. Rodermond, M.R. Sprick, K. Kemper, D.J. Richel, G. Stassi, and J.P. Medema. Wnt activity defines colon cancer stem cells and is regulated by the microenvironment. Nat Cell Biol, 2010. 12(5): p. 468-76.

[57] Zellmer, V.R. and S. Zhang. Evolving concepts of tumor heterogeneity. Cell Biosci, 2014. 4: p. 69.

[58] Holzel, M., A. Bovier, and T. Tuting. Plasticity of tumour and immune cells: a source of heterogeneity and a cause for therapy resistance? Nat Rev Cancer, 2013. 13(5): p. 365-76.

[59] Schreiber, R.D., L.J. Old, and M.J. Smyth. Cancer immunoediting: integrating immunity's roles in cancer suppression and promotion. Science, 2011. 331(6024): p. 1565-70.

[60] Santisteban, M., J.M. Reiman, M.K. Asiedu, M.D. Behrens, A. Nassar, K.R. Kalli, P. Haluska, J.N. Ingle, L.C. Hartmann, M.H. Manjili, D.C. Radisky, S. Ferrone, and K.L. Knutson. Immune-induced epithelial to mesenchymal transition in vivo generates breast cancer stem cells. Cancer Res, 2009. 69(7): p. 2887-95.

[61] Roesch, A., A. Paschen, J. Landsberg, I. Helfrich, J.C. Becker, and D. Schadendorf. Phenotypic tumour cell plasticity as a resistance mechanism and therapeutic target in melanoma. Eur J Cancer, 2016. 59: p. 109-12.

[62] Noman, M.Z., M. Hasmim, Y. Messai, S. Terry, C. Kieda, B. Janji, and S. Chouaib. Hypoxia: a key player in antitumor immune response. A review in the Theme: Cellular Responses to Hypoxia. Am J Physiol Cell Physiol, 2015. 309(9): p. C569-79.

[63] Guise, C.P., A.M. Mowday, A. Ashoorzadeh, R. Yuan, W.H. Lin, D.H. Wu, J.B. Smaill, A.V. Patterson, and K. Ding. Bioreductive prodrugs as cancer therapeutics: targeting tumor hypoxia. Chin J Cancer, 2014. 33(2): p. 80-6.

[64] Wilson, W.R. and M.P. Hay. Targeting hypoxia in cancer therapy. Nat Rev Cancer, 2011. 11(6): p. 393-410.

[65] Hoelder, S., P.A. Clarke, and P. Workman. Discovery of small molecule cancer drugs: successes, challenges and opportunities. Mol Oncol, 2012. 6(2): p. 155-76.

[66] Xia, Y., H.K. Choi, and K. Lee. Recent advances in hypoxia-inducible factor (HIF)-1 inhibitors. Eur J Med Chem, 2012. 49: p. 24-40.

[67] Rapisarda, A., B. Uranchimeg, D.A. Scudiero, M. Selby, E.A. Sausville, R.H. Shoemaker, and G. Melillo. Identification of small molecule inhibitors of hypoxia-inducible factor 1 transcriptional activation pathway. Cancer Res, 2002. 62(15): p. 4316-24.

[68] Yeo, E.J., Y.S. Chun, Y.S. Cho, J. Kim, J.C. Lee, M.S. Kim, and J.W. Park. YC-1: a potential anticancer drug targeting hypoxia-inducible factor 1. J Natl Cancer Inst, 2003. 95(7): p. 516-25.

[69] Isaacs, J.S., Y.J. Jung, E.G. Mimnaugh, A. Martinez, F. Cuttitta, and L.M. Neckers. Hsp90 regulates a von Hippel Lindau-independent hypoxia-inducible factor-1 alpha-degradative pathway. J Biol Chem, 2002. 277(33): p. 29936-44.

[70] Mabjeesh, N.J., D.E. Post, M.T. Willard, B. Kaur, E.G. Van Meir, J.W. Simons, and H. Zhong. Geldanamycin induces degradation of hypoxia-inducible factor 1alpha protein via the proteosome pathway in prostate cancer cells. Cancer Res, 2002. 62(9): p. 2478-82.

[71] Zagzag, D., M. Nomura, D.R. Friedlander, C.Y. Blanco, J.P. Gagner, N. Nomura, and E.W. Newcomb. Geldanamycin inhibits migration of glioma cells in vitro: a potential role for hypoxia-inducible factor (HIF-1alpha) in glioma cell invasion. J Cell Physiol, 2003. 196(2): p. 394-402.

[72] Welsh, S.J., R.R. Williams, A. Birmingham, D.J. Newman, D.L. Kirkpatrick, and G. Powis. The thioredoxin redox inhibitors 1-methylpropyl 2-imidazolyl disulfide and pleurotin inhibit hypoxia-induced factor 1alpha and vascular endothelial growth factor formation. Mol Cancer Ther, 2003. 2(3): p. 235-43.

[73] Welsh, S., R. Williams, L. Kirkpatrick, G. Paine-Murrieta, and G. Powis. Antitumor activity and pharmacodynamic properties of PX-478, an inhibitor of hypoxia-inducible factor-1alpha. Mol Cancer Ther, 2004. 3(3): p. 233-44.

Chapter 19

Cross-Talk Between Hypoxia and the Tumour via Exosomes

Shayna Sharma, Mona Alharbi, Andrew Lai,
Miharu Kobayashi, Richard Kline, Katrina Wade,
Gregory E. Rice and Carlos Salomon

Additional information is available at the end of the chapter

http://dx.doi.org/10.5772/65688

Abstract

Cancer is one of the leading causes of death worldwide, and this is often attributed to the nonspecific symptoms. Additionally, delayed diagnosis and a lack of treatment options negatively impact prognosis. Recently, the role of extracellular vesicles in cancer progression, specifically, in metastasis and in the capacity of several tumours to invade and colonise specific organs has been established. Reduced oxygen tension due to imbalanced oxygen supply and consumption is termed hypoxia and is one of the most commonly observed features in solid tumours. This is often correlated with poor cancer prognosis. Several reports have established that low oxygen tension (i.e. hypoxia) is a common feature of the tumour microenvironment often enhancing the process of epithelial-to-mesenchymal transition (EMT) in cancer cells, thus promoting tumourigenesis and metastasis. Furthermore, hypoxia increases the number of extracellular vesicles released from cancer cells and also modifies their bioactivity and function. The aim of this chapter is to review the association between the tumour microenvironment and extracellular vesicles (EVs), focusing on a specific subpopulation of EVs of endocytic origin, termed exosomes.

Keywords: exosomes, metastasis, metastatic niche, tumourigenesis, cancer

1. Introduction

The global burden of cancer is on the rise and in 2012 around 14.1 million new cases were reported with 8.2 million deaths attributed to cancer [1]. Cancer can be subdivided into categories depending on the area that is affected, including but not limited to lung cancer, pancreatic cancer and ovarian cancer [2, 3].

Consequently, the development of targeted treatments for a large population is difficult due to the heterogeneity of the tumours. Furthermore, in cases such as ovarian cancer, current treatments, which include the use of platinum-based cytotoxic chemotherapy, antiangiogenic drugs and poly (ADP-ribose) polymerase inhibitors, are only beneficial for patients with early stage disease [2]. However, in patients with more advanced stage disease, there is often recurrence of the disease after treatment due to the development of resistance [2]. Therefore, it is essential that diagnostic procedures be explored.

This paradigm shift from focusing on treatments to focusing on early diagnosis of cancer has brought exosomes to the forefront.

Exosomes are small membranous vesicles that are released following the fusion of multivesicular bodies (MVBs) with the cell membrane. They have multiple characteristics including a cup or spherical shape, maximum diameter of approximately 100 nm, a buoyant density of ~1.12 to ~1.19 g /mL on a sucrose gradient, endosomal origin and the enrichment of late endosomal membrane markers, including TSG101 and proteins from the tetraspanin family (e.g. CD63) [3, 4]. Exosomes are covered in a variety of cell surface receptors and contain several proteins such as cytoskeletal proteins, adhesion molecules and heat-shock proteins. Additionally, they encapsulate diverse miRNA and mRNA, which can impact the bioactivity and functionality of the target cells with which the exosomes interact.

While the role of exosomes during tumour progression remains to be fully established, we postulate that tumour cells release exosomes loaded with specific molecules in response to the microenvironment to prepare for and promote metastasis to specific organs.

2. Exosomes: a specific type of extracellular vesicle

Cells secrete a multitude of EVs of different origin, size, content and function. Recent reports have recognised a specific type of extracellular vesicle termed exosomes. Exosomes are believed to be tumour 'couriers', carrying signals and relocating packages of signalling molecules to initiate processes such as metastasis by preparing the metastatic niche [5, 6].

In contrast to other EVs, which are formed by an inward budding of the plasma membrane, exosomes are secreted through the intraluminal invagination of vesicles termed early endosomes [7]. This leads to the formation of multivesicular bodies (MVBs) which contain intraluminal vesicles (ILVs). These ILVs are then released by the cell through the fusion of the MVB with the cellular membrane. The released ILVs are termed exosomes [4, 5, 8]. Exosomes carry a common set of molecules along with cell-specific components. Therefore, exosomes contain proteins which are associated with the biogenesis of MVBs such as tetraspanins, Rab GTPases and Annexins [9]. The endosomal-sorting complex required for transport (ESCRT) pathway facilitates plasma membrane remodelling and is also believed to have a role in ILV formation

[10]. Research has also shown that other pathways independent of the ESCRT complex also exist, as an MVB is also formed when the ESCRT complexes are repressed [11, 12, 14, 15].

Whilst the biogenesis of exosomes has been well understood and defined in recent literature, a consensus on the method to extract exosomes is yet to be established. However, a detailed discussion of the current methodological approaches is beyond the scope of this chapter [16, 17]. A NanoSight Tracking Analysis (NTA) comparison between exosomes and microvesicles is shown in **Figure 1**.

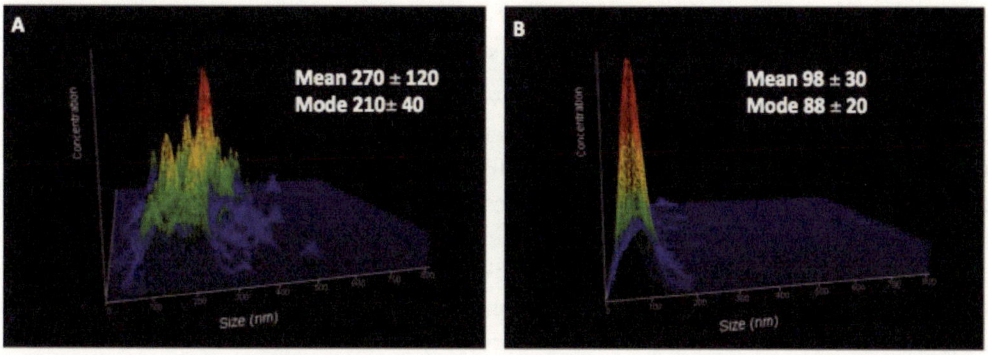

Figure 1. Nanoparticle-tracking analysis using the NanoSight. Representative image of the size distribution of 100,000 g pellet (A) and exosomes (B). The NanoSight instrument measured the rate of Brownian motion of nanoparticles and consists in a light-scattering system that provides a reproducible platform for specific and general nanoparticle characterization (NanoSight Ltd., Amesbury, UK).

Nonetheless, the requirement for a standard isolation procedure is essential as research moves towards examining exosomes as potential therapeutic agents in the context of several diseases such as cancer. Additionally, exosomes are being used to understand the characteristics of the solid tumour, circulating tumour cells and the tumour microenvironment, especially under conditions such as hypoxia.

3. The tumour microenvironment and hypoxia

Under normal conditions, the cellular microenvironment inhibits the development of cancerous cells through tumour interactions thus allowing the environment to annihilate the growth of cancerous cells. The tumour microenvironment comprises endothelial cells (ECs), fibroblasts, perivascular cells and inflammatory cells. These components tend to control the tumourigenic processes—that is, angiogenesis, desmoplasia, lymphangiogenesis and inflammation. Oxygen deficiency in tumour cells, also known as hypoxia, is among the major factors that trigger tumour development and hinder clinical diagnoses [13–15].

An imbalance between oxygen supply and demand causes hypoxic or anoxic conditions. The oxygen supply rate is equivalent to that of metabolic requirements in a normal cell or a tissue.

However, in developed solid tumours, the oxygen consumption rate may fluctuate to adjust for the insufficient oxygen supply, allowing the tissues to develop even in regions with low oxygen levels [15]. Accumulating evidence suggests that up to 60% of locally advanced tumours display hypoxic (≤1% O_2 compared to 2–9% O_2 or 40 mm Hg on average in most mammalian tissues) and/or anoxic (≤0.01% O_2 or undetectable oxygen) areas distributed heterogeneously throughout the tumour and that tumour hypoxia correlates with advanced stages of malignancy [16]. In cancer cells, respective mechanisms are activated to respond to changes in the availability of oxygen. The cells are subjected to lower levels of oxygen and must therefore modify their metabolism, respectively. In such conditions, the hypoxia-inducible factor-1 (HIF-1) transcription factor programme of gene expression changes. This change in expression is assumed to enable the cell to cope with the new environment [17–19].

HIF-1 is a heterodimer complex consisting of two bHLH transcription factors: HIF-1α and HIF-1β [20]. HIF-1α expression is significantly overexpressed in advanced ovarian tumours. O_2-dependent mechanisms primarily regulate HIF-1α degradation. Under normoxic conditions, the O_2-dependent hydroxylation of proline residues in HIF-1α by prolyl hydrolase-domain protein is recognised by the von Hippel-Lindau tumour-suppressor protein and ubiquitinated to be targeted for degradation. Under hypoxic conditions, HIF-1α stabilises and accumulates due to the inhibition of hydroxylation and von Hippel-Lindau protein-mediated ubiquitination, translocates to the nucleus and forms a complex with HIF-1β and a transcriptional co-activator CBP/p300 to activate the transcription of target genes by directly binding to their hypoxia-responsive elements [21].

During hypoxia, HIF-1 activates genes involved in proliferation, cell survival, angiogenesis, vascular tone, metal transport, glycolysis, mitochondrial function, cell growth and survival, and apoptosis and EMT, which all contribute to tumour progression. HIF-1-dependent expression of erythropoietin and angiogenic compounds further enhances the formation of blood vessels and thus facilitates the delivery of oxygenated blood to the hypoxic tissue through the induction of vascular endothelial growth factors (VEGFs). In vitro studies show that increasingly subjecting cancer cells to a hypoxic stimulus results in a gradual increase in VEGF mRNA levels and VEGF protein levels [22, 23].

The addition of HIF-1-induced glycolytic enzymes provides energy as a substrate for oxidative phosphorylation when mitochondria are starved of oxygen [17]. Moreover, due to lower levels of oxygen and nutrients, the ATP level decreases causing a deregulation in the actin cytoskeleton controlled by the down-regulation of Rho proteins. Rho kinase facilitates contractile force generation mediated by actin-myosin by phosphorylating a number of target proteins. Rho/Rho kinase plays a critical role in movement, penetration, cell-cell adhesion, smooth muscle contraction, cytokinesis, mitosis, multiplication, variation, apoptosis and oncogenic transformation within the cell [24–28].

Tumour hypoxia and HIF-1α overexpression have been demonstrated to induce EMT and metastatic phenotypes in cancer cells, yet the crosstalk between the HIF-signalling pathway and EMT is not completely understood [29]. Several studies propose potential molecular mechanisms, such as HIF-1-promoting EMT through the up-regulation of EMT transcriptional factors. Nonetheless, it is known that HIF-1 regulates TWIST expression by binding to their hypoxia-responsive elements. Thus, cells cultured under hypoxia or constitutive HIF-1α expression promoted EMT, whereas the repression of TWIST expression abolished the effect of HIF-1α, shifting the cells back to an epithelial phenotype from the mesenchymal phenotype [29]. HIF-1 expression induced by hypoxia represses E-cadherin-coding genes through SNAI1 and SNAI2 [30–32]. Along with transcriptional factors, hypoxia and HIF-1 activate EMT-associated signalling pathways. Hypoxia also activates the Wnt/β-catenin-signalling pathway by inhibiting GSK3β activation, preventing β-catenin phosphorylation and destruction to increase SNAI1 expression [33]. HIF-1 further interacts with the Notch intracellular domain to increase its transcriptional activity [34].

The Notch-targeted genes HES1 and HEY1 were increased under hypoxic conditions; however, a knockdown of HIF-1α abrogated the hypoxia-induced HES1 and HEY1 expression as well as the SNAI1 expression [35]. Furthermore, HIF-1α targeted lysyl oxidase and lysyl oxidase-like 2 and 3 enzymes, which promote tumour metastasis by mediating cells to matrix adhesion and stabilising SNAI1 activity to induce EMT [36, 37]. Under hypoxia, the consumption of glucose and GLUT1 expression in cancer cells increased as well [17].

It is also well established that bidirectional communication between cancer cells and their tumour microenvironment is essential for cancer progression. For example, most ovarian cancer patients present with ascites—excess fluid in the peritoneal cavity [38]. Ovarian cancer ascites contain molecular factors, including VEGF, cytokines, chemokines and TGF-β, to mediate cellular communication for effective tumourigenesis. Accumulating evidence suggests that cellular communication is not only limited to secretary molecules, but also includes EVs (such as exosomes) that mediate such communication [39]. The nomenclature of EVs is still a matter of debate due to the many terms used (e.g. microvesicles, nanovesicles, shedding vesicles and ectosomes), emphasising the range of EV populations secreted [9].

However, during tumourigenesis, hypoxia serves as a selective agent at various physiological levels. Under hypoxia, a number of transcriptional factors control the cell environment, including Nuclear Factor-kappaB (NF-κB), Activating Transcription Factors (ATFs) and p53s [40–42]. In NF-κB pathways activated by HIF during irregular hypoxia and re-oxygenation [41, 43] and ATF, anoxia drives signalling [44].

Moreover, carbonic anhydrase IX (CAIX) is among the genes in the hypoxic environment of solid tumours that increasingly express themselves. CAIX expression is perceived as causing bladder, ovarian, cervical, colorectal, oral, brain and breast cancers. It enables the balancing of intracellular pH through the extracellular hydration of CO_2 and the production of bicarbonate and protons. The bicarbonate goes back into the cell through bicarbonate transporters and balances the intracellular pH as alkaline, which is favourable for the cell's survival. The protons acidify the extracellular space, thus facilitating the tumour's migratory and invasive behaviour [45–47]. CAIX expression and activity also facilitates the production of Granulocyte-colony stimulating factor (G-CSF),which is in turn required for the transportation of granulocytic Myeloid-derived Suppressor Cells (MDSC) to the metastatic niche—an environment that promotes metastasis. CAIX expression is also required to stimulate NF-κB activity and G-CSF production mediated through hypoxia. The hypoxia-mediated NF-κB activity is triggered by a decrease in the pH level of the culture as well as hypoxia-induced glycolytic activity in the cancer cells [46, 48–50]. The hypoxic areas of tumours usually have lower levels of extracellular pH due to increased metabolic activity [45]. It has been proven that the cells are hampered from acidifying the medium due to a smaller production rate of CAIX in a hypoxic environment [51]. Therefore, hypoxia and the tumour microenvironment are essential factors in regulating disease progression and metastasis.

4. Exosomes, the tumour microenvironment and hypoxia

An evaluation of cancer cells and their microenvironment plays a critical role in hypoxia. Tumour cells under hypoxia secrete molecules that modulate their microenvironment and facilitate tumour angiogenesis and metastasis. Hypoxia is a major hallmark of the tumour environment and is caused when there is a lack of blood supply. The lowered blood supply indicates a lower number of red blood cells being able to reach the tumour cells resulting in decreased oxygen delivery [52]. Moreover, hypoxic tumours have a greater ability to resist standard treatments and the tumour cells are often in a less differentiated or more stem cell-like state [53]. Emerging evidence has shown that exosomes are key membrane vesicles secreted by most cell types under hypoxia. It has also been shown that they have an ability to modulate the tumour microenvironment to ensure adequate nutrition and oxygen supply [54]. There has been an increasing interest in the role of exosomes as a mediator of cell-to-cell communication and its role in ultimately aiding cancer progression.

There have been several processes proposed regarding the release of exosomes into the tumour microenvironment. These processes involve several molecules such as proteins involved in fusion of the multivesicular bodies as well as plasma membrane proteins. Additionally, it has been shown that exosomes present in a cell's environment also regulate exosome release. Riches and colleagues showed that when exosomes were added to the culture medium of cells, the number of exosomes released by the cells decreased evidently [55]. Other proteins that may be involved in increased exosome secretion during hypoxia include the Rab family of proteins, specifically Rab27 as they regulate exosome secretion. The Rab27 protein has two isoforms: Rab27a and Rab27b. Ostrowski and colleagues noted that inhibiting Rab9a, Rab5a, Rab27a, Rab27b and Rab2b led to an inhibition in exosome release [35]. Furthermore, it has been previously shown that the presence of calcium (Ca^{2+}) ionophores can lead to an increase in the release of exosomes [56]. Therefore, although there are several hypotheses, the exact mechanism is still unclear. Thus, the mechanisms underlying exosome release under different tumour microenvironmental conditions such as hypoxia remain to be elucidated. Nonetheless, progress is being made.

The role of exosomes in tumour progression and invasion has been highlighted in literature with a clear correlation being found between the number of hypoxic exosomes released and the aggressiveness of the tumour [57, 58]. A significant increase in the number of exosomes released under hypoxia (1% oxygen) and severe anoxia (0.1% oxygen) was found in a study conducted on three breast cancer cell lines, in which the impact of hypoxia on tumour progression and the release of exosomes was investigated [58]. King and colleagues postulated that the enhancement of exosome release might be mediated by the hypoxia-inducible factor 1 oxygen-sensing pathway (detailed above). They tested their hypothesis by using the HIF hydroxylase inhibitor, Dimethyloxalylglycine (DMOG), to treat the breast cancer cell line, MDA-MB-231 [58]. The role of the DMOG was to trigger an HIF response. This led to a minor although significant rise in the number of exosomes secreted by the cells when quantified by nanoparticle-tracking analysis (NTA). Moreover, when the HIF-1α transcription factor was silenced using siRNA, the increase in exosomes in response to hypoxia was not seen. Therefore, it was concluded that the HIF pathway may have a significant role in the release of exosomes in response to hypoxia. Similar studies were carried out on different cell lines (e.g. leukaemia cell line, K562; human microvascular endothelial cells (HMEC-1); A431 squamous carcinoma; A549 non-small-cell lung (NSCL); H1299 NSCL and HFF-1 foreskin fibroblast cells) to investigate the level of exosomes released under hypoxia and normoxia [57]. The outcome was that the number of exosomes released under hypoxic conditions increased when compared to exosomes released by cells under normoxic conditions in the same amount of time. However, the pathways underlying the hypoxic enhancement of exosome release were unclear [15].

In addition, oncogenic miR-21 was identified at a significant level in exosome fractions [59, 64]. miR-21 is known to down-regulate programmed cell death 4 (PDCD4) expression by directly targeting its 3′-untranslated region. Moreover, it was found that exosomes isolated from peritoneal effusions (ovarian cancer) contained low PDCD4 expression, whereas oncogenic miR-21 was highly expressed compared to exosomes isolated from non-neoplastic peritoneal effusions [59]. The use of exosomal miR-21 as a biomarker for cancer diagnosis has been suggested in several studies as it exists in almost all bodily fluids, is stable and is protected from degradation [60]. Exosomal miR-21 has an effect on a number of signalling pathways which promote metastatic capacity and proliferation. It has been found that miR-21 suppresses phosphatase and tensin homolog expression and promotes the growth and migration of tumour cells [61]. miR-21 also regulates cellular functions by influencing signal transduction, proliferation, carcinogenesis, differentiation and immune response [62–64]. These observations provide key evidence that elevated exosome release under hypoxia is a critical factor affecting tumour proliferation.

Tumour-derived exosomes have the ability to transfer oncogenic activity among tumour cells. Human glioma cells can horizontally transfer an oncogenic form of epidermal growth factor variant III (EGFRvIII) to glioma cells lacking EGFRvIII [65]. The transfer results in an increased expression of the pro-survival gene and a reduction in the cell cycle inhibitor, increasing anchorage-independent growth capacity [65]. An interesting possibility that exosomes are key factors that affect the neighbouring cells is provided by these studies.

Exosomes facilitate communication among tumour cells and contribute to the development of a favourable microenvironment for tumour progression by enhancing processes such as angiogenesis. Angiogenesis is promoted by the activation of endothelial cells through tumour-derived exosomes, and is followed up by the activation of myofibroblasts, a source of matrix-remodelling protein [66, 67]. Tumour-derived exosomes trigger fibroblast to myofibroblast differentiation [68]. In addition to fibroblasts, exosomes can trigger conversion of mesenchymal stem cells from the tumour stroma and adipose tissue to myofibroblasts [69]. The exosomes also contribute to the formation of pre-metastatic niches by educating the bone marrow-derived cells (BMDC). BMDCs when combined with exosomes derived from highly and poorly metastatic melanoma cells accelerated primary tumour growth and also increased the magnitude and number of metastases [6]. Additionally, evidence has shown that exosomes interact with immune cells to suppress antitumour responses and skew them towards the pro-tumourigenic phenotype [70]. Exosomes from hypoxic endothelial cells (EC) show up-regulation of collagen crosslinking activity by activation of lysyl oxidase-like 2 [71]. Lysyl oxidase-like 2 (LOXL2) has been linked to extracellular matrix (ECM) remodelling, angiogenesis, cell proliferation, migration, transcription regulation, fibroblast activation, EMT and metastatic niche formation through a number of processes [36, 72, 73]. The tumour cells can communicate with multiple different cell types via exosomes. Therefore, it is highly likely that this leads to a complex network of interactions.

The reaction of the target cells upon treatment with exosomes depends on the exosomal composition, which has been previously described as being diverse, and the transfer of encapsulated molecules [4, 67]. This ability of exosomes to protect and transfer molecules has led to the hypothesis that they could be used as potential tumour biomarkers or as a non-invasive tumour biopsy.

5. *In vivo* biodistribution of exosomes

Functional characterisation of exosomes often involves the use of an *in vivo* mouse model. Such experiments can give the biodistribution and pharmacokinetic parameters of the exosomes tested, which is important for understanding exosome trafficking and their physiological roles [74].

The starting point at which exosomes are to be isolated varies based on the experimental goals. In studies investigating the role of tumour-derived exosomes in cancer progression, exosomes were isolated from various cancer cell lines such as breast cancer, pancreatic cancer, gastric cancer and colorectal cancer [75]. Another area of interest is the potential use of exosomes as therapeutic carriers of antitumour microRNA or chemotherapy agents [76, 77]. This may allow for improved tissue targeting, increasing the potency of the delivered drug [78]. Exosomes are often isolated from cell-conditioned media with differential centrifugation being the most common method of enriching exosomes [75–77, 79, 80]. Most of the exosome isolation protocols involved low-speed centrifugation steps to remove cells and cell debris followed by high-speed centrifugation at 100,000 g and a washing step of the pellet with a final centrifugation. In a study by Alvarez-Erviti et al. [77], exosomes were derived from cultured dendritic cells, which was chosen based on data demonstrating that dendritic cell-derived exosomes contained immune-stimulating components such as major histocompatibility complex (MHC) class I and class II molecules in addition to T-cell-stimulating molecule, CD86 [81]. Studies also showed that isolated exosomes can be loaded with exogenous RNA or chemotherapy drugs by different methods, including electroporation and sonication [77, 78].

To enable the *in vivo* tracking of exosomes, they can be labelled post isolation with a lipophilic membrane dye such as Paul Karl Horan (PKH), DiOC18 (DIR) or DiIC18 (Dil) [75, 80, 82]. An alternative method of generating labelled exosomes is by transfecting donor cells with a construct encoding for a fluorescence-membrane fusion protein. In this approach, a membrane-bound variant of bioluminescence reporter, Gaussia luciferase, is transfected into the donor cells, producing luciferase-labelled exosomes [82, 83]. A major difference between the two labelling approaches is the time and expertise required. The post-isolation membrane dye labelling is quick (~1 h), whereas the transfection of cells requires additional time (~2 weeks) and expertise in vector and viral cloning and transfection [79, 84]. Additionally, a study by Lai et al [83] reported quicker rates of clearance of transfected luciferase-labelled exosomes compared to the dye-labelled exosomes. The authors attributed this difference to the possibility of the highly stable dyes being an artefact instead of indicating intact exosomal presence.

Exosomes injected into mice are commonly quantified using the Coomassie dye (Bradford)-based method, or copper-based chemistry such as the Bicinchoninic Acid Assay (BCA) [75–77, 82–85]. The yield of exosomes obtained often ranges from 6 to 12 $\mu g/10^6$-cultured dendritic cells, 69.2 $\mu g/2–5 \times 10^7$ of HEK293 and 2–4 $ug/10^6$ HEK cells [76, 77, 79]. There is some ambiguity in the quantification of exosomal protein concentration in these studies. Presumably, the exosomes were first lysed pre-quantification as without lysing the exosomes, only the membrane-bound proteins would be quantified. Another method of determining the required number of exosomes is to use the number of exosomes per gram of animal weight. Techniques such as NTA are used to quantify the number of exosomal particles and their size distribution [85, 90]. Importantly, in order to translate the use of exosomes into a clinical setting, standardising the dose of exosomes injected is critical. Given that isolated exosomes from current techniques such as ultracentrifugation are heterogeneous in size when observed using NTA [85], it is likely that the difference in size translates to differences in total protein concentration. Therefore, methods that quantify the total protein content within exosomes such as the Bradford/BCA assays are a better means of measuring the protein content and thus exosomal dose.

For biodistribution and tissue-uptake studies, the dose of injected exosomes ranged from 4 to 10 μg per mouse [75, 82]. Alternatively, a dosing range of 1.5×10^{10} particles/gram body weight (p/g), 1.0×10^{10} p/g and 0.25×10^{10} p/g was used [85]. In studies where exosomes were used as a potential therapeutic siRNA carrier, the dose of exosomes chosen was much higher, at 150 μg/mouse [77]. An explanation of a higher dose employed could be that systemically administered exosomes are rapidly cleared from the bloodstream, with evidence to suggest that macrophages play a role in exosome clearance [80]. Therefore, the higher dose was chosen to induce a measurable response.

Once the labelled exosomes are administered, the duration of monitoring ranged from 10 min to 6 h for biodistribution studies, which met the goal of tracking the localisation of exosomes over time [82, 83]. It was demonstrated that injected exosomes localised primarily in the liver and lungs [82, 85]. Moreover, it was shown recently that particular integrin expression on tumour-derived exosomes could be used to predict organ-specific metastasis [75]. In particular, exosomes expressing $\alpha 6 \beta 4$ and $\alpha 6 \beta 1$ were linked with lung metastasis, while exosomal integrin $\alpha v \beta 5$ was associated with liver metastasis. For exosomes which carried modified cargo, such as siRNA targeting the abundant GAPDH, the effect induced by the cargo was measured 3 days post injection [77]. This study showed the possibility of using exosome-mediated delivery of potentially therapeutic siRNA to induce a gene-specific knockdown.

In summary, *in vivo* characterisation is an important step in gaining an understanding of the physiological pathways that exosomes are involved in. Further research will strengthen the proposal of using exosomes as a therapeutic carrier and potential diagnostic tool.

6. New approaches to elucidate the role of exosomes in cancer

Identification of biomarkers to detect cancer during its early stages has the potential to improve patient outcomes significantly with exosomes currently being considered. As exosomes are released and circulate in the peripheral circulation, they can be collected from diverse biofluids through minimally invasive procedures from the blood and non-invasive procedures from saliva and urine. Through the isolation and purification process, exosomes are separated from highly abundant proteins present in bodily fluids [56]. Furthermore, cancer-derived exosomes can be specifically distinguished from exosomes originating from other cells by the expression of markers such as CD24 and EpCAM [86]. Storage of exosomes does not significantly affect their protein and miRNA contents thus highlighting their high stability [87]. Most importantly, the release and content of exosomes reflect the tumour state and their microenvironment [88].

Encapsulation of cellular proteins and RNA molecules into exosomes makes exosomes an enriched source of tumour markers, which provides an insight into the originating tumour cells. miRNAs are evolutionarily conserved regulating several cellular processes such as cell differentiation, proliferation and apoptosis [89]. These cellular processes are often altered in cancer-enhancing cellular transformation and tumourigenesis by impaired miRNA biogenesis; therefore, miRNA profiles can differentiate cancer tissues from benign tissues [90]. A complete miRNA-profiling study in epithelial ovarian cancer (EOC) has identified aberrantly expressed miRNA in different subtypes of EOC compared to normal ovaries [91]. Ovarian tumour-derived exosomes isolated from patient sera exhibited similar miRNA profiles to originating tumour cells and the exosome concentration was positively correlated with the progression of disease, highlighting the diagnostic potential of exosomal miRNA [92]. High exosomal miR-21, miR-23b and miR-29a expression of ovarian cancer patient effusion correlated with poor progression-free survival and poor overall survival was related to high expression of miR-21 suggesting their use as prognostic markers [93].

A recent study established the role of EOC-derived exosomes in mediating the activation of macrophages to a tumour-associated macrophage (TAM) state [94]. They also demonstrated that SKOV-3 cells when grown with conditioned media from the transformed macrophages were more likely to migrate and proliferate.

Additional studies have proposed the use of exosomes as both diagnostic biomarkers and therapeutic agents [95]. It has been proposed that exosomes be used to transport antitumour complexes such as drugs to the tumour cells, thus providing a form of targeted therapy.

Furthermore, it has been shown that decreasing exosome production by blocking Rab27a (responsible for exosome release) can also reduce primary tumour growth [96].

Compared to the currently available detection methods, the use of exosomes as biomarkers will involve minimally invasive procedures and as the exosomal content reflects the originating cancer cells and their microenvironment, they will have greater specificity. This will decrease the need for surgical interventions and deaths from surgical complications as a result of false-positive results [97].

Author details

Shayna Sharma[1], Mona Alharbi[1], Andrew Lai[1], Miharu Kobayashi[1], Richard Kline[2], Katrina Wade[2], Gregory E. Rice[1,2] and Carlos Salomon[1,2*]

*Address all correspondence to: c.salomongallo@uq.edu.au

1 Exosome Biology Laboratory, Centre for Clinical Diagnostics, University of Queensland Centre for Clinical Research, Royal Brisbane and Women's Hospital, The University of Queensland, Brisbane, QLD, Australia

2 Department of Obstetrics and Gynecology, Maternal-Fetal Medicine, Ochsner Clinic Foundation, New Orleans, LA, USA

References

[1] Ferlay, J., et al., Cancer incidence and mortality worldwide: sources, methods and major patterns in GLOBOCAN 2012. Int J Cancer, 2015. 136(5): p. E359–86.

[2] Jayson, G.C., et al., Ovarian cancer. The Lancet, 2014. 384(9951): p. 1376-1388.

[3] Salomon, C., et al., Exosomal signaling during hypoxia mediates microvascular endothelial cell migration and vasculogenesis. PLoS One, 2013. 8(7): p. e68451.

[4] Rice, G.E., et al., The effect of glucose on the release and bioactivity of exosomes from first trimester trophoblast cells. J Clin Endocrinol Metab, 2015. 100(10): p. E1280–8.

[5] Brinton, L.T., et al., Formation and role of exosomes in cancer. Cell Mol Life Sci, 2014. 72(4): p. 659-671.

[6] Peinado, H., et al., Melanoma exosomes educate bone marrow progenitor cells toward a pro-metastatic phenotype through MET. Nature Med, 2012. 18(6): p. 883–91.

[7] Salomon, C., et al., Exosomes are fingerprints of originating cells: potential biomarkers for ovarian cancer. Research and Reports in Biochemistry, 2015. 5(15): p. 101-109.

[8] Johnstone, R.M., et al., Vesicle formation during reticulocyte maturation. Association of plasma membrane activities with released vesicles (exosomes). J Biol Chem, 1987. 262(19): p. 9412–20.

[9] Théry, C., Zitvogel, L. and Amigorena, S., Exosomes: composition, biogenesis and function. Nat Rev Immunol, 2002. 2(8): p. 569–79.

[10] Colombo, M., et al., Analysis of ESCRT functions in exosome biogenesis, composition and secretion highlights the heterogeneity of extracellular vesicles. J Cell Sci, 2013. 126(Pt 24): p. 5553–65.

[11] Stuffers, S., et al., Multivesicular endosome biogenesis in the absence of ESCRTs. Traffic, 2009. 10(7): p. 925–37.

[12] Trajkovic, K., et al., Ceramide triggers budding of exosome vesicles into multivesicular endosomes. Science, 2008. 319(5867): p. 1244–7.

[13] Finger, E.C. and Giaccia, A.J., Hypoxia, inflammation, and the tumor microenvironment in metastatic disease. Cancer Metastasis Rev, 2010. 29(2): p. 285–93.

[14] Chan, D.A. and Giaccia, A.J., Hypoxia, gene expression, and metastasis. Cancer Metastasis Rev, 2007. 26(2): p. 333–9.

[15] Vaupel, P. and Mayer, A., Hypoxia in cancer: significance and impact on clinical outcome. Cancer Metastasis Rev, 2007. 26(2): p. 225–39.

[16] Favaro, E., et al., Gene expression and hypoxia in breast cancer. Genome Medicine, 2011. 3(8): p. 55.

[17] Papandreou, I., et al., HIF-1 mediates adaptation to hypoxia by actively downregulating mitochondrial oxygen consumption. Cell Metabolism, 2006. 3(3): p. 187–97.

[18] Ke, Q. and Costa, M., Hypoxia-inducible factor-1 (HIF-1). Mol Pharmacol, 2006. 70(5): p. 1469–80.

[19] Zhou, J., et al., Tumor hypoxia and cancer progression. Cancer Lett, 2006. 237(1): p. 10–21.

[20] Semenza, G.L., Targeting HIF-1 for cancer therapy. Nat Rev Cancer, 2003. 3(10): p. 721–32.

[21] Harris, A.L., Hypoxia – A key regulatory factor in tumour growth. Nat Rev Cancer, 2002. 2(1): p. 38–47.

[22] Zhu, P., et al., The proliferation, apoptosis, invasion of endothelial-like epithelial ovarian cancer cells induced by hypoxia. Journal of Experimental and Clinical Cancer Research, 2010. 29(1): p. 124.

[23] Ziello, J.E., Jovin, I.S. and Huang, Y., Hypoxia-Inducible factor (HIF)-1 regulatory pathway and its potential for therapeutic intervention in malignancy and ischemia. Yale J Biol Med, 2007. 80(2): p. 51–60.

[24] Rědowicz, M.J., Rho-associated kinase: involvement in the cytoskeleton regulation. Arch Biochem Biophys, 1999. 364(1): p. 122–24.

[25] Leong, H.S. and Chambers, A.F., Hypoxia promotes tumor cell motility via RhoA and ROCK1 signaling pathways. Proc Natl Acad Sci, 2014. 111(3): p. 887–8.

[26] Street, C.A. and Bryan, B.A., Rho kinase proteins—pleiotropic modulators of cell, survival and apoptosis. Anticancer Res, 2011. 31(11): p. 3645–57.

[27] Gilkes, D.M., et al., Hypoxia-inducible factors mediate coordinated RhoA-ROCK1 expression and signaling in breast cancer cells. Proc Natl Acad Sci, 2014. 111(3): p. E384–93.

[28] Horiuchi, A., et al., Up-regulation of small GTPases, RhoA and RhoC, is associated with tumor progression in ovarian carcinoma. Lab Investig, 2003. 83(6): p. 861–70.

[29] Yang, M.H., et al., Direct regulation of TWIST by HIF-1alpha promotes metastasis. Nat Cell Biol, 2008. 10(3): p. 295–305.

[30] Kurrey, N.K., et al., Snail and slug mediate radioresistance and chemoresistance by antagonizing p53-mediated apoptosis and acquiring a stem-like phenotype in ovarian cancer cells. Stem Cells, 2009. 27(9): p. 2059–68.

[31] Imai, T., et al., Hypoxia attenuates the expression of E-cadherin via up-regulation of SNAIL in ovarian carcinoma cells. Am J Pathol, 2003. 163(4): p. 1437–47.

[32] Zhang, Y., Fan, N. and Yang, J., Expression and clinical significance of hypoxia-inducible factor 1alpha, Snail and E-cadherin in human ovarian cancer cell lines. Mol Med Rep, 2015. 12(3): p. 3393–9.

[33] Cannito, S., et al., Redox mechanisms switch on hypoxia-dependent epithelial-mesenchymal transition in cancer cells. Carcinogenesis, 2008. 29(12): p. 2267–78.

[34] Haase, V.H., Oxygen regulates epithelial-to-mesenchymal transition: insights into molecular mechanisms and relevance to disease. Kidney Int, 2009. 76(5): p. 492–9.

[35] Ostrowski, M., et al., Rab27a and Rab27b control different steps of the exosome secretion pathway. Nat Cell Biol, 2010. 12(1): p. 19–30; sup pp 1–13.

[36] Peinado, H., et al., A molecular role for lysyl oxidase-like 2 enzyme in Snail regulation and tumor progression. EMBO J, 2005. 24(19): p. 3446–58.

[37] Erler, J.T., et al., Lysyl oxidase is essential for hypoxia-induced metastasis. Nature, 2006. 440(7088): p. 1222–6.

[38] Kipps, E., Tan, D.S. and Kaye, S.B., Meeting the challenge of ascites in ovarian cancer: new avenues for therapy and research. Nat Rev Cancer, 2013. 13(4): p. 273–82.

[39] Kahlert, C. and Kalluri, R., Exosomes in tumor microenvironment influence cancer progression and metastasis. J Mol Med (Berl), 2013. 91(4): p. 431–7.

[40] Graeber, T.G., et al., Hypoxia induces accumulation of p53 protein, but activation of a G1-phase checkpoint by low-oxygen conditions is independent of p53 status. Mol Cell Biol, 1994. 14(9): p. 6264–77.

[41] Cummins, E.P., et al., Hypoxic regulation of NF-kappaB signaling. Methods Enzymol, 2007. 435: p. 479–92.

[42] Köditz, J., et al., Oxygen-dependent ATF-4 stability is mediated by the PHD3 oxygen sensor. Blood, 2007. 110(10): p. 3610–17.

[43] Ameri, K., et al., Induction of activating transcription factor 3 by anoxia is independent of p53 and the hypoxic HIF signalling pathway. Oncogene, 2007. 26(2): p. 284–9.

[44] Ameri, K., et al., Anoxic induction of ATF-4 through HIF-1–independent pathways of protein stabilization in human cancer cells. Blood, 2004. 103(5): p. 1876–82.

[45] Gatenby, R.A. and Gillies, R.J., Why do cancers have high aerobic glycolysis? Nat Rev Cancer, 2004. 4(11): p. 891–9.

[46] Chafe, S.C., et al., Carbonic anhydrase IX promotes myeloid-derived suppressor cell mobilization and establishment of a metastatic niche by stimulating G-CSF production. Cancer Res, 2015. 75(6): p. 996–1008.

[47] McDonald, P.C., et al., Recent developments in targeting carbonic anhydrase IX for cancer therapeutics. Oncotarget, 2012. 3(1): p. 84–97.

[48] Perkins, N.D., The diverse and complex roles of NF-κB subunits in cancer. Nat Rev Cancer, 2012. 12(2): p. 121–32.

[49] Xu, L. and Fidler, I.J., Acidic pH-induced elevation in interleukin 8 expression by human ovarian carcinoma cells. Cancer Res, 2000. 60(16): p. 4610–6.

[50] Fukumura, D., et al., Hypoxia and acidosis independently up-regulate vascular endothelial growth factor transcription in brain tumors in vivo. Cancer Res, 2001. 61(16): p. 6020–4.

[51] Lou, Y., et al., Targeting tumor hypoxia: suppression of breast tumor growth and metastasis by novel carbonic anhydrase IX inhibitors. Cancer Res, 2011. 71(9): p. 3364–76.

[52] Kumar, V. and Gabrilovich, D.I., Hypoxia-inducible factors in regulation of immune responses in tumour microenvironment. Immunology, 2014. 143(4): p. 512–9.

[53] Kim, Y., et al., Hypoxic tumor microenvironment and cancer cell differentiation. Curr Mol Med, 2009. 9(4): p. 425–34.

[54] Dorayappan, K.D.P., et al., The biological significance and clinical applications of exosomes in ovarian cancer. Gynecologic oncology, 2016. 142(1): p. 199-205.

[55] Riches, A., et al., Regulation of exosome release from mammary epithelial and breast cancer cells – A new regulatory pathway. Eur J Cancer, 2014. 50(5): p. 1025–34.

[56] Colombo, M., Raposo, G. and Théry, C., Biogenesis, secretion, and intercellular interactions of exosomes and other extracellular vesicles. Annu Rev Cell Dev Biol, 2014. 30: p. 255–89.

[57] Park, J.E., et al., Hypoxic tumor cell modulates its microenvironment to enhance angiogenic and metastatic potential by secretion of proteins and exosomes. Mol Cell Proteomics: MCP, 2010. 9(6): p. 1085–99.

[58] King, H.W., Michael, M.Z. and Gleadle, J.M., Hypoxic enhancement of exosome release by breast cancer cells. BMC Cancer, 2012. 12(1): p. 1–10.

[59] Cappellesso, R., et al., Programmed cell death 4 and microRNA 21 inverse expression is maintained in cells and exosomes from ovarian serous carcinoma effusions. Cancer Cytopathol, 2014. 122(9): p. 685–93.

[60] Shi, J., Considering exosomal miR-21 as a biomarker for cancer. J Clin Med, 2016. 5(4): p. 42.

[61] Meng, F., et al., MicroRNA-21 regulates expression of the PTEN tumor suppressor gene in human hepatocellular cancer. Gastroenterology, 2007. 133(2): p. 647–58.

[62] Taylor, D.D. and Gercel-Taylor, C., MicroRNA signatures of tumor-derived exosomes as diagnostic biomarkers of ovarian cancer. Gynecol Oncol, 2008. 110(1): p. 13–21.

[63] Ratner, E.S., et al., MicroRNA signatures differentiate uterine cancer tumor subtypes. Gynecol Oncol, 2010. 118(3): p. 251–7.

[64] Bartel, D.P., MicroRNAs: target recognition and regulatory functions. Cell, 2009. 136(2): p. 215–33.

[65] Kucharzewska, P., et al., Exosomes reflect the hypoxic status of glioma cells and mediate hypoxia-dependent activation of vascular cells during tumor development. Proc Natl Acad Sci, 2013. 110(18): p. 7312–7.

[66] Vong, S. and Kalluri, R., The role of stromal myofibroblast and extracellular matrix in tumor angiogenesis. Genes Cancer, 2011. 2(12): p. 1139–45.

[67] Zhuang, G., et al., Tumour-secreted miR-9 promotes endothelial cell migration and angiogenesis by activating the JAK-STAT pathway. EMBO J, 2012. 31(17): p. 3513–23.

[68] Webber, J., et al., Cancer exosomes trigger fibroblast to myofibroblast differentiation. Cancer Res, 2010. 70(23): p. 9621–30.

[69] Cho, J.A., et al., Exosomes from breast cancer cells can convert adipose tissue-derived mesenchymal stem cells into myofibroblast-like cells. Int J Oncol, 2012. 40(1): p. 130–8.

[70] Filipazzi, P., et al. Recent advances on the role of tumor exosomes in immunosuppression and disease progression. in Seminars in cancer biology. 2012. 22(4): p. 342-349.

[71] Jong, O.G., et al., Exosomes from hypoxic endothelial cells have increased collagen crosslinking activity through up-regulation of lysyl oxidase-like 2. Journal of cellular and molecular medicine, 2016. 20(2): p. 342-350.

[72] Hollosi, P., et al., Lysyl oxidase-like 2 promotes migration in noninvasive breast cancer cells but not in normal breast epithelial cells. Int J Cancer, 2009. 125(2): p. 318–27.

[73] Barker, H.E., et al., Tumor-secreted LOXL2 activates fibroblasts through FAK signaling. Mol Cancer Res, 2013. 11(11): p. 1425–36.

[74] Choi, H. and Lee, D.S., Illuminating the physiology of extracellular vesicles. Stem Cell Res Ther, 2016. 7: p. 55.

[75] Hoshino, A., et al., Tumour exosome integrins determine organotropic metastasis. Nature, 2015. 527(7578): p. 329–35.

[76] Ohno, S.-I., et al., Systemically injected exosomes targeted to EGFR deliver antitumor microRNA to breast cancer cells. Mol Ther, 2013. 21(1): p. 185–91.

[77] Alvarez-Erviti, L., et al., Delivery of siRNA to the mouse brain by systemic injection of targeted exosomes. Nat Biotech, 2011. 29(4): p. 341–5.

[78] Kim, M.S., et al., Development of exosome-encapsulated paclitaxel to overcome MDR in cancer cells. Nanomed: Nanotechnol Biol Med, 2016. 12(3): p. 655–64.

[79] El-Andaloussi, S., et al., Exosome-mediated delivery of siRNA in vitro and in vivo. Nat Protocols, 2012. 7(12): p. 2112–26.

[80] Imai, T., et al., Macrophage-dependent clearance of systemically administered B16BL6-derived exosomes from the blood circulation in mice. J Extracell Ves, 2015. 4: p. 10.3402/jev.v4.26238.

[81] Zitvogel, L., et al., Eradication of established murine tumors using a novel cell-free vaccine: dendritic cell derived exosomes. Nat Med, 1998. 4(5): p. 594–600.

[82] Takahashi, Y., et al., Visualization and in vivo tracking of the exosomes of murine melanoma B16-BL6 cells in mice after intravenous injection. J Biotechnol, 2013. 165(2): p. 77–84.

[83] Lai, C.P., et al., Dynamic biodistribution of extracellular vesicles in vivo using a multimodal imaging reporter. ACS Nano, 2014. 8(1): p. 483–94.

[84] Tian, T., et al., Dynamics of exosome internalization and trafficking. J Cell Physiol, 2013. 228(7): p. 1487–95.

[85] Wiklander, O.P.B., et al., Extracellular vesicle in vivo biodistribution is determined by cell source, route of administration and targeting. Journal of Extracellular Vesicles, 2015. 4: p. 26316.

[86] Im, H., et al., Label-free detection and molecular profiling of exosomes with a nano-plasmonic sensor. Nat Biotechnol, 2014. 32(5): p. 490–5.

[87] Sarker, S., et al., Placenta-derived exosomes continuously increase in maternal circulation over the first trimester of pregnancy. J Transl Med, 2014. 12: p. 204.

[88] Kobayashi, M., et al., Ovarian cancer cell invasiveness is associated with discordant exosomal sequestration of Let-7 miRNA and miR-200. J Transl Med, 2014. 12: p. 4.

[89] Paranjape, T., Slack, F.J. and Weidhaas, J.B., MicroRNAs: tools for cancer diagnostics. Gut, 2009. 58(11): p. 1546–54.

[90] Kumar, M.S., et al., Impaired microRNA processing enhances cellular transformation and tumorigenesis. Nat Genet, 2007. 39(5): p. 673–7.

[91] Iorio, M.V., et al., MicroRNA signatures in human ovarian cancer. Cancer Res, 2007. 67(18): p. 8699–707.

[92] Taylor, D.D. and Gercel-Taylor, C., MicroRNA signatures of tumor-derived exosomes as diagnostic biomarkers of ovarian cancer. Gynecol Oncol, 2008. 110(1): p. 13–21.

[93] Vaksman, O., et al., Exosome-derived miRNAs and ovarian carcinoma progression. Carcinogenesis, 2014. 35(9): p. 2113–20.

[94] Ying, X., et al., Epithelial ovarian cancer-secreted exosomal miR-222-3p induces polarization of tumor-associated macrophages. Oncotarget, 2016. 7(28): p. 43076-43087.

[95] Tickner, J.A., et al., Functions and therapeutic roles of exosomes in cancer. Front Oncol, 2014. 4: p. 127.

[96] Bobrie, A., et al., Rab27a supports exosome-dependent and -independent mechanisms that modify the tumor microenvironment and can promote tumor progression. Cancer Res, 2012. 72(19): p. 4920–30.

[97] Moyer, V.A., Screening for ovarian cancer: U.S. Preventive Services Task Force reaffirmation recommendation statement. Ann Intern Med, 2012. 157(12): p. 900–4.

Chapter 20

A Novel Hypoxia Imaging Endoscopy System

Kazuhiro Kaneko, Hiroshi Yamaguchi and
Tomonori Yano

Additional information is available at the end of the chapter

http://dx.doi.org/10.5772/66091

Abstract

Measurement of tumor hypoxia is required for the diagnosis of tumor and the evaluation of therapeutic outcome. Currently, invasive and noninvasive techniques being exploited for tumor hypoxia measurement include polarographic needle electrodes, immunohistochemical (IHC) staining, magnetic resonance imaging (MRI), radionuclide imaging (positron emission tomography [PET] and single-photon emission computed tomography [SPECT]), optical imaging (bioluminescence and fluorescence), and hypoxia imaging endoscopy. This review provides a summary of the modalities available for assessment of tissue oxygenation as well as a discussion of current arguments for and against each modality, with a particular focus on noninvasive hypoxia imaging with emerging agents and new imaging technologies intended to detect molecular events associated with tumor hypoxia.

Keywords: Hypoxia imaging endoscopy, innovation of endoscopy

1. Introduction

In the 1950s, hypoxia research began, and many clinical trials have been reported. Hypoxia of tumor affects outcomes after radiotherapy. But hypoxia has also been shown to be a poor prognostic factor after chemotherapy and surgery. These findings are attributed to chronic hypoxia. Hypoxic tumors are more likely to recur loco-regionally than well-oxygenated tumors regardless of whether surgery or radiation therapy is the primary local treatment. However, the common oxygen measurement used in these reports was polarographic needle electrodes inserted directly into specific sections of tumor tissue. In this method, hypoxia was measured in only pinpointed area for the tumor. In other words, there was no modality used in which the hypoxia imaging results were visible in real time and which reflected the hypoxic state in the whole tumor. Therefore, hypoxia imaging is expected to allow direct visualization of the biological and functional changes in cancer.

Hypoxia is a histopathological condition in which cells in tissues suffer from lack of oxygen for their normal metabolism. An oxygen saturation (StO_2) of arterial blood is almost 100% and that of venous blood is approximately 70%. In contrast, the StO_2 in half of cancers is 50–60% at the highest. Hypoxia takes hold as a tumor becomes large enough to disrupt the balance of oxygen supply and consumption in the area. Approximately, 50–60% of advanced cancer forming solid tumor may show hypoxic and/or anoxic conditions exhibiting heterogeneous distribution in the inside of tumor [1]. Hypoxia proliferates rapidly in solid tumors, and their intratumoral vessels with significantly structural abnormalities are distributed spatially with dilated, tortuous, saccular, and heterogeneous figures. As a result, this distribution leads to perfusion-limited delivery of O_2 [2]. There are mainly two types of hypoxia regarding solid tumor and tissue around tumor. One is perfusion-limited O_2 delivery type, the so-called acute hypoxia, which leads to ischemic condition, however, it is often transient. Another type is diffusion-limited hypoxia, the so-called chronic hypoxia, which can also be caused by an increase in diffusion distances, so that cells far away (>70 μm) from a nutritive blood vessel receive less oxygen (and nutrients) than needed [1]. Regarding hypoxia-induced proteome and/or genome changes, cell cycle arrest, differentiation, apoptosis, and necrosis are found in solid tumor. In contrast, hypoxia-induced changes of proteome may progress tumor growth because of mechanisms enabling cells to overcome nutritive deprivation, to escape from the hostile environment and to favor unrestricted growth. Furthermore, continuous hypoxia can also bring cellular changes as a more aggressive phenotype [3]. Since the presence of hypoxic status in solid tumors was first reported in 1953 to be among the factors associated with treatment failure following radiation therapy [4], tumor hypoxia has drawn attention as a pivotal event in tumor invasion, angiogenesis, apoptosis, metastasis [1], resistance to chemotherapy [5], surgery, and resistance to radiotherapy [6]. In tumor diagnosis and treatment planning, it is crucial to have a grasp of the degree and extent of tumor hypoxia involved prior to the start of treatment.

2. Clinical importance for measurement of tumor hypoxic state

A variety of techniques are being proposed to assess tumor hypoxia, which can be broadly categorized into direct measurements and indirect measurements according to different principles and the ability to quantify tissue oxygenation. Direct measurements, including polarographic needle electrode, phosphorescence imaging, near-infrared spectroscopy (NIRS), blood oxygen level dependent (BOLD) and ^{19}F magnetic resonance imaging (MRI) and electron paramagnetic resonance (EPR) imaging, can detect oxygen partial pressure (pO_2), oxygen concentration, or oxygen percentage. Recently, a hypoxia imaging endoscopy that can derive the oxygen saturation (StO_2) was developed in endoscopic fields. Indirect measurements, including measuring exogenous and endogenous hypoxia markers, can provide parameters related to oxygenation.

Many clinical trials have been performed using direct and indirect measurement methods. It is now known that hypoxia affects outcome after radiotherapy, with poor prognosis in hypoxic cancers. Next, hypoxia has also been shown to be a poor prognostic factor after chemotherapy and surgery. Furthermore, hypoxic tumors are more likely to recur loco-regionally than well-oxygenated tumors regardless of whether surgery or radiation therapy was the primary local treatment.

3. Direct measurements for hypoxia

3.1. Polarographic needle electrodes for direct tumor tissue

The invasive polarographic needle electrodes have been widely employed since the 1990s to assess tumor oxygen status and to measure pO_2 in both human and animal studies [7, 8]. As the gold standard modality, their use has been extended not only to lymph node metastases but to more accessible tumors, which include head and neck cancer, cervical cancer, soft tissue sarcomas of the extremities, astrocytic brain tumors, lung cancer, pancreatic cancer, prostate cancer, and lymph node metastases [8–12]. With the average median pO_2 before treatment of 11.2 mmHg (range 0.4–60 mmHg) [7], these measured values help prediction of the tumor response to treatment [13] and tumor metastatic potential [14]. The polarographic needle electrode is currently available under CT guidance for evaluating tumor pO_2 in deep-seated organs as well as for assessing overall tumor oxygen status [15] with the caveat, however, that insertion of an electrode into the tumor leads to disruption of tissues, thus rendering it difficult to distinguish the necrotic areas and to establish the patterns of hypoxia involved. Furthermore, the use of the modality not only calls for great expertise but is associated with large interobserver variability.

4. Noninvasive imaging of hypoxia

While the polarographic needle electrode and immunohistochemical (IHC) staining can provide a relatively accurate estimation of tumor oxygenation, being subject to selection bias, provide only a partial, but not complete, picture of the entire tumor site [16]. This has led to an increasing interest in the use of noninvasive functional and molecular imaging modalities, which is capable of yielding a large amount of high-quality experimental data per protocol by increasing the number of quantitative data collections and by guiding tissue sampling and allowing a rapid and effective combination of analyses to be conducted [17].

Several imaging modalities have been developed, to date, to allow direct or indirect measurement of tumor oxygenation, with a few of these remaining less mature for clinical application. Of these, EPR spectroscopy, which involves the use of unpaired electron species to obtain images and spectra, is currently being explored in animals as a means to provide a quantitative measure of tissue oxygenation [18]. Although this modality has considerable potential to be developed as a tumor oximeter, i.e., in monitoring changes after tumor oxygenation [19], a suitable paramagnetic marker with low toxicity for human remains yet to become available. The need for appropriate EPR instrumentation in the clinical setting also prevents this promising modality from becoming widespread [20]. Photoacoustic tomography (PAT) is also available for imaging blood oxygenation using the differential optical contrast between O_2Hb and dHb. PAT has been implemented for imaging cerebral blood oxygenation of rats *in vivo*, demonstrating that PAT is capable of capturing the changes from hyperoxia to hypoxia [21], while no study reported on its clinical application.

4.1. Magnetic resonance imaging

BOLD-MRI is shown to have potential as a diagnostic modality for tumor hypoxia [22]. Hemoglobin occurs as deoxyhemoglobin in oxygen-deficient states, where not oxyhemoglobin but paramagnetic deoxyhemoglobin can increase the transverse relaxation of the surrounding protons [23]. BOLD-MRI employs deoxyhemoglobin-derived endogenous signals as image contrast to depict changes in oxygenation in blood. Decreased oxygenation in blood results in decreased signal intensity in T2-weighted images, and this correlation between the BOLD-MRI signal and vascular oxygenation allows pO_2 to be directly estimated. This has indeed led to numerous studies being conducted to investigate carbogen breathing in mice, oxygenation in tumor models [24], and kidney function in patients [22, 25, 26] using the modality as a noninvasive technique with high spatial and temporal resolution [22]. As with phosphorescence and near-infrared fluorescence imaging, the major disadvantage of BOLD-MRI is that it reflects change in oxygen tension in vasculature but not those in tissues. Again, not being a quantitative method, it may easily be affected by multiple factors such as flow effects, hematocrit, pH, and temperature [27].

^{19}F MRI involves the use of two types of markers, i.e., perfluorocarbons (PFCs) and fluorinated nitroimidazoles as contrast agents, which are not used in conventional T1-weighted MRI. While being highly hydrophobic, PFCs are highly oxygen soluble [28]. Due to the linear relationship between the ^{19}F spin lattice relaxation rate of PFCs and the dissolved oxygen concentration, the ^{19}F-based oximetry allows vascular oxygenation to be measured *in vivo* [29]. PFCs investigated to date include hexafluorobenzene (HFB) [30] and perfluoro-15-crown-5-ether (PF15C5) [31, 32], which are injectable intravenously or intratumorally. ^{19}F MRI is increasingly employed to detect changes in tumor oxygenation that occur in response to treatments that are radio-sensitizing and oxygen-augmenting [33]. The disadvantages of ^{19}F MRI are that flow artifacts affect the measurements and that, with some contrast agents, oxygen sensitivity is easily influenced by such conditions as temperature, dilution, pH, common proteins, and blood [34]. Following intravenous injection, most PFC contrast agent is extensively ingested by the reticuloendothelial system (RES) and their slow clearance may cause adverse reactions. Their intratumoral injection may also raise concern over its associated risk, e.g., embolism associated with accidental injection of PFC emulsion into the tumoral vein [35]. One major drawback of the nitroimidazole derivatives is their central nervous system (CNS) toxicity profile, with misonidazole shown to be associated with neuropathy and acute toxicity on the CNS [33].

"Vessel architectural imaging" (VAI) has recently been proposed as a new paradigm in MRI providing a basis for vessel caliber estimation [36] by incorporating an overlooked temporal shift in the MR signal, thus generating, unlike any other noninvasive imaging modality, new information on vessel type and function. Indeed, this new modality allowed an oral pan-vascular endothelial growth factor (pan-VEGF) receptor kinase inhibitor to be evaluated for its therapeutic efficacy in glioblastoma patients [37], demonstrating using VAI that anti-VEGF therapy not only normalizes tumor vasculature and alleviates edema but also prolongs survival in these patients.

4.2. Positron emission tomography

Efforts have recently been directed toward developing contrast agents for noninvasive hypoxia imaging with positron emission tomography (PET) and single-photon emission computed tomography (SPECT). Organic molecular markers labeled with positron-emitting radioisotopes are employed in PET imaging to allow the extent of tumor hypoxia to be measured. Commonly used radioisotopes include ^{18}F, ^{124}I, and $^{60/64}$Cu and the molecular markers to be labeled with these isotopes include 2-nitroimidazoles, e.g., fluoromisonidazole (FMISO), EF5, and fluoroetanidazole (FETA), nucleoside conjugates, e.g., iodoazomycin arabinoside (IAZA), and Cu(II)-diacetyl-bis (N4-methylthiosemicarbazone) (Cu-ATSM) [38–40]. These markers are shown not only to bind maximally to severely hypoxic cells to form such stable adducts as are detectable with a PET scanner but to provide a clear demarcation of hypoxic cells *in vivo* through their rapid reoxidization and removal from normal cells.

Of the first-generation nitroimidazoles, ^{18}F-labeled misonidazole (^{18}F-FMISO) is the most commonly used as being sensitive only to the presence of hypoxia in viable cells [41]. It is reported that a hypoxic state defined as <10 mmHg is required to induce significant ^{18}FMISO uptake [42]. ^{18}F-FMISO uptake is shown to vary widely depending on the type of patients and tumors, whereas ^{18} F-FMISO is shown to allow hypoxia to be detected in various tumors such as glioma, head and neck cancer, renal tumor, and non-small cell lung cancer [42–44]. A clinical trial of glioblastoma multiforme patients [45] demonstrated increased ^{18}F-FMISO uptake and retention on both post-treatment FMISO and FDG images, suggesting that reoxygenation did not take place. It is reported that the distribution of oxygen and hypoxia was increased and decreased, respectively, in non-small cell lung carcinomas following treatment, as assessed by sequential FMISO imaging [46]. Given that no correlation is shown between patient diagnosis and degree of decrease in FMISO uptake and retention, in selectively boosting the radiation dose to hypoxic subvolumes, there appears to be a larger role for serial imaging during treatment than for baseline volume measurement. Again, pretreatment FMISO uptake/retention and survival has been shown to be correlated and allow treatment failure to be predicted [45, 47]. However, ^{18}F-FMISO may not be readily available for use in other cancers [42, 48].

The second-generation nitroimidazoles include 18F-fluorerythronitroimidazole (FETNIM) [49, 50], FETA [51], and EF5 [52, 53], which are more water soluble and not readily susceptible to degradation by most oxidizing mechanisms in place in humans. ^{18}F-EF5 was tested in clinical trials for its feasibility as an imaging agent for hypoxia [54] and was shown to be hypoxia-specific, with its increased uptake shown to be correlated with the extent of tumor and high risk of metastasis in cancer patients [52], suggesting its usefulness in identifying high-risk candidates for clinical trials evaluating the influence of early chemotherapy on the occurrence of metastasis [55]. ^{18}F-FAZA has great promise as an imaging agent for tumor hypoxia due to its faster diffusion into cells and faster clearance from normal tissues than ^{18}F-FMISO [56]. PET imaging using ^{18}F-FMISO demonstrated very high tracer uptake in all seven patients with high-grade gliomas evaluated, showing the potential of ^{18}F-FMISO as an imaging agent in assessing hypoxia in this tumor type [57].

4.3. Phosphorescence imaging

Phosphorescence imaging with injection of porphyrin complex (Oxyphor) into the vasculature also allows tumor vascular pO_2 to be measured [58, 59]. Recently, a general approach has been proposed through which to construct phosphorescent nanosensors with tunable spectral characteristics, varying degrees of quenching, and a high oxygen selectivity [60]. These probes are shown to exhibit excellent performance in measuring vascular pO_2 in the rat brain with *in vivo* microscopy [60]. NIRS are also available for analysis of tumor oxygenation *in vivo* based on recorded spectral changes by hemoglobin in the vasculature [61–63]. Kim and Liu [64] demonstrated in an animal study that NIRS is associated with comparable efficacy to that with electrode measurements in evaluating tumor hypoxia. They showed that either carbogen (95% CO_2 and 5% O_2) or 100% oxygen inhalation could improve the vascular oxygen level of rat breast tumors. However, both phosphorescence imaging and NIRS are not readily translatable into clinical applications due to their low spatial resolution, light scattering, limited path length, low sensitivity, and susceptibility to environmental influence.

4.4. Visible light spectroscopy

In the search for noninvasive, continuous modalities for monitoring ischemia, electrical bioimpedance cardiac output monitoring has been proposed but shown to be incompatible with the thermodilution methods [65, 66]. Again, while near-infrared spectroscopy (NIRS) [67] is shown to respond to both hypoxemia [68, 69] and ischemia [70–72], its clinical use has been limited to large organs, such as the brain [73, 74, 85–87] with its broad normal ranges reported to be between 48% and 88% [75, 76]. Similarly, wide normal ranges are reported for sublingual capnography [77–79]. Also available, albeit invasive are polarographic oximetry probes [80] and fiber-enabled pulmonary catheters.

Visible light spectroscopy (VLS) appears to be similar to NIRS on some counts [81] with its mean VLS StO2 shown to be not significantly different from NIRS StO2 reported in human studies [67–76]. Again, the fractional contribution of venous blood to the cerebral NIRS signal has been reported to be 0.84 ± 0.21 ranging from 0.60 to 1.00 [82–84]. Using central venous and pulse oximetry saturation as estimates for local venous and arterial saturation, it is shown to be not significantly different at 0.89 ± 0.04. It is suggested that the two modalities cover similar microvascular compartments.

http://dx.doi.org/10.5772/66091

At the same time, VLS is shown to be superior to NIRS in monitoring tissues that lend themselves to monitoring, thus suggesting a more versatile role for VLS in patient treatment [81]. The NIRS light sources and detectors require to be spaced 2–5 cm apart or more to illuminate and monitor a large, homogenous tissue volume (>30 ml), thus making NIRS with its long and bulky sensors unsuitable for monitoring tissue regions, e.g., thin tissues such as gastrointestinal mucosa or small tumors. In contrast, the visible light used in VLS is shown to be strongly absorbed by tissue and VLS measurement to be highly localized thus making VLS unsuitable for transcranial use or use over thick skin dominated by surface tissue properties. Using VLS, a rapid real-time drop in tumor oxygenation was detected during local ischemia following clamping or epinephrine administration [85], with the tissue oximetry performed during endoscopy demonstrating a significantly lower tissue oxygenation (StO_2) in tumors (46% ± 22%) than in normal mucosa (72% ± 4%) ($P < 0.0001$). Thus, VSL tissue oximetry may be able to distinguish neoplastic tissue with a high specificity to aid in the endoscopic detection of gastrointestinal tumors. Again, of note, chronic gastrointestinal ischemia was also detected using the same method [86] (**Figure 1**).

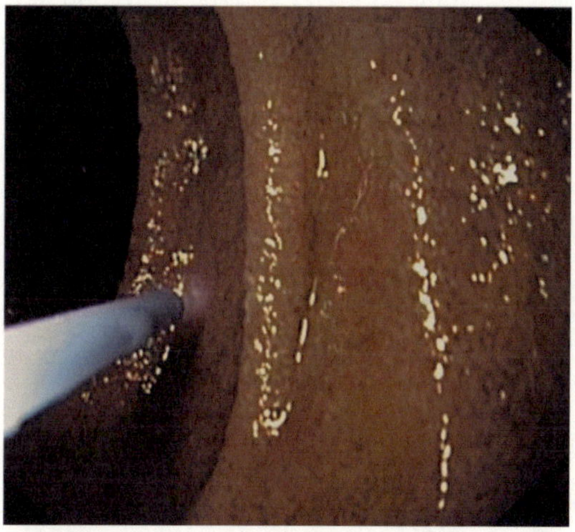

Figure 1. VLS measurements using a fiber-optic catheter-based VLS oximeter. The catheter is passed through the accessory channel of the endoscope and positioned about 1–5 mm above the mucosa.

5. Hypoxia imaging endoscopy with no phosphor

Kaneko et al. [87] reported hypoxia imaging endoscopy equipped with a laser light source. In this system, signals from the laser light passed through the processor were calculated as StO_2. The measurement range of StO_2 was from 0% to 100% in contactless of tumor or normal mucosa under endoscopic observation. Display imaging was performed with the use of laser light alone without phosphor, provided a display of overlay and pseudocolor images. The laser light used was not near-infrared but ranged within visible light wavelengths. In principle, this utilized the difference in absorption coefficient between oxyhemoglobin and deoxyhemoglobin. Two challenges were identified, however, in deriving the StO_2 of tissue in alimentary tracts from differences in absorption spectra between oxyhemoglobin and deoxyhemoglobin using small numbers of wavelengths. First, there is not only a small difference in optical absorption spectra in the visible light region but also a narrow bandwidth between isosbestic points. Second, the reflectance of a tissue depends on hematocrit (Hct) as well as StO_2, given that light absorption increases as hemoglobin density increases.

An imaging system equipped with laser diodes of 445 and 473 nm and a white fluorescent pigment body was therefore developed. Hypoxia imaging with this system rendered visible an alimentary tract tumor in real time and allowed the whole tumor to be visualized. With the tumor surface and normal mucosa rendered visible, no heterogeneity was seen with the use of this system. In the first-in-human clinical trial, early cancers of the esophagus, stomach, and colorectum were detected as hypoxic areas (**Figure 2**). Furthermore, colorectal adenomas with histologically low-grade atypia were also detected as hypoxic areas and no complications were reported in the patients with visualization of these tumors in real-time hypoxia imaging which involved only laser light without injection or oral administration of phosphor. As mentioned above, it will be expected that the hypoxia imaging endoscopy is shown to be superior to VLS or NIRS in measuring StO_2 of surface of tumor and normal mucosa.

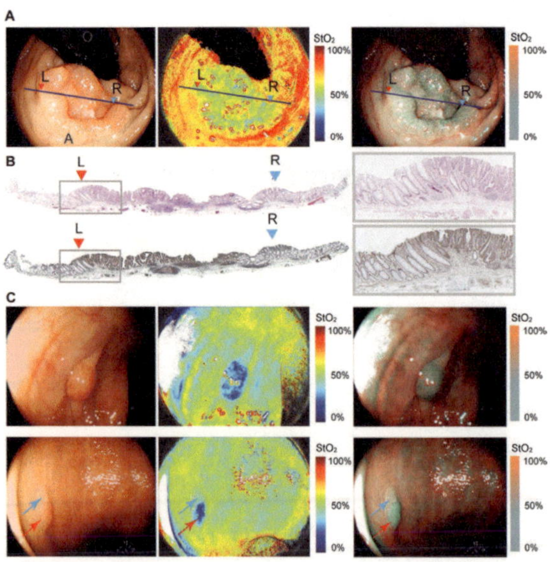

Figure 2. StO_2 maps obtained in human subject research. (A) White light image by endoscopic observation in rectal adenocarcinoma (left). Line (L-R) corresponds to cross section of pathological diagnosis. StO_2 map visualized by laser endoscope system (middle: pseudocolor StO_2 image; right: StO_2 overlay image). (B) Cross-sectional appearance stained with H&E (upper) and HIF1 alpha antibody (lower) corresponding to the hypoxic area visualized with StO_2 map. (C) Endoscopic images of a colorectal adenoma (upper) showing clear hypoxia: white light image (upper left), pseudocolor StO_2 map (upper middle) and overlayed image (upper right). Another case of a colonic lesion (lower) consisting of an adenoma (red arrow) and a hyperplasia (blue arrow): white light image (lower left), pseudocolor StO_2 map (lower middle) and overlayed image (lower right). Only the adenoma was detected as hypoxia.

6. Indirect hypoxia evaluation

Proteins and genes whose expression is associated with hypoxia have potential as endogenous molecular markers of hypoxia and have been explored over the years; meanwhile, hypoxia-specific agents have also been explored and shown to be useful in monitoring hypoxia [88]. Immunohistochemical (IHC) staining for hypoxia marker adducts in situ is also available to provide indirect quantitative information on the relative oxygenation of tissue at a cellular resolution. IHC approaches have a role to play particularly *in vitro* studies, including assays of human biopsy specimens. Given the complex biology of tumor hypoxia for which no single marker is expected to have a strong prognostic power in clinical practice, efforts have been directed toward combining various markers to create a prognostic profile of hypoxia [89].

6.1. Hypoxia-inducible factor 1

Optical imaging has had an important role to play in evaluating hypoxia, especially in biopsy specimens. With the introduction of transgenes with the hypoxia responsive element as promoter sequences coupled to reporter genes, e.g., luciferase reporter gene [90, 91] or green fluorescent protein (GFP) [92], a number of modalities have been developed to allow HIF-1 activity to be directly measured. Of these, a HIF-1-dependent promoter-regulated luciferase reporter gene, shown to produce a 100-fold increased luciferase response to hypoxia, has been used to evaluate anti-hypoxia therapy for its efficacy in animals [93]. Again, an imaging probe has been developed for HIF-1-active cells using a PTD-ODD fusion protein. given that, being involved in the same ODD control as HIF-1α, PTD-ODD fusion proteins are thought likely to be co-localized with HIF-1α [93–96]. First developed as a model probe, PTD-ODD-enhanced GFP-labeled with near-infrared fluorescent dye Cy5.5 was shown to permeate cell membrane with high efficiency, with its stability controlled in an oxygen concentration-dependent manner; to accumulate in hypoxic tumor cells with HIF-1 activity, thus allowing the hypoxic tumor cells with HIF-1 activity to be imaged in contrast to the surrounding cells under aerobic conditions [96]. Bioluminescence imaging has also been used to noninvasively depict HIF-1α as it is upregulated *in vivo* following chemotherapy, suggesting that this modality may prove useful in the evaluation of emerging anti-HIF-1 therapeutics [97]. While these imaging tools have a role to play in elucidating the biology of hypoxia and mechanisms of tumor response to therapy, heterogeneous gene responses to HIF-1 pose challenges to these HIF-1-targeted modalities. Furthermore, only weak correlation has been shown between HIF-1α expression and oxygen electrode or PET imaging measurements [98, 99], thus throwing in doubt the value of HIF-1α quantification as a measure of hypoxia.

6.2. Carbonic anhydrase IX

Downstream of HIF-1, carbonic anhydrase 9 (CA IX), a member of the CA family known to exist in cytosolic, membrane-associated, mitochondrial, and secreted carbonic anhydrases (CAs), may represent an alternative target [100]. A membrane-associated enzyme involved in the respiratory gas exchange and acid-base balance, CA IX is shown to be found less abundantly in normal tissue and only in gastric mucosa, small intestine, and muscle. Under hypoxic conditions, CA IX is shown to be overexpressed in different types of cancer [101], with the staining pattern shown to be more generalized in VHL-associated tumors and focal-perinecrotic in non-VHL-associated tumors [102].

CA IX has been imaged with fluorescent-labeled sulfonamides in a tumor xenograft model to allow hypoxic and (re)-oxygenated cells to be distinguished [103], which demonstrated that CA IX required exposure to hypoxia for its binding and retention—a finding confirmed by an *in vivo* imaging study [103]. In renal-cell carcinoma xenografts, a G250 monoclonal antibody against CA IX was shown to significantly inhibit tumor growth [104]. Again, phase II clinical trials employed G250-based radioimmunoimaging to detect primary and metastatic lesions as well as to guide radioimmunotherapy after labeling G250 with therapeutic radioisotopes, which included ^{177}Lu, ^{90}Y, or ^{186}Re [105]. High-affinity human monoclonal antibodies (A3 and CC7) specific to human CA IX were developed using phage display technology [106] and these reagents may have a role to play in a wide range of settings, including noninvasive imaging of hypoxia and drug delivery [106]. In this regard, combining CA IX and a proliferation marker may prove helpful in identifying proliferating cells under hypoxic conditions [107, 108], while no correlation is shown between the amount of CA IX and direct oxygen measurement with a needle electrode [109].

Furthermore, hypoxia markers have been identified and shown to be induced by hypoxia and expressed in human tumors, including VEGF and GLUTs, both of which are upregulated by increased activity of HIF-1 under hypoxic conditions [110]. Imaging strategies targeting these proteins have also been explored for their ability to assess tumor vasculature and proliferation, while the relationship between pO_2 values and protein expression levels remains unclear [111].

7. Heterogeneity of tumor

Tissue oxygenation is shown to be highly heterogeneous due to the presence of both highly oxygenated arterial vascular regions and poorly oxygenated tissues and cells. Spatial and temporal heterogeneity also contribute to the complexity of the issue. Heterogeneity is thus a major factor in hypoxia measurement that affects our ability to stratify patients and predict outcomes using the imaging technologies available, and its biological implications need to be further explored, and effective approaches to assessing heterogeneity remain to be established. Hypoxia imaging endoscopy allowed early cancers of the pharynx, esophagus, stomach, and colorectum to be captured in whole for the first time [87], with no heterogeneity found in nearly all early cancers or colorectal neoplasia detected. Given that tissue heterogeneity may vary between early, advanced, and metastatic tumors, however, it remains crucial to elucidate tissue heterogeneity as it is associated with tumor progression.

http://dx.doi.org/10.5772/66091

8. Future of hypoxia measuring methods

Given the wide variety of techniques available for assessing hypoxia, e.g., polarographic needle electrodes, IHC staining, PET, MRI, optical imaging with NIR fluorescence or bioluminescence, visible light spectroscopy, and hypoxia imaging endoscopy, it remains critically important to determine their relative advantages and disadvantages for clinical application. Improvements in hypoxia measuring techniques will hinge primarily on which techniques are chosen and how these techniques are applied in the clinic. Clearly, the best of these are expected to be sensitive to the biological sequel of hypoxia, and the ideal one expected to be clinically safe, readily available, minimally invasive, and free from radiation exposure, while at the same time providing high resolution and ease of use. In addition, NIR over 1000 nm wavelength, the so-called biological window, will be promising, because this wavelength area is good for tissue permeability due to reducing both light scattering and infrared absorption [112].

In the endoscopic fields of alimentary tracts, the existing diagnosis for neoplasia is based on the morphologic features of the tumor. However, imaging of a tumor focused on its function or metabolism yields a novel set of data. Hypoxia imaging endoscope system equipped with a laser source allows oxygen saturation to be shown with two types of overlay and pseudocolor images displayed one on top of the other [87]. Available for handling similarly to conventional endoscopy, this modality is easy to treat with and completely safe without being invasive. Of the large number of patients with cancers in the alimentary tract, such as oral cavity, esophagus, stomach, and colorectum in the world, a majority with advanced cancer patients receives chemotherapy, radiotherapy, and combination therapy. In this regard, this modality is expected to allow not only hypoxic states but also hyperoxic states of tumor to be detected in these patients, thus contributing to selection of therapy or drug as well as evaluation of their therapeutic efficacy. Furthermore, this modality will serve as a screening method facilitating detection of early cancer. Advances in research into hypoxia and intratumoral microvessels of tumor with this endoscopic modality are expected and lead to development of new drugs. Thus, the proposed laser source-equipped hypoxia endoscope system appears to have the potential to redraw the endoscopic landscape.

9. Conclusions and perspectives

Tumor hypoxia assessment allows cancer patients to be followed up early after treatment initiation and drug resistance and radioresistance to be predicted. Current insights into the molecular mechanisms of hypoxia have indeed led to novel probes being developed for noninvasive imaging of hypoxia. Again, real-time hypoxic imaging in digestive endoscopy was obtained using such laser light as remains within visible light wavelengths, with no use of any probes. For innovation of endoscopy, it was elucidated that most of all early cancers and precursor lesions have already been to hypoxic state. This is a cutting edge finding. This imaging technology highlights a novel aspect of cancer biology as a potential biomarker which may come to be widely used in cancer diagnosis and treatment effect prediction. These approaches appear to have great promise and further studies on the predictive value of hypoxia measurement in tumors may help identify independent predictive marker of hypoxia as well as optimal parameters for assessing hypoxia. It remains to be clarified whether these new agents may help reduce hypoxic disease or whether they are available for hypoxia imaging.

Author details

Kazuhiro Kaneko[1], Hiroshi Yamaguchi[2] and Tomonori Yano[1*]

*Address all correspondence to: toyano@east.ncc.go.jp

1 Division of Science and Technology for Endoscopy, National Cancer Center Hospital East, Chiba, Japan

2 Imaging Technology Center, FUJIFILM Corporation, Tokyo, Japan

References

[1] Vaupel P, Mayer A (2007) Hypoxia in cancer: significance and impact on clinical outcome. Cancer Metastasis Rev 26:225–239

[2] Fukumura D, Jain RK (2007) Tumor microvasculature and microenvironment: targets for anti-angiogenesis and normalization. Microvasc Res 74:72–84

[3] Vaupel P, Mayer A, Hockel M (2004) Tumor hypoxia and malignant progression. Methods Enzymol 381:335–354

[4] Gray LH, Conger AD, Ebert M, Hornsey S, Scott OCA (1953) The concentration of oxygen dissolved in tissues at the time of irradiation as a factor in radiotherapy. Br J Radiol 26:638–648

[5] Matthews NE, Adams MA, Maxwell LR, Gofton TE, Graham CH (2001) Nitric oxide-mediated regulation of chemosensitivity in cancer cells. J Natl Cancer Inst 93:1879–1885

[6] Nordsmark M, Bentzen SM, Rudat V et al (2005) Prognostic value of tumor oxygenation in 397 head and neck tumors after primary radiation therapy. An international multi-center study. Radiother Oncol 77:18–24

[7] Brizel DM, Sibley GS, Prosnitz LR, Scher RL, Dewhirst MW (1997) Tumor hypoxia adversely affects the prognosis of carcinoma of the head and neck. Int J Radiat Oncol Biol Phys 38:285–289

[8] Hockel M, Vorndran B, Schlenger K, Baussmann E, Knapstein PG (1993) Tumor oxygenation: a new predictive parameter in locally advanced cancer of the uterine cervix. Gynecol Oncol 51:141–149

[9] Nordsmark M, Loncaster J, Chou SC et al (2001) Invasive oxygen measurements and pimonidazole labeling in human cervix carcinoma. Int J Radiat Oncol Biol Phys 49:581–586

[10] Nordsmark M, Overgaard J (2000) A confirmatory prognostic study on oxygenation status and loco-regional control in advanced head and neck squamous cell carcinoma treated by radiation therapy. Radiother Oncol 57:39–43

[11] Evans SM, Judy KD, Dunphy I et al (2004) Hypoxia is important in the biology and aggression of human glial brain tumors. Clin Cancer Res 10:8177–8184

[12] Powell ME, Collingridge DR, Saunders MI et al (1999) Improvement in human tumour oxygenation with carbogen of varying carbon dioxide concentrations. Radiother Oncol 50:167–171

[13] Gatenby RA, Moldofsky PJ, Weiner LM (1988) Metastatic colon cancer: correlation of oxygen levels with I-131 F(ab')2 uptake. Radiology 166:757–759

[14] Brizel DM, Scully SP, Harrelson JM et al (1996) Radiation therapy and hyperthermia improve the oxygenation of human soft tissue sarcomas. Cancer Res 56:5347–5350

[15] Pauwels EK, Mariani G (2007) Assessment of tumor tissue oxygenation: agents, methods and clinical significance. Drug News Perspect 20:619–626

[16] Massoud TF, Gambhir SS (2007) Integrating noninvasive molecular imaging into molecular medicine: an evolving paradigm. Trends Mol Med 13:183–191

[17] Willmann JK, van Bruggen N, Dinkelborg LM, Gambhir SS (2008) Molecular imaging in drug development. Nat Rev Drug Discov 7:591–607

[18] Swartz HM, Clarkson RB (1998) The measurement of oxygen *in vivo* using EPR techniques. Phys Med Biol 43:1957–1975

[19] Matsumoto K, English S, Yoo J et al (2004) Pharmacokinetics of a triarylmethyl-type paramagnetic spin probe used in EPR oximetry. Magn Reson Med 52:885–892

[20] Krohn KA, Link JM, Mason RP (2008) Molecular imaging of hypoxia. J Nucl Med 49(Suppl 2):129S–148S

[21] Wang X, Xie X, Ku G, Wang LV, Stoica G (2006) Noninvasive imaging of hemoglobin concentration and oxygenation in the rat brain using high-resolution photoacoustic tomography. J Biomed Opt 11:024015

[22] Padhani A (2010) Science to practice: what does MR oxygenation imaging tell us about human breast cancer hypoxia? Radiology 254:1–3

[23] Howe FA, Robinson SP, McIntyre DJ, Stubbs M, Griffiths JR (2001) Issues in flow and oxygenation dependent contrast (FLOOD) imaging of tumours. NMR Biomed 14:497–506

[24] Stubbs M (1999) Application of magnetic resonance techniques for imaging tumour physiology. Acta Oncol 38:845–853

[25] Tumkur SM, Vu AT, Li LP, Pierchala L, Prasad PV (2006) Evaluation of intra-renal oxygenation during water diuresis: a time-resolved study using BOLD MRI. Kidney Int 70:139–143

[26] O'Connor JP, Naish JH, Parker GJ et al (2009) Preliminary study of oxygen-enhanced longitudinal relaxation in MRI: a potential novel biomarker of oxygenation changes in solid tumors. Int J Radiat Oncol Biol Phys 75:1209–1215

[27] Mason RP (2006) Non-invasive assessment of kidney oxygenation: a role for BOLD MRI. Kidney Int 70:10–11

[28] Thomas SR, Pratt RG, Millard RW et al (1996) *In vivo* PO_2 imaging in the porcine model with perfluorocarbon F-19 NMR at low field. Magn Reson Imaging 14:103–114

[29] Mason RP, Shukla H, Antich PP (1993) *In vivo* oxygen tension and temperature: simultaneous determination using 19F NMR spectroscopy of perfluorocarbon. Magn Reson Med 29:296–302

[30] Zhao D, Ran S, Constantinescu A, Hahn EW, Mason RP (2003) Tumor oxygen dynamics: correlation of *in vivo* MRI with histological findings. Neoplasia 5:308–318

[31] van der Sanden BP, Heerschap A, Simonetti AW et al Characterization and validation of noninvasive oxygen tension measurements in human glioma xenografts by 19F-MR relaxometry. Int J Radiat Oncol Biol Phys 44:649–658

[32] McNab JA, Yung AC, Kozlowski P (2004) Tissue oxygen tension measurements in the Shionogi model of prostate cancer using 19F MRS and MRI. Magma 17:288–295

[33] Davda S, Bezabeh T (2006) Advances in methods for assessing tumor hypoxia *in vivo*: implications for treatment planning. Cancer Metastasis Rev 25:469–480

[34] Yu JX, Kodibagkar VD, Cui W, Mason RP (2005) 19F: a versatile reporter for non-invasive physiology and pharmacology using magnetic resonance. Curr Med Chem 12:819–848

[35] Hunjan S, Zhao D, Constantinescu A et al (2001) Tumor oximetry: demonstration of an enhanced dynamic mapping procedure using fluorine-19 echo planar magnetic resonance imaging in the Dunning prostate R3327-AT1 rat tumor. Int J Radiat Oncol Biol Phys 49:1097–1108

[36] Emblem KE, Mouridsen K, Bjornerud A et al (2013) Vessel architectural imaging identifies cancer patient responders to anti-angiogenic therapy. Nat Med; doi:10.1038/nm.3289

[37] Batchelor TT, Sorensen AG, di Tomaso E et al (2007) AZD2171, a pan-VEGF receptor tyrosine kinase inhibitor, normalizes tumor vasculature and alleviates edema in glioblastoma patients. Cancer Cell 11:83–95

[38] Rasey JS, Koh WJ, Evans ML et al (1996) Quantifying regional hypoxia in human tumors with positron emission tomography of [18F] fluoromisonidazole: a pretherapy study of 37 patients. Int J Radiat Oncol Biol Phys 36:417–428

[39] Lehtio K, Eskola O, Viljanen T et al (2004) Imaging perfusion and hypoxia with PET to predict radiotherapy response in head-and-neck cancer. Int J Radiat Oncol Biol Phys 59:971–982

[40] Souvatzoglou M, Grosu AL, Roper B et al (2007) Tumour hypoxia imaging with [18F] FAZA PET in head and neck cancer patients: a pilot study. Eur J Nucl Med Mol Imaging 34:1566–1575

[41] Koh WJ, Rasey JS, Evans ML et al (1992) Imaging of hypoxia in human tumors with [F-18] fluoromisonidazole. Int J Radiat Oncol Biol Phys 22:199–212

[42] Lee ST, Scott AM (2007) Hypoxia positron emission tomography imaging with 18f-fluoromisonidazole. Semin Nucl Med 37:451–461

[43] Gagel B, Reinartz P, Demirel C et al (2006) [18F] fluoromisonidazole and [18F] fluorodeoxyglucose positron emission tomography in response evaluation after chemo-/radiotherapy of non-small-cell lung cancer: a feasibility study. BMC Cancer 6:51

[44] Eschmann SM, Paulsen F, Reimold M et al (2005) Prognostic impact of hypoxia imaging with 18F-misonidazole PET in non-small cell lung cancer and head and neck cancer before radiotherapy. J Nucl Med 46:253–260

[45] Rajendran JG, Mankoff DA, O'Sullivan F et al (2004) Hypoxia and glucose metabolism in malignant tumors: evaluation by [18F] fluoromisonidazole and [18F] fluorodeoxyglucose positron emission tomography imaging. Clin Cancer Res 10:2245–2252

[46] Koh WJ, Bergman KS, Rasey JS et al (1995) Evaluation of oxygenation status during fractionated radiotherapy in human nonsmall cell lung cancers using [F-18] fluoromisonidazole positron emission tomography. Int J Radiat Oncol Biol Phys 33:391–398

[47] Rajendran JG, Wilson DC, Conrad EU et al (2003) [18F] FMISO and [18F] FDG PET imaging in soft tissue sarcomas: correlation of hypoxia, metabolism and VEGF expression. Eur J Nucl Med Mol Imaging 30:695–704

[48] Bentzen L, Keiding S, Nordsmark M et al (2003) Tumour oxygenation assessed by 18F-fluoromisonidazole PET and polarographic needle electrodes in human soft tissue tumours. Radiother Oncol 67:339–344

[49] Lehtio K, Oikonen V, Gronroos T et al (2001) Imaging of blood flow and hypoxia in head and neck cancer: initial evaluation with [15O] H_2O and [18F] fluoroerythronitroimidazole PET. J Nucl Med 42:1643–1652

[50] Yang DJ, Wallace S, Cherif A et al (1995) Development of F-18-labeled fluoroerythronitroimidazole as a PET agent for imaging tumor hypoxia. Radiology 194:795–800

[51] Barthel H, Wilson H, Collingridge DR et al (2004) *In vivo* evaluation of [18F] fluoroetanidazole as a new marker for imaging tumour hypoxia with positron emission tomography. Br J Cancer 90:2232–2242

[52] Ziemer LS, Evans SM, Kachur AV et al (2003) Noninvasive imaging of tumor hypoxia in rats using the 2-nitroimidazole 18F-EF5. Eur J Nucl Med Mol Imaging 30:259–266

[53] Evans SM, Kachur AV, Shiue CY et al (2000) Noninvasive detection of tumor hypoxia using the 2-nitroimidazole [18F] EF1. J Nucl Med 41:327–336

[54] Komar G, Seppanen M, Eskola O et al (2008) 18F-EF5: a new PET tracer for imaging hypoxia in head and neck cancer. J Nucl Med 49:1944–1951

[55] Evans SM, Fraker D, Hahn SM et al (2006) EF5 binding and clinical outcome in human soft tissue sarcomas. Int J Radiat Oncol Biol Phys 64:922–927

[56] Kumar P, Emami S, Kresolek Z et al (2009) Synthesis and hypoxia selective radiosensitization potential of beta-2-FAZA and beta-3-FAZL: fluorinated azomycin beta-nucleosides. Med Chem 5:118–129

[57] Postema EJ, McEwan AJ, Riauka TA et al (2009) Initial results of hypoxia imaging using 1-alpha-D: -(5-deoxy-5-[18F]-fluoroarabinofuranosyl)-2-nitroimidazole (18F-FAZA). Eur J Nucl Med Mol Imaging 36:1565–1573

[58] Rumsey WL, Vanderkooi JM, Wilson DF (1988) Imaging of phosphorescence: a novel method for measuring oxygen distribution in perfused tissue. Science 241:1649–1651

[59] Vinogradov SA, Grosul P, Rozhkov V et al (2003) Oxygen distributions in tissue measured by phosphorescence quenching. Adv Exp Med Biol 510:181–185

[60] Lebedev AY, Cheprakov AV, Sakadzic S et al (2009) Dendritic phosphorescent probes for oxygen imaging in biological systems. ACS Appl Mater Interfaces 1:1292–1304

[61] Pennekamp CW, Bots ML, Kappelle LJ, Moll FL, de Borst GJ (2009) The value of near-infrared spectroscopy measured cerebral oximetry during carotid endarterectomy in perioperative stroke prevention. A review. Eur J Vasc Endovasc Surg 38:539–545

[62] Jobsis FF (1977) Non-invasive, infra-red monitoring of cerebral O_2 sufficiency, blood volume, HbO_2-Hb shifts and blood flow. Acta Neurol Scand Suppl 64:452–453

[63] Hull EL, Conover DL, Foster TH (1999) Carbogen-induced changes in rat mammary tumour oxygenation reported by near infrared spectroscopy. Br J Cancer 79:1709–1716

[64] Kim JG, Liu H (2008) Investigation of biphasic tumor oxygen dynamics induced by hyperoxic gas intervention: the dynamic phantom approach. Appl Opt 47:242–252

http://dx.doi.org/10.5772/66091

[65] Barry BN, Mallick A, Bodenham AR, Vucevic M (1997) Lack of agreement between bioimpedance and continuous thermodilution measurement of cardiac output in intensive care unit patients. Crit Care 1:71–74

[66] Imhoff M, Lehner JH, Lohlein D (2000) Noninvasive whole-body electrical bioimpedance cardiac output and invasive thermodilution cardiac output in high-risk surgical patients. Crit Care Med 28:2812–2818

[67] Kurth CD, Steven JM, Benaron D, Chance B (1993) Near-infrared monitoring of the cerebral circulation. J Clin Monit 9:163–170

[68] Watkin SL, Spencer SA, Dimmock PW, Wickramasinghe YA, Rolfe P (1999) A comparison of pulse oximetry and near infrared spectroscopy (NIRS) in the detection of hypoxaemia occurring with pauses in nasal airflow in neonates. J Clin Monit Comput 15:441–447

[69] El-Desoky AE, Jiao LR, Havlik R, Habib N, Davidson BR, Seifalian AM (2000) Measurement of hepatic tissue hypoxia using near infrared spectroscopy: comparison with hepatic vein oxygen partial pressure. Eur Surg Res 32:207–214

[70] Fortune PM, Wagstaff M, Petros AJ (2001) Cerebro-splanchnic oxygenation ratio (CSOR) using near infrared spectroscopy may be able to predict splanchnic ischaemia in neonates. Intensive Care Med 27:1401–1407

[71] Fukui D, Urayama H, Tanaka K, Kawasaki S (2002) Use of near-infrared spectroscopic measurement at the buttocks during abdominal aortic surgery. Circ J 66:1128–1131

[72] DeBlasi RA, Quaglia E, Gasparetto A, Ferrari M (1992) Muscle oxygenation by fast near infrared spectrophotometry (NIRS) in ischemic forearm. Adv Exp Med Biol 316:163–172

[73] Shin'oka T, Nollert G, Shum-Tim D, du Plessis A, Jonas RA (2000) Utility of near-infrared spectroscopic measurements during deep hypothermic circulatory arrest. Ann Thorac Surg 69:578–583

[74] Vernieri F, Rosato N, Pauri F, Tibuzzi F, Passarelli F, Rossini PM (1999) Near infrared spectroscopy and transcranial Doppler in monohemispheric stroke. Eur Neurol 41:159–162

[75] Kurth CD, Steven JL, Montenegro LM, Watzman HM, Gaynor JW, Spray TL, Nicolson SC (2001) Cerebral oxygen saturation before congenital heart surgery. Ann Thorac Surg 72:187–192

[76] Misra M, Stark J, Dujovny M, Widman R, Ausman JI (1998) Transcranial cerebral oximetry in random normal subjects. Neurol Res 20:137–141

[77] Marik PE (2001) Sublingual capnography: A clinical validation study. Chest 120:923–927

[78] Povoas HP, Weil MH, Tang W, Sun S, Kamohara T, Bisera J (2001) Decreases in mesenteric blood flow associated with increases in sublingual pCO_2 during hemorrhagic shock. Shock 15:398–402

[79] Know, now. Sublingual CO_2. CapnoProbe Sublingual (SL) System brochure. Pleasanton, California, Nellcor Puritan Bennett, 2002, p 4

[80] Movsas B, Chapman JD, Hanlon AL, Horwitz EM, Pinover WH, Greenberg RE, Stobbe C, Hanks GE (2001) Hypoxia in human prostate carcinoma: An Eppendorf PO_2 study. Am J Clin Oncol 24:458–461

[81] Benaron DA, Parachikov IH, Friedland S et al (2004) Continuous, noninvasive, and localized microvascular tissue oximetry using visible light spectroscopy. Anesthesiology 100(6)

[82] Brun NC, Moen A, Borch K, Saugstad OD, Greisen G (1997) Near-infrared monitoring of cerebral tissue oxygen saturation and blood volume in newborn piglets. Am J Physiol 273(part 2):H682–H686

[83] Watzman HM, Kurth CD, Montenegro LM, Rome J, Steven JM, Nicolson SC (2000) Arterial and venous contributions to near-infrared cerebral oximetry. Anesthesiology 93:947–953

[84] Fantini S (2002) A haemodynamic model for the physiological interpretation of *in vivo* measurements of the concentration and oxygen saturation of haemoglobin. Phys Med Biol 47:N249–N257

[85] Maxim PG, Carson JJ, Benaron DA et al (2005) Optical detection of tumors *in vivo* by light tissue oximetry. Technol Cancer Res Treat 4:227–234.

[86] Noord DV, Sana A, Benaron DA et al (2011) Endoscopic visible light spectroscopy: a new, minimally invasive technique to diagnose chronic GI ischemia. Gastrointest Endosc 73:291–298

[87] Kaneko K, Yamaguchi H, Saito T et al (2014) Hypoxia imaging endoscopy equipped with laser light source from preclinical live animal study to first-in-human subject research. PLoS One 9(6):e99055. doi:10.1371/journal.pone.0099055

[88] Bussink J, Kaanders JH, van der Kogel AJ (2003) Tumor hypoxia at the micro-regional level: clinical relevance and predictive value of exogenous and endogenous hypoxic cell markers. Radiother Oncol 67:3–15

[89] Koukourakis MI, Bentzen SM, Giatromanolaki A et al (2006) Endogenous markers of two separate hypoxia response pathways (hypoxia inducible factor 2 alpha and carbonic anhydrase 9) are associated with radiotherapy failure in head and neck cancer patients recruited in the CHART randomized trial. J Clin Oncol 24:727–735

[90] Shibata T, Giaccia AJ, Brown JM (2000) Development of a hypoxia-responsive vector for tumor-specific gene therapy. Gene Ther 7:493–498

[91] Payen E, Bettan M, Henri A et al (2001) Oxygen tension and a pharmacological switch in the regulation of transgene expression for gene therapy. J Gene Med 3:498–504

[92] Vordermark D, Shibata T, Brown JM (2001) Green fluorescent protein is a suitable reporter of tumor hypoxia despite an oxygen requirement for chromophore formation. Neoplasia 3:527–534

[93] Harada H, Kizaka-Kondoh S, Hiraoka M (2005) Optical imaging of tumor hypoxia and evaluation of efficacy of a hypoxia-targeting drug in living animals. Mol Imaging 4:182–193

[94] Harada H, Hiraoka M, Kizaka-Kondoh S (2002) Antitumor effect of TAT-oxygen-dependent degradation-caspase-3 fusion protein specifically stabilized and activated in hypoxic tumor cells. Cancer Res 62:2013–2018

[95] Harada H, Kizaka-Kondoh S, Hiraoka M (2006) Mechanism of hypoxia-specific cytotoxicity of procaspase-3 fused with a VHL-mediated protein destruction motif of HIF-1alpha containing Pro564. FEBS Lett 580:5718–5722

[96] Harada H, Kizaka-Kondoh S, Li G et al (2007) Significance of HIF-1-active cells in angiogenesis and radioresistance. Oncogene 26:7508–7516

[97] Viola RJ, Provenzale JM, Li F et al (2008) *In vivo* bioluminescence imaging monitoring of hypoxia-inducible factor 1alpha, a promoter that protects cells, in response to chemotherapy. AJR Am J Roentgenol 191:1779–1784

[98] Mayer A, Wree A, Hockel M et al (2004) Lack of correlation between expression of HIF-1alpha protein and oxygenation status in identical tissue areas of squamous cell carcinomas of the uterine cervix. Cancer Res 64:5876–5881

[99] Lehmann S, Stiehl DP, Honer M et al (2009) Longitudinal and multimodal *in vivo* imaging of tumor hypoxia and its downstream molecular events. Proc Natl Acad Sci USA 106:14004–14009

[100] Potter CP, Harris AL (2003) Diagnostic, prognostic and therapeutic implications of carbonic anhydrases in cancer. Br J Cancer 89:2–7

[101] Ivanov S, Liao SY, Ivanova A et al (2001) Expression of hypoxia-inducible cell-surface transmembrane carbonic anhydrases in human cancer. Am J Pathol 158:905–919

[102] Wykoff CC, Beasley NJ, Watson PH et al Hypoxia-inducible expression of tumor-associated carbonic anhydrases. Cancer Res 60:7075–7083

[103] Dubois L, Lieuwes NG, Maresca A et al (2009) Imaging of CA IX with fluorescent labelled sulfonamides distinguishes hypoxic and (re)-oxygenated cells in a xenograft tumour model. Radiother Oncol 92:423–428

[104] van Dijk J, Uemura H, Beniers AJ et al Therapeutic effects of monoclonal antibody G250, interferons and tumor necrosis factor, in mice with renal-cell carcinoma xenografts. Int J Cancer 56:262–268

[105] Stillebroer AB, Oosterwijk E, Oyen WJ, Mulders PF, Boerman OC (2007) Radiolabeled antibodies in renal cell carcinoma. Cancer Imaging 7:179–188

[106] Ahlskog JK, Schliemann C, Marlind J et al (2009) Human monoclonal antibodies targeting carbonic anhydrase IX for the molecular imaging of hypoxic regions in solid tumours. Br J Cancer 101:645–657

[107] Hoogsteen IJ, Marres HA, Wijffels KI et al (2005) Colocalization of carbonic anhydrase 9 expression and cell proliferation in human head and neck squamous cell carcinoma. Clin Cancer Res 11:97–106

[108] Kim SJ, Shin HJ, Jung KY et al (2007) Prognostic value of carbonic anhydrase IX and Ki-67 expression in squamous cell carcinoma of the tongue. Jpn J Clin Oncol 37:812–819

[109] Mayer A, Hockel M, Vaupel P (2005) Carbonic anhydrase IX expression and tumor oxygenation status do not correlate at the microregional level in locally advanced cancers of the uterine cervix. Clin Cancer Res 11:7220–7225

[110] Macheda ML, Rogers S, Best JD (2005) Molecular and cellular regulation of glucose transporter (GLUT) proteins in cancer. J Cell Physiol 202:654–662

[111] Jonathan RA, Wijffels KI, Peeters W et al (2006) The prognostic value of endogenous hypoxia-related markers for head and neck squamous cell carcinomas treated with ARCON. Radiother Oncol 79:288–297

[112] Anderson RR, Parrish JA (1981) The optics of human skin. J Invest Dermat 77:13–19

Chapter 21

Hypoxia and its Emerging Therapeutics in Neurodegenerative, Inflammatory and Renal Diseases

Deepak Bhatia, Mohammad Sanaei Ardekani,
Qiwen Shi and Shahrzad Movafagh

Additional information is available at the end of the chapter

http://dx.doi.org/10.5772/66089

Abstract

Hypoxia is a common underlying condition of many disease states. Hypoxia can occur with ischemia, a lack of blood flow to tissues, or independent of ischemia as in acute lung injury, anemia, and carbon monoxide poisoning. Hypoxia may be observed in patients with diseases such as obstructive sleep apnea, cerebrovascular diseases, systemic hypertension, cardiovascular diseases, chronic obstructive pulmonary disease (COPD), pulmonary hypertension and congestive heart failure (CHF), inflammatory disease states, and acute and chronic renal diseases. In the past decade, research has shown hypoxic signaling to be involved in a range of responses from adaptation of the body to reduced oxygen to pathogenesis of disease. Hypoxic signaling intermediates orchestrate a whole host of responses from angiogenesis, glycolysis, and erythropoiesis to inflammation and remodeling, which could be beneficial or harmful to the hosting organ. The length of exposure to low oxygen pressure as well as the existing signaling pathways within different cells dictates their benefit or disadvantage from hypoxic signaling. Therefore, activation or inhibition of hypoxic intermediates could serve as novel therapeutic strategies. In this chapter, we review the role of hypoxic signaling in neurodegenerative, inflammatory, and renal disease states and the emerging therapeutic approaches involving hypoxic signaling.

Keywords: hypoxia, hypoxia-inducible factor, neurodegenerative disease, Parkinson's disease, Alzheimer's disease, ischemia/reperfusion, inflammation, epigenetics, microRNA, inflammatory bowel disease, rheumatoid arthritis, acute kidney injury, chronic kidney disease, erythropoiesis, anemia, allograft rejection

1. Hypoxia and neurodegenerative diseases

1.1. Introduction

Neurodegenerative diseases are defined by the progressive loss of specific neuronal cell population and protein misfolding and aggregate. Reduced oxygen supply has been detected during the aging process as well as the pathogenesis of neurodegenerative diseases. Besides, diseases associated with a lowering of systemic oxygen levels predispose individuals to neurodegenerative diseases. Although the connection between hypoxia and neurodegeneration has been well established, the exact role of hypoxia in neurodegenerative diseases has yet to be elucidated.

This section summarizes current identified clues linking hypoxia to the onset and progression of neurodegenerative diseases, including neurotoxic effects, altered signaling transduction and protein expression, and abnormal epigenetic modification. Furthermore, the following discussion emphasizes on the detrimental impacts of cerebral oxygen deficiency on three major neurodegenerative diseases: Alzheimer's disease (AD), Parkinson's disease (PD), and amyotrophic lateral sclerosis (ALS).

1.1.1. Hypoxia and Alzheimer's disease

AD is characterized by progressive impairments in memory and cognitive function. The hallmark features of AD are extracellular plaques whose major components are amyloid β peptide (Aβ) and intracellular neurofibrillary tangles constituted by hyperphosphorylated tau protein. Other changes identified in AD brains are loss of synapses and neurons, proliferation of reactive astrocytes, and microglial activation. The incidence of AD in the United States is 11% among the population aged over 65 years and approximately 32% among those 85 years and older (Alzheimer's Association, 2015) [1]. Apparently, aging is the most significant risk factor for AD, since the risk of developing AD doubles every 5 years after the age of 65 years. Other factors, including environmental neurotoxins/metals, gene mutations, susceptibility polymorphisms, cardiovascular diseases, traumatic brain injury, and ischemia/hypoxia, also potentially prompt the development of AD.

Although the exact mechanisms and triggers initiating AD remain unclear, both clinical and preclinical studies suggest that hypoxia should be considered as an important risk factor in AD pathogenesis. Chronic cerebral hypoperfusion and glucose hypometabolism appearing decades before cognitive dysfunction promote the initiation and progression of cognitive decline and AD [2]. Patients after cerebral hypoxia or ischemia are more susceptible to developing dementia. Cerebral blood flow (CBF) reduction decreases the synthesis of proteins necessary for memory and learning and contributes likely to neuritic injury, neuronal death, and the onset and progression of dementia [3]. Correspondingly, significantly reduced resting CBF is distinguished in AD patients and is also present in the early stages of AD pathogenesis [4].

Generally, hypoxia modifies Aβ production and tau phosphorylation at numerous points (**Figure 1**). Aβ is a cleavage product generated through the sequential actions of β- and γ-secretases on amyloid precursor protein (APP). Hypoxia can stimulate Aβ generation and senile plaque formation in AD through increasing the expression of β- and γ-secretases along with the localization of γ-secretase from cell body to axon [5]. Furthermore, hypoxia elevates the levels of APP and presenilin-1 (PS-1), a main component of γ-secretase complex, in vivo [6]. The expression of neprilysin (NEP), an enzyme responsible for Aβ degeneration, is reduced during hypoxia [7]. Rats exposed to hypoxic stress display tau hyperphosphorylation in the hippocampus as well as memory deficit, and Aβ-induced tau phosphorylation is raised through calpain upon hypoxia exposure [8, 9]. The activity of protein phosphatase 2A (PP2A) is compromised in AD and is believed to be a cause of tau neurofibrillary. Brain hypoxia generates an acidic environment that promotes the cleavage of I_2^{PP2A}, a potent inhibitor of PP2A, by activating asparaginyl endopeptidase, thus giving rise to tau hyperphosphorylation [10].

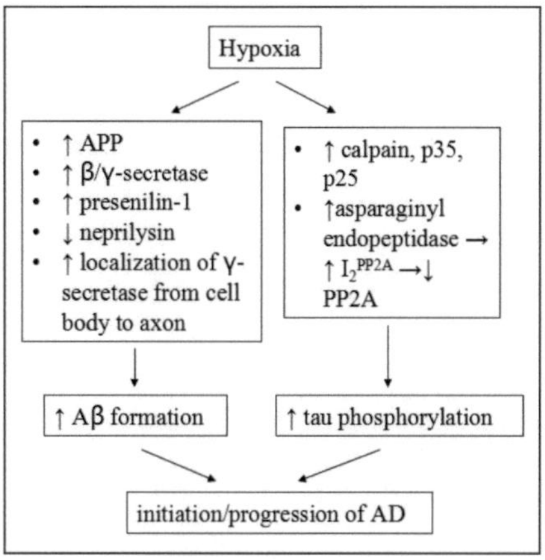

Figure 1. The molecular mechanisms of hypoxic predisposition to AD.

1.1.2. Hypoxia and Parkinson's disease

The clinical features of PD include classical motor symptoms (bradykinesia, rigidity, postural instability, resting tremor) and non-motor symptoms (dementia, sleep disorder, depression, autonomic dysfunction), resulting from a continuous degeneration and loss of dopaminergic neurons in the substantia nigra (SN) and the presence of intracytoplasmic proteinaceous inclusions called Lewy bodies (LB) [11].

α-Synuclein (α-syn), a major constituent of LB, is the pathological hallmark of PD. Hypoxic brain injury is a potential cause of PD, as it enhances α-synuclein expression and aggregation [12]. ATP13A2 (PARK9) mutations have been found in postmortem PD patients, declaring its relevance to PD pathogenesis [13]. Although the exact molecular mechanism remains unknown, it turns out that hypoxia upregulates ATP13A2 transcription via HIF-1 alpha (HIF-1α) in dopaminergic cells [14]. Hypoxia changes the localization of intracellular hemoglobin whose overexpression is correlated with an increased risk of PD [15]. In addition, subnormal sensitivity to hypoxia has been noticed in PD patients even at an early stage of diseases, probably leading to the exacerbation of respiratory failure in PD [16].

1.1.3. Hypoxia and amyotrophic lateral sclerosis

ALS, also known as Lou Gehrig's disease, is a progressive and fetal disease resulted from damaged motor neurons in the spinal cord, brain stem, and motor cortex. The incidence rate of ALS worldwide is estimated to be 2 in 100,000 people, and in the United States, about 5000 persons are diagnosed with ALS every year [17]. ALS risk is influenced by physical activity, smoking habit, type of diet, and exposure to agriculture chemicals and heavy metals. Occupations that may cause intermittent hypoxia, such as fire fighter, double the risk of ALS, and genetic impairment in reaction to hypoxia predisposes motor neuron to death [18].

Hypoxia is not only a causative factor of ALS but also accelerates the progression of ALS. Motor neurons under hypoxic conditions fail to survive and undergo degeneration [19]. $SOD1^{G93A}$ mutant mice, an ALS animal model, have experienced aggravation in motor neuronal loss, neuromuscular weakness and possibly cognitive deficiency, with higher level of oxidative stress and inflammation after chronic intermittent hypoxia [20]. Chronic sustained hypoxic condition induces the activation of apoptosis-related genes such as caspase 3, apoptosis-inducing factor (AIF), and cytochrome C in motor neurons from the spinal cord of ALS mice, facilitating the progression of ALS [21].

1.2. The mechanism of hypoxia-induced injury in neural cells

Cellular and molecular pathways underlying hypoxia-induced neurotoxicity and cell death are multifaceted and complex, including a number of cross-talked mechanisms. Ensuing hypoxia stimulates the production and release of proteins mediating oxidative stress, inflammation, apoptosis, mitochondrial metabolism, metal homeostasis, synaptic transmission, and autophagy, contributing to neuronal death (**Figure 2**).

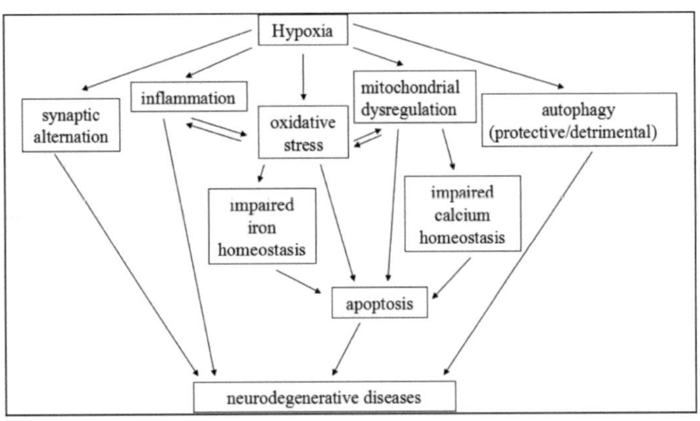

Figure 2. Different pathogenic mechanisms linking hypoxia to neurodegenerative diseases.

1.2.1. Hypoxia-promoted oxidative stress

Oxidative stress has been implicated in hypoxic injury and neurodegenerative diseases. It occurs due to the disruption of oxidative balance and excessive production of reactive oxygen species (ROS) and reactive nitrogen species (RNS), including hydrogen peroxide (H_2O_2), nitric oxide (NO), superoxide (O_2^-), and the highly reactive hydroxyl radicals (·OH) [22]. The production of ROS and RNS is increased under hypoxic condition, probably because there is no acceptor for the electrons available. During hypoxic events, high levels of free radicals are produced through mitochondrial complex III, and the antioxidant status is depleted, thus leading to oxidative damage of vital cellular components. For instance, neuroblastoma cells exposed to hypoxia have augmented production of free radicals accompanied by a concomitant decrease in reduced glutathione (GSH) content, glutathione reductase (GR), glutathione peroxidase (GPx), and superoxide dismutase (SOD) activities, further inciting apoptotic death [22].

Increased oxidative stress is believed to be associated with neurological disorders and classical neuropathy. Reduced antioxidant capacity is a trait of AD. The activation of NO/NOS signaling system by cerebral ischemia in aged rats triggers hippocampal Aβ production through β-secretase 1 (BACE1) pathway, implying RNS is a bridge linking hypoxia to AD [23]. In retinal ganglion cells (RGEs) derived from rats, hypoxia exposure triggers Aβ formation, intracellular ROS accumulation, and following cell death, suggesting the involvement of Aβ in hypoxia-induced retinal degeneration in AD [24]. In PD, the promotion of ROS formation is highly correlated to mutant α-syn phosphorylation at serine 129 (Ser129), possibly preceding cell degeneration [25]. Agents with antioxidant property ameliorate neurodegenerative situation, including natural compounds and iron chelators.

1.2.2. Hypoxia-altered ionic homeostasis

Impaired cellular homeostasis of metals can be triggered by hypoxic conditions, resulting in neurodegeneration through various mechanisms, such as oxidative stress, inflammation, and aberrant expression of metalloproteins.

Calcium dyshomeostasis is a fundamental mechanism in the pathogenesis of neurodegenerative diseases. The interaction between γ-aminobutyric acid (GABA) and calcium-dependent neurotransmission as well as calcium-dependent neuronal metabolism also reveals the role of Ca^{2+} in neuronal degeneration. Ca^{2+} acts as an intracellular messenger, controlling not only transsynaptic signal transmission but also cellular metabolism by reaching the mitochondria [26]. Hypoxia can disrupt Ca^{2+} entry and signaling in various cell types. In hypoxic human neuroblastoma cells, the storage of intracellular Ca^{2+}, Na^+/Ca^{2+} exchange, and capacitative Ca^{2+} entry are boosted, indicating adaptive cellular remodeling in response to prolonged hypoxia [27]. Similarly, chronic hypoxia enhances capacitative Ca^{2+} entry and mitochondria Ca^{2+} content in the primary culture of rat type-I cortical astrocytes [28]. In terms of AD, chronic hypoxia potentiates posttranscriptional trafficking of L-type Ca^{2+} channels that may result from the interaction between Aβ and Ca^{2+} channel subunit [29].

Iron can be released from storage protein in the brain under hypoxic circumstances, and disruption of intracellular free iron homeostasis is an early event upon hypoxic stimulation in oligodendrocytes that contain enriched iron and ferritin [30]. Progressive hypoxia dramatically activates the synthesis of ferritin, a major iron-binding protein, in oligodendrocytes, and this induction may require ROS formation as it can be enhanced by co-treatment with H_2O_2 [31]. Intracellular free iron has neurotoxic effects. Iron promotes Aβ aggregation in vitro [32], and iron-Aβ interaction exhibits toxic effects through ROS [33]. Iron also binds to tau, but interestingly, its effect on tau relies on the oxidation state. Fe^{3+} induces the aggregation of hyperphosphorylated tau and reduces the phosphorylation of tau, whereas Fe^{2+} exerts an opposite action [34]. As for PD, abnormal accumulation of iron results in α-syn aggregation by promoting its synthesis and inhibiting its degradation [35].

1.2.3. Hypoxia-disrupted mitochondrial functions

The consequences of mitochondrial dysfunction cover oxidative stress, intracellular Ca^{2+} dysregulation, apoptosis, and metabolic failure, aggravating the deleterious effect.

Respiratory chain reprogramming is the first stage in the development of hypoxia-triggered mitochondrial disorders, converting complex I electron transport chain (ETC) to complex II succinate oxidation. The activation of succinate is regarded as a protective and compensatory mechanism in response to oxygen shortage and preserves the aerobic energy production [36]. Otherwise, the dysregulation of complex I during oxygen deficiency may lead neurons to acute degeneration, characterized by decreased membrane potential, loss of ATP, and respiration disorders caused by abnormal oxidation of nicotinamide adenine dinucleotide (NADH) [37]. The study of mitochondrial genes informs that hypoxia upregulates genes involved in glycolytic pathways, indicating a shift in energy production from oxidative phosphorylation to glycolysis, which converts glucose to pyruvate and eventually lactate. This shift is supported by the observation of elevated brain extracellular lactate concentration in traumatic brain injury (TBI) patients. A cerebral microdialysis study discloses that the neurons in TBI patient are unable to utilize lactate produced by astrocyte through tricarboxylic acid (TCA) cycle, leading to increased lactate/pyruvate ratio [38]. In addition, the ketogenic capacity of cultured astroglia and neurons is augmented under hypoxia, probably because of the susceptibility of pyruvate dehydrogenase to oxygen deprivation [39].

Many rare mitochondrial diseases are actually models of neurodegeneration, such as Leber's hereditary optic neuropathy (LHON) and autosomal dominant optic atrophy (ADOA), and abnormal mitochondrial function has been discovered in several age-related neurodegenerative diseases. Suppression of complex I potentiates tau phosphorylation, pointing out the role of mitochondrial dysfunction in the formation of tangles in AD [40]. During prolonged exposure to hypoxia, ROS production, Aβ accumulation, and Ca^{2+} dyshomeostasis are enhanced through regulation on ETC [41]. The SN of PD patients has reduced activity of mitochondrial complex I, and inhibitors of complex I produce neurological changes similar to PD [42].

1.2.4. Hypoxia-mediated apoptotic cascades

Cerebral hypoxia results in increased activities of caspase-9, caspase-8, and caspase-3 in the cerebral cortex of newborn piglets and enhances cytochrome C expression and caspase-3 activity followed by the induction of apoptosis in neuroblastoma cells. NO induced by hypoxia exerts proapoptotic property through elevating the expression of proteins such as Bax and Bad, leading to APAF-1 activation and consequential activation of caspase-9 and caspase-3, and, on the other hand, through downregulating antiapoptotic proteins of the B-cell lymphoma-2 (Bcl-2) family [22, 43] . Exposure of primary neuron cells from ALS mice to chronic sustained hypoxia results in enhanced cellular apoptosis, suggesting hypoxia could accelerate ALS via neuronal apoptosis [21]. Angiogenin (ANG) is a potent inducer of neovascularization and is responsive to hypoxia. Silence of ANG promotes hypoxic injury-induced motor neuron apoptosis, while exogenous overexpression of ANG has an antiapoptotic function. Mutation of ANG has been identified in ALS patients, proposing the importance of ANG in ALS pathogenesis [44].

Blockage of apoptosis can be neuroprotective. Rasagiline and its derivatives, a group of highly potent irreversible monoamine oxidase (MAO) B inhibitor, exert their anti-Parkinson feature by preventing apoptotic cascades. They activate Bcl-2 and protein kinase C (PKC) and inhibit proapoptosis FAS and Bax against neuronal apoptosis [45]. Treatment of 0.5% isoflurane, an inhaled anesthetic, attenuates caspase-3 activation, BACE upregulation, and Bcl-2 reduction caused by hypoxia in H4 human neuroglioma cells, hinting the neuroprotective effect of isoflurane in AD [46].

1.2.5. Hypoxia-modified synaptic signaling

Synaptic transmission in the central nervous system (CNS) is extremely sensitive to hypoxia, since it requires 30–50% of cerebral oxygen. Decrease in synaptic efficacy occurs very early during hypoxia and is possibly the first response of neurons to ischemic insult.

Oxygen-sensitive ion channels and voltage-gated Ca^{2+} and K^+ channel are activated in response to hypoxia, bringing about changes in excitation and inhibition of neuronal and glial cells [47]. Under hypoxic circumstance, there is an accumulation of adenosine in the extracellular space, due to the increased catabolism of adenosine triphosphate (ATP) into adenosine monophosphate (AMP) [48]. Adenosine is a neurotransmitter inhibiting synaptic transmission, and its effect is mediated by adenosine A1 receptor. The mechanism is that receptor activation stimulates inwardly rectifying K^+ channels, substantially inhibiting Ca^{2+} channels, phospholipase C activation, and the release of neurotransmitters including glutamate, dopamine, serotonin, and acetylcholine [49].

P2Y1 receptor is a G-protein-coupled ATP receptor activated by ATP released from neurons and astrocytes during neuronal activity or under pathophysiological conditions such as hypoxia, brain injury, and AD [50]. Emerging evidence shows that P2Y1 receptor obstructs the release of neurotransmitters and modulates synaptic plasticity in the brain, especially in the prefrontal cortex, hippocampus, and cerebellum, leading to impaired cognitive process [50]. P2Y1 receptors are localized with AD features such as neurofibrillary tangles and neuritic plaques, suggesting the altered distribution of P2Y1 in AD brains [51]. Astrocytic hyperactivity consisting of single-cell transients and Ca^{2+} waves has been observed around Aβ plaques. P2Y1 receptors are strongly expressed by reactive astrocytes, and blockade of P2Y1 receptors can reduce astrocytic hyperactivity back to normal [52].

1.2.6. Hypoxia and autophagy

In general, autophagy is regarded as a survival mechanism, but under severe hypoxia/ischemia, autophagy may cause self-digestion and eventual cell death due to its overactivation [53]. The morphological characteristics of autophagic-programmed cell death have been observed in both mice and rats with cerebral ischemia [54, 55].

Enormous studies indicate autophagy dysfunction in AD. Autophagic vacuoles (AVs) are significantly accumulated in the brain of AD patients compared to normal brain, possibly leading to lysosomal enzyme dysfunction [56]. The cross talk between autophagy and tau aggregation indicates the change of autophagic function in the pathogenesis of AD. Autophagy initially degrades tau to protect neurons; however, hyperphosphorylation of tau results in autophagic dysfunction, which substantially exacerbates AD via inducing tau aggregation [57, 58]. Remarkably, hypoxia induces autophagic activation through AMPK-mTOR signaling, resulting in more Aβ production and AD aggravation in vitro [56].

Defective autophagy has been implicated in PD [59], and several mutations in PD are strongly relevant to autophagy dysregulation, such as PTEN-induced putative kinase 1 (PINK1) [60]. Autophagy in ALS prevents neurons from degeneration, and inhibition of autophagy aggravates motor neuron viability, since the aggregates composed of intermediate filaments and insoluble forms of proteins can be cleared by autophagy pathway [61].

1.3. The role of hypoxia-sensitive transcription factors in neurodegenerative diseases

Several transcription factors are responsive to hypoxia and subsequently alter gene expression and cellular activity. The signaling pathways relevant to these transcription factors have been indicated in the development of neurodegenerative diseases. Therefore, these transcription factors may provide a link between hypoxic environment and neurodegeneration. The following discussion will include HIF-1, the most well-studied hypoxia-inducible gene, and two other redox-sensitive transcription factors, nuclear factor-kappa B (NF-κB) and NF-E2-related factor 2 (Nrf2).

1.3.1. Hypoxia-inducible factor-1

Hypoxia-inducible factor-1 (HIF-1) is a transcriptional activator involved in oxygen hemostasis, regulating the expression of genes and the activation of signaling pathways that participate in angiogenesis, erythropoiesis, neovascularization, iron metabolism, glucose metabolism, cell proliferation, apoptosis, and cell cycle control (**Figure 3**).

http://dx.doi.org/10.5772/66089

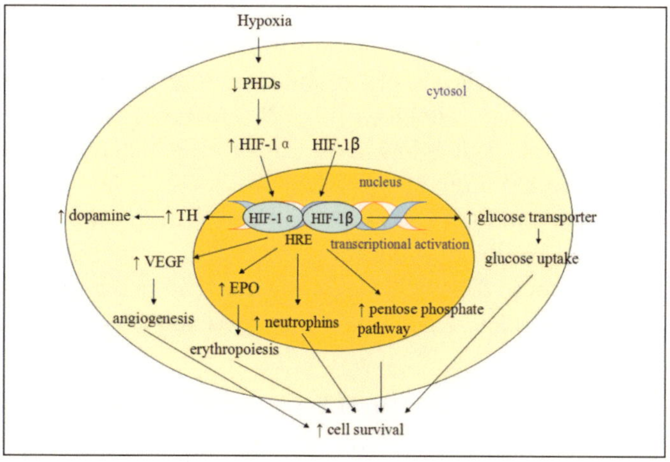

Figure 3. The neuroprotective role of HIF-1α activation in hypoxia.

In AD, HIF-1α upregulates neuronal glucose transporters such as GLUT-1 and GLUT-3 and facilitates glucose uptake, thus providing increased oxygen supply to hypoxic tissues [62]. It also contributes to cell survival by inducing the key enzymes in pentose phosphate pathway, including glucose-6-phosphate dehydrogenase and 6-phosphogluconate dehydrogenase [63]. HIF-1α also connects hypoxia to amyloidogenic processing of APP through transcriptionally upregulating BACE1 and eventually increases Aβ formation [64].

The protective role of HIF-1 in PD has been demonstrated by its ability to increase dopamine synthesis and dopaminergic neuron growth. Tyrosine hydroxylase (TH) is the rate-limiting enzyme of dopamine synthesis in dopaminergic neurons, and interestingly, it contains an HRE [65]. HIF-1 elevated in response to hypoxia increases TH expression in rat brain stem, and HIF-1α conditional knockout mice exhibit reduced expression of TH and aldehyde dehydrogenase in SN [57]. HIF-1 activation may defend against dysregulation of brain iron homeostasis and mitochondria in PD. Iron accumulation has been observed in the SN of PD patients and is considered as a culprit of ROS generation and intracellular α-syn aggregation [66]. Moreover, the neurotransmitter dopamine is a metal reductant that reduces the oxidation state of metals such as Fe^{3+} and subsequently results in elevated oxidative stress [67]. Deferoxamine (DFO), an iron chelator, prevents neurotoxicity in MPTP-treated mice through upregulation of HIF-1α protein expression, leading to declined expression of proteins such as α-syn, divalent metal transporter with iron-responsive element (DMT1 + IRE) and transferrin receptor (TFR), and elevated expression of HIF-1 target genes, including TH, vascular endothelial growth factor (VEGF), and growth associated protein 43 (GAP43) [68].

HIF-1 activation during hypoxia should be beneficial to ALS. HIF-1-VEGF pathway can induce angiogenesis and increase blood supply to motor neurons. VEGF overexpression delays motor neuron loss and impairment in $SOD1^{G93A}$ mutant mice and prolongs the survival of mice [69]. Deletion of HRE in VEGF promoter region abolishes hypoxia-increased VEGF expression, causing motor neuron degeneration [70]. Additionally, HIF-1-erythropoietin (EPO) pathway is suggested to be a new therapeutic target for ALS. EPO treatment in SOD1^{G93A} mice postpones the onset and progression of motor deterioration and modulates the immune-inflammatory response through reducing the levels of pro-inflammatory cytokines and enhancing the expression of anti-inflammatory cytokines [71, 72]. However, both above pathways are impaired in ALS. The level of VEGF is low in the CSF of early ALS patients, and likewise, the expression of VEGF in the CSF from hypoxemic ALS patients is lower than that in the CSF from normoxemic ALS patients [73, 74]. EPO protein level is declined in the surrounding glial cells of SOD1^{G93A} mice, and in the anterior horn cells (AHCs) from SOD1^{G93A} mice, impaired cytoplasmic-nuclear transport of HIF-1α has appeared since the presymptomatic stage, indicating the abnormality in HIF-1 pathway might precede motor neuron degradation [75, 76].

The well-studied group of agents targeting HIF-1 is iron chelators. The neuroprotective and neurorestorative activities of M30, an iron chelator with brain-selective monoamine oxidase (MAO) AB inhibitory function, share a same pathway, the activation of HIF-1, in different neurodegenerative diseases. M30 elevates HIF-1 to regulate neurotrophins BDNF, GDNF, VEGF, and EPO in PD, and meanwhile, it delays the onset of ALS in SOD1^{G93A} mutant mice through HIF-1 upregulation [77, 78]. In APP/PS1 AD mice model, M30 treatment upregulates HIF-1α in the frontal cortex, resulting in the beneficial modulation of target glycolytic gene expression, such as aldolase A, enolase-1, and GLUT-1 [79].

Taken together, HIF-1 is a key player protecting neuron cells against hypoxia and oxidative stress, as well as a reasonable therapeutic target against major neurodegenerative diseases, since its participation in the pathogenesis of neurodegeneration has been well identified.

1.3.2. Nuclear factor-kappa B

Nuclear factor-kappa B (NF-κB) is analogous to HIF-1 in structure, function, and mechanism of activation and plays a critical role in inflammation, immune response, synaptic transmission, neuronal plasticity, and apoptosis [80]. In resting state, NF-κB is complexed with the inhibitory subunit I-κB; however, under physiological or pharmacological stimulus such as oxidative stress, I-kappa B (I-κB) is degraded, leading to translocation of NF-κB from cytoplasm to nucleus to modulate gene transcription. NF-κB and I-κB proteins comprise a growing family of structurally related transcription factors, and functional NF-κB complexes are present in generally all cell types in the nervous system, such as neurons, astrocytes, microglia, and oligodendrocytes [81, 82]. In neurons, the most common variants consist of p50, p65/RelA, and I-κB subunits.

As a redox-sensitive transcription factor, the mobilization and upregulation of NF-κB have been reported in hypoxia and ischemia-reperfusion damage. Hypoxic-ischemic brain damage (HIBD) upregulates the expression of NF-κB and the NO content in rat cortex cells, suggesting the involvement of NF-κB/nNOS pathway during the recovery of HIBD-induced neuron damage [83]. The role of NF-κB in neonatal HIBD depends on the duration of hypoxia. Early activation of NF-κB is detrimental, and at that time point, treatment of NF-κB inhibitor, TAT-NBD, exhibits significant therapeutic outcomes, whereas late NF-κB activation enhances antiapoptotic pathway and contributes to endogenous neuroprotection [84]. The overall effect

http://dx.doi.org/10.5772/66089

of NF-κB activation seems to facilitate ischemic neuronal degeneration, but still, the effect can be either neuroprotective or deleterious depending on the cell type and the strength of signal [85]. The suppression of NF-κB or I-κB in neuron can reduce infarct size after stroke, and the inhibition of NF-κB caused by Ginkgolide B has protective effects on ischemic stroke [86, 87].

NF-κB activation has been observed in neurons and astroglia of brain sections from AD patients but only in cells surrounding early plaques, suggesting that the induction of NF-κB activity by Aβ is partially responsible for the aberrant gene expression in diseased nervous tissue [88]. In addition, intraperitoneal injection of sodium hydrosulfide (NaHS), a donor of H_2S whose level is reduced in the hippocampus of Aβ-injected rats, inhibits MAPK/NF-κB pathway and dramatically mitigates cognitive decline and neuroinflammation [83]. Another novel drug for AD, Gx-50, exerts anti-inflammatory effects against Aβ-triggered microglial overactivation in AD mice model via inhibition of NF-κB signaling [89].

Increased NF-κB activation has been reported in dopaminergic neurons of SN from PD patients, as well as in astrocytes of spinal cords from ALS patients [90]. Compounds inhibiting NF-κB translocation in microglia such as vinyl sulfone compound (VSC2) downregulate the expression of inducible NOS (iNOS) and TNF-α, leading to anti-inflammatory and antioxidant events in PD animal model [91]. NF-κB is also involved in microglia-induced motor neuron death in ALS. Deletion of NF-κB signaling in microglia rescues motor neuron from microglia-mediated death and extends survival in ALS mice by impairing pro-inflammatory microglial activation [92].

Collectively, NF-κB is responsive to the injury of nervous system in both acute and chronic neurodegenerative conditions. Agents suppressing NF-κB activation have been tested in animal models of neurodegenerative conditions, but their usage should be considered cautiously because of the involvement of NF-κB in learning and memory.

1.3.3. NF-E2-related factor 2

NF-E2-related factor 2 (Nrf2) is a basic leucine zipper (bZIP) transcription factor that is ubiquitously expressed in a wide range of tissues and cell types. It heterodimerizes with small Maf or Jun proteins and binds to the antioxidant response element (ARE) in the promoter region of target genes in response to oxidative stress [93]. Nrf2 knockout mice are susceptible to oxidative stress and neurodegeneration without obvious phenotypic defects [94].

The upregulation of Nrf2 exerts neuroprotective action during hypoxia/ischemia. Hypoxia preconditioning on rat brain against severe hypoxia or ischemia insult is through upregulating Nrf2 and HO-1 expression and alleviating oxidative stress damage [95]. rhEPO administration in ischemic rat activates Keap-Nrf2/ARE pathway to decrease H_2O_2 concentration and to protect brain tissue [96]. Similarly, in oxygen-deficient astrocytes, sulfiredoxin-1, an endogenous antioxidant protein, ameliorates oxidative stress via Nrf2/ARE pathway to prevent the brain from ischemic injury [97].

The expression level of Nrf2 is significantly decreased in the hippocampal neurons from AD patients [98]. The beneficial effect of Nrf2 upregulation in AD is evidenced by the finding that Nrf2 is able to induce NDP52, an autophagy adaptor protein, which facilitates the clearance of phosphorylated tau in neurons [99]. Examination of postmortem brain samples from PD patients reveals that NQO1 and p62 whose expression is associated with Nrf2 are partly sequestered in LB, demonstrating the impaired Nrf2 signaling in PD, and pharmacological activation of Nrf2 defends PD by protecting nigral dopaminergic neurons against α-syn toxicity and decreasing astrocytosis and microgliosis [100]. Correspondingly, in ALS mice model, WN1316, a novel acylaminoimidazole, boosts the activity of Nrf2 to protect motor neurons against oxidative injury and repress glial inflammation, microgliosis, and astrocytosis [101].

The Nrf2 signaling pathway is an attractive therapeutic target for neurodegenerative diseases, and thus, the chemopreventive agents aiming at Nrf2 might be suitable candidates against the development and progression of neurodegeneration.

1.4. Epigenetic modification

Epigenetics is the study of heritable and nonheritable changes in gene expression without changes to the underlying DNA sequence. Currently, at least three systems, DNA methylation, histone medication, and noncoding RNA (ncRNA)-associated gene silencing, are identified in epigenetic changes. A large body of evidence documents that hypoxia triggers epigenetic alternation that contributes to the initiation and aggravation of neurodegeneration.

1.4.1. Modification of DNA and histone

DNA methylation and histone modification are two important epigenetic mechanisms altering the transcription of genes. The methylation of CpG island in the promoter region results in the silence of gene expression, whereas demethylation undergoes the opposite direction. The posttranslational modification (PTM) of histone includes acetylation, methylation, and phosphorylation that are regulated by pairs of enzymes, impacting gene expression via altering chromatin structure or recruiting histone modifiers.

Short-term hypoxia causes long-lasting changes in genomic DNA methylation in hippocampal neuronal cells and subsequent alternation in the expression of a number of genes participating in neural growth and development [102]. Chronic hypoxia-mediated downregulation of NEP in mouse primary cortical and hippocampal neurons is through G9a histone methyltransferase and histone deacetylase 1 (HDAC1) other than methylation of gene promoter [103]. Cultured astrocytes under ischemia-hypoxia (IH) condition show hypermethylation of global DNA and hypoacetylation of histone H3/H4, manifesting epigenetic reprogramming induced by hypoxia [104]. Chronic hypoxia exaggerated the neuropathology and cognitive impairment in AD mice through decreasing the expression of DNA methyltransferase 3b (DNMT3b) to prevent the methylation of γ-secretase promoter [105].

Epigenetic modifications are reversible that make it a promising candidate for therapy. Valproic acid is a neuroprotective agent showing HDAC inhibitory property. It prevents the decrease of H3-Ace in the NEP promoter regions in prenatal hypoxia-induced AD neuropathology, upregulating NEP to improve learning deficits and decrease Aβ level [106].

1.5. Conclusion

This section reviews the major consequences of hypoxia in the CNS and the contribution of individual consequence to the pathogenesis of several neurodegenerative diseases. However, the cross-link among these consequences and how they may predispose hypoxic patients to neurodegeneration remain to be determined, as well as the communication between neurons and glia in response to hypoxic environment. Different types of hypoxia, acute, chronic, sustained, or intermittent, may vary in terms of their effects on neural cells. Therefore, further investigation is required. The prevention of hypoxic condition is clearly helpful for the reduction of neurodegeneration, and the molecules targeted by hypoxia provide therapeutic strategies and interventions against common neurodegenerative diseases.

2. Hypoxia and the inflammatory diseases

2.1. Introduction

Inflammatory diseases are pathological conditions associated with local or systemic activation and persistent activity of inflammatory mediators, leading to cellular, tissue, or organ damage. The inflammatory cascade leads to increased vascular leakage, recruitment of leukocytes, increased generation and secretion of local and systemic inflammatory cytokines and chemokines, and activation and proliferation of innate and adaptive immune cell members. Ultimately, the inflammatory response leads to destruction of target molecules as well as their hosting cells and tissues, which could lead to pathological conditions such as inflammatory bowel disease and rheumatoid arthritis.

Hypoxia and inflammation have been extensively studied, and the two conditions seem to have a complex interrelated relationship. In general, hypoxia induces the inflammatory response via activation of cytokines and inflammatory cells, while inflammatory states are complemented with severe hypoxia and induction of hypoxic signaling intermediates [107, 108]. A key mediator of hypoxic signaling in inflammation is HIF-1. Aside from low oxygen tension, recent evidence shows that various oxygen-independent pathways regulate HIF-1α transcription and translation under normoxia. For example, endogenous nitric oxide has been shown to stabilize HIF-1α under normoxia [109–111]. Angiotensin II is another factor that increases HIF-1α transcription and translation under normoxia, and angiotensin receptor blockade has shown to independently reduce HIF-1α levels under hypoxic injury [112, 113]. Other nonhypoxic HIF-1 regulatory molecules are via growth factors, thrombin, bacterial lipopolysaccharide (LPS), interleukins, and tumor necrosis factor-α (TNF-α) [114]. In general transcriptional and translational regulation of HIF-1α occurring as a secondary mode of HIF-1 regulation may aggravate or hinder the hypoxic response of the protein.

It has been noted that during hypoxemic states the levels of inflammatory cytokines such as IL-1, IL6, and TNF-α increase in serum [107, 115, 116]. Activation of macrophages and other innate and adaptive immune cell members is also shown to be induced by HIF-1 under hypoxia via activation of Toll-like receptor (TLR) signaling [117, 118]. Likewise, ischemia reperfusion is associated with recruitment of polymorphonuclear (PMN) leukocytes and vascular leakage [116, 119, 120]. This response is shown to be mediated via several endothelial cell surface glycoproteins and receptors and secondary activation of signaling via HIF-1–induced adenosine generation and NF-κB [116, 119].

It is noteworthy that ischemia and hypoxia are observed in inflamed tissues due to occlusion of blood flow via inflammatory cells [108]. As a result, signaling via inflammatory intermediates has been shown to potentiate hypoxic signaling via HIF-1. Macrophages in specific have been shown to release cytokines that stabilize and increase the activity of HIF-1 [111, 121]. Ultimately, transcriptional activation of factors such as VEGF by HIF-1 seems to increase angiogenesis and blood flow restoration to the site of inflammation.

Activation of HIF-1 further assures energy supply and survival of myeloid cells as well as bactericidal capacity of macrophages [122, 123]. Among the signaling pathways induced by HIF-1 in macrophages are mediators such as NF-κB, TNF-α, and nitric oxide that play key roles in the inflammatory capacity of the myeloid cells [111, 121, 123]. Interestingly, HIF-1α stabilization in turn positively regulates the production of inflammatory cytokines such as TNF-α, and therefore, through a positive feedback mechanism, inflammation and hypoxic signaling potentiate one another [123]. In the following sections, detailed mechanisms of this interaction will be discussed. Furthermore, the role of hypoxia and HIF molecules in arthritic and inflammatory bowel disease (IBD) pathophysiology and potential therapeutic targets relating to hypoxic signaling will be examined.

2.2. Hypoxic signaling and key inflammatory intermediates

2.2.1. TNF-α

TNF-α is a key mediator of the inflammatory response. It has been shown that HIF-1a stabilization and DNA-binding activity are enhanced by TNF-α [111]. Interaction of TNF-α and HIF-1 is rather complex. Physiologically, the stabilization of HIF-1a by TNF-α is thought to be mediated by activated macrophages [121]. Accumulation of HIF-1α via the TNF-α is via a mechanism independent from hypoxic accumulation or transcriptional activation of HIF-1α. Several studies have investigated the mechanism of HIF-1α stabilization via TNF-α, and among such mechanisms, NF-κB signaling seems to be the key mediator of this process [124, 125]. Studies by Zhou et al. have shown that TNF-α leads to accumulation of ubiquitinated form of HIF-1α, which is normally one of HIF-1α degradation steps. This interaction was mediated through increased NF-κB transcription [124]. They also noted that transfection of cells with p50/p65 members of NF-κB family leads to normoxic accumulation of HIF-1α in the absence of TNF-α [124]. Interestingly it has also been shown that reactive oxygen species (ROS) such as H_2O_2 or SO^- interfere with TNF-α–mediated accumulation of HIF-1α [126]. Aside from protein accumulation, additional studies have shown increased translation of HIF-1α via TNF-α that is also mediated via NF-κB through upregulation of an antiapoptotic protein Bcl-2 [127].

2.2.2. *Nuclear factor-kappa β*

NF-κB is a family of transcription factors involved in development, proliferation, survival, and antimicrobial response of innate and adaptive immune system cells. Numerous extensive studies have been conducted to elucidate the very complex role of NF-κB in the immune response [128]. The NF-κB family is composed of five related transcription factors, which can form homodimers or heterodimer complexes with DNA-binding activity. These identified members are p50, p52, RelA (p65), RelB, and c-Rel [128]. NF-κB complexes are inactive in the cytoplasm and are bound to an inhibitory protein called I-κB. Once NF-κB signaling is activated, the I-κB proteins are degraded, which then allow the transcription factors to translocate to the nucleus [128]. In the innate immune response, NF-κB is activated secondary to Toll-like receptor (TLR) activation. Toll-like receptors are pattern recognition receptors (PRR), which help immune cells recognize and combat pathogenic components. There are 11 identified mammalian TLRs with various coupled signaling pathways. TLRs are expressed in the cytosol as well as on the plasma membrane of immune cells [128]. Upon ligand binding, TLR signaling leads to recruitment of specific adaptor proteins and second messenger molecules, which in turn activate several transcription factors. Among such signaling pathways are mediators that result in degradation of I-κB proteins and activation of NF-κB [128]. NF-κB in turn induces gene expression of cytokines and other proteins involved in bactericidal activity against pathogens. NF-κB activation and signaling are also involved in adaptive immunity. T-cell and B-cell receptor activation and signaling activate NF-κB, which in turn activates antiapoptotic proteins and increases transcription of cytokines that ensure survival, proliferation, and differentiation of B and T cells [128].

2.2.3. *Hypoxia and the cross talk between HIF-1 and NF-κB*

It has been shown that NF-κB is directly activated under hypoxic conditions [129, 130]. Although the mechanism of NF-κB activation under hypoxia remains to be an extensive area of research, it has been shown that I-κB tyrosine residues are phosphorylated under hypoxia [129]. More recent studies suggest phosphorylation and inactivation of I-κB under hypoxia occur secondary to activation of transforming growth factor beta-activated kinase-1 (TAK1) and I-kappa B kinase (IKK) complex, primarily responsible for in I-κB degradation resulting in NF-κB activation [130–133]. Additionally, it has been shown that O_2-dependent prolyl hydroxylases (PHDs) that are involved in HIF-1 inactivation also play a role in proline hydroxylation of IKKβ and NF-κB repression [133]. Thus, during hypoxia loss of PHD activity would activate NF-κB.

Although hypoxic activation of NF-κB is to be better understood, a large body of convincing evidence shows a critical role for NF-κB in induction of HIF-1. Activation of NF-κB leads to induction of HIF-1α gene expression and basal HIF-1α mRNA, and protein levels are dependent upon NF-κB subunit expression levels [134, 135]. Several studies have explored the mechanism of regulation of HIF-1 by NF-κB [124, 127, 134, 136, 137]. It has been shown that NF-κB induces expression and increases protein levels of HIF-1α both in hypoxia and normoxia [124, 134, 137]. Indeed, certain studies suggest that HIF-1α gene expression under hypoxia is dependent upon intact NF-κB signaling pathway [134, 137]. These studies also provide mechanistic evidence into the regulation of HIF-1α gene expression via binding of several NF-κB subunits to the HIF-1α promoter region [134, 135]. Thus, secondary to direct activation of HIF-1 under hypoxic conditions, interaction of NF-κB additionally contributes to this process by increasing basal levels of HIF-1α protein.

Respective regulation of NF-κB by HIF-1 has also been reported in the literature [114, 138, 139]. These studies suggest direct activation of NF-κB via HIF-1 signaling in inflammatory cells. Among suggested mechanisms are increased expression of TLR2 and TLR6 leading to activation of NF-κB, hyperphosphorylation of IKKβ, and phosphorylation of serine residues of p65 subunit of NF-κB leading to its translocation to nucleus and transcriptional activity [117, 138, 139].

Overall, hypoxia and signaling via NF-κB and HIF-1 are closely linked and, respectively, regulate one another to enhance the inflammatory response.

2.3. Hypoxia and inflammatory bowel disease (IBD)

IBD is associated with loss of intestinal mucosal barrier, inflammation of mucosa, and increased incidence of bacterial infections [140]. IBD is categorized as ulcerative colitis (UC) and Crohn's disease (CD). Both conditions are associated with severe inflammation and breakdown of intestinal mucosal barrier and chronic gastrointestinal discomfort. Current therapeutic approaches to IBD include anti-inflammatory agents mostly targeted at TNF-α and immune cell members.

Hypoxia has been shown to be a critical component of inflammation in IBD. Surgical specimens of intestinal mucosa of IBD patients show increased expression of HIF-1 and HIF-2 [141]. Increased vascular proliferation and density has been noted in intestines of IBD patients secondary to hypoxia-induced VEGF activity [142]. Additionally microvascular abnormality and loss of endothelial nitric oxide production are seen in IBD mucosa [143].

The intestinal mucosa is exposed to fluctuating levels of oxygen. On the one hand, the intestinal lumen is nearly anoxic, and oxygen pressure is generally low on the luminal side of the mucosa. On the other hand, the rate of perfusion of the subendothelium is dependent upon meal intake, and PO_2 changes dramatically from high to low in between meals. The shift in oxygen tension in the mucosal layer renders it resistant to hypoxic states. This could be in part due to basal activity of hypoxic signaling intermediates such as HIF-1 in the intestinal mucosal. Indeed, HIF-1α–null mice in the intestinal epithelium show diminished mucosal protection and increased clinical symptoms in murine model of colitis [144]. HIF-1–induced epithelial protection is shown to be due to induction of several proteins such as mucin, p-glycoprotein, and ecto-5′-nucleotidase (CD73), an enzyme that converts AMP to adenosine (A_2B) receptor [140]. Adenosine production during hypoxia has shown to decrease vascular leakage and neutrophil accumulation and thus plays an anti-inflammatory role [120]. In a case-control cohort study, patients with polymorphisms in CD39, a vascular and immune cell ecto-nucleotidase that converts extracellular ATP and ADP to AMP, had increased susceptibility to Crohn's disease [145]. Therefore, HIF-1 signaling via adenosine is a key step in protection against IBD inflammation (**Figure 4**).

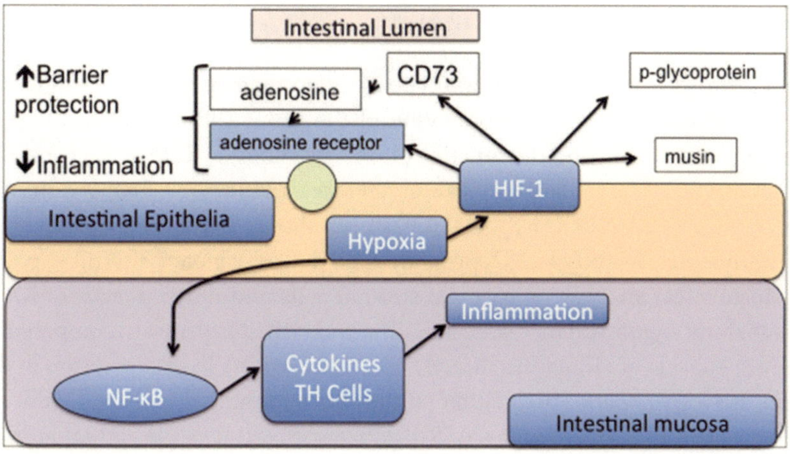

Figure 4. Hypoxia and IBD pathogenesis.

Aside from HIF-1, NF-κB is also involved in inflammatory events of IBD [146, 147]. Nuclear levels of NF-κB p65 have long been seen in lamina propria biopsies of patients with Crohn's disease [148]. Activation of NF-κB in mucosal macrophages leads to induction of pro-inflammatory cytokines such as TNF-α, IL-1, and IL-6, which mediate mucosal tissue damage [149]. NF-κB activation in intestinal mucosa also plays a role in differentiation of T-helper cells, which also play a role in IBD inflammation (**Figure 4**) [149]. In addition to pro-inflammatory activity, some studies have shown a protective role for NF-κB [146]. Loss of β or γ subunits of the IKK complex leads to colitis and apoptosis of intestinal mucosa [150, 151]. Additionally, polymorphisms of TLR4 and TLR5, which are involved in NF-κB activation, have been strongly associated with IBD in canines [152]. The protective role of NF-κB in IBD is thought to be in terms of maintaining mucosal barrier and integrity. Overall, NF-κB seems to play a dual role in IBD.

Due to the protective role of HIF-1 in models of colitis, it has been proposed that induction of HIF-1 could serve as a potential therapeutic target for treatment of IBD. The common pharmacological method of HIF-1 induction is via inhibition of PHD enzymes, which break down the HIF-1α subunit in the presence of oxygen. In vitro pharmacological inhibition of PHD using 2-oxoglutarate analogs as co-substrates of PHDs or dimethyloxaloglycine, has shown to stabilize HIF-1α [153–155]. In these studies PHD inhibitors decreased clinical symptoms in murine models of colitis and thus present promising therapeutic targets for IBD [153, 155, 156]. As mentioned previously blockade of PHDs can also lead to NF-κB activation. Using PHD inhibitors has thus been suggested to have dual benefits in treatment of IBD.

NF-κB activity, however, is associated with increased inflammation, and therefore, inhibition of NF-κB has also been examined and shows promise in treatment of IBD [149]. Selective NF-κB inhibitors, antisense oligonucleotides against NF-κB, and targeting DNA-binding activity of NF-κB using decoy oligodeoxynucleotides have been among the strategies tested that have produced promising results in murine models of colitis and IBD [157, 158].

2.4. Hypoxia and rheumatoid arthritis (RA)

Rheumatoid arthritis is the most common type of inflammatory arthritis. As an autoimmune disorder, RA is characterized as inflammation of the synovium, loss of cartilage, and bone erosion leading to joint pain and dysfunction [159]. The synovial fluid in RA is infiltrated with fibroblasts, immune cells, and angiogenesis of new vasculature [159, 160]. Additionally, a key feature of synovial fluid in RA is hypoxia. It has been shown that the synovium of knee joints of RA patients has significantly less O_2 pressure than that of osteoarthritis (OA) patients [161]. Immunohistochemical analysis of synovial stromal cells and macrophages of RA- and OA-affected joints show significant increases in HIF1α and HIF2α expression compared to normal. Additionally, the levels of HIFs were directly correlated with VEGF expression in the stromal cell lining in these specimens [162]. Other studies have identified HIF-2α significantly upregulated in fibroblast-like synoviocytes of RA and associated IL-6 upregulation in these cells [163]. These and other similar studies imply HIF signaling as the orchestrator of synovial inflammation and secondary joint damage [159, 164, 165]. A large number of HIF-activated inflamamtory mediators have been identified in RA synovial fluid including but not limited to stromal cell–derived factor 1 (SDF-1), VEGF, TNF-α, IL-1β, and IL-8 [166]. Various TLRs are also expressed in synovial tissue and macrophages, which further activate NF-κB pathway and increase expression of other inflammatory proteins [167]. Not surprisingly, HIF-dependent pathways have also been implicated in TLR expressions in many tissues including synovial cells [117, 118]. Finally, recruitment of CXCR4+ lymphocytes and matrix metalloproteinases (MMPs) in the synovial fibroblasts involved in cartilage destruction has also shown to be HIF-1 mediated and NF-κB mediated [168, 169]. Overall, a large body of evidence implicates hypoxia and HIF signaling as a key underlying mechanism in pathogenesis of RA (**Figure 5**).

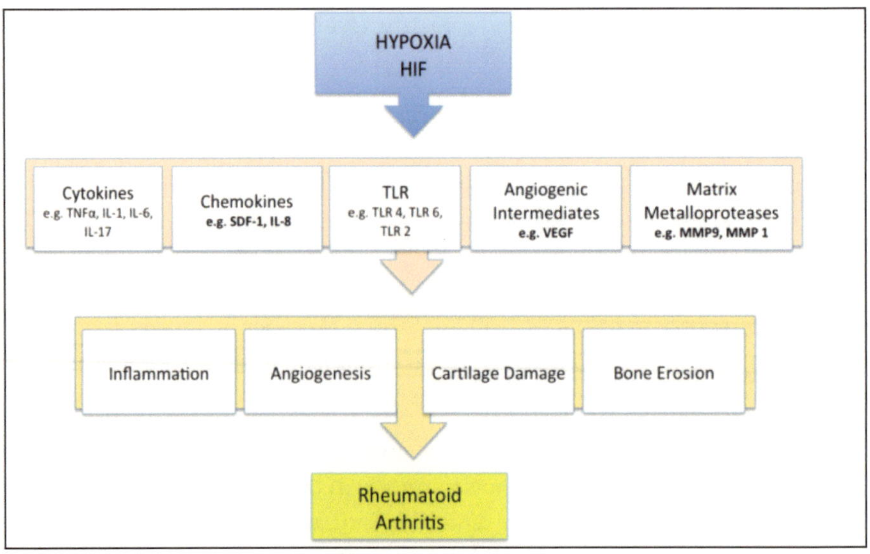

Figure 5. Hypoxia and pathogenesis of rheumatoid arthritis.

As discussed above, hypoxia- and HIF-mediated signaling is highly pro-inflammatory and destructive in RA. The key approach to treatment of RA is thus inhibition of HIF signaling. Many HIF inhibitors have been tested in cancer that may show promise in treatment of RA [170]. The limiting factor in administering HIF inhibitors is pharmacokinetic availability of these compounds in the synovial space as well as specific targetting of joints rather than systemic therapy. Gene targetting of HIF molecules using antisense oligonucleotides targetting HIF-1α mRNA has also been tested, which may show efficacy in RA treatment [159]. Additional approaches including anti-VEGF antibodies or anti-VEGF receptor molecules have been tested in models of arthritis and have shown efficacy in delaying onset and severity of RA in animal models [159, 171]. These strategies remain to be clinically tested yet show great promise in novel therapeutics of RA.

2.5. Conclusion

Section 2 discussed the complex relationship between hypoxia and inflammatory process and highlighted the key intermediates and pathways involved in this relationship. The discovery of hypoxic-inflammatory pathways has led to a greater understanding of inflammatory and autoimmune diseases such as IBD and RA and the use of novel pharmacological approaches targetting HIF and hypoxic signaling intermediates in these conditions. So far, these agents have been mostly studied in cancer clinical trials. Additional clinical studies are needed to examine the safety and efficacy of new HIF-modulating agents in treatment of inflammatory disease states.

3. Hypoxia and renal diseases

3.1. Introduction

Approximately 26 million Americans have some evidence of chronic kidney disease (CKD) and are at risk to develop kidney failure. The number of Americans with end-stage renal diseases (ESRD) is expected to grow to 785,000 by 2020 (currently 485,000). The annual cost of treating ESRD is currently over $32 billion. It is estimated that healthcare system can save up to $18.5 to $60.6 billion by reducing rate of progression of chronic kidney disease (CKD) by 10–30% over the next decade.

In acute setting acute kidney injury (AKI) has been shown to be associated with bad outcome, for instance, mortality rate of hospitalized patients with AKI increases more than fourfold [172]. Due to high medical and economic impact of AKI and CKD, finding new therapeutic tools in treatment of CKD is becoming of an increasing importance.

Hypoxia-inducible factor (HIF) has become the focus of medical community as a putative target because its augmentation is likely to ease the burden of kidney disease. The following sections discuss the evidence regarding the role of HIF molecules in various kidney pathologies and potential therapeutic approaches with respect to the HIF system.

3.1.1. Pathophysiology

Kidneys have a rich blood supply. In fact human kidneys receive 20% of cardiac output, while they weigh less than 1% of the total body weight. However, renal medulla, physiologically, has low oxygen tension and hence is very sensitive to hypoxia.

Hypoxia is the final common pathway to irreversible renal damage and eventually ESRD [173]. Since Fine et al. introduced chronic hypoxia hypothesis for the first time, it has been confirmed in several studies [174]. Also, hypoxia plays a role in pathogenesis of AKI as well as transformation of AKI to CKD.

Three phases of cell damage have been recognized following hypoxic insult to kidneys (by ligation of a branch of renal artery) [175]:

- Phase I: 1–6 h post hypoxic damage; in this phase parenchymal cells still appear viable.
- Phase II or intermediate phase: 1–3 days following insult; in this phase tissue damage is completed.
- Phase III or late phase: after 3 days; when tissue repair and remodeling are initiated.

In order to survive hypoxemia or regional hypoxia, the kidneys adopt a set of sophisticated defense mechanisms, which include expression of HIF. HIF is the cornerstone of adaptation to hypoxia. This master regulator of the cellular response to hypoxia orchestrates several hundred target genes affecting metabolism, the cell cycle, and inflammation [176]. The hypoxia-inducible transcription factors have been extensively studied in the kidneys [177]. HIF-1α is mainly expressed in tubular cells, while HIF-2α is found in peritubular, interstitial, endothelial, and glomerular regions [178]. Likewise, PHD1 and PHD3 are mostly present in glomeruli, and PHD1, PHD2, and PHD3 express more in the distal tubules than in the proximal tubules [179].

Numerous studies have found critical roles for HIF molecules in hypoxic adaptation of the kidneys as well as pathophysiology of various kidney diseases [177]. Given the fact HIF is the key step in renal response to hypoxia targeting HIF and its regulatory mechanisms is a plausible approach to prevent and treat hypoxic insults to kidney. In quest for novel therapeutic tools for treatment and prevention of kidney diseases, HIF-related pathways have shown promising results.

3.2. HIF in acute kidney injury

AKI is defined by rapid decline in renal function. AKI has multitude of causes. One of the most common causes of AKI is ischemia as a result of decreased renal perfusion, which leads to acute tubular necrosis (ATN) [180]. With renal ischemia several mechanisms in small arterioles will perpetuate regional hypoxia (**Figure 6**); these mechanisms include:

a. Decreased generation of nitric oxide (vasodilator) by endothelial cells [181]

b. Enhanced reactivity to endogenous mediators of vasoconstriction [182]

c. Small vessel occlusion due to activation of coagulation system interaction between the endothelium and leukocytes [183]

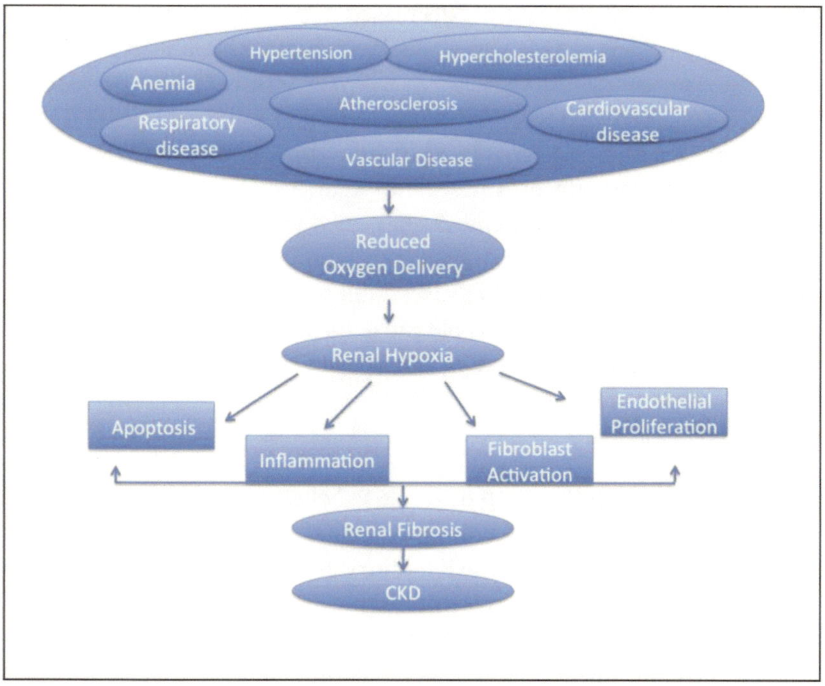

Figure 6. Diagram summarizing the interrelation between different factors causing hypoxia and CKD.

It has been shown that after renal ischemic attack, the number of capillaries in the medulla will decrease, which in turn leads to chronic ischemia, fibrosis, and progression to CKD [184]. Therefore, AKI is a risk factor for development of CKD. At the same time, patients with CKD have more incidence of AKI. In fact the most important risk factor of AKI is CKD [185]. AKI carries high risk of mortality; among patients older than 66 years with a first AKI hospitalization, the in-hospital mortality rate in 2013 was up to 14.4% (2015 USRDS Annual Data Report). Mortality rate in patients with AKI admitted to intensive care unit may surpass 50%. These data obviated the need for finding new therapies in AKI focused on renal hypoxia.

The key hypoxic intermediates mostly studied in animal models of AKI are HIF-1 and HIF-2. Rosenberger et al. showed that upregulation of HIF-1α occurs up to 7 days following ligation of a branch of the renal artery. HIF-2α expression has also been noted but to a lesser degree than HIF-1α and was confined to resident and infiltrating peritubular cells in the cortex [186]. Numerous studies have shown the involvement of HIF proteins in protection against acute renal injury [177]. Induction of HIF-1 or its target genes have shown to reduce injury secondary to various types of acute renal insult [187, 188].

3.2.1. HIF in contrast-induced nephropathy

The exact mechanism of contrast-induced nephropathy (CIN) remains elusive. Among possible mechanisms are renal vasoconstriction and decreased vasodilatation, which leads to tubular hypoxemia, decreased mitochondrial function and generation of reactive oxygen species (ROS), increased prostaglandins, decreased NO levels, and increased oxygen consumption due to osmotic demand of contrast media on tubular Na/K ATPase, all of which lead to medullary cell damage [189, 190]. Clearly, a direct link with hypoxia and CIN exists. Reversible renal vasoconstriction has been demonstrated in animal studies [191]. In an animal study, Rosenberger et al. induced renal hypoxia by a combination of COX inhibition, radiocontrast material, and blockade of nitric oxide synthase. In this study generalized HIF induction (tubules, interstitium, and endothelial cells) initiated within minutes of regional renal hypoxia. They showed medullary thick ascending limb (TAL) of Henle had less HIF expression, which may explain the higher susceptibility of this region to hypoxia [175]. These findings render regional hypoxia a plausible cause for CIN pathophysiology and a potential role for preventative HIF induction therapy in this condition.

3.2.2. Ischemic acute kidney injury

Ischemic injury in thick ascending limb of Henle is believed to play a pivotal role in pathogenesis of AKI due to regional renal low oxygen tension. Activation of HIF-1 has shown to be protective in models of ischemia-reperfusion injury. Schley and his colleagues showed that deletion of the von Hippel-Lindau (*VHL*) protein in thick ascending limb (TAL) of Henle preserved its function following ischemia-reperfusion. Notably, this study demonstrated better recovery in *VHL*-knocked-out animals by showing higher number of proliferating cells [192]. Furthermore, preconditional activation of HIF-1 via carbon monoxide or PHD1 inhibitor has shown to ameliorate the degree of renal ischemic damage in rat models of ischemia-reperfusion injury [188]. Others have shown activation of HIF-1 via cobalt chloride leads to reduction of tubulointerstitial damage secondary to acute renal injury in rats [187].

3.3. HIF in chronic kidney disease (CKD)

Chronic renal hypoxia causes apoptosis and also differentiation of tubular cells to myofibroblasts. Under hypoxic condition renal fibroblasts will also get activated. These together will lead to progressive renal failure and eventually ESRD. Glomerulosclerosis as a result of chronic high blood pressure or high blood sugar can also cause tubular ischemia by impairing tubular perfusion.

Several pharmacological means of reducing renal hypoxia are already widely available for use in daily clinical practice. Treatment with erythropoietin (EPO)-stimulating agents has been shown to slow down the progression of CKD [193]. Renin-angiotensin system (RAS) blockade can also be protective against hypoxia. RAS blockade will improve perfusion of peritubular capillaries by decreasing tone of efferent arteriols in parent glomerulus [194]. Yu et al. studied the effect of HIF activation (via a nonselective PHD inhibitor, L-mimosine) in rats with CKD. Animals underwent subtotal nephrectomy. In this study they demonstrated HIF activation can have different (beneficial or deleterious) effects on renal tissue. It was also shown that function of remnant kidney is also dependent upon the timing of HIF activation. Early activation of HIF in CKD caused increased fibrosis (rise in mRNA of collagen type III) and inflammation, while late activation of HIF showed anti-fibrotic effects [195].

3.3.1. *HIF in diabetic nephropathy*

Diabetic kidney disease (diabetic nephropathy (DN)) is the leading cause of ESRD. Hyperglycemia and resultant hyperfiltration will increase renal oxygen consumption. Eighty percent of the total renal oxygen consumption is related to sodium-potassium pump in cortical proximal tubule. Diabetes causes decreased renal oxygen tension by increasing oxygen consumption. Inoue et al. by using diffusion-weighted (DW) and blood oxygen level-dependent (BOLD) MRI showed tissue hypoxia in diabetic kidneys [196]. Palm et al. also demonstrated lower parenchymal oxygen tension along with higher oxygen consumption in diabetic rats [197]. In the setting of hypoxia, paradoxically, the activity of HIF-1α seems to be decreased or altered in diabetic rat kidneys [198, 199]. Polymorphism of pro582ser in HIF-1α gene, which results in altered response of HIF-1α to low oxygen, is associated with increased incidence of diabetic nephropathy in diabetic patients [199]. It appears from this evidence that HIF-1α-protective activity in the kidney is compromised in the setting of diabetes. This is further supported by the finding that pharmacologic activation of HIF pathway decreases renal damage in diabetic rats by decreasing proteinuria, improving tubulointerstitial damage and normalizing glomerular hyperfiltration [200]. There is thus indication for the use of HIF-1–activating approaches in prevention of diabetic nephropathy.

3.4. HIF in anemia of kidney disease

HIF plays a role in anemia of CKD and ESRD. Erythropoietin is secreted from human kidneys after birth. The kidney accounts for ~90% of the total EPO production in the adult human [201]. Renal erythropoietin-producing cells are fibroblasts in peritubular capillaries in the cortex and outer medulla [202].

Kidneys are the perfect choice to be responsible for erythropoietin secretion due to their regional low oxygen tension. Any minute changes in renal oxygen tension will lead to adjustments of serum hematocrit. In subcellular level HIF binds to the EPO enhancer, the hypoxia-responsive element, and activates the transcription of EPO. Renal EPO synthesis is regulated by HIF-2 [203]. HIF-2 exerts its multipronged effect by increasing EPO production, increasing iron absorption, and also increasing maturation of erythroid progenitors in the bone marrow. Studies indicate that in ESRD patients erythropoietin concentration is below normal due to dysfunctional EPO-producing cells (not due to cell death) [204]. Erythropoietin-producing cells in renal fibrosis remain alive and preserve their plasticity: although the exact mechanism of erythropoietin production in ESRD remains elusive, it is possible plasticity of erythropoietin-producing cells plays a role when signals for HIF pathway are augmented. Pathways to stabilize or even augment HIF response will mimic the state of hypoxia, which will lead to erythropoietin production; this is considered a novel therapeutic tool in our armamentarium to treat anemia of CKD. HIF stabilizers inhibit PHDs, which will subsequently cause accumulation of HIF, and as a result erythropoietin production ensues.

In 2010 a phase 1 clinical trial revealed PHD inhibitor (FG-2216) led to increased EPO production and plasma EPO levels in patients with ESRD [205]. In a phase 2-b study of nondialysis-dependent patients with chronic kidney disease, related anemia treatment with an oral PHD inhibitor (Roxadustat) was shown to increase EPO level and correct anemia. Clinical response was independent of iron intake (oral or IV) [206].

3.5. HIF in renal transplant

As of January 2016, there are 100,791 people waiting for renal transplants in the United States. Every 14 min a patient is added to the kidney transplant waiting list. In 2012, the probability of 1-year graft survival was 92% and 97% for deceased and living donor kidney transplant recipients, respectively. The estimated US average charges for a kidney transplant in 2011 is $262,900. This data emphasizes on the need for exploring new ways to save and preserve more allografts.

In the process of renal transplantation, harvested organ is subjected to hypoxia. Hypoxia-reperfusion occurs during organ procurement, preservation, and after implantation. Ischemia-Reperfusion injury (IRI) has prognostic implications for the allograft and kidney recipient. As mentioned before HIF has been shown to be a renoprotective agent and may alter transplantation outcome.

Conde et al. found HIF-1α increases in human proximal tubular cells (in vitro) after hypoxia and also during reoxygenation period. A similar biphasic pattern was observed in IRI model in SD rats (en vivo). The en vivo part of the study proved that HIF-1α induction during reperfusion phase was required for survival of proximal tubule cells and expedited recovery. Conde and his colleagues also studied human allograft biopsies (7–15 days post-transplant): HIF-1α expression was more robust in proximal tubule cells with minimal ischemic damage. Again, this finding indicate a protective role of HIF in IRI. AN interesting finding in this study was demonstration of the role of Akt/mTOR signaling in HIF-1α induction. Using rapamycin (mTOR inhibitor) during reoxygenation period prevented HIF-1α stabilization [207].

Renal ischemia-reperfusion injury is an important factor in determination of the fate of a renal allograft. Immunological response is potentiated under ischemia-reperfusion. CD4+ T cells play the main role in pathogenesis of IRI and natural killer (NK) cells are part of the immediate response to IRI. Regulatory family differentially affect the immune response to the of HIF affect allograft's during ischemia-reperfusion. While HIF-1α plays a crucial role in T-cell survival and function , HIF-2α has a protective function in T-cell mediated renal IRI [208]. In an animal study, Zhang et al. showed the role of HIF-2α in mitigating NK T-cell–mediated cytotoxicity in IRI. In this study HIF-2α and adenosine A2A receptor (adora2a) worked in concert with each other (so-called hypoxia-adenosinergic immunosuppression) to restrict NK T-cell activation [209]. This finding is of clinical importance as pharmacologic activation of HIF-2α can potentially limit allograft IRI and subsequently improve the outcome of renal transplantation.

3.6. Conclusion

The overwhelming clinical and economical impact of renal disease and the limited therapeutic options available have placed a great demand on finding additional therapeutic ap-

http://dx.doi.org/10.5772/66089

proaches. The evidence discussed in this section suggests a widespread role of hypoxia and HIF signaling in a range of acute and chronic renal diseases and a clear indication for HIF-targeted therapies. It appears that HIF-1 activity is protective in acute renal injury, while prolonged activity of HIF-1 may lead to worsened outcomes in CKD. The protective versus deleterious roles of HIF-1 thus complicate the use of HIF-1–targeted approaches. On the other hand, HIF-2 therapies may be more promising especially in terms of anemia of kidney disease and renal allograft rejection. In either case, additional clinical research is needed in the use and efficacy of both HIF-1 and HIF-2 therapies in prevention or treatment of various renal diseases.

Author details

Deepak Bhatia[1], Mohammad Sanaei Ardekani[2], Qiwen Shi[3] and Shahrzad Movafagh[1*]

*Address all correspondence to: smovafag@su.edu

1 Bernard J Dunn School of Pharmacy, Shenandoah University, VA, USA

2 Kidney and Hypertension Specialists, VA, USA

3 Collaborative Innovation Center of Yangtza River Delta Region Green Pharmaceuticals, Zhejiang University of Technology, Hangzhou, Zhejiang

References

[1] Alzheimer's Disease Facts and Figures, "2015 Alzheimer's Disease Facts and Figures," Alzheimer's Association, Facts and Figure, 2015. https://www.alz.org/facts/downloads/facts_figures_2015.pdf

[2] Daulatzai MA. Cerebral hypoperfusion and glucose hypometabolism: Key pathophysiological modulators promote neurodegeneration, cognitive impairment, and Alzheimer's disease. J Neurosci Res. 2016 Jun 27; PubMed PMID: 27350397.

[3] R. D. Bell, and B. V. Zlokovic, "Neurovascular mechanisms and blood-brain barrier disorder in Alzheimer's disease," *Acta Neuropathol. (Berl.)*, Vol. 118, No. 1, pp. 103–113, Jul. 2009.

[4] C. Carvalho *et al.*, "Role of mitochondrial-mediated signaling pathways in Alzheimer disease and hypoxia," *J. Bioenerg. Biomembr.*, Vol. 41, No. 5, pp. 433–440, Oct. 2009.

[5] N. Gertsik, D. Chiu, and Y. M. Li, "Complex regulation of γ-secretase: from obligatory to modulatory subunits," *Front. Aging Neurosci.*, Vol. 6, p. 342, 2014.

[6] I. F. Smith, J. P. Boyle, K. N. Green, H. A. Pearson, and C. Peers, "Hypoxic remodelling of Ca^{2+} mobilization in type I cortical astrocytes: involvement of ROS and pro-amyloidogenic APP processing," *J. Neurochem.*, Vol. 88, No. 4, pp. 869–877, Feb. 2004.

[7] L. Fisk, N. N. Nalivaeva, J. P. Boyle, C. S. Peers, and A. J. Turner, "Effects of hypoxia and oxidative stress on expression of neprilysin in human neuroblastoma cells and rat cortical neurones and astrocytes," *Neurochem. Res.*, Vol. 32, No. 10, pp. 1741–1748, Oct. 2007.

[8] L. Gao, S. Tian, H. Gao, and Y. Xu, "Hypoxia increases Aβ-induced tau phosphorylation by calpain and promotes behavioral consequences in AD transgenic mice," *J. Mol. Neurosci. MN*, Vol. 51, No. 1, pp. 138–147, Sep. 2013.

[9] C. E. Zhang, X. Yang, L. Li, X. Sui, Q. Tian, W. Wei, J. Wang, and G. Liu, "Hypoxia-induced tau phosphorylation and memory deficit in rats," *Neurodegener Dis.*, Vol. 14, No. 3, pp. 107–116, Nov. 2014.

[10] G. Basurto-Islas, I. Grundke-Iqbal, Y. C. Tung, F. Liu, and K. Iqbal, "Activation of asparaginyl endopeptidase leads to Tau hyperphosphorylation in Alzheimer disease," *J. Biol. Chem.*, Vol. 288, No. 24, pp. 17495–17507, Jun. 2013.

[11] P. Srivanitchapoom, S. Pandey, and M. Hallett, "Drooling in Parkinson's disease: a review," *Parkinsonism Relat. Disord.*, Vol. 20, No. 11, pp. 1109–1118, Nov. 2014.

[12] T. Chen *et al.*, "δ-Opioid receptor activation reduces α-synuclein overexpression and oligomer formation induced by MPP(+) and/or hypoxia," *Exp. Neurol.*, Vol. 255, pp. 127–136, May 2014.

[13] C. Vilariño-Güell *et al.*, "ATP13A2 variability in Parkinson disease," *Hum. Mutat.*, Vol. 30, No. 3, pp. 406–410, Mar. 2009.

[14] Q. Xu *et al.*, "Hypoxia regulation of ATP13A2 (PARK9) gene transcription," *J. Neurochem.*, Vol. 122, No. 2, pp. 251–259, Jul. 2012.

[15] F. Shephard, O. Greville-Heygate, S. Liddell, R. Emes, and L. Chakrabarti, "Analysis of mitochondrial haemoglobin in Parkinson's disease brain," *Mitochondrion*, Vol. 29, pp. 45–52, Jul. 2016.

[16] H. Onodera, S. Okabe, Y. Kikuchi, T. Tsuda, and Y. Itoyama, "Impaired chemosensitivity and perception of dyspnoea in Parkinson's disease," *Lancet Lond. Engl.*, Vol. 356, No. 9231, pp. 739–740, Aug. 2000.

[17] S. Zarei *et al.*, "A comprehensive review of amyotrophic lateral sclerosis," *Surg. Neurol. Int.*, Vol. 6, p. 171, Nov. 2015.

[18] N. Vanacore, P. Cocco, D. Fadda, and M. Dosemeci, "Job strain, hypoxia and risk of amyotrophic lateral sclerosis: results from a death certificate study," *Amyotroph. Lateral Scler. Off. Publ. World Fed. Neurol. Res. Group Mot. Neuron Dis.*, Vol. 11, No. 5, pp. 430–434, Oct. 2010.

[19] V. Subramanian, B. Crabtree, and K. R. Acharya, "Human angiogenin is a neuroprotective factor and amyotrophic lateral sclerosis associated angiogenin variants affect neurite extension/pathfinding and survival of motor neurons," *Hum. Mol. Genet.*, Vol. 17, No. 1, pp. 130–149, Jan. 2008.

[20] S. M. Kim *et al.*, "Intermittent hypoxia can aggravate motor neuronal loss and cognitive dysfunction in ALS mice," *PloS One*, Vol. 8, No. 11, p. e81808, Nov. 2013.

[21] R. Xu *et al.*, "Linking hypoxic and oxidative insults to cell death mechanisms in models of ALS," *Brain Res.*, Vol. 1372, pp. 133–144, Feb. 2011.

[22] S. K. S. Sarada, P. Himadri, D. Ruma, S. K. Sharma, T. Pauline, and Mrinalini, "Selenium protects the hypoxia induced apoptosis in neuroblastoma cells through upregulation of Bcl-2," *Brain Res.*, Vol. 1209, pp. 29–39, May 2008.

[23] S. Li, W. Wang, C. Wang, and Y. Y. Tang, "Possible involvement of NO/NOS signaling in hippocampal amyloid-beta production induced by transient focal cerebral ischemia in aged rats," *Neurosci. Lett.*, Vol. 470, No. 2, pp. 106–110, Feb. 2010.

[24] J. Li *et al.*, "Hypoxia induces beta-amyloid in association with death of RGC-5 cells in culture," *Biochem. Biophys. Res. Commun.*, Vol. 410, No. 1, pp. 40–44, Jun. 2011.

[25] R. Perfeito, D. F. Lázaro, T. F. Outeiro, and A. C. Rego, "Linking alpha-synuclein phosphorylation to reactive oxygen species formation and mitochondrial dysfunction in SH-SY5Y cells," *Mol. Cell. Neurosci.*, Vol. 62, pp. 51–59, Sep. 2014.

[26] J. W. Błaszczyk, "Parkinson's disease and neurodegeneration: GABA-collapse hypothesis," *Front. Neurosci.*, Vol. 10, p. 269, 2016.

[27] I. F. Smith, J. P. Boyle, P. F. Vaughan, H. A. Pearson, and C. Peers, "Effects of chronic hypoxia on Ca(2+) stores and capacitative Ca(2+) entry in human neuroblastoma (SH-SY5Y) cells," *J. Neurochem.*, Vol. 79, No. 4, pp. 877–884, Nov. 2001.

[28] I. F. Smith, L. D. Plant, J. P. Boyle, R. A. Skinner, H. A. Pearson, and C. Peers, "Chronic hypoxia potentiates capacitative Ca^{2+} entry in type-I cortical astrocytes," *J. Neurochem.*, Vol. 85, No. 5, pp. 1109–1116, Jun. 2003.

[29] J. L. Scragg, I. M. Fearon, J. P. Boyle, S. G. Ball, G. Varadi, and C. Peers, "Alzheimer's amyloid peptides mediate hypoxic up-regulation of L-type Ca^{2+} channels," *FASEB J. Off. Publ. Fed. Am. Soc. Exp. Biol.*, Vol. 19, No. 1, pp. 150–152, Jan. 2005.

[30] G. M. Bishop and S. R. Robinson, "Quantitative analysis of cell death and ferritin expression in response to cortical iron: implications for hypoxia-ischemia and stroke," *Brain Res.*, Vol. 907, No. 1–2, pp. 175–187, Jul. 2001.

[31] Y. Qi, T. M. Jamindar, and G. Dawson, "Hypoxia alters iron homeostasis and induces ferritin synthesis in oligodendrocytes," *J. Neurochem.*, Vol. 64, No. 6, pp. 2458–2464, Jun. 1995.

[32] P. W. Mantyh *et al.*, "Aluminum, iron, and zinc ions promote aggregation of physiological concentrations of beta-amyloid peptide," *J. Neurochem.*, Vol. 61, No. 3, pp. 1171–1174, Sep. 1993.

[33] M. Nakamura *et al.*, "Three histidine residues of amyloid-beta peptide control the redox activity of copper and iron," *Biochemistry* (*Mosc.*), Vol. 46, No. 44, pp. 12737–12743, Nov. 2007.

[34] A. Yamamoto *et al.*, "Iron (III) induces aggregation of hyperphosphorylated tau and its reduction to iron (II) reverses the aggregation: implications in the formation of neurofibrillary tangles of Alzheimer's disease," *J. Neurochem.*, Vol. 82, No. 5, pp. 1137–1147, Sep. 2002.

[35] P. Dusek, P. M. Roos, T. Litwin, S. A. Schneider, T. P. Flaten, and J. Aaseth, "The neurotoxicity of iron, copper and manganese in Parkinson's and Wilson's diseases," *J. Trace Elem. Med. Biol. Organ Soc. Miner. Trace Elem. GMS*, Vol. 31, pp. 193–203, 2015.

[36] L. D. Lukyanova, E. L. Germanova, T. A. Tsybina, and G. N. Chernobaeva, "Energotropic effect of succinate-containing derivatives of 3-hydroxypyridine," *Bull. Exp. Biol. Med.*, Vol. 148, No. 4, pp. 587–591, Oct. 2009.

[37] L. D. Lukyanova and Y. I. Kirova, "Mitochondria-controlled signaling mechanisms of brain protection in hypoxia," *Front. Neurosci.*, Vol. 9, p. 320, 2015.

[38] K. L. H. Carpenter, I. Jalloh, and P. J. Hutchinson, "Glycolysis and the significance of lactate in traumatic brain injury," *Front. Neurosci.*, Vol. 9, pp. 112, 2015.

[39] S. Takahashi, T. Iizumi, K. Mashima, T. Abe, and N. Suzuki, "Roles and regulation of ketogenesis in cultured astroglia and neurons under hypoxia and hypoglycemia," *ASN Neuro*, Vol. 6, No. 5, 2014.

[40] S. Melov *et al.*, "Mitochondrial oxidative stress causes hyperphosphorylation of tau," *PloS One*, Vol. 2, No. 6, p. e536, 2007.

[41] S. T. Brown, J. L. Scragg, J. P. Boyle, K. Hudasek, C. Peers, and I. M. Fearon, "Hypoxic augmentation of Ca^{2+} channel currents requires a functional electron transport chain," *J. Biol. Chem.*, Vol. 280, No. 23, pp. 21706–21712, Jun. 2005.

[42] A. H. V. Schapira, "Mitochondria in the aetiology and pathogenesis of Parkinson's disease," *Lancet Neurol.*, Vol. 7, No. 1, pp. 97–109, Jan. 2008.

[43] P. Khurana, Q. M. Ashraf, O. P. Mishra, and M. Delivoria-Papadopoulos, "Effect of hypoxia on caspase-3, -8, and -9 activity and expression in the cerebral cortex of newborn piglets," *Neurochem. Res.*, Vol. 27, No. 9, pp. 931–938, Sep. 2002.

[44] J. Sebastià *et al.*, "Angiogenin protects motoneurons against hypoxic injury," *Cell Death Differ.*, Vol. 16, No. 9, pp. 1238–1247, Sep. 2009.

[45] S. Mandel, O. Weinreb, T. Amit, and M. B. H. Youdim, "Mechanism of neuroprotective action of the anti-Parkinson drug rasagiline and its derivatives," *Brain Res. Brain Res. Rev.*, Vol. 48, No. 2, pp. 379–387, Apr. 2005.

[46] C. Pan, Z. Xu, Y. Dong, Y. Zhang, J. Zhang, S. McAuliffe, Y. Yue, T. Li, and Z. Xie, "The potential dual effects of anesthetic isoflurane on hypoxia-induced caspase-3 activation and increases in β-site amyloid precursor protein-cleaving enzyme levels," *Anesth. Analg.*, Vol. 113, No. 1, pp. 145–152, Jul. 2011.

[47] G. Mukandala, R. Tynan, S. Lanigan, and J. J. O'Connor, "The effects of hypoxia and inflammation on synaptic signaling in the CNS," *Brain Sci.*, Vol. 6, No. 1, 2016.

[48] A. Görlach, "Control of adenosine transport by hypoxia," *Circ. Res.*, Vol. 97, No. 1, pp. 1–3, Jul. 2005.

[49] D. Boison, "Adenosine kinase, epilepsy and stroke: mechanisms and therapies," *Trends Pharmacol. Sci.*, Vol. 27, No. 12, pp. 652–658, Dec. 2006.

[50] S. J. Guzman and Z. Gerevich, "P2Y receptors in synaptic transmission and plasticity: therapeutic potential in cognitive dysfunction," *Neural Plast.*, Vol. 2016, p. 1207393, 2016.

[51] D. Moore, S. Iritani, J. Chambers, and P. Emson, "Immunohistochemical localization of the P2Y1 purinergic receptor in Alzheimer's disease," *Neuroreport*, Vol. 11, No. 17, pp. 3799–3803, Nov. 2000.

[52] A. Delekate, M. Füchtemeier, T. Schumacher, C. Ulbrich, M. Foddis, and G. C. Petzold, "Metabotropic P2Y1 receptor signalling mediates astrocytic hyperactivity *in vivo* in an Alzheimer's disease mouse model," *Nat. Commun.*, Vol. 5, p. 5422, 2014.

[53] M. Xu, and H. Zhang, "Death and survival of neuronal and astrocytic cells in ischemic brain injury: a role of autophagy," *Acta Pharmacol. Sin.*, Vol. 32, No. 9, pp. 1089–1099, Sep. 2011.

[54] F. Adhami *et al.*, "Cerebral ischemia-hypoxia induces intravascular coagulation and autophagy," *Am. J. Pathol.*, Vol. 169, No. 2, pp. 566–583, Aug. 2006.

[55] A. P. Qin *et al.*, "Autophagy was activated in injured astrocytes and mildly decreased cell survival following glucose and oxygen deprivation and focal cerebral ischemia," *Autophagy*, Vol. 6, No. 6, pp. 738–753, Aug. 2010.

[56] Z. Liu *et al.*, "The ambiguous relationship of oxidative stress, tau hyperphosphorylation, and autophagy dysfunction in Alzheimer's disease," *Oxid. Med. Cell. Longev.*, Vol. 2015, p. 352723, 2015.

[57] T. Hamano *et al.*, "Autophagic-lysosomal perturbation enhances tau aggregation in transfectants with induced wild-type tau expression," *Eur. J. Neurosci.*, Vol. 27, No. 5, pp. 1119–1130, Mar. 2008.

[58] D. Heras-Sandoval, J. M. Pérez-Rojas, J. Hernández-Damián, and J. Pedraza-Chaverri, "The role of PI3K/AKT/mTOR pathway in the modulation of autophagy and the clearance of protein aggregates in neurodegeneration," *Cell. Signal.*, Vol. 26, No. 12, pp. 2694–2701, Dec. 2014.

[59] E. Janda, C. Isidoro, C. Carresi, and V. Mollace, "Defective autophagy in Parkinson's disease: role of oxidative stress," *Mol. Neurobiol.*, Vol. 46, No. 3, pp. 639–661, Dec. 2012.

[60] E. Kesidou, R. Lagoudaki, O. Touloumi, K. N. Poulatsidou, and C. Simeonidou, "Autophagy and neurodegenerative disorders," *Neural Regen. Res.*, Vol. 8, No. 24, pp. 2275–2283, Aug. 2013.

[61] F. Madeo, T. Eisenberg, and G. Kroemer, "Autophagy for the avoidance of neurodegeneration," *Genes Dev.*, Vol. 23, No. 19, pp. 2253–2259, Oct. 2009.

[62] Q. Ke and M. Costa, "Hypoxia-inducible factor-1 (HIF-1)," *Mol. Pharmacol.*, Vol. 70, No. 5, pp. 1469–1480, Nov. 2006.

[63] S. Guo, M. Miyake, K. J. Liu, and H. Shi, "Specific inhibition of hypoxia inducible factor 1 exaggerates cell injury induced by *in vitro* ischemia through deteriorating cellular redox environment," *J. Neurochem.*, Vol. 108, No. 5, pp. 1309–1321, Mar. 2009.

[64] X. Zhang *et al.*, "Hypoxia-inducible factor 1alpha (HIF-1alpha)-mediated hypoxia increases BACE1 expression and beta-amyloid generation," *J. Biol. Chem.*, Vol. 282, No. 15, pp. 10873–10880, Apr. 2007.

[65] P. O. Schnell, M. L. Ignacak, A. L. Bauer, J. B. Striet, W. R. Paulding, and M. F. Czyzyk-Krzeska, "Regulation of tyrosine hydroxylase promoter activity by the von Hippel-Lindau tumor suppressor protein and hypoxia-inducible transcription factors," *J. Neurochem.*, Vol. 85, No. 2, pp. 483–491, Apr. 2003.

[66] O. Weinreb, S. Mandel, M. B. H. Youdim, and T. Amit, "Targeting dysregulation of brain iron homeostasis in Parkinson's disease by iron chelators," *Free Radic. Biol. Med.*, Vol. 62, pp. 52–64, Sep. 2013.

[67] F. A. Zucca *et al.*, Interactions of iron, dopamine and neuromelanin pathways in brain aging and Parkinson's disease. Prog Neurobiol. 2015 Oct 9;PubMed PMID: 26455458; NIHMSID: NIHMS729596; PubMed Central PMCID: PMC4826627.

[68] C. Guo *et al.*, "Deferoxamine-mediated up-regulation of HIF-1α prevents dopaminergic neuronal death via the activation of MAPK family proteins in MPTP-treated mice," *Exp. Neurol.*, Vol. 280, pp. 13–23, Jun. 2016.

[69] Y. Wang *et al.*, "Vascular endothelial growth factor overexpression delays neurodegeneration and prolongs survival in amyotrophic lateral sclerosis mice," *J. Neurosci. Off. J. Soc. Neurosci.*, Vol. 27, No. 2, pp. 304–307, Jan. 2007.

[70] B. Oosthuyse *et al.*, "Deletion of the hypoxia-response element in the vascular endothelial growth factor promoter causes motor neuron degeneration," *Nat. Genet.*, Vol. 28, No. 2, pp. 131–138, Jun. 2001.

[71] J. F. Grunfeld, Y. Barhum, N. Blondheim, J. M. Rabey, E. Melamed, and D. Offen, "Erythropoietin delays disease onset in an amyotrophic lateral sclerosis model," *Exp. Neurol.*, Vol. 204, No. 1, pp. 260–263, Mar. 2007.

[72] M. Y. Noh, K. A. Cho, H. Kim, S. M. Kim, and S. H. Kim, "Erythropoietin modulates the immune-inflammatory response of a SOD1(G93A) transgenic mouse model of amyotrophic lateral sclerosis (ALS)," *Neurosci. Lett.*, Vol. 574, pp. 53–58, Jun. 2014.

[73] D. Devos *et al.*, "Low levels of the vascular endothelial growth factor in CSF from early ALS patients," *Neurology*, Vol. 62, No. 11, pp. 2127–2129, Jun. 2004.

[74] C. Moreau *et al.*, "Paradoxical response of VEGF expression to hypoxia in CSF of patients with ALS," *J. Neurol. Neurosurg. Psychiatry*, Vol. 77, No. 2, pp. 255–257, Feb. 2006.

[75] Y. Nagara *et al.*, "Impaired cytoplasmic-nuclear transport of hypoxia-inducible factor-1α in amyotrophic lateral sclerosis," *Brain Pathol. Zurich Switz.*, Vol. 23, No. 5, pp. 534–546, Sep. 2013.

[76] K. Sato *et al.*, "Impaired response of hypoxic sensor protein HIF-1α and its downstream proteins in the spinal motor neurons of ALS model mice," *Brain Res.*, Vol. 1473, pp. 55–62, Sep. 2012.

[77] L. Kupershmidt, O. Weinreb, T. Amit, S. Mandel, M. T. Carri, and M. B. H. Youdim, "Neuroprotective and neuritogenic activities of novel multimodal iron-chelating drugs in motor-neuron-like NSC-34 cells and transgenic mouse model of amyotrophic lateral sclerosis," *FASEB J. Off. Publ. Fed. Am. Soc. Exp. Biol.*, Vol. 23, No. 11, pp. 3766–3779, Nov. 2009.

[78] M. B. H. Youdim, "M30, a brain permeable multitarget neurorestorative drug in post nigrostriatal dopamine neuron lesion of parkinsonism animal models," *Parkinsonism Relat. Disord.*, Vol. 18 Suppl. 1, pp. S151–S154, Jan. 2012.

[79] D. Mechlovich, T. Amit, O. Bar-Am, S. Mandel, M. B. H. Youdim, and O. Weinreb, "The novel multi-target iron chelator, M30 modulates HIF-1α-related glycolytic genes and insulin signaling pathway in the frontal cortex of APP/PS1 Alzheimer's disease mice," *Curr. Alzheimer Res.*, Vol. 11, No. 2, pp. 119–127, Feb. 2014.

[80] N. G. Bazan, R. Palacios-Pelaez, and W. J. Lukiw, "Hypoxia signaling to genes: significance in Alzheimer's disease," *Mol. Neurobiol.*, Vol. 26, No. 2–3, pp. 283–298, Dec. 2002.

[81] M. P. Mattson and S. Camandola, "NF-kappaB in neuronal plasticity and neurodegenerative disorders," *J. Clin. Invest.*, Vol. 107, No. 3, pp. 247–254, Feb. 2001.

[82] Q. Shi and G. E. Gibson, "Oxidative stress and transcriptional regulation in Alzheimer disease," *Alzheimer Dis. Assoc. Disord.*, Vol. 21, No. 4, pp. 276–291, Dec. 2007.

[83] H. Liu *et al.*, "Sodium hydrosulfide attenuates beta-amyloid-induced cognitive deficits and neuroinflammation via modulation of MAPK/NF-κB pathway in rats," *Curr. Alzheimer Res.*, Vol. 12, No. 7, pp. 673–683, 2015.

[84] C. H. Nijboer, C. J. Heijnen, F. Groenendaal, M. J. May, F. van Bel, and A. Kavelaars, "A dual role of the NF-kappaB pathway in neonatal hypoxic-ischemic brain damage," *Stroke J. Cereb. Circ.*, Vol. 39, No. 9, pp. 2578–2586, Sep. 2008.

[85] M. Srinivasan and D. K. Lahiri, "Significance of NF-κB as a pivotal therapeutic target in the neurodegenerative pathologies of Alzheimer's disease and multiple sclerosis," *Expert Opin. Ther. Targets*, Vol. 19, No. 4, pp. 471–487, Apr. 2015.

[86] E. L. Pagé *et al.*, "Induction of hypoxia-inducible factor-1alpha by transcriptional and translational mechanisms," *J. Biol. Chem.*, Vol. 277, No. 50, pp. 48403–48409, Dec. 2002.

[87] A. Görlach and S. Bonello, "The cross-talk between NF-kappaB and HIF-1: further evidence for a significant liaison," *Biochem. J.*, Vol. 412, No. 3, pp. e17–e19, Jun. 2008.

[88] B. Kaltschmidt, M. Uherek, B. Volk, P. A. Baeuerle, and C. Kaltschmidt, "Transcription factor NF-kappaB is activated in primary neurons by amyloid beta peptides and in neurons surrounding early plaques from patients with Alzheimer disease," *Proc. Natl. Acad. Sci. U. S. A.*, Vol. 94, No. 6, pp. 2642–2647, Mar. 1997.

[89] S. Shi *et al.*, "Gx-50 reduces β-amyloid-induced TNF-α, IL-1β, NO, and PGE2 expression and inhibits NF-κB signaling in a mouse model of Alzheimer's disease," *Eur. J. Immunol.*, Vol. 46, No. 3, pp. 665–676, Mar. 2016.

[90] S. Hunot *et al.*, "Nuclear translocation of NF-kappaB is increased in dopaminergic neurons of patients with Parkinson disease," *Proc. Natl. Acad. Sci. U. S. A.*, Vol. 94, No. 14, pp. 7531–7536, Jul. 1997.

[91] J. A. Lee *et al.*, "A novel compound VSC2 has anti-inflammatory and antioxidant properties in microglia and in Parkinson's disease animal model," *Br. J. Pharmacol.*, Vol. 172, No. 4, pp. 1087–1100, Feb. 2015.

[92] A. E. Frakes *et al.*, "Microglia induce motor neuron death via the classical NF-κB pathway in amyotrophic lateral sclerosis," *Neuron*, Vol. 81, No. 5, pp. 1009–1023, Mar. 2014.

[93] J. W. Kaspar, S. K. Niture, and A. K. Jaiswal, "Nrf2:INrf2 (Keap1) signaling in oxidative stress," *Free Radic. Biol. Med.*, Vol. 47, No. 9, pp. 1304–1309, Nov. 2009.

[94] P. Shelton and A. K. Jaiswal, "The transcription factor NF-E2-related factor 2 (Nrf2): a protooncogene?," *FASEB J. Off. Publ. Fed. Am. Soc. Exp. Biol.*, Vol. 27, No. 2, pp. 414–423, Feb. 2013.

[95] L. Shu *et al.*, "The neuroprotection of hypoxic preconditioning on rat brain against traumatic brain injury by up-regulated transcription factor Nrf2 and HO-1 expression," *Neurosci. Lett.*, Vol. 611, pp. 74–80, Jan. 2016.

[96] H. Meng, J. Guo, H. Wang, P. Yan, X. Niu, and J. Zhang, "Erythropoietin activates Keap1-Nrf2/ARE pathway in rat brain after ischemia," *Int. J. Neurosci.*, Vol. 124, No. 5, pp. 362–368, May 2014.

[97] Y. Zhou *et al.*, "Sulfiredoxin-1 attenuates oxidative stress via Nrf2/ARE pathway and 2-Cys Prdxs after oxygen-glucose deprivation in astrocytes," *J. Mol. Neurosci.*, Vol. 55, No. 4, pp. 941–950, Apr. 2015.

[98] B. Sheng *et al.*, "Impaired mitochondrial biogenesis contributes to mitochondrial dysfunction in Alzheimer's disease," *J. Neurochem.*, Vol. 120, No. 3, pp. 419–429, Feb. 2012.

[99] C. Jo, S. Gundemir, S. Pritchard, Y. N. Jin, I. Rahman, and G. V. W. Johnson, "Nrf2 reduces levels of phosphorylated tau protein by inducing autophagy adaptor protein NDP52," *Nat. Commun.*, Vol. 5, p. 3496, 2014.

[100] I. Lastres-Becker *et al.*, "Repurposing the NRF2 activator dimethyl fumarate as therapy against synucleinopathy in Parkinson's disease," *Antioxid. Redox Signal.*, Vol. 25, No. 2, pp. 61–77, Jul. 2016.

[101] S. Tanaka, T. Tanaka, and M. Nangaku, "Hypoxia as a key player in the AKI-to-CKD transition," *Am. J. Physiol. Ren. Physiol.*, Vol. 307, No. 11, pp. F1187–F1195, Dec. 2014.

[102] I. Hartley *et al.*, "Long-lasting changes in DNA methylation following short-term hypoxic exposure in primary hippocampal neuronal cultures," *PloS One*, Vol. 8, No. 10, p. e77859, 2013.

[103] Z. Wang *et al.* Hypoxia-induced down-regulation of neprilysin by histone modification in mouse primary cortical and hippocampal neurons. PLoS One. 2011 Apr 29;6(4):e19229. PubMed PMID: 21559427; PubMed Central PMCID: PMC3084787.

[104] Q. Yang, X. Wu, J. Sun, J. Cui, and L. Li, "Epigenetic features induced by ischemia-hypoxia in cultured rat astrocytes," *Mol. Neurobiol.*, Vol. 53, No. 1, pp. 436–445, Jan. 2016.

[105] H. Liu, H. Qiu, J. Yang, J. Ni, and W. Le, "Chronic hypoxia facilitates Alzheimer's disease through demethylation of γ-secretase by downregulating DNA methyltransferase 3b," *Alzheimers Dement. J. Alzheimers Assoc.*, Vol. 12, No. 2, pp. 130–143, Feb. 2016.

[106] Z. Wang, X. J. Zhang, T. Li, J. Li, Y. Tang, and W. Le, "Valproic acid reduces neuritic plaque formation and improves learning deficits in APP(Swe)/PS1(A246E) transgenic mice via preventing the prenatal hypoxia-induced down-regulation of neprilysin," *CNS Neurosci. Ther.*, Vol. 20, No. 3, pp. 209–217, Mar. 2014.

[107] H. K. Eltzschig and P. Carmeliet, "Hypoxia and inflammation," *N. Engl. J. Med.*, Vol. 364, No. 7, pp. 656–665, Feb. 2011.

[108] C. Murdoch, M. Muthana, and C. E. Lewis, "Hypoxia regulates macrophage functions in inflammation," *J. Immunol.*, Vol. 175, No. 10, pp. 6257–6263, Nov. 2005.

[109] S. Movafagh, S. Crook, and K. Vo, "Regulation of hypoxia-inducible factor-1a by reactive oxygen species: new developments in an old debate," *J. Cell. Biochem.*, Vol. 116, No. 5, pp. 696–703, May 2015.

[110] B. Brüne, and J. Zhou, "Hypoxia-inducible factor-1α under the control of nitric oxide," in *Methods Enzymol.*, Vol. 435, Helmut Sies and Bernhard Brüne, Ed. Academic Press, pp. 463–478, 2007.

[111] K. B. Sandau, J. Zhou, T. Kietzmann, and B. Brüne, "Regulation of the hypoxia-inducible factor 1α by the inflammatory mediators nitric oxide and tumor necrosis factor-α in contrast to desferroxamine and phenylarsine oxide," *J. Biol. Chem.*, Vol. 276, No. 43, pp. 39805–39811, Oct. 2001.

[112] S. Inamoto *et al.*, "Angiotensin-II receptor blocker exerts cardioprotection in diabetic rats exposed to hypoxia," *Circ. J. Off. J. Jpn. Circ. Soc.*, Vol. 70, No. 6, pp. 787–792, Jun. 2006.

[113] G. Hartmann *et al.*, "High altitude increases circulating interleukin-6, interleukin-1 receptor antagonist and c-reactive protein," *Cytokine*, Vol. 12, No. 3, pp. 246–252, Mar. 2000.

[114] H. K. Eltzschig and C. D. Collard, "Vascular ischaemia and reperfusion injury," *Br. Med. Bull.*, Vol. 70, pp. 71–86, 2004.

[115] J. Kuhlicke, J. S. Frick, J. C. Morote-Garcia, P. Rosenberger, and H. K. Eltzschig, "Hypoxia inducible factor (HIF)-1 coordinates induction of toll-like receptors TLR2 and TLR6 during hypoxia," *PloS One*, Vol. 2, No. 12, Dec. 2007.

[116] B. Crifo and C. T. Taylor, "Crosstalk between toll-like receptors and hypoxia-dependent pathways in health and disease," *J. Investig. Med.*, Vol. 64, No. 2, pp. 369–375, Feb. 2016.

[117] H. K. Eltzschig *et al.*, "Endothelial catabolism of extracellular adenosine during hypoxia: the role of surface adenosine deaminase and CD26," *Blood*, Vol. 108, No. 5, pp. 1602–1610, Sep. 2006.

[118] L. F. Thompson *et al.*, "Crucial role for ecto-5'-nucleotidase (CD73) in vascular leakage during hypoxia," *J. Exp. Med.*, Vol. 200, No. 11, pp. 1395–1405, Dec. 2004.

[119] J. Zhou, J. Fandrey, J. Schümann, G. Tiegs, and B. Brüne, "NO and TNF-α released from activated macrophages stabilize HIF-1α in resting tubular LLC-PK1 cells," *Am. J. Physiol. Cell Physiol.*, Vol. 284, No. 2, pp. C439–C446, Feb. 2003.

[120] T. Cramer *et al.*, "HIF-1α is essential for myeloid cell-mediated inflammation," *Cell*, Vol. 112, No. 5, pp. 645–657, Mar. 2003.

[121] C. Peyssonnaux *et al.*, "HIF-1α expression regulates the bactericidal capacity of phagocytes," *J. Clin. Invest.*, Vol. 115, No. 7, pp. 1806–1815, Jul. 2005.

[122] J. Zhou, T. Schmid, and B. Brüne, "Tumor necrosis factor-α causes accumulation of a ubiquitinated form of hypoxia inducible factor-1α through a nuclear factor-κB-dependent pathway," *Mol. Biol. Cell*, Vol. 14, No. 6, pp. 2216–2225, Jun. 2003.

[123] D. H. Shin, S. H. Li, S. W. Yang, B. L. Lee, M. K. Lee, and J. W. Park, "Inhibitor of nuclear factor-kappaB alpha derepresses hypoxia-inducible factor-1 during moderate hypoxia by sequestering factor inhibiting hypoxia-inducible factor from hypoxia-inducible factor 1alpha," *FEBS J.*, Vol. 276, No. 13, pp. 3470–3480, Jul. 2009.

[124] J. J. Haddad, and S. C. Land, "A non-hypoxic, ROS-sensitive pathway mediates TNF-alpha-dependent regulation of HIF-1alpha," *FEBS Lett.*, Vol. 505, No. 2, pp. 269–274, Sep. 2001.

[125] J. Zhou, M. Callapina, G. J. Goodall, and B. Brüne, "Functional integrity of nuclear factor kappaB, phosphatidylinositol 3'-kinase, and mitogen-activated protein kinase signaling allows tumor necrosis factor alpha-evoked Bcl-2 expression to provoke internal ribosome entry site-dependent translation of hypoxia-inducible factor 1alpha," *Cancer Res.*, Vol. 64, No. 24, pp. 9041–9048, Dec. 2004.

[126] M. S. Hayden, A. P. West, and S. Ghosh, "NF-κB and the immune response," *Oncogene*, Vol. 25, No. 51, pp. 6758–6780, 2006.

[127] A. C. Koong, E. Y. Chen, and A. J. Giaccia, "Hypoxia causes the activation of nuclear factor κB through the phosphorylation of IκBα on tyrosine residues," *Cancer Res.*, Vol. 54, No. 6, pp. 1425–1430, Mar. 1994.

[128] N. S. Kenneth and S. Rocha, "Regulation of gene expression by hypoxia," *Biochem. J.*, Vol. 414, No. 1, pp. 19–29, Aug. 2008.

[129] A. Melvin, S. Mudie, and S. Rocha, "Mechanism of hypoxia-induced NFκB," *Cell Cycle*, Vol. 10, No. 6, pp. 879–882, Mar. 2011.

[130] A. Adhikari, M. Xu, and Z. J. Chen, "Ubiquitin-mediated activation of TAK1 and IKK," *Oncogene*, Vol. 26, No. 22, pp. 3214–3226, 2007.

[131] E. P. Cummins *et al.*, "Prolyl hydroxylase-1 negatively regulates IκB kinase-β, giving insight into hypoxia-induced NFκB activity," *Proc. Natl. Acad. Sci. U. S. A.*, Vol. 103, No. 48, pp. 18154–18159, Nov. 2006.

[132] P. van Uden, N. S. Kenneth, and S. Rocha, "Regulation of hypoxia-inducible factor-1α by NF-κB," *Biochem. J.*, Vol. 412, No. 3, pp. 477–484, Jun. 2008.

[133] R. S. BelAiba *et al.*, "Hypoxia up-regulates hypoxia-inducible factor-1α transcription by involving phosphatidylinositol 3-kinase and nuclear factor κB in pulmonary artery smooth muscle cells," *Mol. Biol. Cell*, Vol. 18, No. 12, pp. 4691–4697, Dec. 2007.

[134] C. T. Taylor and E. P. Cummins, "The role of NF-kappaB in hypoxia-induced gene expression," *Ann. N. Y. Acad. Sci.*, Vol. 1177, pp. 178–184, Oct. 2009.

[135] S. F. Fitzpatrick *et al.*, "An intact canonical NF-κB pathway is required for inflammatory gene expression in response to hypoxia," *J. Immunol. Baltim. Md 1950*, Vol. 186, No. 2, pp. 1091–1096, Jan. 2011.

[136] M. Scortegagna *et al.*, "HIF-1α regulates epithelial inflammation by cell autonomous NFκB activation and paracrine stromal remodeling," *Blood*, Vol. 111, No. 7, pp. 3343–3354, Apr. 2008.

[137] S. R. Walmsley *et al.*, "Hypoxia-induced neutrophil survival is mediated by HIF-1α-dependent NF-κB activity," *J. Exp. Med.*, Vol. 201, No. 1, pp. 105–115, Jan. 2005.

[138] C. T. Taylor, and S. P. Colgan, "Hypoxia and gastrointestinal disease," *J. Mol. Med.*, Vol. 85, No. 12, pp. 1295–1300, Nov. 2007.

[139] A. Giatromanolaki *et al.*, "Hypoxia inducible factor 1α and 2α overexpression in inflammatory bowel disease," *J. Clin. Pathol.*, Vol. 56, No. 3, pp. 209–213, Mar. 2003.

[140] A. Kapsoritakis *et al.*, "Vascular endothelial growth factor in inflammatory bowel disease," *Int. J. Colorectal Dis.*, Vol. 18, No. 5, pp. 418–422, May 2003.

[141] O. A. Hatoum, D. G. Binion, and D. D. Gutterman, "Paradox of simultaneous intestinal ischaemia and hyperaemia in inflammatory bowel disease," *Eur. J. Clin. Invest.*, Vol. 35, No. 10, pp. 599–609, Oct. 2005.

[142] J. Karhausen, G. T. Furuta, J. E. Tomaszewski, R. S. Johnson, S. P. Colgan, and V. H. Haase, "Epithelial hypoxia-inducible factor-1 is protective in murine experimental colitis," *J. Clin. Invest.*, Vol. 114, No. 8, pp. 1098–1106, Oct. 2004.

[143] D. J. Friedman *et al.*, "From the cover: CD39 deletion exacerbates experimental murine colitis and human polymorphisms increase susceptibility to inflammatory bowel disease," *Proc. Natl. Acad. Sci. U. S. A.*, Vol. 106, No. 39, pp. 16788–16793, Sep. 2009.

[144] M. E. Spehlmann and L. Eckmann, "Nuclear factor-kappa B in intestinal protection and destruction," *Curr. Opin. Gastroenterol.*, Vol. 25, No. 2, pp. 92–99, Mar. 2009.

[145] A. Wullaert, "Role of NF-κB activation in intestinal immune homeostasis," *Int. J. Med. Microbiol.*, Vol. 300, No. 1, pp. 49–56, Jan. 2010.

[146] S. Schreiber, S. Nikolaus, and J. Hampe, "Activation of nuclear factor κB in inflammatory bowel disease," *Gut*, Vol. 42, No. 4, pp. 477–484, Apr. 1998.

[147] I. Atreya, R. Atreya, and M. F. Neurath, "NF-kappaB in inflammatory bowel disease," *J. Intern. Med.*, Vol. 263, No. 6, pp. 591–596, Jun. 2008.

[148] L. W. Chen, L. Egan, Z. W. Li, F. R. Greten, M. F. Kagnoff, and M. Karin, "The two faces of IKK and NF-κB inhibition: prevention of systemic inflammation but increased local injury following intestinal ischemia-reperfusion," *Nat. Med.*, Vol. 9, No. 5, pp. 575–581, May 2003.

[149] F. R. Greten *et al.*, "IKKbeta links inflammation and tumorigenesis in a mouse model of colitis-associated cancer," *Cell*, Vol. 118, No. 3, pp. 285–296, Aug. 2004.

[150] A. Kathrani *et al.*, "Polymorphisms in the TLR4 and TLR5 gene are significantly associated with inflammatory bowel disease in German shepherd dogs," *PloS One*, Vol. 5, No. 12, p. e15740, 2010.

[151] I. Schlemminger *et al.*, "Analogues of dealanylalahopcin are inhibitors of human HIF prolyl hydroxylases," *Bioorg. Med. Chem. Lett.*, Vol. 13, No. 8, pp. 1451–1454, Apr. 2003.

[152] D. R. Mole *et al.*, "2-Oxoglutarate analogue inhibitors of HIF prolyl hydroxylase," *Bioorg. Med. Chem. Lett.*, Vol. 13, No. 16, pp. 2677–2680, Aug. 2003.

[153] E. P. Cummins *et al.*, "The hydroxylase inhibitor dimethyloxalylglycine is protective in a murine model of colitis," *Gastroenterology*, Vol. 134, No. 1, pp. 156–165, Jan. 2008.

[154] A. Robinson, S. Keely, J. Karhausen, M. E. Gerich, G. T. Furuta, and S. P. Colgan, "Mucosal protection by hypoxia-inducible factor (HIF) prolyl hydroxylase inhibition," *Gastroenterology*, Vol. 134, No. 1, pp. 145–155, Jan. 2008.

[155] M. F. Neurath, S. Pettersson, K. H. Meyer zum Büschenfelde, and W. Strober, "Local administration of antisense phosphorothioate oligonucleotides to the p65 subunit of NF-kappa B abrogates established experimental colitis in mice," *Nat. Med.*, Vol. 2, No. 9, pp. 998–1004, Sep. 1996.

[156] S. Fichtner-Feigl, I. J. Fuss, J. C. Preiss, W. Strober, and A. Kitani, "Treatment of murine Th1- and Th2-mediated inflammatory bowel disease with NF-kappa B decoy oligonucleotides," *J. Clin. Invest.*, Vol. 115, No. 11, pp. 3057–3071, Nov. 2005.

[157] S. Hua and T. H. Dias, "Hypoxia-Inducible Factor (HIF) as a Target for Novel Therapies in Rheumatoid Arthritis," Front. Pharmacol., vol. 7:184, Jun. 2016.

[158] U. Müller-Ladner, C. Ospelt, S. Gay, O. Distler, and T. Pap, "Cells of the synovium in rheumatoid arthritis. Synovial fibroblasts," *Arthritis Res. Ther.*, Vol. 9, No. 6, p. 223, 2007.

[159] Y. A. Lee *et al.*, "Synovial proliferation differentially affects hypoxia in the joint cavities of rheumatoid arthritis and osteoarthritis patients," *Clin. Rheumatol.*, Vol. 26, No. 12, pp. 2023–2029, Dec. 2007.

[160] A. Giatromanolaki *et al.*, "Upregulated hypoxia inducible factor-1α and -2α pathway in rheumatoid arthritis and osteoarthritis," *Arthritis Res. Ther.*, Vol. 5, No. 4, pp. R193–R201, 2003.

[161] J. H. Ryu *et al.*, "Hypoxia-inducible factor-2α is an essential catabolic regulator of inflammatory rheumatoid arthritis," *PLoS Biol.*, Vol. 12, No. 6, p. e1001881, Jun. 2014.

[162] M. J. del Rey *et al.*, "Human inflammatory synovial fibroblasts induce enhanced myeloid cell recruitment and angiogenesis through a hypoxia-inducible transcription factor 1α/vascular endothelial growth factor–mediated pathway in immunodeficient mice," *Arthritis Rheum.*, Vol. 60, No. 10, pp. 2926–2934, Oct. 2009.

[163] U. Fearon, M. Canavan, M. Biniecka, and D. J. Veale, "Hypoxia, mitochondrial dysfunction and synovial invasiveness in rheumatoid arthritis," *Nat. Rev. Rheumatol.*, Vol. 12, No. 7, pp. 385–397, May 2016.

[164] C. M. Quiñonez-Flores, S. A. González-Chávez, and C. Pacheco-Tena, "Hypoxia and its implications in rheumatoid arthritis," *J. Biomed. Sci.*, Vol. 23, No. 1, p. 62, 2016.

[165] Q. Q. Huang, and R. M. Pope, "Role of toll like receptors in rheumatoid arthritis," *Curr. Rheumatol. Rep.*, Vol. 11, No. 5, pp. 357–364, Oct. 2009.

[166] G. Li *et al.*, "Interleukin-17A promotes rheumatoid arthritis synoviocytes migration and invasion under hypoxia by increasing MMP2 and MMP9 expression through NF-κB/HIF-1α pathway," *Mol. Immunol.*, Vol. 53, No. 3, pp. 227–236, Mar. 2013.

[167] G. Li *et al.*, "Anti-invasive effects of celastrol in hypoxia-induced fibroblast-like synoviocyte through suppressing of HIF-1α/CXCR4 signaling pathway," *Int. Immunopharmacol.*, Vol. 17, No. 4, pp. 1028–1036, Dec. 2013.

[168] C. Wigerup, S. Påhlman, and D. Bexell, "Therapeutic targeting of hypoxia and hypoxia-inducible factors in cancer," *Pharmacol. Ther.*, Vol. 164, pp. 152–169, Aug. 2016.

[169] M. De Bandt *et al.*, "Blockade of vascular endothelial growth factor receptor I (VEGF-RI), but not VEGF-RII, suppresses joint destruction in the K/BxN model of rheumatoid arthritis," *J. Immunol. Baltim. Md 1950*, Vol. 171, No. 9, pp. 4853–4859, Nov. 2003.

[170] H. E. Wang, P. Muntner, G. M. Chertow, and D. G. Warnock, "Acute kidney injury and mortality in hospitalized patients," *Am. J. Nephrol.*, Vol. 35, No. 4, pp. 349–355, May 2012.

[171] M. Nangaku, "Chronic hypoxia and tubulointerstitial injury: a final common pathway to end-stage renal failure," *J. Am. Soc. Nephrol. JASN*, Vol. 17, No. 1, pp. 17–25, Jan. 2006.

[172] L. G. Fine, D. Bandyopadhay, and J. T. Norman, "Is there a common mechanism for the progression of different types of renal diseases other than proteinuria? Towards the unifying theme of chronic hypoxia," *Kidney Int. Suppl.*, Vol. 75, pp. S22–S26, Apr. 2000.

[173] C. Rosenberger *et al.*, "Cellular responses to hypoxia after renal segmental infarction," *Kidney Int.*, Vol. 64, No. 3, pp. 874–886, Sep. 2003.

[174] C. J. Schofield and P. J. Ratcliffe, "Oxygen sensing by HIF hydroxylases," *Nat. Rev. Mol. Cell Biol.*, Vol. 5, No. 5, pp. 343–354, May 2004.

[175] M. Nangaku and K. U. Eckardt, "Hypoxia and the HIF system in kidney disease," *J. Mol. Med. Berl. Ger.*, Vol. 85, No. 12, pp. 1325–1330, Dec. 2007.

[176] K. U. Eckardt, W. Bernhardt, C. Willam, and M. Wiesener, "Hypoxia-inducible transcription factors and their role in renal disease," *Semin. Nephrol.*, Vol. 27, No. 3, pp. 363–372, May 2007.

[177] J. Schödel *et al.*, "HIF-prolyl hydroxylases in the rat kidney: physiologic expression patterns and regulation in acute kidney injury," *Am. J. Pathol.*, Vol. 174, No. 5, pp. 1663–1674, May 2009.

[178] K. Nash, A. Hafeez, and S. Hou, "Hospital-acquired renal insufficiency," *Am. J. Kidney Dis. Off. J. Natl. Kidney Found.*, Vol. 39, No. 5, pp. 930–936, May 2002.

[179] O. Kwon, S. M. Hong, and G. Ramesh, "Diminished NO generation by injured endothelium and loss of macula densa nNOS may contribute to sustained acute kidney injury after ischemia-reperfusion," *Am. J. Physiol. Renal Physiol.*, Vol. 296, No. 1, pp. F25–F33, Jan. 2009.

[180] J. V. Bonventre and L. Yang, "Cellular pathophysiology of ischemic acute kidney injury," *J. Clin. Invest.*, Vol. 121, No. 11, pp. 4210–4221, Nov. 2011.

[181] J. V. Bonventre, and A. Zuk, "Ischemic acute renal failure: an inflammatory disease?," *Kidney Int.*, Vol. 66, No. 2, pp. 480–485, Aug. 2004.

[182] D. P. Basile, "The endothelial cell in ischemic acute kidney injury: implications for acute and chronic function," *Kidney Int.*, Vol. 72, No. 2, pp. 151–156, Jul. 2007.

[183] L. S. Chawla, P. W. Eggers, R. A. Star, and P. L. Kimmel, "Acute kidney injury and chronic kidney disease as interconnected syndromes," *N. Engl. J. Med.*, Vol. 371, No. 1, pp. 58–66, Jul. 2014.

[184] C. Rosenberger *et al.*, "Up-regulation of HIF in experimental acute renal failure: evidence for a protective transcriptional response to hypoxia," *Kidney Int.*, Vol. 67, No. 2, pp. 531–542, Feb. 2005.

[185] M. Matsumoto *et al.*, "Induction of renoprotective gene expression by cobalt ameliorates ischemic injury of the kidney in rats," *J. Am. Soc. Nephrol.*, Vol. 14, No. 7, pp. 1825–1832, Jul. 2003.

[186] W. M. Bernhardt, *et al.*, "Preconditional activation of hypoxia-inducible factors ameliorates ischemic acute renal failure," *J. Am. Soc. Nephrol.*, Vol. 17, No. 7, pp. 1970–1978, Jul. 2006.

[187] P. C. Y. Wong, Z. Li, J. Guo, and A. Zhang, "Pathophysiology of contrast-induced nephropathy," *Int. J. Cardiol.*, Vol. 158, No. 2, pp. 186–192, Jul. 2012.

[188] P. B. Persson, P. Hansell, and P. Liss, "Pathophysiology of contrast medium-induced nephropathy," *Kidney Int.*, Vol. 68, No. 1, pp. 14–22, Jul. 2005.

[189] L. G. Cantley, K. Spokes, B. Clark, E. G. McMahon, J. Carter, and F. H. Epstein, "Role of endothelin and prostaglandins in radiocontrast-induced renal artery constriction," *Kidney Int.*, Vol. 44, No. 6, pp. 1217–1223, Dec. 1993.

[190] G. Schley *et al.*, "Hypoxia-inducible transcription factors stabilization in the thick ascending limb protects against ischemic acute kidney injury," *J. Am. Soc. Nephrol.*, Vol. 22, No. 11, pp. 2004–2015, Nov. 2011.

[191] C. Gouva, P. Nikolopoulos, J. P. A. Ioannidis, and K. C. Siamopoulos, "Treating anemia early in renal failure patients slows the decline of renal function: a randomized controlled trial," *Kidney Int.*, Vol. 66, No. 2, pp. 753–760, Aug. 2004.

[192] K. Manotham *et al.*, "Evidence of tubular hypoxia in the early phase in the remnant kidney model," *J. Am. Soc. Nephrol.*, Vol. 15, No. 5, pp. 1277–1288, May 2004.

[193] X. Yu *et al.*, "The balance of beneficial and deleterious effects of hypoxia-inducible factor activation by prolyl hydroxylase inhibitor in rat remnant kidney depends on the timing of administration," *Nephrol. Dial. Transplant. Off. Publ. Eur. Dial. Transpl. Assoc. Eur. Ren. Assoc.*, Vol. 27, No. 8, pp. 3110–3119, Aug. 2012.

[194] T. Inoue *et al.*, "Noninvasive evaluation of kidney hypoxia and fibrosis using magnetic resonance imaging," *J. Am. Soc. Nephrol. JASN*, Vol. 22, No. 8, pp. 1429–1434, Aug. 2011.

[195] F. Palm, J. Cederberg, P. Hansell, P. Liss, and P. O. Carlsson, "Reactive oxygen species cause diabetes-induced decrease in renal oxygen tension," *Diabetologia*, Vol. 46, No. 8, pp. 1153–1160, Aug. 2003.

[196] H. Thangarajah *et al.*, "The molecular basis for impaired hypoxia-induced VEGF expression in diabetic tissues," *Proc. Natl. Acad. Sci. U. S. A.*, Vol. 106, No. 32, pp. 13505–13510, Aug. 2009.

[197] H. F. Gu *et al.*, "Impact of the hypoxia-inducible factor-1 α (HIF1A) Pro582Ser polymorphism on diabetes nephropathy," *Diabetes Care*, Vol. 36, No. 2, pp. 415–421, Feb. 2013.

[198] L. Nordquist *et al.*, "Activation of hypoxia-inducible factors prevents diabetic nephropathy," *J. Am. Soc. Nephrol. JASN*, Vol. 26, No. 2, pp. 328–338, Feb. 2015.

[199] M. J. Koury, M. C. Bondurant, S. E. Graber, and S. T. Sawyer, "Erythropoietin messenger RNA levels in developing mice and transfer of 125I-erythropoietin by the placenta," *J. Clin. Invest.*, Vol. 82, No. 1, pp. 154–159, Jul. 1988.

[200] S. Yamazaki *et al.*, "A mouse model of adult-onset anaemia due to erythropoietin deficiency," *Nat. Commun.*, Vol. 4, p. 1950, 2013.

[201] Y. Solak *et al.*, "Novel masters of erythropoiesis: hypoxia inducible factors and recent advances in anemia of renal disease," *Blood Purif.*, pp. 160–167, 2016.

[202] Y. Sato and M. Yanagita, "Renal anemia: from incurable to curable," *AJP Ren. Physiol.*, Vol. 305, No. 9, pp. F1239–F1248, Nov. 2013.

[203] W. M. Bernhardt *et al.*, "Inhibition of prolyl hydroxylases increases erythropoietin production in ESRD," *J. Am. Soc. Nephrol. JASN*, Vol. 21, No. 12, pp. 2151–2156, Dec. 2010.

[204] R. Provenzano *et al.*, "Oral hypoxia-inducible factor prolyl hydroxylase inhibitor roxadustat (FG-4592) for the treatment of anemia in patients with CKD," *Clin. J. Am. Soc. Nephrol. CJASN*, Vol. 11, No. 6, pp. 982–991, Jun. 2016.

[205] E. Conde *et al.*, "Hypoxia inducible factor 1-alpha (HIF-1 alpha) is induced during reperfusion after renal ischemia and is critical for proximal tubule cell survival," *PloS One*, Vol. 7, No. 3, p. e33258, 2012.

[206] D. Lukashev *et al.*, "Cutting edge: hypoxia-inducible factor 1alpha and its activation-inducible short isoform I.1 negatively regulate functions of CD4+ and CD8+ T lymphocytes," *J. Immunol. Baltim. Md 1950*, Vol. 177, No. 8, pp. 4962–4965, Oct. 2006.

[207] J. Zhang *et al.*, "Hypoxia-inducible factor-2α limits natural killer T cell cytotoxicity in renal ischemia/reperfusion injury," *J. Am. Soc. Nephrol.*, Vol. 27, No. 1, pp. 92–106, Jan. 2016.